Robotic-Assisted Minimally Invasive Surgery

Shawn Tsuda · Omar Yusef Kudsi

Editors

Robotic-Assisted Minimally Invasive Surgery

A Comprehensive Textbook

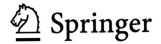 Springer

Editors
Shawn Tsuda
School of Medicine
Department of Surgery
University of Nevada
Las Vegas, NV
USA

Omar Yusef Kudsi
Department of General Surgery
Tufts University School of Medicine
Boston, MA
USA

ISBN 978-3-319-96865-0   ISBN 978-3-319-96866-7   (eBook)
https://doi.org/10.1007/978-3-319-96866-7

Library of Congress Control Number: 2018958625

This Springer imprint is published by the registered company Springer Nature Switzerland AG
The registered company address is: Gewerbestrasse 11, 6330 Cham, Switzerland

Preface

Robotic-Assisted Minimally Invasive Surgery: A Comprehensive Textbook is a one-of-a-kind book which covers all fields of surgery that currently use robotic platforms to facilitate a minimally invasive approach to procedures. The advantages of robotic surgery including improvements in instrumentation, three-dimensional optics, and computer-assisted motion have jump-started the implementation of more than 4000 systems worldwide and over 7000 peer-reviewed research studies. A textbook that comprehensively covers this evolution of surgery is timely and necessary.

The target audience for this book spans a wide breadth, including surgeons using, or planning to use, robotic platforms; general, specialty, and gynecologic residents; medical students; nurses; surgical technologists; hospital administrators; and even patients seeking to understand more about their options for the robotic-assisted surgical management of disease.

Most texts on the topic of robotic surgery are limited to a specific field. *Robotic-Assisted Minimally Invasive Surgery: A Comprehensive Textbook* in addition to the background, training, and economics of robotic surgery covers procedural details of general surgery, gynecology, urology, cardiothoracic surgery, plastics, otolaryngology, military surgery, and future robotic platforms. Included are disease-specific procedures that have been described and published in the peer-reviewed medical literature. Each chapter includes a literature review, preoperative planning, setup, procedural steps, and postoperative care of each surgical disease that has been managed with robotics.

Established experts and pioneers in the area of robotic surgery authored the chapters of this book. The latest knowledge and techniques are presented in a concise manner, with figures and photos to supplement the text. For the fastest-growing method of surgery across all fields, *Robotic-Assisted Minimally Invasive Surgery: A Comprehensive Textbook* is the authoritative resource.

Las Vegas, NV, USA   Shawn Tsuda, MD, FACS
Boston, MA, USA   Omar Yusef Kudsi, MD, MBA, FACS

Contents

Contributors

Abbas E. Abbas, MD, MS, FACS Thoracic Medicine and Surgery, Temple University Hospital, Philadelphia, PA, USA

Micahel Argenziano, MD Department of Surgery, New-York Presbyterian Hospital, New York, NY, USA

Michael M. Awad, MD, PhD, FACS Department of Surgery, Section of Minimally Invasive Surgery, Barnes-Jewish Hospital, Saint Louis, MO, USA

Bilgi Baca, MD Department of General Surgery, Acibadem Mehmet Ali Aydinlar University, School of Medicine, Istanbul, Turkey

Charles T. Bakhos, MD, MS, FACS Thoracic Medicine and Surgery, Temple University Hospital, Philadelphia, PA, USA

Conrad Ballecer, MD, MS Department of Surgery, Abrazo Arrowhead Hospital, Peoria, AZ, USA

Ovunc Bardakcioglu, MD FACS FASCRS Department of Surgery, University of Nevada Las Vegas Medicine, Las Vegas, NV, USA

Richard C. Baynosa, MD, FACS Division of Plastic Surgery, Plastic Surgery Residency Program, UNLV School of Medicine, Las Vegas, NV, USA

Eren Berber, MD, FACS Department of Endocrine Surgery, Cleveland Clinic, Cleveland, OH, USA

Costas Bizekis, MD Division of Thoracic Surgery, New York University Medical Center, New York, NY, USA

Jeffrey A. Cadeddu, MD Department of Urology, University of Texas Southwestern, Dallas, TX, USA

Abdullah Erdem Canda, MD Koc University, School of Medicine, Department of Urology, Istanbul, Turkey

Robert Cerfolio, MD Department of Cardiothoracic Surgery, New York University NYU Langone Health, New York, NY, USA

Myriam Curet, MD Intuitive Surgical, Inc., Sunnyvale, CA, USA

Peter S. Dahlberg, MD, PhD Department of Surgery, Allina Health, United Hospital, St. Paul, MN, USA

Giovanni Dapri, MD, PhD, FACS Saint-Pierre University Hospital, European School of Laparoscopic Surgery, Department of Gastrointestinal Surgery, Brussels, Belgium

Scott C. DeRoo, MD Cardiothoracic Surgery, Columbia University/New-York Presbyterian Hospital, New York, NY, USA

Erica Dolph Department of Surgery, Center for Advanced Surgical Technology, University of Nebraska Medical Center, Omaha, NE, USA

Matthew Dong, MD, MPH Department of Surgery, The Mount Sinai Hospital, New York, NY, USA

Darrell Downs, BS Surgical Surgery, Florida Hospital Tampa, Tampa, FL, USA

Kemal Ener, MD Umraniye Training and Research Hospital, Department of Urology, Istanbul, Turkey

Jared Rocky Funston, MD Department of Surgery, Huntington Hospital, Pasadena, CA, USA

Antonio R. Gargiulo, MD Department of Obstetrics, Gynecology and Reproductive Biology, Harvard Medical School, Center for Infertility and Reproductive Surgery, Brigham and Women's Hospital, Boston, MA, USA

Center for Robotic Surgery, Brigham and Women's Hospital, Boston, MA, USA

William Gerull, BA Department of Surgery, Section of Minimally Invasive Surgery, Barnes-Jewish Hospital, Saint Louis, MO, USA

Fahri Gokcal, MD Department of Surgery, Good Samaritan Medical Center, Brockton, MA, USA

University of Health Sciences Istanbul Bakirkoy Dr. Sadi Konuk Training and Research Hospital Bakirkoy, Istanbul, Turkey

Daniel Groves, MD Department of Urology, Cleveland Clinic, Akron, OH, USA

Elizabeth M. Hechenbleikner, MD Department of General Surgery, Mount Sinai Hospital, New York, NY, USA

Department of General Surgery, Garlock Division of Surgery, Mount Sinai Hospital, New York, NY, USA

Daniel M. Herron, MD Department of Surgery, The Mount Sinai Hospital, New York, NY, USA

Juan José Hidalgo Diaz Department of Hand Surgery, SOS Main, CCOM, University Hospital of Strasbourg, FMTS, University of Strasbourg, Illkirch, France

Brian P. Jacob, MD Department of General Surgery, Mount Sinai Hospital, New York, NY, USA

Icahn School of Medicine at Mount Sinai, Laparoscopic Surgical Center of New York, New York, NY, USA

Brett A. Johnson, MD Department of Urology, University of Texas Southwestern, Dallas, TX, USA

Bora Kahramangil, MD Department of Endocrine Surgery, Cleveland Clinic, Cleveland, OH, USA

Daniel M. Kirgan, MD Department of Surgery, Division of Surgical Oncology, UNLV School of Medicine, Las Vegas, NV, USA

Crystal Krause, PhD Department of Surgery, Center for Advanced Surgical Technology, University of Nebraska Medical Center, Omaha, NE, USA

Jayram Krishnan, DO Department of Urology, Cleveland Clinic, Akron, OH, USA

Omar Yusef Kudsi, MD, MBA, FACS Department of Surgery, Good Samaritan Medical Center, Tufts University School of Medicine, Boston, MA, USA

Robert B. Lim, MD Uniformed Services University of the Health Sciences, Bethesda, MD, USA

Department of Surgery, Tripler Army Medical Center, Honolulu, HI, USA

Philippe Liverneaux, MD, PhD Department of Hand Surgery, SOS Main, CCOM, University Hospital of Strasbourg, FMTS, University of Strasbourg, Illkirch, France

Joshua MacDavid, MD UNLV School of Medicine, Department of Surgery, University Medical Center, Las Vegas, NV, USA

Christopher Francis McNicoll, MD, MPH, MS Department of Surgery, University of Nevada, Las Vegas School of Medicine, Las Vegas, NV, USA

Heidi J. Miller, MD, MPH Department of Surgery, University of New Mexico, Albuquerque, NM, USA

Kyle Miller, MD, MBA Intuitive Surgical, Inc., Sunnyvale, CA, USA

Brian Minh Nguyen, MD San Diego, CA, USA

Yuri W. Novitsky, MD Department of Surgery, Columbia University, New York, NY, USA

Dmitry Oleynikov, MD Department of Surgery, University of Nebraska Medical Center, Omaha, NE, USA

Department of Surgery, Center for Advanced Surgical Technology, University of Nebraska Medical Center, Omaha, NE, USA

Sean B. Orenstein, MD, FACS Oregon Health & Science University, Department of Surgery, Division of Gastrointestinal and General Surgery, Portland, OR, USA

Volkan Ozben, MD Department of General Surgery, Acibadem Mehmet Ali Aydinlar University, School of Medicine, Istanbul, Turkey

Ankit D. Patel, MD Department of General and GI Surgery, Emory University, Atlanta, GA, USA

Jasmine Pedroso, MD MPH Obstetrics and Gynecology, MountainView Hospital, Centennial Hills Hospital, Las Vegas, NV, USA

Roman V. Petrov, MD, PhD, FACS Thoracic Medicine and Surgery, Temple University Hospital, Philadelphia, PA, USA

Alexander S. Rosemurgy, MD Department of Surgery, Florida Hospital Tampa, Tampa, FL, USA

Sharona B. Ross, MD Department of Surgery, Florida Hospital Tampa, Tampa, FL, USA

Nicola Santelmo, MD Department of Thoracic Surgery, University Hospital of Strasbourg, FMTS, Strasbourg, France

Peter Michael Santoro, MD, FACS Department of Surgery, Christiana Care Health System, Wilmington, DE, USA

Benjamin E. Schneider, MD Minimally Invasive and Bariatric Surgery, Department of Surgery, University of Texas Southwestern, Dallas, TX, USA

Keri Seymour, DO Department of Surgery, Duke University Medical Center, Durham, NC, USA

Anushi Shah, MD General Surgery, Maricopa Medical Center, Phoenix, AZ, USA

Shinil K. Shah, DO Department of Surgery, McGovern Medical School, University of Texas Health Science Center at Houston, Houston, TX, USA

Michael E. DeBakey Institute for Comparative Cardiovascular Science and Biomedical Devices, Texas A&M University, College Station, TX, USA

Beth-Ann Shanker, MD Department of Surgery, Saint Joseph's Mercy Hospital Ann Arbor, Ypsilanti, MI, USA

Mark S. Sneider, MD, FACS Department of Surgery, Allina Health, United Hospital, St. Paul, MN, USA

Mark K. Soliman, MD, FACS Colon and Rectal Surgery, Colon and Rectal Clinic of Orlando, Orlando, FL, USA

Charles R. St. Hill, MD, MSc Department of Surgery, Division of Surgical Oncology, UNLV School of Medicine, Las Vegas, NV, USA

Jamil Stetler, MD Department of General Surgery, Emory University, Atlanta, GA, USA

Erica Stockwell, DO Las Vegas Minimally Invasive Surgery, WellHealth Quality Care, a DaVita Medical Group, Las Vegas, NV, USA

Iswanto Sucandy, MD Department of Surgery, Florida Hospital Tampa, Tampa, FL, USA

Ranjan Sudan, MD Department of Surgery, Duke University Health System, Duke University Medical Center, Durham, NC, USA

Thomas Swope, MD, FACS Center for Minimally Invasive Surgery, Mercy Medical Center, Baltimore, MD, USA

Anthony R. Tascone, MD Department of Surgery, Christiana Care Health System, Wilmington, DE, USA

Sandeep S. Vijan, MBBS, FACS Sangre de Cristo Surgical Associates P.C., Parkview Medical Center, Pueblo, CO, USA

K. Warren Volker, MD, PhD Las Vegas Minimally Invasive Surgery, WellHealth Quality Care, a DaVita Medical Group, Las Vegas, NV, USA

Peter A. Walker, MD Department of Surgery, McGovern Medical School, University of Texas Health Science Center at Houston, Houston, TX, USA

Health First Medical Group, Rockledge, FL, USA

Benjamin Wei, MD Division of Thoracic Surgery, New York University Medical Center, New York, NY, USA

Erik B. Wilson, MD Department of Surgery, McGovern Medical School, University of Texas Health Science Center at Houston, Houston, TX, USA

Yanghee Woo, MD, FACS Department of Surgery, City of Hope National Medical Center, Duarte, CA, USA

Fred Xavier, MD, PhD Orthopedic Surgery, Biomedical Engineering, Cincinnati, OH, USA

Spine Surgery, Dalhousie University, Halifax, NS, Canada

Anusak Yiengpruksawan, MD, FACS, FRCST (Hon.) The Valley Minimally Invasive and Robotic Surgery Center, The Valley Hospital, Ridgewood, NJ, USA

Minimally Invasive Surgery Unit, Department of Surgery, Faculty of Medicine, Siriraj Hospital, Mahidol University, Bangkok, Thailand

Michael Zervos, MD Division of Thoracic Surgery, New York University Medical Center, New York, NY, USA

Department of Cardiothoracic Surgery, New York University NYU Langone Medical Center, New York, NY, USA

Ahmed Zihni, MD Department of Surgery, Section of Minimally Invasive Surgery, Barnes-Jewish Hospital, Saint Louis, MO, USA

Part I

Surgical Robots

Kyle Miller and Myriam Curet

Company Background

Intuitive Surgical, Inc., with corporate headquarters in Sunnyvale, California, pioneered the rapidly expanding field of robotic-assisted minimally invasive surgery. Founded in 1995, the company initially aimed for adoption in cardiac surgery with its introduction of the *da Vinci®* Surgical System. However, as history would demonstrate, urologists were the first group to widely adopt robotic-assisted minimally invasive approaches for prostatectomies leading to a revolution in the field of surgery [1]. Intuitive Surgical now supports and serves customers throughout the USA and world, providing technology innovation in cardiac, thoracic, gynecology, colorectal, otolaryngology, urology, pediatric, and general surgery disciplines.

When Intuitive was first founded, the vision for the product revolved around four key specifications or product pillars for a surgical robotic system: (i) a reliable, fail-safe surgical device, (ii) a system providing intuitive control of the instrumentation, (iii) dexterous manipulation with six degrees of freedom, and (iv) three-dimensional stereo vision. The goal for the company with its formation was to provide surgeons with a minimally invasive approach while regaining key benefits of open surgery that were lost with the invention and adoption of laparoscopic surgery: virtual transposition of the surgeon's eyes and hands onto the surgical workspace. The *da Vinci®* System was appropriately named during the company's first month of existence for the renowned renaissance polymath, Leonardo da Vinci, given his lasting contributions in the fields of science, art, anatomy, and engineering.

The technology was initially licensed from SRI International, IBM, and MIT providing a foundation for the *da Vinci®* Surgical System. Dr. Fred Moll, Rob Younge, and John Freund co-founded Intuitive Surgical in 1995 by licensing telepresence surgery technology from SRI and began by hiring

three engineers. The company developed two generations of technology prototypes (Lenny and Mona) that would be utilized in the first set of animal and human trials [2]. The Lenny prototype was completed and taken to animal trials during the summer of 1996 for a period of 6–9 months to demonstrate safety and feasibility around intuitive motion mapping and dexterity with six degrees of freedom with the wristed architecture. From this prototype, the team learned an extraordinary amount from the initial in vivo experiments. With lessons from the Lenny prototype, the Mona prototype was born with dramatic redesigns and improvement with the patient-side manipulators, interchangeable architecture, master-slave interface, and setup mechanisms [2]. The Mona prototype (Fig. 1.1), named after Leonardo's timeless masterpiece, the Mona Lisa, would be the first prototype tested in humans. These prototypes eventually led to the launch of Intuitive's flagship product, the *da Vinci®* Surgical System. The company began marketing the *da Vinci®* Surgical System initially in Europe in

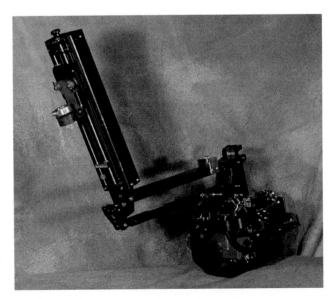

Fig. 1.1 da Vinci® Mona prototype. (With permission ©2018 Intuitive Surgical, Inc.)

K. Miller (✉) · M. Curet
Intuitive Surgical, Inc., Sunnyvale, CA, USA
e-mail: kyle.miller@intusurg.com

© Springer Nature Switzerland AG 2019
S. Tsuda, O. Y. Kudsi (eds.), *Robotic-Assisted Minimally Invasive Surgery*, https://doi.org/10.1007/978-3-319-96866-7_1

Fig. 1.2 Zeus prototype.
(With permission ©2018
Intuitive Surgical, Inc.)

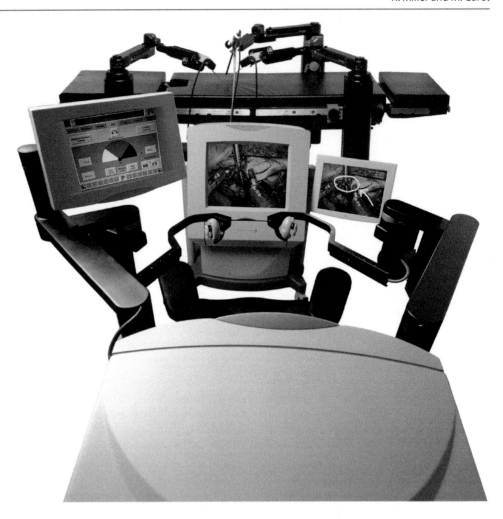

1999. A month after the company's initial public offering in June of 2000, Intuitive received FDA clearance for applications in general surgery with clearance for thoracic and urological procedures a year later [3].

In the initial pursuit to launch a robotic-assisted surgical system, a competitor emerged with Computer Motion, makers of the Zeus Surgical System (Fig. 1.2). Launched in 1997, the Zeus system utilized a voice-controlled endoscopic manipulator aimed at providing laparoscopic surgeons with improved precision and tremor filtration. Competition between the two companies led to Zeus focusing primarily on adoption by traditional laparoscopists, and the Intuitive *da Vinci*® System marketed toward open surgeons. Various patent infringement lawsuits were filed between the two companies with a legal battle starting to impact growth for both start-up surgical robotic companies. In 2003, the two companies elected to merge. Following the merger, the *da Vinci*® System became the company's single system offering [3, 4].

In 2003, a fourth arm was added to the patient-side cart in the creation of the *da Vinci*® Standard System (Fig. 1.3) in order to provide the surgeon with more control in exposure and traction. In addition to a new arm, the instrumentation

available on the system expanded from 6 to over 50 units. With continued improvements, the *da Vinci S*® product was released in 2006 (Fig. 1.4) with a focus on refining the ergonomics of the patient-side cart, which reduced the setup time by half [2]. With the *da Vinci S*® System, the side arms were lighter and smaller, improving the range of motion. Visualization improved with high-definition video, and TilePro™ was added for data interaction.

da Vinci Si® System (Fig. 1.5) was released in 2009 and focused on improvement for the surgeon console and vision cart building upon the patient cart improvements made in the *da Vinci S*® System [2]. With *da Vinci Si*® System, a higher-resolution 3D monitor was introduced along with improvements in ergonomic adjustability for the surgeon console. A wide-screen, higher-resolution touchscreen monitor was implemented into the vision cart. And finally, the *da Vinci Si*® System was developed to integrate two surgeon consoles to operate in unison with a patient-side cart. The introduction of the instrument "give-and-take" feature enabled advanced surgeon training and collaboration.

da Vinci Xi® System (Fig. 1.6) was introduced into the market in 2014 [2]. Advancements for the *da Vinci Xi*® System

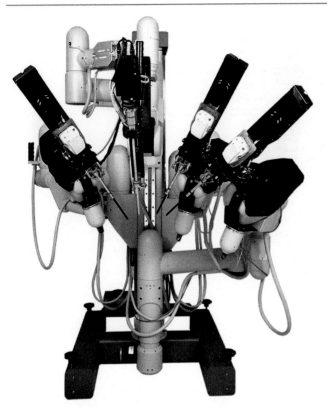

Fig. 1.3 da Vinci® standard patient cart. (With permission ©2018 Intuitive Surgical, Inc.)

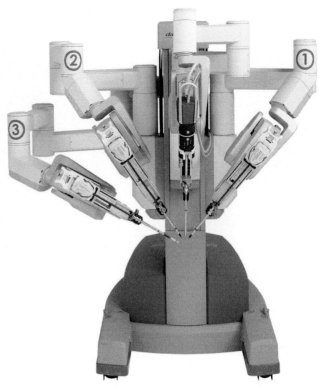

Fig. 1.5 *da Vinci Si*® patient cart. (With permission ©2018 Intuitive Surgical, Inc.)

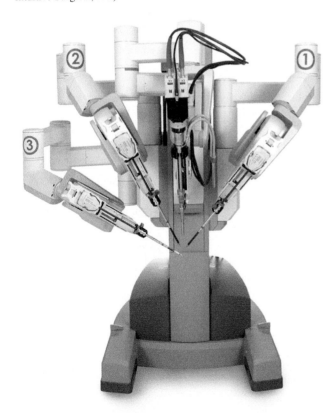

Fig. 1.4 da Vinci S® patient cart. (With permission ©2018 Intuitive Surgical, Inc.)

included redesigned kinematics for the patient cart that allowed for seamless deployment, roll-up, and docking steps to maximize workspace during an operation. Whereas the *da Vinci Si*® System relied upon orientation of the cart to plan for workspace, the *da Vinci Xi*® System's novel gantry system enabled wider tolerances and clearances with deployment and docking.

Finally, *da Vinci X*™ System (Fig. 1.7) entered the market in 2017 [5]. The *da Vinci X*® System integrates the thinner, enhanced arms of *da Vinci Xi*® System and positions them onto the cart like the *da Vinci Si*® model. The *da Vinci X*® System retains several *da Vinci Xi*® features including voice and laser guidance, 3DHD vision, and the surgeon-side console. The aim of the *da Vinci X* System is to provide access to advanced technologies associated with the *da Vinci Xi*® System at a more affordable entry point. The company has received both CE Marking and FDA 510(k) clearance for the *da Vinci X*® System.

Four Generations of *da Vinci* Systems

Intuitive Surgical has produced five surgical robotic systems including the *da Vinci*® Standard System, the *da Vinci S*® System, the *da Vinci Si*® System, the *da Vinci Xi*® System, and the *da Vinci X*® System. The company is also anticipating launch of *the da Vinci SP*® (Single-Port) System. The *da Vinci Si*® Surgical System and the *da Vinci Xi*® Surgical System are

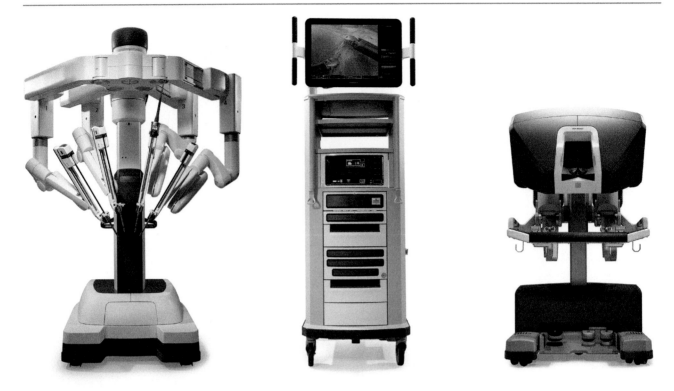

Fig. 1.6 da Vinci Xi® patient cart. (With permission ©2018 Intuitive Surgical, Inc.)

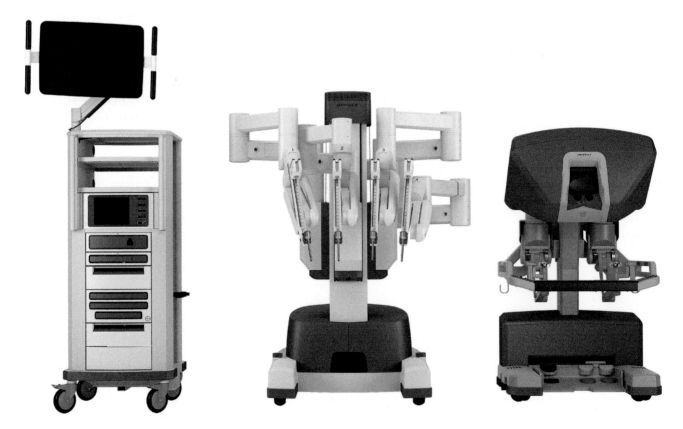

Fig. 1.7 da Vinci X® patient cart. (With permission ©2018 Intuitive Surgical, Inc.)

widely adopted with the latest addition to the family – the *da Vinci X®* Surgical System – released in 2017. Each of the *da Vinci Si®*, *da Vinci X®*, and *da Vinci Xi®* Systems features two control consoles that can be used in tandem, the addition of an integrated laser technology for fluorescent imaging and the capability of single-site technology.

Global Presence

As of June 2017, the company has more than 4000 *da Vinci®* Surgical Systems installed throughout the world including the USA (2624), Europe (678), and Asia (520) [6]. There were approximately 750,000 *da Vinci®* procedures performed in 2016 with more than four million procedures performed with a *da Vinci®* System since the company's inception. The company remains dedicated to advancing the field of robotic surgery to provide for comprehensive patient care, reduction in length of stay, reduced complications, fewer readmissions, and lower infection rates [6]. The company offers surgeons' technical training on its robotic platforms while also utilizing skill simulators with modules allowing surgeons to improve their skills outside of their clinical practice. To date, there are more than 13,000 peer-reviewed publications on the *da Vinci®* Surgical System with more than 1700 comparative studies performed on *da Vinci®* procedures. The clinical library related to *da Vinci®* procedures is increasing at a current rate of approximately 90–110 publications per month. In addition to the company's product pillars, the company is now focusing on enhanced imaging, intelligent systems, less invasive approaches, data analytics, and optimized learning.

Regulatory

The *da Vinci®* Surgical System is classified by the Food and Drug Administration (FDA) as a Class II device. At the time of this publication, the *da Vinci®* Surgical System has clearance for urologic surgical procedures, general laparoscopic surgical procedures, inguinal hernia procedures, gynecologic laparoscopic surgical procedures, transoral otolaryngology surgical procedures restricted to benign and malignant tumors classified as T1 and T2 and for benign base of tongue resection procedures, general thoracoscopic surgical procedures, and thoracoscopically assisted cardiotomy procedures. The system can be employed with adjunctive mediastinotomy to perform coronary anastomosis during cardiac revascularization. The system is indicated for adult and pediatric use except for transoral otolaryngology surgical procedures. The *da Vinci®* Surgical Systems are cleared through a Conformité Européene (CE) mark for a variety of indications throughout Europe and have obtained regulatory approvals in Asia and other parts of the world.

da Vinci **Platform**

The *da Vinci®* System is based on three distinct subsystems: (i) the surgeon-side cart, (ii) the vision cart, and (iii) the patient-side cart. A competent surgical team is required to perform surgery, and several team members in the operating theater interact with the *da Vinci®* System and its subsystems during the phases of a robotic-assisted operation: draping and sterile field preparation, system setup, roll-up to patient bedside, deployment, docking, operation, undocking, and stowing along with reprocessing and sterilization of the instrumentation and accessories. While the most visible part of the *da Vinci®* System is the mechatronic arms, the robotic-assisted surgical system is based on a vast platform enabling the surgeon to perform robotic-assisted surgery. This platform includes advanced instrumentation: monopolar, bipolar, and ultrasonic energy, vessel sealers, intelligent stapling systems featuring *SmartClamp* technology, and dozens of additional instruments and accessories. In addition, the *da Vinci®* Surgical System utilizes a stereoscopic three-dimensional endoscope to guide surgical operations. The advanced imaging system has *Firefly™* near-infrared imaging technology enabling the surgeon to see vasculature and tissue perfusion with the aid of intravenous administration of indocyanine green (ICG). More recent advances in the *da Vinci®* platform include the integrated table motion feature of the *da Vinci Xi®* System, which allows the system to directly communicate with the TRUMPF Medical advanced operating table, the *TruSystem™* 7000dV (TRUMPF Medizin Systeme, Saalfeld, Germany). When utilizing this feature, the *da Vinci Xi®* System and TRUMPF table are synchronized so that the surgical team can reposition the operating table while maintaining the patient's anatomical orientation relative to the robotic arms.

da Vinci Xi® **Subsystems: Surgical Console**

The *surgical console* (Fig. 1.8) is the central control component of the *da Vinci Xi®* System. The system includes the master controllers, the 3D high-definition stereo viewer, central touch pad, left and right pods, and the footswitch panel. The surgeon operates while seated comfortably at the console which is outside of the sterile field allowing for controlled movement of the robotic arms, 3D endoscope, and *EndoWrist®* instrumentation. The real-time anatomical workspace is streamed through the stereo viewer.

The *master controllers* are the manual control units for the surgeon which allow for seamless translation of the surgeon's hand, wrist, and finger movements into precise, real-time movements of the surgical instrumentation. The movement of the designated instrument within the surgical

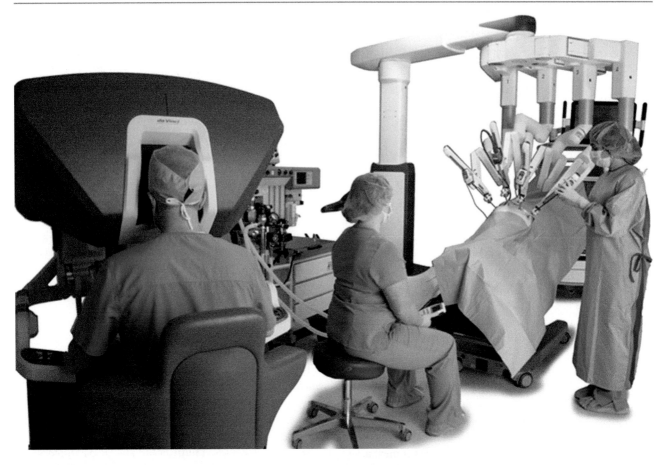

Fig. 1.8 da Vinci Xi® surgical console. (With permission ©2018 Intuitive Surgical, Inc.)

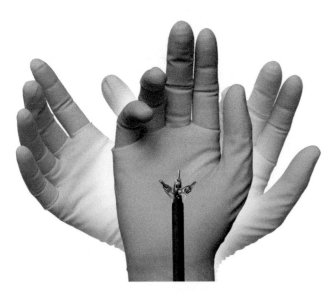

Fig. 1.9 Automorphic master control. (With permission ©2018 Intuitive Surgical, Inc.)

field mimics that of the surgeon's hand, wrist, thumb, and index or middle finger, supporting the anthropomorphic principle (Fig. 1.9). Clutch buttons that disengage the master

controllers from the robotic instrumentation enable repositioning without robotic arm or instrument movement.

The *stereo viewer* is the central visual element of the *da Vinci®* Surgical System allowing for 3D high-definition viewing of the anatomical workspace. The surgeon has several advanced features including a full-screen mode and multi-image mode or *TilePro™* which displays the image of the surgical field along with additional images, such as patient imaging. The images displayed to the surgeon in the stereo viewer are duplicated on the vision cart monitor visible to all operating room staff.

da Vinci Xi® **Subsystems: Patient Cart**

The patient-side cart (Fig. 1.10) is positioned adjacent to the patient during the operation. The *da Vinci Xi®* patient cart allows the camera and instrumentation to be introduced into the surgical field while providing tremor stabilization during the procedure. The patient compartment is comprised of setup joints and four robotic arms. The setup joints of the *da Vinci®* patient cart allow for human-like movements of the robotic arms. They are utilized to position the arms during sterile drap-

Fig. 1.10 da Vinci Xi®
patient cart. (With permission
©2018 Intuitive Surgical,
Inc.)

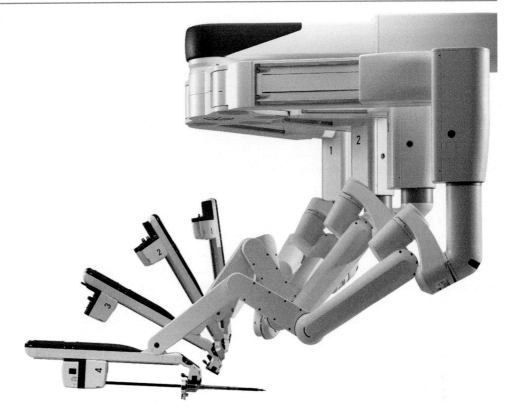

ing and to establish remote centers which optimize the range of motion of the *da Vinci®* instrumentation. The instrument arms of the patient cart provide the interface for the *EndoWrist®* instrumentation and the camera. All robotic arms are covered with sterile drapes with sterile adapters providing for mounting of the camera and instrumentation. Installation, removal, and exchange of the camera as well as the instruments are performed by a trained bedside assistant. The *EndoWrist®* instruments are mounted onto the robotic arms for use during procedures. Their innovative design enables seven degrees of freedom and full articulation of the wrist architecture allowing for dexterity in a minimally invasive setting [2].

The *da Vinci Single-Site®* instrumentation kit (Fig. 1.11) has been designed to enable intuitive control of the *da Vinci Xi®* system through a single skin incision site of 2–2.5 cm. The kit includes a five-lumen port that provides access for an endoscope, two curved single-site cannulae that cross at the level of the abdominal wall, an accessory port, and insufflation adaptor. The *da Vinci Xi®* System detects the specialized *da Vinci Single-Site®* instrumentation and reassigns the surgeon's hands with the correct instrument to provide intuitive control.

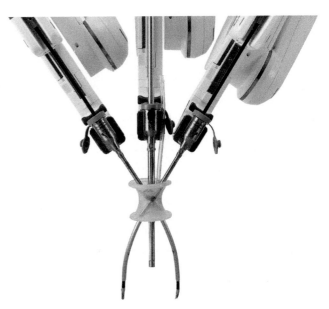

Fig. 1.11 da Vinci Xi® Single-Site. (With permission ©2018 Intuitive Surgical, Inc.)

da Vinci Xi® **Subsystems: Vision Cart**

The vision cart is the system's central processing and vision equipment that contains a touchscreen monitor enabling operating room personnel to view video and control central functions of the system. The vision cart contains a microphone and speakers for two-way communication with the surgeon operator along with space for the electrosurgical generator and insufflator units. The vision cart also houses the *da Vinci Xi®* core, which is the system's central connect hub where all system, auxiliary equipment, and audiovisual connections are routed.

The vision cart allows for integration of the *da Vinci Firefly®Firefly* imaging feature. A laser light source is used to excite fluorophores at wavelengths around 800 nm. This emitted light is captured by the *da Vinci®* endoscope giving the surgeon the ability to see vasculature and tissue perfusion with the aid of ICG injected into the blood stream which binds to plasma proteins in the patient's blood stream.

The Next Addition to the *da Vinci®* Family: *da Vinci SP®* System

The *da Vinci SP®* (Single-Port) System,[1] which is currently under development and not yet commercially available, introduces articulated instruments and camera through a single incision with a diameter of approximately 2.5 cm. This design allows the entire array of instruments to enter a single cannula along parallel axes, as opposed to the single-site system. The articulated instruments and camera are snake-like robots that can be manipulated independently to provide better surgical access after entering the body. This makes *da Vinci SP®* suitable for procedures that require natural orifice endoluminal access, such as transoral and transanal procedures.

Future of Robotic-Assisted Surgery

Intuitive Surgical seeks to enhance product offerings through an enhanced platform that surgeons can leverage for their operations. The future of robotic-assisted surgery is promising in regard to surgical access, vision, emerging competition, and intelligent systems.

In the area of surgical access, there was a strong push for natural orifice transluminal endoscopic surgery (NOTES) in 2005 [7]. The feasibility of performing transcolonic, transvaginal, and transgastric procedures was established; however, a clear patient benefit was initially lacking with these approaches, and the technological limitations of the available flexible platforms remained challenging. Novel procedures including peroral esophageal myotomy (POEM) arose from NOTES as did a renewed interest in flexible, advanced catheter systems [8]. We expect this field to continue its progression in the future with the launch of the *da Vinci SP®* System, which will focus on endoluminal applications in transoral, transanal, and urological procedures.

In the area of vision, advancements in visualization techniques are being driven by the gaming industry and virtual reality technology. In a recent survey of robotic urology surgeons, 87% of surgeons felt that there is a role for augmented reality as a navigation tool in robotic-assisted surgery [9]. Further, Mitchell and Herrell reported in 2014 that advances in molecular imaging are likely to find a use in robotic-assisted surgery with the advent of molecular markers [10].

In regard to competition, multiple surgical robotic companies are following the pathway forged by Intuitive as the field of surgery continues to embrace robotic- and computer-assisted surgery. TransEnterix, Inc., has filed a FDA 510(k) application in 2017 for its Senhance™ system with an emphasis on haptic force feedback [11]. Titan Medical, Inc., is looking to enter the market with its SPORT™ surgical system featuring multi-articulated instruments [12]. Verb Surgical, Inc., is building its digital surgery prototype in collaboration with Ethicon Endo-Surgery, Inc., and Verily Life Sciences [13]. Multiple others including Cambridge Medical Robotics Ltd., Avatera Medical, Medtronic, Inc., and Meere Company will also look to have product offerings in the future.

Autonomous surgery continues to be a topic of debate with numerous regulatory concerns. With technological advancement in the near term, there is value in a surgeon remaining in the feedback loop; however, supervised automation of specific surgical tasks remains an active area of scientific exploration [14]. The field of surgical robotics will soon see the implementation of advanced data analytics and machine learning. The integration of intelligent systems will support clinical decision-making while helping to define surgeon performance. Intuitive Surgical, Inc., is looking forward to the future as we strive to make surgery more effective, less invasive, and easier on surgeons, patients, and their families.

References

1. Thaly R, Shah K, Patel VR. Applications of robots in urology. J Robot Surg. 2007;1(1):3–17.
2. So DM, Hanuschik M, Kreaden U. Chap. 7 : The da vinci surgical system. In: Rosen J, Hannaford B, Satava RM, editors. Surgical robotics – systems, applications, and visions. 1st ed: Springer; 2011.
3. [Internet]. 2017 [cited 2017 Jul 1]; Available from: https://www.fda.gov/downloads/MedicalDevices/NewsEvents/WorkshopsConferences/UCM454811.pdf.
4. Intuitive Surgical Inc. Form 8-K filing with the United States Securities and Exchange Commission (SEC). June 20, 2003.
5. [Internet]. 2017 [cited 2017 Jul 1]; Available from: https://www.accessdata.fda.gov/scripts/cdrh/cfdocs/cfpmn/pmn.cfm?ID=K171294.
6. [Internet]. 2017. [cited 2017 Jul 1]; Available from: Investor presentation download http://phx.corporate-ir.net/phoenix.zhtml?c=122359&p=irol-irhome.
7. Atallah S, Martin-Perez B, Keller D, et al. Natural orifice transluminal endoscopic surgery. Br J Surg. 2015;102:e73–92.
8. Wong I, Law S. Peroral endoscopic myotomy (POEM) for treating esophageal motility disorders. Ann Transl Med. 2017;5(8):192.

---

[1]As of July 2017, the *da Vinci SP* System is not 510(k) cleared, and the safety or effectiveness of the product has not been established. The *da Vinci SP* System is not currently for sale in the USA.

9. Hughes-Hallett A, Mayer EK, et al. The current and future use of imaging in urological robotic surgery: a survey of the European Association of Robotic Urological Surgeons. Int J Med Robot Comput Assist Surg. 2015;11(1):8–14.

10. Mitchell CR, Herrell SD. Image-guided surgery and emerging molecular imaging: advances to complement minimally invasive surgery. Urol Clin N Am. 2014;41(4):567–80.

11. [Internet]. 2017 [cited 2017 Jul 1]; Available from: http://www.transenterix.com/overview/.

12. [Internet]. 2017 [cited 2017 Jul 1]; Available from: http://www.titanmedicalinc.com/technology/.

13. [Internet]. 2017 [cited 2017 Jul 1]; Available from: http://www.verbsurgical.com/about/.

14. Azizian M, Khoshnam M, et al. Visual servoing in medical robotics: a survey. Part I: endoscopic and direct vision imaging – techniques and applications. Int J Med Robot Comput Assist Surg. 2014;10(3):263–74.

Robotic Simulation Training

Ahmed Zihni, William Gerull, and Michael M. Awad

Introduction

Robot-assisted laparoscopic surgery continues to expand among surgical modalities in a variety of specialties [1–5]. With this expansion, it is increasingly important to provide surgical trainees with adequate training to include robot-assisted surgery in their independent practices. Additionally, just as assessment of basic laparoscopic skills has become a prerequisite of graduation from general surgical training, assessment of robotic fundamentals may also become a requirement of surgical training [6, 7]. Finally, robotics is a new and evolving dimension of surgery that holds promise to expand into nearly every surgical subspecialty and become an important modality that many fully trained surgeons will have to learn. For these reasons, developing training strategies and formalized curricula for robot-assisted surgery is a critical task for today's surgical educators.

Robot-assisted surgery represents a unique platform with many differences from standard laparoscopy and open surgery. Current robotic systems function through a communication system in which surgical tasks are performed by a platform at the patient bedside, while the surgeon exerts direct control over this platform using a console, removed from direct contact with the patient. The surgeon's console allows the surgeon to control the laparoscopic camera and to "clutch" instruments, making it possible to use their full length, while the console masters are kept at a comfortable distance from the surgeon. The surgeon may also employ more than two working arms at a time by swapping control among three engaged instruments. Additionally, different instruments can be changed out by an assistant at the patient bedside when necessary. This multifaceted construct presents many training challenges [8, 9]. The added distance between the surgeon console and robotic cart requires robotic

surgery trainees, assistants, and operating room staff to gain proficiency at positioning and docking the robot to the patient ports. The added distance also requires the operating surgeon to learn to perform procedures without haptic feedback. The use of clutching, extra instruments for retraction and exposure, and camera driving by the surgeon, rather than an assistant, makes robot-assisted procedures less analogous to their laparoscopic or open counterparts. Several studies have detailed these aspects of robotic surgery, showing that laparoscopic and surgical skills are not portable across platforms and that robot-assisted surgery has a significant learning curve, even for experienced surgeons [10–14]. These findings highlight the importance of incorporating dedicated robotic training curricula, particularly simulation-based curricula, into robot-assisted surgical training.

Simulation represents an ideal strategy for robotic surgical training and is a core component of various emerging robotic training curricula [6, 7, 15, 16]. In this chapter, we will review the principles of simulation as they pertain to surgical training, the simulation models currently available, and the instruments available for assessment of training progress and competence.

Simulation

Simulation involves the modeling of a real-world process for a variety of purposes including training, education, testing and assessment, research, predictive analytics, process improvement, investigation, and entertainment. The development and study of simulation is a rapidly expanding field, particularly with the development of more powerful computer systems that can process increasingly complex simulated systems. Many of the broad uses of simulation are applicable in the healthcare setting; however, our focus is on simulation as a training, education, and assessment tool in robotic surgery. In this context, there are three classifications of simulation that form a conceptual framework for discussing specific simulated systems and training models.

A. Zihni · W. Gerull · M. M. Awad (✉)
Department of Surgery, Section of Minimally Invasive Surgery, Barnes-Jewish Hospital, Saint Louis, MO, USA
e-mail: awadm@wustl.edu

© Springer Nature Switzerland AG 2019
S. Tsuda, O. Y. Kudsi (eds.), *Robotic-Assisted Minimally Invasive Surgery*, https://doi.org/10.1007/978-3-319-96866-7_2

Fidelity

The fidelity of a simulation describes how accurately the simulation represents the intended reality. A low-fidelity simulation is usually a stylized or simplified depiction of a system [17]. In surgical training simulations, which are almost universally interactive, the interactions between a user and a low-fidelity simulation can still produce meaningful outputs. Low-fidelity simulations are often used to practice basic sub-tasks within a more complex process or to engage with the conceptual framework of a process rather than its practical function. High-fidelity simulations more closely mirror the process being simulated. They accurately depict a task for a trainee; therefore, as the fidelity of a task performance simulator increases, so does the ability of simulated performance to predict actual task performance.

Setting

The setting of a simulation can vary, and this is of importance when it comes to training for high-fidelity complex tasks. A live setting, in the surgical context, would be a simulation exercise that takes place in the operating room, the surgical ward, or another setting using the equipment, teams, and procedures that would be used in the real-world process. This form of simulation is commonly seen in operating room training drills, emergency response exercises, and team building programs. A laboratory simulation is one in which the simulated scenario takes place in a setting contrived for this purpose. Surgical skills labs, virtual reality environments, and animal or cadaveric operative models all represent laboratory simulations.

Computerization

Advanced computer modeling has revolutionized simulation and has led to the development of virtual reality simulators for surgical training [18]. In these simulations, a virtual environment is simulated by a computer program, and the user interacts with the virtual environment to perform the training task using various means. In contrast, physical simulations involve more traditional practical simulation models.

Models

Didactics

In discussing models of simulation for robotic surgical training, it is important to begin by discussing didactic training. While many of these didactic curricula would not necessarily be considered simulation, formal education in the concepts and theory of robotic surgery is an important foundation for further training. A variety of didactic models exist for the training of robotic surgeons. Many surgical training institutions employ an ad hoc model in which robotic surgery is mentioned in lectures or written coursework within a broader surgical training curriculum, but a robotic-specific curriculum is never taught. For fully trained surgeons who are learning robotic surgery, a similar model takes the form of informal proctoring sessions with colleagues. This lack of structured robotic training at multiple training levels combined with the increased importance of robotic surgery has spurred the development of formal robotic didactic curricula. Intuitive Surgical, Inc., has developed a set of training modules that are accessible online and cover theoretical and technical topics related to robotic surgery [19]. This online program forms the didactic core of robotic surgery curricula at several training institutions. In recent years, several textbooks and atlases of robotic surgery have been published that may be incorporated into the reading lists of residencies and fellowships.

Practical Simulation

Simulations in a practical environment include all real-world or laboratory simulations that do not involve virtual reality, which make up a large proportion of robotic training. The advantages of these simulations are that they can be very high-fidelity, can involve entire care teams instead of one individual learner, and can avoid the need to purchase dedicated simulation equipment. Additionally, the Society of American Gastrointestinal and Endoscopic Surgeons (SAGES) has published a consensus document on robotic surgery which included recommended guidelines for credentialing surgeons to perform robot-assisted surgery. For attending surgeons who were not formally trained in robotic surgery, the consensus group recommended hands-on experience in a dry lab environment as a necessity prior to embarking on actual surgery using a surgical robot [20].

One of the critical aspects of this form of simulation is in the room and robot setup. Robotic surgical cases require a precise sequence of actions to appropriately prepare the robotic platform prior to the case. This sequence includes how to drape the robot, position the patient appropriately for robotic surgery, and dock the robot to the patient once surgery has been initiated. These actions differ from the typical workflow of a laparoscopic or open surgical case and can often lead to a significant time expenditure in the operating room, which has been shown to reliably diminish as surgeons progress along the robotic surgery learning curve. Often, robotic training entails a hands-on simulated setup in a simulation lab with a robotic surgery platform or in an actual robotic operating room at a time when the room is not in use. The learner is coached in the basics of preparation for robotic surgery, including draping the robot, maneuvering the arms into place, docking, and swapping instruments. A similar, more complex form of simulation is team-based simulation focused on communication and problem-solving within a team during robotic surgery [21].

Basic console use is another area of robotic surgery often taught in a lab environment using a dedicated training robot or a robotic platform in the OR during a time when it is not in use. In addition, introductory-level robotic training courses are available around the country for surgeons at the senior trainee and attending levels to become familiar with robotic technology. In this environment, the learner is proctored in basic console use including console setup, camera control, and clutching.

Low-fidelity dry lab simulations have long been a mainstay of training in open and laparoscopic surgery and in recent years have been widely adapted for use with robotic platforms. Simple suturing and knot-tying boards, made from a variety of materials, are used by learners to practice basic operative skills outside of the operating room [22]. These tools are widely used in medical student and intern "boot camp" programs to teach fundamental skills prior to clinical immersion. Suture boards, including several robot-specific variants, have been used to similarly practice basic operative skills such as tissue handling, suturing, and knot tying, during robot-assisted surgery. A very broad array of box-based simulators have been developed for laparoscopic surgery. These constructs are based on a system in which a camera and laparoscopic instruments are introduced into a box, simulating a body cavity, to perform a task within. The tasks performed are generally low-fidelity simulations of common surgical actions like tissue manipulation, dissection, targeting and grasping objects, and intracorporeal suturing. The most important of these simulations are the required tasks in the Fundamentals of Laparoscopic Surgery (FLS) program developed by SAGES and the American College of Surgeons (ACS) [23]. This program also includes a didactic curriculum focused on laparoscopic surgery, and general surgery residents are required to pass a written exam and a skills assessment based on the FLS tasks to take the American Board of Surgery (ABS) qualifying exam for certification. Therefore, the FLS tasks and performance goals are almost universally known in surgical training programs nationwide and have been very extensively validated in a broad evidence-based research studies [23–27]. With the advent of robotic surgery, most FLS tasks were found to be easily adaptable to the robotic platform and were found to be similarly useful in developing and assessing surgical skills on the robotic platform. FLS-based tasks were used as a task performance model in many early studies on robotic surgical skills acquisition, ergonomics, and performance evaluation [23, 28–30].

They remain an important educational tool for robotic surgeons around the country. Additionally, the Fundamentals of Robotic Surgery (FRS) program, an educational project funded by the Department of Defense and Intuitive Surgical, Inc., was modeled on FLS and has developed a didactic curriculum, written examination, and trainer box-based performance assessment for proficiency certification in robotic surgery. An analogous virtual reality-based robotic surgery proficiency examination has also been developed, and validation studies comparing the two assessments are currently underway [7].

High-fidelity *in vivo*, explant, and cadaveric models are important simulation models for robotic surgery. These models allow a surgeon to practice live surgery on an animal model or use a cadaver or ex vivo model to perform surgery on true-to-life human anatomy. A simulation lab must be equipped not only with a robotic surgical platform but also with the capability to safely perform animal or cadaveric procedures for this form of simulation, making it a complex and expensive model. It is, however, the highest fidelity form of simulation for the manipulation of tissue, the interaction between the robotic platform and physical specimen, and the considerations related to operating within a living model. A large body of literature supports the use of animal and cadaveric models for robotic surgical simulation. These models are particularly useful in the development and propagation of new techniques and in expanding the indications of the robotic platform to surgical specialties and procedures where it previously had not been used [15, 26, 31, 32].

Virtual Reality Simulation

The use of virtual reality (VR) in surgical simulation represents a leap forward in simulation technology. VR holds promise for profound future advances as the technology continues to develop. Strictly speaking, VR refers to any computer-generated environment that is designed to give the user the sensation of being present within the environment rather than observing the environment. Current VR technology is usually based on a headset which projects binocular video to generate a three-dimensional image, utilizes headphones or speakers to produce three-dimensional sound, and incorporates gyroscopes and other motion sensors to track the motion of the headset to generate corresponding sensory inputs. In this way the user is immersed in the virtual setting through the sound and visual senses. Since VR has found its broadest application in video gaming, these systems often include handpieces or controllers that allow for interaction with the virtual environment. This basic construct theoretically allows interaction with any virtual environment and could be used to simulate open surgery, laparoscopic surgery, robotic surgery, or endoscopic surgery. It could also be used to simulate real surgical procedures under various conditions in living patients or clinical interactions outside of the operating room. In addition, VR systems allow for tracking of a variety of parameters that are very difficult to track in practical simulation models, such as economy of motion and simulated tension on tissues [33–35]. Finally, VR technology has the potential for allowing unique interactions between educators and learners [15, 28, 31]. For example, VR systems can allow a learner to visualize and emulate the exact actions of an expert performing a task. VR also allows for the possibility of telementoring, in which a remote expert can interact with and direct a learner or a group of learners within a virtual environment.

The potential of VR technology for surgical training and research is enormous, but currently its use is held back by the limits of graphics processing, haptic technology, and artificial intelligence. Robotic surgery, however, represents an ideal use for VR simulation. Current robotic VR simulators employ a console very similar to actual robotic surgery consoles, with computer-generated images projected into its eyepieces. The user can interact with objects in the VR environment using console handpieces just as they would during live robotic surgery. Since robotic surgical systems do not provide the user with haptic feedback from the surgical field, the VR system does not have to simulate haptics, eliminating one of the major hurdles in true-to-life surgical simulation. Additionally, the VR environment is projected into a console rather than a free-floating headset, eliminating the disorientation and vertigo that can be associated with VR environments. However, given the computational limit of modern computers, a high-fidelity simulation of complex surgical operations is not yet available on robotic VR platforms. Instead, the most commonly used VR simulators are equipped with training modules that simulate basic surgical tasks such as camera driving, targeting and transferring objects, pattern cutting, suturing and knot tying, basic use of surgical energy, and tissue manipulation [6, 33]. Metrics are collected via modules that are graded by difficulty, task completion time, motion parameters, and various faults, with a defined performance goal set for passing the module. This metrics collection feature allows learners to track their own performance and educators to design curricula using a set of modules that learners must complete to achieve basic proficiency. Several such curricula have been proposed, and several groups are currently at work validating VR-based curricula for robotic surgery and associating their use with surgeon and patient outcomes [6, 16, 34, 36].

Assessment

Most uses of surgical simulation involve assessment tools to determine utility of the simulation and evaluate the progression of users during the simulation. Two broad categories of learner assessment with wide application in surgical simulation are subjective and objective assessments.

Subjective Assessment

Subjective assessments are those that depend on the perspective of the user interacting with the simulation. These assessment tools are important for understanding how individuals perceive their interactions within a simulation and are useful for designing and improving simulated constructs. Subjective assessment tools can be simple surveys specific to a particular simulation, which provide focused and relevant data but are often not generalizable. Other subjective assessment tools are designed and validated for broad applicability to almost any task, such as the NASA task load index (NTLX), a survey instrument that assesses various domains of workload during task performance [16, 21, 23].

Objective Assessment

A variety of objective evaluations on user performance have been applied to robotic simulation. The most important of these is the performance evaluation necessary to achieve certification in the Fundamentals of Robotic Surgery (FRS) program. Objective evaluation of learners by mentoring surgeons is also necessary, and several tools have been developed for this purpose. Our group developed a robot-specific adaptation of the Ottawa Surgical Competency Operating Room Evaluation (RO-SCORE), and several other similar evaluation tools have been reported in the literature [16, 37–41]. VR simulators also provide a variety of metrics on performance time, motion, and task quality. These objective measures of task performance can be interpreted to track performance and identify specific parameters for improvement. Finally, our group and others have used objective ergonomic measures, as quantified by surface electromyography (sEMG), to quantify physical stress during task performance on simulated tasks and live operative procedures [23, 42, 43].

Conclusion

Surgical simulation tools are increasingly important in training, research, and skills assessment. They hold particular importance in robotic surgery, where simulation is central to educational curricula, skills assessment, and certification criteria. As VR technology continues to progress, it promises to revolutionize surgical simulation even further. Future research into robotic surgical simulation will be necessary to describe the effects of advanced simulation models and curricula on patient and surgeon outcomes.

References

1. Menaker SA, Shah SS, Snelling BM, Sur S, Starke RM, Peterson EC. Current applications and future perspectives of robotics in cerebrovascular and endovascular neurosurgery. J Neurointerv Surg. 2017;10(1):78–82.

2. Nelson RJ, Chavali JSS, Yerram N, Babbar P, Kaouk JH. Current status of robotic single-port surgery. Urol Ann. 2017;9(3):217–22.

3. Schiff L, Tsafrir Z, Aoun J, Taylor A, Theoharis E, Eisenstein D. Quality of communication in robotic surgery and surgical outcomes. JSLS. 2016;20(3):00026.

4. Falkenback D, Lehane CW, Lord RV. Robot-assisted oesophageal and gastric surgery for benign disease: antireflux operations and Heller's myotomy. ANZ J Surg. 2015;85(3):113–20.

5. Chang EHE, Kim HY, Koh YW, Chung WY. Overview of robotic thyroidectomy. Gland Surg. 2017;6(3):218–28.

6. Connolly M, Seligman J, Kastenmeier A, Goldblatt M, Gould JC. Validation of a virtual reality-based robotic surgical skills curriculum. Surg Endosc. [Journal Article Research Support, Non-U.S. Gov't Validation Studies]. 2014;28(5):1691–4.

7. Smith R, Patel V, Satava R. Fundamentals of robotic surgery: a course of basic robotic surgery skills based upon a 14-society consensus template of outcomes measures and curriculum development. Int J Med Robot. 2014;10(3):379–84.

8. Lee MR, Lee GI. Does a robotic surgery approach offer optimal ergonomics to gynecologic surgeons?: a comprehensive ergonomics survey study in gynecologic robotic surgery. J Gynecol Oncol. 2017;28(5):e70.

9. Raza SJ, Froghi S, Chowriappa A, Ahmed K, Field E, Stegemann AP, et al. Construct validation of the key components of fundamental skills of robotic surgery (FSRS) curriculum – a multi-institution prospective study. J Surg Educ. 2014;71(3):316–24.

10. Efanov M, Alikhanov R, Tsvirkun V, Kazakov I, Melekhina O, Kim P, et al. Comparative analysis of learning curve in complex robot-assisted and laparoscopic liver resection. HPB (Oxford). 2017;19(9):818–24.

11. Goldenberg MG, Goldenberg L, Grantcharov TP. Surgeon performance predicts early continence after robot-assisted radical prostatectomy. J Endourol. 2017;31(9):858–63.

12. Lee S, Son T, Kim HI, Hyung WJ. Status and prospects of robotic gastrectomy for gastric cancer: our experience and a review of the literature. Gastroenterol Res Pract. 2017;2017:7197652.

13. Raimondi P, Marchegiani F, Cieri M, Cichella A, Cotellese R, Innocenti P. Is right colectomy a complete learning procedure for a robotic surgical program? J Robot Surg. 2017;12(1):147–55.

14. Zelhart M, Kaiser AM. Robotic versus laparoscopic versus open colorectal surgery: towards defining criteria to the right choice. Surg Endosc. 2017;32(1):24–38.

15. Badash I, Burtt K, Solorzano CA, Carey JN. Innovations in surgery simulation: a review of past, current and future techniques. Ann Transl Med. 2016;4(23):453.

16. Zihni AM, Ray S, Declue A, Tiemann D, Wang R, Liang Z, Awad MM. Operative performance outcomes of a simulator-based robotic surgical skills curriculum. Houston: Society of American Gastrointestinal and Endoscopic Surgeons; 2017.

17. Brackney DE, Priode K. Back to reality: the use of the presence questionnaire for measurement of fidelity in simulation. J Nurs Meas. 2017;25(2):66–73.

18. Brown K, Mosley N, Tierney J. Battle of the bots: a comparison of the standard da Vinci and the da Vinci surgical skills simulator in surgical skills acquisition. J Robot Surg. 2016;11(2):159–62.

19. Intuitive Surgical, Inc. da Vinci training. Sunnyvale: Intuitive Surgical, Inc; 2017. [cited 2017 06/01]; Available from: https://www.intuitivesurgical.com/training/.

20. Herron DM. A consensus document on robotic surgery. Los Angeles: Society of American Gastrointestinal and Endoscopic Surgeons; 2007. [cited 2017 06/01]; Available from: https://www.sages.org/publications/guidelines/consensus-document-robotic-surgery/.

21. Sexton K, Johnson A, Gotsch A, Hussein AA, Cavuoto L, Guru KA. Anticipation, teamwork and cognitive load: chasing efficiency during robot-assisted surgery. BMJ Qual Saf. 2018;27(2):148–54.

22. Seeley MA, Kazarian E, King B, Biermann JS, Carpenter JE, Caird MS, et al. Core concepts: orthopedic intern curriculum boot camp. Orthopedics. 2016;39(1):e62–7. Epub 2016 Jan 5. https://doi.org/10.3928/01477447-20151228-03.

23. Zihni AM, Ohu I, Cavallo JA, Ousley J, Cho S, Awad MM. FLS tasks can be used as an ergonomic discriminator between laparoscopic and robotic surgery. Surg Endosc. 2014;28(8):2459–65.

24. Cullinan DR, Schill MR, DeClue A, Salles A, Wise PE, Awad MM. Fundamentals of laparoscopic surgery: not only for senior residents. J Surg Educ. 2017;74(6):e51–4.

25. Franklin BR, Placek SB, Wagner MD, Haviland SM, O'Donnell MT, Ritter EM. Cost comparison of fundamentals of laparoscopic surgery training completed with standard fundamentals of laparoscopic surgery equipment versus low-cost equipment. J Surg Educ. 2017;74(3):459–65.

26. Nemani A, Ahn W, Cooper C, Schwaitzberg S, De S. Convergent validation and transfer of learning studies of a virtual reality-based pattern cutting simulator. Surg Endosc. 2017;32(3):1265–72.

27. Zendejas B, Ruparel RK, Cook DA. Validity evidence for the fundamentals of laparoscopic surgery (FLS) program as an assessment tool: a systematic review. Surg Endosc. 2016;30(2):512–20.

28. Lum MJ, Rosen J, Lendvay TS, Wright AS, Sinanan MN, Hannaford B. TeleRobotic fundamentals of laparoscopic surgery (FLS): effects of time delay – pilot study. Conf Proc IEEE Eng Med Biol Soc. 2008;2008:5597–600.

29. Stefanidis D, Hope WW, Scott DJ. Robotic suturing on the FLS model possesses construct validity, is less physically demanding, and is favored by more surgeons compared with laparoscopy. Surg Endosc. 2011;25(7):2141–6.

30. Panait L, Shetty S, Shewokis PA, Sanchez JA. Do laparoscopic skills transfer to robotic surgery? J Surg Res. 2014;187(1):53–8.

31. Forgione A, Guraya SY. The cutting-edge training modalities and educational platforms for accredited surgical training: a systematic review. J Res Med Sci. 2017;22:51.

32. Schlottmann F, Murty NS, Patti MG. Simulation model for laparoscopic foregut surgery: The University of North Carolina foregut model. J Laparoendosc Adv Surg Tech A. 2017;27(7):661–5.

33. Alzahrani T, Haddad R, Alkhayal A, Delisle J, Drudi L, Gotlieb W, et al. Validation of the da Vinci surgical skill simulator across three surgical disciplines: a pilot study. Can Urol Assoc J. 2013;7(7–8):E520–9.

34. Raison N, Ahmed K, Fossati N, Buffi N, Mottrie A, Dasgupta P, et al. Competency based training in robotic surgery: benchmark scores for virtual reality robotic simulation. BJU Int. 2016;119(5):804–11.

35. Yang K, Zhen H, Hubert N, Perez M, Wang XH, Hubert J. From dV-trainer to real robotic console: the limitations of robotic skill training. J Surg Educ. 2017;74(6):1074–80.

36. Hogg ME, Tam V, Zenati M, Novak S, Miller J, Zureikat AH, et al. Mastery-based virtual reality robotic simulation curriculum: the first step toward operative robotic proficiency. J Surg Educ. 2016;74(3):477–85.

37. Dubin AK, Smith R, Julian D, Tanaka A, Mattingly P. A comparison of robotic simulation performance on basic virtual reality skills: simulator subjective vs. objective assessment tools. J Minim Invasive Gynecol. 2017;24(7):1184–9.

38. Frederick PJ, Szender JB, Hussein AA, Kesterson JP, Shelton JA, Anderson TL, et al. Surgical competency for robot-assisted hysterectomy: development and validation of a

robotic hysterectomy assessment score (RHAS). J Minim Invasive Gynecol. 2017;24(1):55–61.

39. Liu M, Purohit S, Mazanetz J, Allen W, Kreaden US, Curet M. Assessment of robotic console skills (ARCS): construct validity of a novel global rating scale for technical skills in robotically assisted surgery. Surg Endosc. 2017;32(1):526–35.

40. Mills JT, Hougen HY, Bitner D, Krupski TL, Schenkman NS. Does robotic surgical simulator performance correlate with surgical skill? J Surg Educ. 2017;74(6):1052–6.

41. Vargas MV, Moawad G, Denny K, Happ L, Misa NY, Margulies S, et al. Transferability of virtual reality, simulation-based, robotic suturing skills to a live porcine model in novice surgeons: a single-blind randomized controlled trial. J Minim Invasive Gynecol. 2017;24(3):420–5.

42. Zihni AM, Cavallo JA, Ray S, Ohu I, Cho S, Awad MM. Ergonomic analysis of primary and assistant surgical roles. J Surg Res. 2016;203(2):301–5.

43. Zihni AM, Ohu I, Cavallo JA, Cho S, Awad MM. Ergonomic analysis of robot-assisted and traditional laparoscopic procedures. Surg Endosc. 2014;28(12):3379–84.

Robotic Resident and Fellow Surgery Training

3

Jamil Stetler and Ankit D. Patel

Introduction

Robotic surgery has been growing for over a decade and has even become the preferred approach for certain surgical procedures. Currently, the only commercially available system in the United States is manufactured by Intuitive Surgical and marketed under the da Vinci ® platform. It is now estimated that one in four US hospitals has at least one da Vinci robot [1]. Over half a million worldwide da Vinci robotic procedures were performed in 2014, which is a 178% increase compared to 2009, with majority of these cases being performed in the United States [1]. This growth has been seen across most specialties, and in fact, general surgery is one of the fastest growing specialties using robotic technology. Approximately 140,000 robotic surgeries were performed in general surgery in 2015, which is 31% more than in 2014 [2]. Therefore, whether residents decide to work in an academic-, a private-, or a hospital-based practice, there is a high likelihood that they will have exposure to this technology during their careers. With its adoption and growth across the country, residency programs need to incorporate robotic training into their curriculums.

The addition of new techniques/technology into resident training is not new. For example, the boom of laparoscopy in the 1990s heralded new training paradigms and curriculum for residents. During the adoption period of laparoscopy, there were similar barriers and concerns about its impact on surgical resident training and whether residents would have adequate exposure to open surgical approaches. Now, majority of cases that were routinely performed in an open fashion are predominately offered in a minimally invasive form which has improved patient recovery, decreased postoperative pain, shortened hospital length of stay, reduced overall cost, and reduced postoperative complication rates. With its growth and acceptance, it became a cornerstone of general surgery resident training. The Fundamentals of Laparoscopic Surgery ® (FLS) program was born from this and is now a validated curriculum being used at all general surgery residencies; the American Board of Surgery has added it as a requirement for general surgery trainees [3, 4].

Today, general surgery widely accepts laparoscopy; however, some of the same negative past sentiments toward laparoscopy are now repeating themselves toward the emerging popularity of robotic surgery and are likely slowing the inevitable widespread adoption of this technology. To date, there is no standardized robotic surgery training curriculum. However, in the future, there will likely be fundamental robotic skill requirements for graduating general surgery residents just as there are for laparoscopy. Robotic surgery curricula do exist, and examples include da Vinci Surgery Community (Intuitive Surgical Inc., Sunnyvale, CA, www.davincisurgerycommunity.com), Fundamentals of Robotic Surgery (FRS, http://frsurgery.org/), or individual residency programs that have adopted their own curriculum [5, 6]. Prior studies have validated and identified unique skills/tasks that are required to perform robotic operations and have developed comprehensive proficiency-based robotic training curriculum; however, there are some challenges, namely, access to the platform and cost to incorporating these models into training curriculum [7].

Challenges to Resident Robotic Training

Access

Many residency programs have a robotic platform at their institution. However, resident access to the platform at each institution varies widely. Additionally, not every institution has general surgery attendings that routinely use the device

J. Stetler
Department of General Surgery, Emory University, Atlanta, GA, USA

A. D. Patel (✉)
Department of General and GI Surgery, Emory University, Atlanta, GA, USA
e-mail: Apatel7@emory.edu

for their procedures, and at institutions where the use of robotics in general surgery is growing, these new users are still going through their learning curve, which may limit teaching to the residents. Farivar, B et al. conducted a national survey of residents at 240 ACGME-approved surgery training programs in 2013, of which only 193 residents responded [8]. However, they noted that 96% of their responders had robot systems at their institution, with 63% of the respondents reporting that they participated in robotic cases [8]. Most assisted in ten or fewer robotic cases with the most common exposure consisting of robotic trocar placement, docking, and undocking [8]. Strikingly, only 18% operated at the robotic console [8].

Cost

In an ideal world, residents would be able to train in a simulated setting and/or in the operating room with a dual console platform. However, for most this is not feasible given the additional cost of acquiring a stand-alone robotic simulator (~$85,000–100,000) and a backpack that attaches to a console ($75,000–85,000 not including the console), having a full robotic platform purely for simulation, or having a dual console in the operating room (~$500,000 for additional console). Additionally, unlike in laparoscopy where relatively affordable box trainers can offer simulation to achieve proficiency in fundamental skills, this is not an option for learning robotic surgery.

Duty Hours

The Accreditation Council for Graduate Medical Education (ACGME) implemented the 80-h workweek reforms in 2003, with further restrictions added in 2011. These new constraints resulted in residency programs restructuring their training curriculum and concentrating their training efforts in order to accommodate these changes. As a consequence, some training programs are struggling to meet basic training requirements for general surgery training given the time constraints by the current duty hour restrictions. This has caused some residents to feel undertrained when completing residency and opting for further training in various specialty fellowships. Adding another training requirement on top of the current training model will be difficult and may take away from other training experiences like laparoscopy. Currently, completion of Fundamentals of Laparoscopic Surgery ® (FLS) and Fundamentals of Endoscopic Surgery ® (FES) are required to qualify for general surgery boards, while no robotic requirements exist. Given this, most institutions are likely to prioritize training in these areas.

Impact on Laparoscopy Skills

Implementing robotic surgery training into the general surgery curriculum will likely decrease laparoscopic case volumes as well as directly impacting resident participation in those cases [2]. Mehaffey et al. reviewed all of the patients at their institution who underwent laparoscopic or robotic cholecystectomy, inguinal hernia repair, or ventral hernia repair from 2011 to 2015. They analyzed 2391 cases, of which 162 were performed robotically, over that 5-year period. They found that as robotic surgery was being adopted, there was a decrease in the number of laparoscopic cases being performed [2]. Additionally, they found that less than 20% of robotic cases were being performed primarily by trainees [2]. Furthermore, laparoscopic cases that were usually delegated to junior residents, such as cholecystectomy and hernia repairs, were now covered by chief resident 89% of the time when performed robotically [2]. In summary, they noted a decrease in the number of laparoscopic cases being performed, decreased overall trainee involvement in these cases, and an upward shift in the level of resident performing the operations. Programs implementing robotic surgery into their curriculum will have to balance their residents acquiring the necessary fundamentals of laparoscopy with learning the fundamentals of robotic surgery.

Goals of a Robotic Curriculum

In a general surgery program, trainees performing open or laparoscopic surgery progress in a stepwise fashion from a level of observation to operating independently. The same holds true for robotic surgery training. Trainees should progress from observation, to bedside assisting, to console time, and finally to operating autonomously and teaching their juniors. Prior to this succession, trainees should complete didactic training modules and some form of simulation. The goal of general surgery residency should be to help residents become well versed in the robotic platform components, indications for use, benefits, and limitations of the current technology and develop proficiency in basic robotic skills. Even if the trainees are not planning to use the platform in their practice, they will likely be called upon at some point in their career to assist other services using the robot platform (i.e., urology, gynecology, surgical oncology, etc.) for intraoperative assistance, and it may behoove them to have basic training.

Acquiring Basic Skills

Learning and mastering the principles of general surgical technique are few of the main goals of all general surgery residency training programs. The principles of surgical technique do not change whether the procedure is performed openly, laparoscopically, or robotically. Residents who learn how to perform open or laparoscopic surgery at a high level will be able to accomplish these procedures whether they use a robotic platform or any new emerging technology. Furthermore, majority of basic skills learned in laparoscopy are translatable to robotic surgery. Therefore, trainees at programs with strong laparoscopy training will acquire these skills more easily.

The curriculum we suggest should be based on four components: didactic learning (www.davincisurgerycommunity.com or frsurgery.org), bedside assistant training, simulation (robotic simulator pack or dry lab simulation), and training in the operating room. The online didactics at www.davinci-surgerycommunity.com cover the basics of the Si and Xi systems including the surgeon console controls, patient cart, vision cart, docking, instrument placement and exchange, and safety features. These modules are available free to anyone associated with a training program. After completing all the required modules, the trainee will obtain a certificate of completion. The curriculum available at FRS is very similar and could also be used; however, at this time, completion of those modules does not count toward the equivalency certificate issued by Intuitive.

Bedside assistant training will allow the trainee to learn port placement, patient positioning, and instrument exchange, gain a better understanding of the equipment needed to perform the case, understand how to assist at bedside, observe surgical technique required for various cases, and troubleshoot issues that may arise at bedside, such as arm collisions or errors. The trainee should have bedside training involving all components of the robotic platform in a non-operative setting by an experienced instructor to cover these topics, after which a minimum of 5–10 bedside assistant cases should be completed (this number of bedside assistant cases has been generally accepted by other authors) [9]. At our institution we require ten bedside assistant cases, and the trainee must track and report these cases to the residency program so that they can be filed (Fig. 3.1).

Place stickers from cases in which you were the bedside assistant and participated in inserting trocars, docking the robot, and inserting and exchanging instruments. You need a minimum of 1(cases. Copy this page as needed and turn in completed forms.

Patient Sticker	Date	Attending	Operation

Name

Signature

Fig. 3.1 Bedside assist log

Simultaneously, the trainee should participate in simulation. The type of simulation will vary at every institution based on what resources are available. If a stand-alone simulator or backpack is available, the trainee should complete the simulation program tasks that focus on teaching wrist manipulation, camera movement, instrument clutching, needle manipulation and suturing, fourth arm use, dissection, and application of energy. These tasks should be completed until a level of proficiency has been met or to a set score. At our institution, we require a score of 90% or greater, and the residents must provide documentation of task completion to the residency program (Fig. 3.2). Studies have validated the

simulator and identified the unique skills/tasks that are required to perform robotic operations [7]. Some institutions may have access to a full robotic platform in a dry lab setting which can be used to practice more bedside robotic skills. However, this level of simulation may be cost prohibitive for most training programs.

Finally, the trainee will have the opportunity to gain operative console experience in a supervised fashion by an experienced robotic surgeon. The portions of the case the trainee will be able to complete will be dependent on the attending surgeons and the trainee's level of experience. Just as in open or laparoscopic surgery training, the trainee should have the

Submit when completed:

Module	Date Completed	Score (%)
Camera and Clutching → Camera Targeting 1		
Camera and Clutching → Camera Targeting 2		
Endowrist Manipulation 1→ Pick & Place		
Endowrist Manipulation 1→ Peg Board 1		
Endowrist Manipulation 1→ Peg Board 2		
Energy & Dissection → Energy Switching 1		
Energy & Dissection → Energy Switching 2		
Energy & Dissection → Energy Dissection 1		
Energy & Dissection → Energy Dissection 2		
Needle Control → Needle Targeting		
Needle Control → Thread the Rings		
Needle Driving → Suture Sponge 1		
Needle Driving → Suture Sponge 2		
Needle Driving → Tubes		

Resident:

_____   _____
Name   Signature

Verified by:

_____   _____
Name   Date

Fig. 3.2 Simulator module completion log. Trainee must score ≥90% on each module

opportunity for graduated responsibility and autonomy. The trainee should get exposure to a mixture of common general surgery pathology and systems such as hernia, foregut, biliary, solid organ, and intestinal tract cases. Ideally, cases would be performed using a dual console system, but this is obviously not mandatory as not every program has access to this system. The supervising surgeon will have to assess each residents' capabilities and allow for graduated intraoperative responsibility while being readily available to take over when needed, just as with open and laparoscopic cases. At our institution, we require trainees to track their console surgeon cases. They must document the completion of at least 20 console cases where they performed a significant portion of the case (Fig. 3.3). Residents in their final year of training that have completed the requirements will be evaluated by the supervising robotic surgeons for their last five cases as console surgeon (Fig. 3.4).

A physical curriculum should be provided to the residents, and they will be responsible to complete each step in the curriculum and provide documentation of completion to their education department. If satisfactory, the residents will receive a certificate of completion. Ultimately, privileges for performing robotic surgery will be determined by the trainee's future hospital of employment and their surgical privileges committee. However, having documentation of completion of basic requirements and case logs may aid in acquiring privileges.

Acquiring Advance Skills

High-volume robotic centers may have the case numbers and exposure to robotics for residents to learn more advance procedures. However, at this point in time, the majority of train-

Place stickers from a minimum of 15 cases in which you were the console surgeon and performed a significant portion of the case. Copy this page as needed and turn in completed forms.

Patient Sticker	Date	Attending	Operation

Fig. 3.3 Console surgeon resident case log

_____
Name

_____
Signature

Fig. 3.4 Chief year case log

This form is for residents in their final year who have already performed 15 cases as console surgeon. The evaluation is to be completed by the attending physician and reviewed with the resident at the completion of the case. Make a copy of this form for each case and turn forms in when complete. You must perform this evaluation for at least 5 cases.

Patient Sticker	Resident	Date
	Operation	

Skill	Adequate	More Practice Recommended
Demonstrates understanding of trocar placement and spacing		
Understands principles of docking and is able to dock in a timely fashion		
Uses camera appropriately and is able to focus the camera		
Demonstrates appropriate clutching and maintains hands in a comfortable workspace		
Demonstrates ability to use third arm and switch between instruments		
SAFETY: Does not move instruments that are not in view		
SAFETY: Recognizes tissue response to assess grip strength and handles tissue appropriately		
Demonstrates ability to troubleshoot system and manage collisions		

Please comment on areas of strength:

Please comment on opportunities for improvement:

The resident demonstrates competency on the robotic system.   YES   NO

_____   _____
Attending Name   Attending Signature

ing programs do not have the case volumes to offer this to every general surgery resident. For these trainees who wish to add these capabilities, they may need more advanced training in minimally invasive surgery fellowships, in new robotic surgery fellowships, or in postgraduate case proctoring.

To date there are no standardized national curriculums for robotic surgery, and there are several challenges to implementing robotic surgery curriculums. Each training program will have to assess their access to the platform, caseload, and number of residents in their program to develop the most appropriate curriculum for their situation.

Summary

We are currently in an age of robotic surgery and are seeing its exponential growth across multiple surgical fields. Residents in training are now getting increased exposure to the platform and will likely have to assimilate its use into their future practices,

but there is no standardized curriculum for robotic training. General surgery training programs are now having to develop their own training curriculum to prepare their trainees. As outlined in this chapter, there are several challenges to incorporating these curricula. The goal of a robotic training curriculum should be that trainees become well versed in the robotic components, indications for its use, benefits, and limitations of the current technology and develop proficiency in basic robotic skills. Trainees should progress in a stepwise fashion from a level of observation to operating independently. A complete curriculum should start with some form of didactic learning. Next, trainees should complete bedside assist training with a focus on learning port placement, patient positioning, and instrument exchange, observing surgical technique required for various cases, and troubleshooting issues that may arise at bedside, such as arm collisions or errors. Then, the trainee should complete simulation exercises, whether on the simulator packs or in a dry lab setting. Lastly, the trainee should progress to console surgeon with direct attending supervision. These

Fig. 3.5 Activities by postgraduate years

I. PGY-1/2
   a. Complete online training
   b. Attend a hands-on course
   c. Complete all required modules on the simulator
   d. Observer or bedside assistant for robotic cases
   e. Perform portions of hernia/sleeve cases
   f. Practice on the simulator

2. PGY-3/4
   a. Completed all of the above
   b. Continue practice on the simulator
   c. Perform portions of robotic hernia/foregut operations/cholecystectomies
   d. Perform portions of the mobilization in segmental colectomies

3. PGY-5
   a. Completed all of the above
   b. Perform complete cases
   c. Assist junior residents in robotic procedures

requirements can be dispersed throughout a 5-year general surgery program, with tasks assigned to level appropriate postgraduate years (Fig. 3.5). The trainee should track their progress throughout the curriculum and provide documentation to their programs for filing. At the time of graduation, residents will receive a letter of completion documenting their experience and competency. While all hospitals will have different requirements regarding surgical readiness, documentation of adequate robotic training in residency could ultimately replace any industry-sponsored training.

References

1. ECRI Institute. https://www.ecri.org/Resources/ASG/Robotic_Surgery_Infographic_MS15369_web.pdf. 2015. Accessed 1 Aug 2017.
2. Mehaffey JH, Michaels AD, Mullen MG, Yount KW, Meneveau MO, Smith PW, Friel CM, Schirmer BD. Adoption of robotics in a general surgery residency program: at what cost? J Surg Res. 2017;213:269–73, ISSN 0022–4804, https://doi.org/10.1016/j.jss.2017.02.052. http://www.sciencedirect.com/science/article/pii/S0022480417301026.
3. Fundamentals of Laparoscopic Surgery. http://www.flsprogram.org. Accessed 9 Mar 2017.
4. American Board of Surgery. http://www.absurgery.org/default.jsp?certgsqe_training. Accessed 9 Mar 2017.
5. da Vinci Surgical Community. www.davincisurgerycommunity.com. Accessed 9 Mar 2017.
6. Fundamentals of Robotic Surgery. http://frsurgery.org/. Accessed 9 Mar 2017.
7. Dulan G, et al. Proficiency-based training for robotic surgery: construct validity, workload, and expert levels for nine inanimate exercises. Surg Endosc. 2012;26(6):1516–21.
8. Farivar BS, Flannagan M, Michael Leitman I. General surgery residents' perception of robot-assisted procedures during surgical training. J Surg Educ. 2015;72(2):235–42, ISSN 1931-7204, https://doi.org/10.1016/j.jsurg.2014.09.008. http://www.sciencedirect.com/science/article/pii/S1931720414002591.
9. Winder JS, Juza RM, Sasaki J, et al. Implementing a robotics curriculum at an academic general surgery training program: our initial experience. J Robot Surg. 2016;10:209. https://doi-org.proxy.library.emory.edu/10.1007/s11701-016-0569-9

Medicolegal Issues in Robotic Surgery

4

Elizabeth M. Hechenbleikner and Brian P. Jacob

The Rise of Robotic Surgery

Surgeons' use of robotic platforms to perform surgery is on the rise and will continue to expand globally for years to come before becoming mainstream. The marriage between robotics and surgery continues to evolve and become more durable. Across the 1980s and 1990s, the expansion in minimally invasive surgical procedures was largely limited to laparoscopic technology and instruments. During this time, the emergence of robotic technology was in part ignited by collaborations between NASA and the Stanford Research Institute (SRI) to develop telesurgery models [1]. Subsequently, the US Army funded efforts with the help of the SRI to build mobile vehicle-based robotic surgical arms that were controlled by surgeons at workstations housed at surgical hospitals; these efforts were intended for damage control surgery in wounded soldiers but thus far have only been implemented in animal models [2]. Naturally, military efforts toward expansion of surgical robotics ultimately led to commercialization by early front-runners like Integrated Surgical Systems, Inc., and Computer Motion, Inc. Despite the advent of ROBODOC® for orthopedic surgery and the Aesop® system for laparoscopic camera manipulation, the real juggernaut of robotic surgery is the *da Vinci*® Surgical System launched by Intuitive Surgical, Inc., and approved by the US Food and Drug Administration (FDA) in 2000 for general laparoscopic procedures. With increasingly sophisticated *da Vinci*® models and FDA approval across

multiple surgical specialties, thousands of units have been sold worldwide [3] with over 7000 peer-reviewed publications to date [4].

Stakeholders at Medicolegal Risk in Robotic Surgery

When a patient undergoes a robotic surgery, there are many stakeholders at risk for medicolegal compliance as summarized in Table 4.1.

Available General Surgery Guidelines for Surgical Robotics

Several years after FDA approval of the *da Vinci*® system, the Society of American Gastrointestinal and Endoscopic Surgeons (SAGES) and Minimally Invasive Robotic Association (MIRA) convened an international multidisciplinary group in 2006 (the SAGES-MIRA Robotics Consensus Conference) to establish guidelines and a broad consensus statement on the tenets of implementing robotic surgery [5]. Some of the key areas addressed during this conference were as follows: (1) training and credentialing, (2) appropriate clinical applications, and (3) patient risks. Patient outcomes were briefly addressed across multiple specialties including gynecology, urology, general surgery, and thoracic surgery. Key limitations identified included lack of appropriate training and paucity of outcomes data. Furthermore, some of the patient risks addressed in the consensus statement included the absence of haptic or tactile feedback in current robotic technology, mechanical and electronic device failures, and institutional risks for maintaining robotic systems in accordance with manufacturer recommendations [5].

More recently, the SAGES Technology and Value Assessment Committee (TAVAC) published a consensus statement in 2015 based on a comprehensive literature review of the use of the *da Vinci*® system for gastrointestinal sur-

E. M. Hechenbleikner
Department of General Surgery, Mount Sinai Hospital, New York, NY, USA

Department of General Surgery, Garlock Division of Surgery, Mount Sinai Hospital, New York, NY, USA

B. P. Jacob (✉)
Department of General Surgery, Mount Sinai Hospital, New York, NY, USA

Icahn School of Medicine at Mount Sinai, Laparoscopic Surgical Center of New York, New York, NY, USA

© Springer Nature Switzerland AG 2019
S. Tsuda, O. Y. Kudsi (eds.), *Robotic-Assisted Minimally Invasive Surgery*, https://doi.org/10.1007/978-3-319-96866-7_4

Table 4.1 Stakeholders involved in robotic surgery and their associated responsibility

Stakeholder	Responsibility
Device manufacturer	All device-, instrument-, or implant-related use and safety issues Device-related training of surgeons Device-related training of surgical assistants and operating room staff Device-related training to the hospitals
Primary surgeons and their surgical team (bedside surgical assistants, residents, nurses, staff, etc.)	Safe use of the device and instruments within reasonable acceptable surgical standards Providing preoperative, intraoperative, and postoperative patient care as per one's local acceptable standards Ethical and factual advertising and dissemination of claims Conflict of interest management
Hospital and institutions	All device or implant processing and sterilization issues Providing adequate device maintenance Providing accurate advertising and marketing claims Providing adequate credentialing criteria for all users Providing adequate training to staff, nurses, surgical residents, etc. as appropriate Assuring quality control of outcomes

gery across a variety of surgical specialties including foregut, bariatric, hepatopancreaticobiliary, and colorectal [6]. In general, robotic-assisted surgical approaches had similar outcomes to laparoscopic approaches but frequently had longer operative times and increased costs. The authors concluded that the *da Vinci®* system appeared to have similar morbidity, mortality, and overall benefits when compared to standard laparoscopy but required adequate training and experience. Moreover, future high-quality research is required to better evaluate patient outcomes, satisfaction, and healthcare costs associated with robotic- vs. laparoscopic-assisted surgery.

Global Market Expansion in Surgical Robotics

Since the SAGES-MIRA Robotics Consensus Conference in 2006, the global surgical robotics market has continued to see astronomical growth and expansion. Annual US-based volume for robotic-assisted laparoscopic procedures dramatically increased from roughly 40,000 in 2006 to over 300,000 in 2011 (Fig. 4.1) [7]. By 2025, the surgical robotics market is projected to be worth over $12 billion worldwide with *da Vinci®* robots expected to lead the way with the largest global installation volume across 2016. While gynecologic specialties dominated the market value and case volume in 2016, general surgery cases will likely account for the highest procedural volume by 2025. Hospitals are the leading source of purchasing and installing robotic systems, particularly in North America, with continued growth also being seen in ambulatory surgical centers [8].

Across 2017, the annual revenue for Intuitive Surgical alone was over $3 billion. The majority of the company's revenue was accounted for in instrument and accessory equipment which is intimately associated with overall usage and case volume. The overall 2017 procedure volume for *da Vinci®* systems was almost 900,000, largely due to global increases in urologic procedures as well as US-based general surgery cases [9]. The skyrocketing progress in *da Vinci®* case volume and profits is matched by a very aggressive sales and marketing infrastructure and culture at Intuitive Surgical; with the push to implement this technology, not surprisingly, there has been a rapid rise in adverse safety event reporting along with an increasing numbers of lawsuits [10].

Safety Concerns in Surgical Robotics and the MAUDE Database

In order to evaluate the publicly available information on safety concerns regarding a device, some turn to the MAUDE database. While this database is *NOT* to be used to evaluate the rates of adverse events, the publicly available MAUDE (Manufacturer and User Facility Device Experience) database contains all FDA-mandated and voluntary adverse event reports for medical devices. It is limited in that it is self-reported and clearly will not capture all adverse events.

In a 2016 comprehensive review of the MAUDE database, Alemzadeh et al. reported 10,624 adverse events across a 14-year period (2000–2013) associated with the use of robotic systems in a variety of procedures and surgical sub-specialties [11]. The overwhelmingly majority of these reports were submitted by manufacturers and distributors with an estimated adverse event rate per procedure of <0.6%; Fig. 4.2 demonstrates annual adverse event reports as well as adverse event reports per 100,000 procedures. In addition, 14.4% of adverse events led to serious patient injuries including 144 deaths along with other negative outcomes like device malfunctions which were identified in 76% of overall

Fig. 4.1 Annual US and International Robotic-Assisted Procedure Volumes (2004–2011). (From Cooper et al. [7], with permission of Wolters Kluwer Health, Inc.)

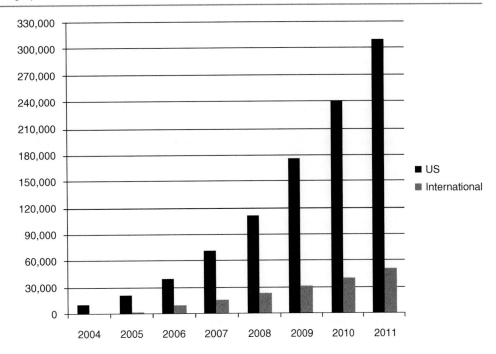

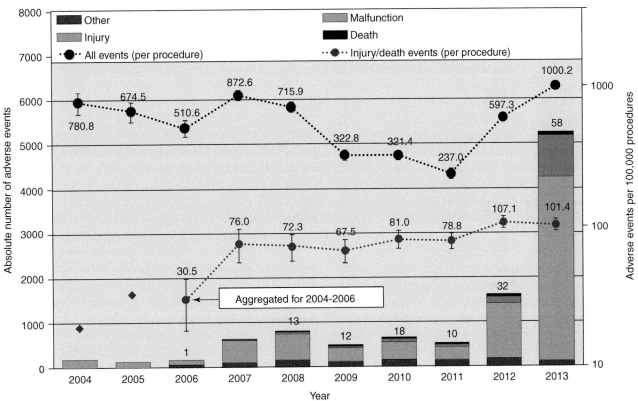

Fig. 4.2 MAUDE database annual adverse event reports and adverse event rates per 100,000 procedures. [a]Numbers written at the top of the bars indicate annual reported deaths. [b]Error bars depict 95% confidence intervals for the proportion estimates for the absolute adverse events as well as the adverse events per 100,000 procedures. (From Alemzadeh et al. [11], with permission)

reported events. From 2006 to 2013, total annual robotic procedure volume increased by 10-fold along with a 32-fold increase in absolute annual adverse event reporting. While the annual estimated adverse event rate per procedure was roughly 0.55% from 2004 to 2011, this nearly doubled to a peak of 1% across 2013; despite this increase, patient injuries and deaths per procedure have fortunately remained relatively stable from 2007 to 2013 [11].

Moreover, studies have demonstrated both underreporting and errors in adverse event reporting in the MAUDE database, including robotic surgery procedures [7, 12]. Cooper et al. cross-referenced MAUDE reports from 2000 to 2012 for *da Vinci*®-related complications with legal and public record databases to look for discrepancies in reporting; the authors determined that a total of eight cases reported to the FDA were either "inaccurate, filed late, or not filed." Across the 13-year study period, 245 injuries were reported including 71 fatalities. The majority of patient deaths were following gynecology, urology, or cardiothoracic cases ($n = 49$, 69%), while only three deaths (4%) were associated with general surgery procedures. In addition, Cooper et al. categorized the top 3 causes of patient deaths as follows: hemorrhage (29.6%), not reported (28.2%), and sepsis (14.1%).

Intuitive Surgical has faced many product liability claims from surgeries performed on *da Vinci*® systems since the mid-2000s. By the end of the 2017 fiscal year, the company was actively named as a defendant in approximately 43 separate product liability lawsuits as well as a larger multi-plaintiff lawsuit involving 55 patients from multiple states related to injuries and/or deaths following procedures performed on *da Vinci*® systems. Some of these lawsuits are seeking damages related to complications from specific instruments, several of which have already been recalled from the market. In addition, inadequate surgeon training and failure to warn hospitals about the risks of inadequate surgery training have been noted. In one trial, Taylor vs. Intuitive Surgical, Inc., that finally concluded in February 2017, the case went all the way to the level of the Washington Supreme Court where they eventually ruled that the lower courts should have told Intuitive that it had a duty to warn the hospital making the robotic device purchase, not just the operating surgeon, about the dangers of robotic-assisted surgeries [13].

Furthermore, Intuitive has reported $16.3 million of pretax expenses toward settling some of these product liability lawsuits in addition to $12.8 million in other related liabilities [14]. To date, there are no studies or reports evaluating direct or indirect healthcare-related costs to patients and/or hospitals as a result of injuries incurred during procedures performed on robotic systems.

Professional Liability and Litigation

The legal principles that impact professional liability are consistent throughout medicine as well as surgery, including surgical robotics. Three key factors often addressed in litigation against surgeons are direct harm or injury to a patient, an error made by the physician, and causality between that error and harm. Surgeons are liable for the safe and effective execution of their practice encompassing everything from indications for a particular procedure to thorough informed consent as well as maintenance of appropriate education and skills-based training with the ultimate goal of preventing harm to patients. Robotic surgery has the added requirement of understanding the practical aspects of operating and troubleshooting the robotic system itself but also acquiring the technical skill for safely operating the device in patients [15].

While the FDA does not act as regulatory organization overseeing the practice of medicine and surgery, it does regulate the marketing and distribution of medical devices like the *da Vinci*® Surgical System [16]. The *da Vinci*® system was ultimately approved as a Class II medical device which is generally defined as a device with the small but real possibility of leading to patient harm; these devices must meet certain manufacturing and engineering as well as medical device reporting standards along with FDA-mandated comprehensive training for all surgeons and hospital teams using the system. The Class II device designation has also allowed Intuitive Surgical to apply for multiple *da Vinci*® 510(K) authorizations from the FDA across a wide variety of surgical procedures and specialties; essentially, these authorizations are "substantial equivalent" designations to laparoscopic surgery for these various procedures [16, 17]. Additionally, medical devices under 510(K) clearances are subject to product liability lawsuits which is of paramount importance in robotic surgery [16].

Litigation related to surgical robotics typically encompasses several different areas of the law including product liability, medical malpractice, and wrongful death. Under product liability law, there are three main claims for how a robotic surgical system or instrument may be defective: a design defect, a manufacturing defect, and a warning defect [18]. Design defects are intrinsic flaws in instrument or systems design, whereas manufacturing defects are flaws during physical construction of these products. Defects in warning are related to inadequate risks reported with the use of instruments or systems, not a problem with the products themselves. In contrast to defects, medical malpractice implies negligence or failure to provide the standard level of care to a patient. Medical malpractice against a surgeon cannot be claimed unless a patient care obligation was required and violated and this violation directly led to an alleged injury [19]. Lastly, wrongful death lawsuits seek compensation for relatives of injured or deceased patients regarding medical and/or funeral costs or the resulting loss of income and/or emotional support [18]. Furthermore, product liability and medical malpractice claims can sometimes overlap from a legal perspective. For example, if patient harm during a robotic-assisted surgery is claimed to be related to the use of a particular instrument, this could in part be the fault of the manufacturer for not providing complete information about the risks related to the use of this instrument as well as a surgeon using the instrument in a way not specifically outlined by the manufacturer [20].

To Blame or Not to Blame: Device, Surgeon, or Institution?

Device-Related and Manufacturer Responsibilities and Failures

Device-related adverse events or failures include things like breaches in the protective components of instruments leading to unintended tissue damage and can occur during laparoscopic- and robotic-assisted surgery. Device or instrument malfunctions are incredibly broad and can lead to a range of negative outcomes from prolonged operating room time to minor patient injury and even death; these failures typically lead to product liability lawsuits whereby Intuitive Surgical would be named as the corporate defendant. While instrument malfunctions are relatively infrequent in robotic surgery, they are well-described and can range widely from a video processor hardware problems to a defective camera, a stapler misfiring, or even damaged pieces on robotic arms or other devices. A 2011 study published in the *American Journal of Obstetrics and Gynecology* demonstrated significantly higher insulation failures in robotic instruments compared to laparoscopic instruments based on extracorporeal voltage tests using a porosity detector [21]. Insulation failures can cause missed thermal bowel injuries and other complications leading to significant patient morbidity and even mortality.

In 2013, Friedman et al.'s analysis of the MAUDE database over a 2-year period (2009–2010) identified 528 adverse event reports associated with 565 device-related failures [22]. The three most common types of report failures were as follows: (1) articulating wrist or instrument tip ($n = 285$), (2) electrosurgical ($n = 174$), and (3) instrument shaft ($n = 76$). Broken instrument jaws or tips were cited the most frequently ($n = 150$) followed by reports that either the "instrument" broke or a part of it fell off ($n = 66$). Ninety percent of electrosurgical failures were arcing incidents with roughly 50% either being directly visualized or leading to thermal tissue injury intraoperatively. Instrument shaft malfunctions were most commonly from cracking or broken-off materials ($n = 36$). Furthermore, Alemzadeh et al. stratified robotic device-related failures from the MAUDE database into five key areas: (1) systems and video/imaging malfunctions, (2) falling of instrument pieces into the patient, (3) electric arcing of instruments, (4) unintentional instrument actions, and (5) miscellaneous [11]. During the 14-year study period, roughly 15% of adverse events were related to damaged or missing instrument parts falling into patients leading to 119 injuries and 1 death as well as added time in the operating room. Electric arcing of instruments was the next most common cause of adverse events at 10.5% ultimately harming about 190 patients followed closely by unintentional instrument actions (i.e., forceful movements) contributing to 10.1% of adverse events along with 52 injuries and 1 death. While systems and video/imaging malfunctions only led to 7.4% of overall adverse events, this was the main category leading to case cancellation altogether as well as converting to other approaches (i.e., laparoscopic, open) [11].

Importantly, manufacturers like Intuitive Surgical are obligated to report any device-related and/or systems-based malfunctions that could have contributed to a patient injury or death via the MAUDE database; device-user facilities including hospitals and ambulatory surgical centers are held to the same standard [23]. In 2013, Intuitive was issued a FDA warning letter for regulatory violations associated with practices that did not comply with reporting mandates for the *da Vinci*® system. The company received multiple complaints and medical device reports (MDRs) from 2010 to 2011 for patient injuries from arcing due to damaged components on certain monopolar instruments and intraoperative cleaning practices for some devices. Ultimately, this was resolved by sending a letter to clients (i.e., hospitals, surgeons) providing a warning in the Instructions for Use against practices with these instruments that could lead to similar injuries. Intuitive, however, did not comply with the required regulatory documentation and design control process to assess for defects in these device and instrument components [24]. The company did eventually take the appropriate action to correct these FDA violations, but it highlights the complexity and consequences of not reporting these device-related malfunctions via the correct channels. For example, if surgeons are provided with a label warning for robotic instrument failures, the burden of ensuring patient safety is shifted toward the operator of these instruments rather than the manufacturer's design input process that could determine a root cause to the malfunction [25].

Surgeon-Related Responsibilities and Failures

Operator or surgeon errors that occur during robotic surgery can be as equally devastating as device-related failures and frequently lead to medical malpractice lawsuits. Some robotic surgery complications may lead to long-term negative outcomes (i.e., wound infection, anastomotic leak, chronic pain, etc.) that are surgeon-dependent and not related to a manufacturer-related device malfunction or institution-based failure. Robotic surgery clearly requires an elevated dependence on verbal communication between the surgeon, scrub technician, circulating nurse, and bedside assistant. While the console is controlled by the primary surgeon, instrument exchanges, needle insertion and retrieval, mesh fixation device deployment, and trocar manipulation are frequently performed by a bedside assistant who may or may not have an equivalent level of training and experience; this has inherent added risks to the patient that are not encountered in standard laparoscopic surgery. That said, bedside assistants are also responsible and at risk for medicolegal lawsuits, even though they often fall under the responsibility of the surgeon or the hospital. Intraoperative complications such as an injury related to an instrument exchange caused by the bedside assistant, for example, would still fall on the responsibility of the primary surgeon; all members of the surgical team must have a heightened sense of awareness of these potential complications during robotic-assisted approaches and ensure appropriate communication and vigilance toward patient safety. The primary surgeon is obligated to oversee all aspects of perioperative technical skill execution as well as clinical decision-making, and any deviations from the standard of care pose a liability risk to the surgeon and surgical team.

For any type of minimally invasive procedure (i.e., laparoscopic or robotic), not all surgeon-driven errors are from technical missteps rather some are related to ethical- and judgment-based problems. Importantly, adverse events reported in the MAUDE database are often due to a combination of causes such as device malfunctions as well as operator issues like inadequate training (i.e., surgeon cannot troubleshoot a non-recoverable systems error during a critical part of a case) or a judgment-based error (i.e., surgeon does not convert to a different approach when a complication occurs causing further injury or prolonging operative time.) According to Alemzadeh et al., roughly 7% of death reports and 7% of patient injury reports manually reviewed in the MAUDE database were related to surgical team errors alone, either by the primary surgeon directly or other surgical staff [11]. It should be mentioned that another responsibility of the surgeon is training other primary surgeons and residents. In general, this responsibility is outside that of the device manufacturer and the institution itself, unless done in coordination with an actual surgeon. This will be further addressed in the next section.

From an ethical standpoint, surgeons must be vigilant about educating their patients regarding the potential device-related, operator-related, and systems-based malfunctions that are unique to robotic surgery. From a legal standpoint, the "prudent physician standard" is the most common standard used for the informed consent process; this standard "establishes what a reasonably prudent physician would typically disclose to patients in similar situations as determined by expert physician testimony." [19] Thus, surgeons must fully disclose why a robotic approach is recommended, their level of experience with such procedures, as well as the potential risks, adverse outcomes, and expected recovery to ensure adherence to the informed consent process. Failure to obtain informed consent is considered medical negligence.

Another ethical dilemma albeit somewhat beyond the scope of this chapter but worth mentioning given the potential impact on robotic surgery lawsuits is conflict of interest (COI). For example, many robotic surgeons are paid directly by the robotic device manufacturer to provide training, proctoring, hands-on labs, speaking engagements, and education to other surgeons. Moreover, a quick review of the publicly available CMS (Centers for Medicare and Medicaid Services) open payment system [26] showed that Intuitive Surgical, Inc., actually spent over 34.7 million dollars in 2016 alone just in education-related payments to surgeons. All individual surgeons are listed in this database, and the amounts they are paid are transparently displayed, as well as the number of times they are paid each year and the number of payments that they disputed. To be clear, we believe that surgeons and industry, in a responsible fashion, can and should work together and foster relationships. In fact, some of these relationships are essential for the evolution and dissemination of safe technique and to improve patient outcomes. However, in a world where surgeons, hospitals, and device manufacturers are also marketing claims directly to patients using a variety of media, the same patients also deserve to know that they have the ability to look up the amounts that their surgeons are getting paid by a device company. While surgeons will always chose a technique that they believe will offer the best outcomes for their patients, by using this database, the patients also can then draw their own conclusions as to whether or not there is a potential COI existing with that surgeon that may potentially lead a surgeon to offer a robotic approach vs. another approach (open or laparoscopic) for surgery. In fact, there is no role for a device manufacturer's reimbursement to that surgeon to get in the way of a safe decision on technique, and it is the responsibility of the surgeon to uphold that value and disclose any potential COI. This transparent disclosure is a form of managing COI. That said, a surgeon is ethically and legally responsible for ensuring that the patient's best interest is at the forefront of all surgical decision-making. Violations of these ethical principles or failure to manage a surgeon's COI appropriately and transparently can contribute to potential legal implications should a lawsuit develop in a particular case.

Institution-Related Responsibilities and Failures

Institutions like hospitals and ambulatory surgical centers have medicolegal responsibilities to assure a safe robotic surgery; these hospital-related responsibilities can be broken down into several large buckets as follows: (1) marketing and advertising responsibilities, (2) patient experience, (3) robotic device processing and maintenance, and (4) staff and resident credentialing and training. Hospitals and institutions (and some surgeons) have increasingly been advertising their robotic services in almost all media available (billboards, newspapers, social media, Internet, and journals). False opinions and claims that are not backed by science yet market directly to patients (social media, Internet, newspapers, billboards, emails) are subject to medicolegal lawsuits. In addition, there has been inherent bias on the part of institutions to market their systems and products directly to patients for financial gain. For example, Jin et al. reported their analysis of robotic surgery claims for 400 US-based hospitals in 2011; ultimately, 37% had robotic surgery content on their homepages, but none disclosed any risks or complications [27]. Schiavone et al. analyzed marketing web content for robotic gynecologic surgery at hospitals with at least 200 beds; 44.4% of hospitals in this study contained such marketing. The authors found that the majority of these hospitals reported superior outcomes with robotic gynecologic surgery and 41% indicated that the robotic approach was "overall better." Furthermore, only 15% of websites reported any evidence-based data, and even fewer (<2%) mentioned any risks or complications associated with the robotic approach [28]. Given the direct-to-consumer promotions of robotic surgery on many hospital websites, patients may get a skewed perception about the safety of robotic surgical approaches which, of course, will vary based on surgeon experience and skill level. Ultimately, hospitals have an ethical responsibility to report accurate and balanced educational content and may ultimately be required to do so by government agencies.

Hospitals are responsible for overseeing and evaluating many aspects of robotic surgery practices including patient experience and satisfaction, maintenance and cleaning of robotic system components, instrument processing and sterilization, as well as training of surgeons and other appropriate staff. For example, instrument processing and sterilization for robotic surgery instruments require special manufacturer-guided cleaning protocols and high-pressure hoses to flush the instruments. Hospitals and other device-user facilities are accountable for training all staff to properly handle and clean robotic instruments, which is complex, time-consuming, and a significant financial burden. A recent study by Saito et al. evaluated the effectiveness of cleaning protocols for robotic-assisted vs. open surgical instruments [29]. The authors compared protein contamination levels on *da Vinci®* system instruments used for urologic and colorectal cases to open instruments used for gastrointestinal surgery. After the initial phase of cleaning with flushing and ultrasonication, robotic instruments were shown to have a significantly higher level of protein contamination. The next phase of cleaning involved three consecutive processing sessions to determine residual protein levels; while the robotic and open surgical instruments demonstrated decreased residual protein levels after each session, the robotic instruments overall still had significantly higher levels of protein contamination. The authors ultimately concluded that cleaning protocols were 97.6% effective for robotic instruments compared to 99.1% for open instruments. Future studies are required to assess the impact of robotic instrument processing and sterilization techniques on clinical outcomes like wound infection and anastomotic leak.

In addition, training and credentialing are critical aspects of maintaining patient safety standards for robotic surgery and are mandatory for primary surgeons as well as the entire surgical team including surgical technicians, circulating nurses, and ancillary staff involved in these cases. Training of surgical technique is the responsibility of the practicing surgeons. The device company is responsible for training all parties on how to use their devices or equipment and is legally responsible to assure their equipment functions as it is intended to function. The companies, themselves, however, are not responsible to train surgical technique. For that matter, it is our opinion that device manufacturer sales representatives who are frequently present in the operating room with surgeons should sustain from teaching surgical technique or offering technical advice to the primary surgeon, the bedside assistant, or any surgical trainees without the consent of that surgeon, as this responsibility falls outside that of the device manufacturer and its employees.

With regard to credentialing, hospitals are individually responsible for establishing credentialing requirements and granting privileges for robotic surgeons and other staff based on documentation of training, experience, and competency. We believe this is a safe process that is vital to patient safety. Hospitals should also provide oversight to assess outcomes, and they should reassess their surgeons at least yearly, if not more often. The minimum FDA surgical robotics requirements for the primary surgeon usually involve a 1- to 2-day training course on the *da Vinci®* system with dry lab and cadaver exercises as well as didactic sessions. Alternatively, hospitals typically require a combination of simulation and didactic training along with cadaver or animal labs, a set number of proctored cases and observation of independent cases to be able to obtain provisional privileges in robotic surgery. Currently there is no uniform consensus among hospitals or other surgical societies on how much training and experience are required to both receive and maintain appropriate credentialing and granting privileges for robotic surgery. In contrast to requirements for measuring competency in laparoscopic surgery, the Accreditation Council for Graduate Medical Education (ACGME) has no established robotics training curriculum for US-based surgical residents; this will clearly change over time. Robotic credentialing and privileging are of serious medicolegal concern for hospitals and surgeons with over 30 states having received negligent credentialing claims in specialties like gynecology [19].

Conclusions

Medicolegal issues in surgical robotics vary widely in their scope and complexity. Device malfunctions, surgeon errors, and inadequate hospital oversight of robotics training all contribute to increasing medicolegal liability risks and, more importantly, can negatively impact patient outcomes. Given the rapid expansion in robotic surgery volume both in the United States and internationally, legal systems are facing unparalleled and complex litigation claims predominantly under product liability and medical malpractice law. For device-related issues, it remains important to ensure accuracy of reporting adverse events associated with robotic surgery in repositories like the MAUDE database; however, many robotic surgery cases with complications that lead to lawsuits will not appear in that database. The rapid expansion of robotic technology must be met by enhanced critical review and analysis of all adverse events and their impact on patient injuries and deaths. More importantly, when it comes to medicolegal responsibility for robotic surgery, each of the stakeholders must recognize their own obligations as well as their own limitations to these responsibilities. Surgeons and their teams, device manufacturers, and hospitals as well as hospital staff must uphold the highest level of care, ethics, and execution of services to deliver on each of their responsibilities to assure a safe patient experience and outcome.

References

1. Lanfranco AR, Castellanos AE, Desai JP, Meyers WC. Robotic surgery: a current perspective. Ann Surg. 2004;239(1):14–21.
2. Satava RM. Surgical robotics: the early chronicles: a personal historical perspective. Surg Laparosc Endosc Percutan Tech. 2002;12(1):6–16.
3. Warren H, Dasgupta P. The future of robotics. Investig Clin Urol. 2017;58:297–8.
4. Intuitive Surgical. Clinical evidence: level of evidence of peer-reviewed publications [Internet]. 2014 [cited 2018 Apr 28]; Available from: https://www.davincisurgerycommunity.com/evidence.
5. Herron DM, Marohn M, The SAGES-MIRA Robotic Surgery Consensus Group. A consensus document on robotic surgery [Internet]. 2007; Available from: https://www.sages.org/publications/guidelines/consensus-document-robotic-surgery/.
6. Tsuda S, Oleynikov D, Gould J, et al. SAGES TAVAC safety and effectiveness analysis: da Vinci ® Surgical System (Intuitive Surgical, Sunnyvale, CA). Surg Endosc. 2015;29(10):2873–84.
7. Cooper MA, Ibrahim A, Lyu H, Makary MA. Underreporting of robotic surgery complications. J Healthc Qual. 2015;37(2):133–8.
8. Reportlinker. Global surgical robotics market to reach $12.6 billion 2025 [Internet]. 2018 [cited 2018 Apr 28]; Available from: https://www.prnewswire.com/news-releases/global-surgical-robotics-market-to-reach-126-billion-2025-300587080.html.
9. Intuitive Surgical. Intuitive Surgical announces preliminary fourth quarter and full year 2017 results [Internet]. 2018 [cited 2018 Apr 24]; Available from: http://investor.intuitivesurgical.com/mobile.view?c=122359&v=203&d=1&id=2325993.
10. Greenberg H. Robotic surgery: growing sales, but growing concerns [Internet]. 2013 [cited 2018 Apr 27]; Available from: https://www.cnbc.com/id/100564517.
11. Alemzadeh H, Raman J, Leveson N, Kalbarczyk Z, Iyer RK. Adverse events in robotic surgery: a retrospective study of 14 years of fda data. PLoS One. 2016;11(4):e0151470.
12. Hauser R, Katsiyiannis W, Gornick C, Almquist A, Kallinen L. Deaths and cardiovascular injuries due to device-assisted implantable cardioverter-defibrillator and pacemaker lead extraction. Europace. 2010;12(3):395–401.
13. Justia. Taylor v. Intuitive Surgical Inc. (Majority and Dissent) [Internet]. 2017 [cited 2018 May 27]; Available from: https://law.justia.com/cases/washington/supreme-court/2017/92210-1.html.
14. Intuitive Surgical. Annual report 2017 [Internet]. 2018; Available from: http://phx.corporate-ir.net/phoenix.zhtml?c=122359&p=irol-sec.
15. Mavroforou A, Michalodimitrakis E, Hatzitheofilou C, Giannoukas A. Legal and ethical issues in robotic surgery. Int Angiol. 2010;29(1):75–9.
16. McLean T. The complexity of litigation associated with robotic surgery and cybersurgery. Int J Med Robot Comput Assist Surg. 2007;3:23–9.
17. Intuitive Surgical. Annual report 2004 [Internet]. 2005; Available from: http://www.annualreports.com/HostedData/AnnualReportArchive/i/NASDAQ_ISRG_2004.pdf.
18. FindLaw. Da Vinci robot surgery lawsuits [Internet]. 2017 [cited 2018 Apr 29]; Available from: https://injury.findlaw.com/product-liability/da-vinci-robot-surgery-lawsuits.html.
19. Lee YL, Kilic GS, Phelps JY. Medicolegal review of liability risks for gynecologists stemming from lack of training in robot-assisted surgery. J Minim Invasive Gynecol. 2011;18(4):512–5.
20. Rozbruch L. Litigation and robotic surgery: product liability or medical malpractice? [Internet]. 2018 [cited 2018 Apr 28]; Available from: https://www.pulj.org/the-roundtable/litigation-robotic-surgery-product-liability-or-medical-malpractice.
21. Espada M, Munoz R, Noble BN, Magrina JF. Insulation failure in robotic and laparoscopic instrumentation: a prospective evaluation. Am J Obstet Gynecol. 2011;205(2):e1–5.
22. Friedman D, Lendvay T, Hannaford B. Instrument failures for the da Vinci surgical system: a Food and Drug Administration MAUDE database study. Surg Endosc. 2013;27(5):1503–8.
23. U.S. Food & Drug Administration. MAUDE – manufacturer and user facility device experience [Internet]. 2018 [cited 2018 May 10]; Available from: https://www.accessdata.fda.gov/scripts/cdrh/cfdocs/cfmaude/search.cfm#fn1.
24. U.S. Food & Drug Administration. Intuitive Surgical, Inc. 7/16/13 [Internet]. 2014 [cited 2018 May 10]; Available from: https://www.fda.gov/ICECI/EnforcementActions/WarningLetters/2013/ucm363260.htm.
25. Greenberg H. FDA: Intuitive Surgical failed to report warning [Internet]. 2013 [cited 2018 Apr 30]; Available from: https://www.cnbc.com/id/100843549.
26. Centers for Medicare & Medicaid Services. Open payments search tool [Internet]. 2018 [cited 2018 May 27]; Available from: https://openpaymentsdata.cms.gov.
27. Jin L, Ibrahim A, Newman N, Makarov D, Pronovost P, Makary M. Robotic surgery claims on United States hospital websites. J Healthc Qual. 2011;33(6):48–52.
28. Schiavone MB, Kuo EC, Naumann RW, et al. The commercialization of robotic surgery: unsubstantiated marketing of gynecologic surgery by hospitals. Am J Obstet Gynecol. 2012;207(174):e1–7.
29. Saito Y, Yasuhara H, Murakoshi S, Komatsu T, Fukatsu K, Uetera Y. Challenging residual contamination of instruments for robotic surgery in Japan. Infect Control Hosp Epidemiol. 2017;38(2):143–6.

Part II

General Surgery

Robotic Hiatal Hernias and Nissen Fundoplication

Fahri Gokcal and Omar Yusef Kudsi

Introduction

Hiatal hernia is defined as the protrusion of the intra-abdominal organs, most commonly the upper portion of the stomach, into the mediastinum through the esophageal hiatus of the diaphragm, and it is a common disorder affecting 10–50% of the population [1, 2]. According to the position of gastroesophageal junction and the content of hernia sac, hiatal hernias are classified into four types: sliding (type I, the most common type), paraesophageal (type II), combined (type III, includes components of types I and II), and giant paraesophageal (type IV, herniation of intra-abdominal organs beside the stomach) (Table 5.1) [2, 3].

The circumferential laxity of the phrenoesophageal ligament (Laimer's membrane) and the dilatation of the diaphragmatic hiatus may cause cephalad migration of the gastroesophageal junction, and this situation may lead an incompetent lower esophageal sphincter [4, 5]. Although hiatal hernias may remain asymptomatic in most individuals and diagnosed incidentally, they are frequently associated with gastroesophageal reflux disease (GERD) resulting from inadequate lower esophageal sphincter.

Surgical management should be considered in case of symptomatic HH or GERD which is refractory to medical therapies such as antiacids and lifestyle modifications. Minimally invasive surgical repair is the preferred approach for the majority of hiatal hernias [3]. With regarding the technique of hiatal hernia repair, it is suggested that the fundoplication should be performed during the repair [3, 6].

F. Gokcal
Department of Surgery, Good Samaritan Medical Center, Brockton, MA, USA

University of Health Sciences Istanbul Bakirkoy Dr. Sadi Konuk Training and Research Hospital Bakirkoy, Istanbul, Turkey

O. Y. Kudsi (✉)
Department of Surgery, Good Samaritan Medical Center, Tufts University School of Medicine, Boston, MA, USA
e-mail: omar.kudsi@tufts.edu

The Nissen fundoplication has been the most widely preferred procedure for the surgical management of GERD and hiatal hernias. It was first described by Dr. Rudolf Nissen (1896–1981) as an antireflux procedure in the late 1950s [7]. In fact, the background of this procedure is based on the operation he performed for a benign cardia ulcer by enforced burying the anastomosis of the transected esophagus in the fundus of the stomach, when he was the chief of Department of Surgery at the Cerrahpasa Hospital in Istanbul, Turkey, in the late 1930s [8, 9]. Since the introduction of laparoscopy, the standard for fundoplication has become a minimally invasive approach. In recent years, minimally invasive surgery is quickly evolving with the guidance of new technology. It is possible to take advantages of the technological facilities, such as the high-definition three-dimensional vision and enhanced manipulation capabilities of the instruments, provided by robotic platform when the surgical procedure requires fine dissection and movements at limited spaced anatomic sites such as Nissen fundoplication.

We have set as the goals of this chapter to provide a brief review of the current literature on robotic HH and GERD surgery and to explain operative steps of robotic Nissen fundoplication.

Literature Review

Since the first robotic surgery system was launched in 2001, many reports have been published demonstrating successfully performed robotic antireflux procedures for symptomatic HH and GERD [10–21]. Majority of these reports were retrospective single institutional series, and the authors represented their experiences. A few studies specifically assessed the role of robotic HH repair; however, there are no prospective randomized trials in this field.

In a report, which was designed in a retrospective nature and representing the largest series (n:61) of robotic-assisted paraesophageal hernia (type II–IV) repair, the authors concluded that the outcomes seemed to be comparable to those achieved by

© Springer Nature Switzerland AG 2019
S. Tsuda, O. Y. Kudsi (eds.), *Robotic-Assisted Minimally Invasive Surgery*, https://doi.org/10.1007/978-3-319-96866-7_5

Table 5.1 The types of hiatal hernias

Types	Hiatal hernias	Gastroesophageal junction	Fundus	
I	Sliding	Migrates above the diaphragm	Remains below the gastroesophageal junction	
II	Paraesophageal (PEH)	Remains in its normal anatomic position	A portion herniates through the diaphragmatic hiatus	

III	Combination of types I and II	Migrates above the diaphragm	Lies above the gastroesophageal junction	
IV	Giant paraesophageal	The presence of a structure other than the stomach (omentum, colon, or small bowel)		

the conventional laparoscopic technique and robotic hiatal hernia repair had a learning curve of about 36 cases [10]. In a case-control trial (CCT) with a total of 42 cases (12 cases robotic, 17 cases conventional laparoscopic, and 13 cases open method) that underwent hiatal hernia (>5 cm) repair, it has been showed that robot-assisted surgery is feasible and can be used safely for paraesophageal hernia. Additionally, it has been emphasized that although robotic surgery is superior to open surgery for paraesophageal hernia repair regarding the operative time, intraoperative complications, and patients' early postoperative course, it is not superior to conventional laparoscopy [11]. Brenkman et al. [12] reported the follow-up results of 40 consecutive patients undergoing robot-assisted laparoscopic hiatal hernia repair (without mesh) followed by Toupet fundoplication (270° posterior). There was only one recurrence (%2.5) in their entire cohort after a median follow-up of 11 months. Also, perioperative outcomes, such as blood loss, operation time, morbidity, and quality of life (QoL) scores, were satisfactory in this study.

Regarding the antireflux surgery, several studies have been published comparing the robot-assisted laparoscopy and conventional laparoscopy. In these studies, it is obviously seen that the Nissen fundoplication is the most commonly preferred fundoplication, if the fundoplication is performed. A retrospective multicenter study, including a large database of 12,079 antireflux operations (9572 patients laparoscopic, 2168 open, and 339 robotic), showed that both robotic and laparoscopic Nissen fundoplication techniques were superior to open surgery as demonstrated by their short-term outcomes, length of stay, and intensive care unit admissions. When they compared open costs to robotic costs, the former were higher, and this was related to length of stay, complications, and ICU admissions [13].

In a prospective non-randomized trial, Melvin et al. [14] reported no differences in clinical outcomes when comparing laparoscopic to robotic approaches; however, it has been found that there was a significant difference in mean operating time (102 ± 31 min. Laparoscopic versus 134 ± 19 min. robotic). There are four major randomized controlled trials on antireflux surgery, comparing laparoscopic fundoplication to robot-assisted fundoplication by the aid of the da Vinci® Surgical System [15–18]. Both approaches were shown to be equally safe, with no appreciable difference in conversion or complication rates, postoperative symptoms, quality of life, or functional assessments. In contrast to other studies, Muller-Stich et al. [15] are the only group reporting that the duration of operation was significantly shorter for the robotic surgery (88 ± 18 min, setup, 23 ± 5 versus 102 ± 19 min; setup, 20 ± 3). This situation may be related to performing of all operations by well-experienced one surgeon in robotic surgery and a well-trained surgical team.

In a meta-analysis, which includes 6 RCTs for a total of 221 patients, 111 were allocated to the conventional laparoscopic Nissen fundoplication group and 110 to the robot-assisted. Regarding operation complications, Wang et al. [19] showed that there were no significant differences in intraoperative incidents (small capsule tear of the liver and spleen, pneumothorax, minor bleeding, stomach perforation, and minor technical incidents) (RR = 0.81, $P = 0.62$), dysphagia (RR = 0.83, $P = 0.58$), and flatulence (RR = 1.26, $P = 0.56$). There was no significant difference on postoperative anti-secretory medication administration rates between both groups (RR = 0.43, $P = 0.12$). No differences in patient satisfaction were found (RR = 1.02, $P = 0.74$). Although the hiatal dissection time was similar between both groups, as well as the time from incision to closure of the skin, the fundoplication time was shorter in the conventional laparoscopic group (95% CI 2.33–4.00; $P = 0.00001$). Also, the operative costs (total operative costs and costs of hospital stay) appeared to be higher in the robot-assisted group (95% CI -4.61–17.39; $P = 0.00001$).

In a systematic review and meta-analysis, Mi et al. [20] included 11 studies (7 RTCs, 4 CCTs) to compare robot-assisted including da Vinci, Aesop, and Mona surgical systems (n: 198) and conventional laparoscopic (n: 335) fundoplication. When the rates of complications were analyzed separately as perioperative (pneumothorax, blood loss, relevant organ injury, and conversion) and postoperative (pneumonia, dysphagia, flatulence, and urinary tract infection) with 7 of the 11 studies, there was no significant difference between the 2 approaches with regard to perioperative complication rate (OR = 0.67, 95% CI = 0.30–1.48, $P = 1.00$). Although the postoperative complication rates of both approaches were showed approximately the same in 6 of the 11 studies which were included in the review, the main meta-analysis with fixed-effect model indicated a significant reduction of 65% in the relative odds of complication rates for the robotic approach (OR = 0.35, 95% CI = 0.13, 0.93, $P = 0.04$). There was no statistically significant difference between both approaches regarding the length of the hospital stay (95% CI = −0.25, 0.26, $P = 0.97$). The meta-analysis was not performed for the effective operating time, which was defined as the time between the introduction of the laparoscopic instrument and the completion of the last skin suture, since there was heterogeneity between the two approaches. However, total operating time was longer by 24.5 min in the robotic approach, and the authors explained this elongation as mostly due to the setup time, the time-consuming trocar placement, the unadapted optical system, and camera motion interrupting the surgeon's procedure. In terms of costs, the 4 of 11 studies investigated cost and the results showed statistically difference for both operative and total costs ($P = 0.01$ and $P = 0.003$). Authors emphasized that there was no article focused on costs of long-term outcomes, and high investment and maintenance fees, as well as disposable instruments cost made for this difference between both groups.

On the other hand, in the most recent meta-analysis on robotic Nissen fundoplication, it was reported that some of previously published meta-analyses have methodological errors such as inclusion criteria bias and subgroup analyses errors. The authors have carried out their own meta-analyses with 5 RCTs, including total of 160 patients. There were no significant differences between two groups regarding total operation times, effective operation times, the incidence of reoperations, hospital stay, and in-hospital costs due to the fact that meta-analyses demonstrated significant heterogeneity. In terms of intraoperative conversion and postoperative dysphagia within 1 month, even though meta-analysis demonstrated no significant heterogeneity, there were no significant differences between groups. Regarding intraoperative and postoperative complication, no meta-analysis was introduced because of the incompletion of data [21].

Overall, the conflicting results of the current literature make new prospective multicenter trials necessary to better understand the precise advantages and disadvantages of robotic-assisted laparoscopic surgery for HH and GERD as compared to the conventional laparoscopic approach.

Robot-Assisted Nissen Fundoplication

Hiatal hernias are frequently found incidentally during the diagnostic workup of symptomatic reflux. Antireflux surgery is an alternative modality for the management of patients with proven GERD, with or without a sliding HH. But, repairing of sliding hernia is not necessary in the absence of reflux disease. The following list of criteria represents generally accepted indications for Nissen fundoplication:

- Typical symptoms for GERD, persistent atypical reflux symptoms, or extra-esophageal manifestations (e.g., asthma, hoarseness, cough chest pain, aspiration)
- Symptom-reflux relationship, esophagitis (in the past before PPI), and acid reflux (documented by pH-metry, impedance, or esophagogastroduodenoscopy (EGD))
- Failure of medical management (persistent symptoms despite optimal medical therapy with PPI, incomplete response to PPI, or need for PPI dosage increase)
- Complications related to GERD (e.g., Barrett's esophagus, bleeding, etc.)
- Mixed and paraesophageal hernia
- Patient preference (e.g., unwillingness to long-term medical therapy because of reduced quality of life, financial concerns, or intolerance to pharmacotherapy)
- Sufficient esophageal motility to overcome the outflow resistance composed by the valve
- Recurrent reflux or complications after previous antireflux surgical therapy

Preoperative Planning

The proper preoperative workup consists of EGD, pH monitoring, manometry, and barium esophagram in order to appropriately delineate the extent of the disease. EGD can accurately evaluate the anatomy of the esophagus and the gastroesophageal junction, the presence and size of hiatal hernia, and the degree of esophagitis if there is. pH monitoring is necessary to confirm the presence of acid reflux. This is particularly important for patients with atypical GERD symptoms where pH monitoring can be used to calculate the DeMeester score (percentage of time of esophageal acid exposure to pH < 4.0) and verify the presence of acid reflux. It is imperative to document the existence of reflux disease in patients with classic symptoms of heartburn and regurgitation. Erosive esophagitis or Barrett's metaplasia symptoms are not reliable guides to the presence of disease [22].

Esophageal manometry can reveal esophageal motility disorders. Based on this information, the surgeon is able to decide the optimal surgical approach and to determine if a complete or partial fundoplication is to be performed. Computed tomography (CT) scan may be useful for patients who have paraesophageal hernia and antireflux surgery history. Barium esophagram is performed to outline the anatomy of the esophagus and abnormalities such as a hiatal hernia, diverticulum, stricture, or luminal mass. It also helps in assessing esophageal length. Presence of a large (>5 cm) hiatal hernia suggests the presence of a shortened esophagus and may change the choice of the operation [23].

Patient Selection

The appropriate patient selection is one of the most important factors that impacts on outcomes after successfully surgical treatment of GERD and HH. The presence of dysphagia, obesity, and psychiatric history should also be taken into consideration in patients who have met the abovementioned criteria. In patients who present with dysphagia and GERD, the causes of dysphagia must be investigated, and the situations such as tumors, diverticula, and esophageal motor disorders must be excluded since they require different treatments. Furthermore, even if symptoms of dysphagia improve after fundoplication, the existence of preoperative dysphagia presumably effects on long-term clinical outcomes in a negative way [24]. Paying attention to the preoperative dysphagia is also important to determine the degree of fundoplication which can optimize reflux control while minimizing adverse sequela of postoperative dysphagia.

In the surgical treatment of GERD, morbid obesity is occasionally a challenging condition to surgeons because of technical difficulties. Not only morbid obesity is a significant independent risk factor for development of GERD and HH, but also it increases the failure rate of antireflux surgery. A study has demonstrated that while obese patients (BMI 30–34.9 kg/m^2) have similar outcomes to other patients, the morbidly obese individuals (BMI > 35 kg/m^2) have a higher failure rate [25]. If a morbid obese patient presents with GERD, he/she must be informed about potential risks of his/her condition. The possible benefits of a bariatric procedure as a dual targeted treatment for GERD instead of an antireflux procedure alone should be discussed to obtain both the weight loss and the relief of reflux symptoms [26]. It is a necessity to note that it does not mean that the morbid obesity is alone contraindication for antireflux procedures despite the fact that the failure incidence of operation may be higher than in the normal-weight individuals [27]. Patients should be attentively educated on the potential risks and benefits of their choice in order to obtain an informed decision about their healthcare.

A history of psychiatric disorders is another risk of failure for antireflux surgery outcomes. A study that has focused on preoperative prediction of long-term outcomes showed that a history of psychiatric illness trended toward a higher failure rate, although it did not reach statistical significance ($p = 0.06$). The patients who have history of psychiatric disorders were found to be more unsatisfied with their outcomes ($P < 0.01$), and a higher percentage of them complained of severe symptoms. However, a correlation was not found between a history of psychiatric illness and reoperation rates, and complaints of severe symptoms [25].

Patient Preparation

In preparation for surgery, the patient is being kept nothing by mouth (NPO) after midnight the night before the operation. If any esophageal dysmotility accompanied with GERD is found with preoperative workup studies, it might be beneficial for the patient to be placed on a clear liquid diet for 24–48 h prior to the operation, to minimize the amount of retained food in the esophageal lumen. This reduces the risk of aspiration upon endotracheal intubation and facilitates the performance of intraoperative EGD if required.

Setup

Patient Positioning, Docking of the Robot and Room Setup

The patient is positioned in a supine on the surgical table as the arms in abduction secured on padded arm boards. After induction of general anesthesia with orotracheal intubation, the peripheral lines are placed, and standard operative protocols are utilized including antibiotic proflaxy, body hair clipping, and placement of sequential compression devices if indicated. Foley catheterization is not generally required except prolonged case expectation. Nasogastric tube is placed. The patient should be fully secured to the surgical table to prevent slipping off and should be properly padded to obstruct robotic arm collision during operation. A heater device is placed on the upper chest and arms.

The steps that up to patient-side cart docking can be done in the temporary location of the surgical table, and the surgical table can be relocated to actual location just prior to the "docking" depending on the model of the robotic system and available space of operating room. The undocked patient-side cart (prepared and draped) is positioned at the site of the patient's head. Once asepsis has been achieved via chlorhexidine, the surgical drapes are placed over patient providing the entire abdominal area uncover.

Afterward, the head side of surgical table is slightly raised up to obtain a reverse Trendelenburg position (head up approximately >30°) which will help in displacing the organs from the hiatus and optimize the exposure of the working area. Additional adjustments of the surgical table might need to be applied to facilitate the anesthesiologist's workup. Patient position should be finalized prior to docking of the patient-side cart and must remain constant during operation. After ensuring trocar placement safely and properly, the patient-side cart is advanced by an assistant (with closely guided by the surgeon) into correct position, and the docking process is completed after connecting trocars and robotic arms. Of note, with the Si system, the patient-side cart must be positioned at the head side of the operating table to achieve "in-line" rule, whereas with the Xi system, the patient-side cart can be positioned at the patient's side as this platform includes an overhead boom allowing the arms to rotate as a group into any orientation. This allows for direct approach to the patient by the anesthesia team. Once the camera arm is docked and the camera inserted, the surgeon points the scope at the target anatomy and the system will automatically position the boom to ensure an optimal arm configuration for the procedure.

The console and vision cart are located safely away from the robot to allow for adequate movement of the arms and adequate space for the anesthesia team. The monitor is either at the foot of the table or mounted on the wall. This setup can be modified depending on what the operating room will allow. According to our room setup, anesthesiologist takes place at the patient's left side after relocating surgical table, and the scrub nurse works at the patient's right side.

Procedure

Access and Trocar Position

Correct placement of the ports is of utmost importance in robotic surgery. Four trocars for robotic arms and an additional trocar (depends on surgeon preference), for the purpose of retraction of the liver left lobe to expose the gastroesophageal junction, are usually enough in robotic Nissen fundoplication. Pneumoperitoneum can be achieved in a number of techniques. Access to the abdominal cavity through an open technique (Hasson's) at the position of planned first trocar is a valid entry option. However, our preference is that after pneumoperitoneum is established by inserting a Veress needle at Palmer's point, 1–2 cm below the left costal margin at the left midclavicular line, the initial port is inserted in the abdominal cavity. Alternatively, it may be obtained by optical trocar by using 0° camera.

Particular attention must be paid to achieving adequate distance between each trocar and surgical target so that not robotic arms collision and extensive troublesome. For this purpose, commonly applied rule is that a minimum of 8 cm of distance be maintained between each trocar and an ideal distance of 10–20 cm is suggested between the trocars and the surgical target. In this scenario, xiphoid can be used as a landmark for being ~5 cm below of diaphragmatic hiatus. A sterilized ruler may be used to confirm correct distance between trocars. Our approach is the following: the position of supra umbilical port is 12 cm caudal to the xiphoid and 2 cm to the patient's right. For patients who have larger abdomen, port is placed 15 cm caudal to the xiphoid and 2 cm to the right. The distance might need to be readjusted especially if the procedure includes a large hiatal hernia repair. The two trocars for the robotic arms are placed on the same horizontal line and 8 cm lateral to the camera port in the left and right upper quadrant close to the midclavicular line. The third trocar for the third robotic arm is inserted in the left anterior axillary line. The liver retractor is positioned so as not to obstruct the robotic arm. The right upper quadrant or epigastric region can be used for the liver retractor trocar (Fig. 5.1).

Operative Steps

Robotic Nissen fundoplication consists of mainly three steps: hiatal dissection, restoration of the esophageal hiatus, and circumferential wrapping of fundus.

Hiatal dissection begins with the developing a window at the lesser omentum (Fig. 5.2a). For this, anterior epigastric fat pad is retracted with a Cadiere grasper, and the stomach is pulled downward and toward the left lower quadrant, and so the gastrohepatic ligament is exposed. The gastrohepatic ligament is divided along the edge of the caudate lobe using the monopolar scissors. The dissection plane is moved cephalad until the junction between the right crus of the hiatus and the phrenoesophageal ligament (Laimer's membrane) is encountered (Fig. 5.2b). It is important to take extra care for the anterior vagus nerve and especially the nerve of Latarjet and any aberrant left hepatic arteries. The right anterior phrenoesophageal ligament and the peritoneum overlying

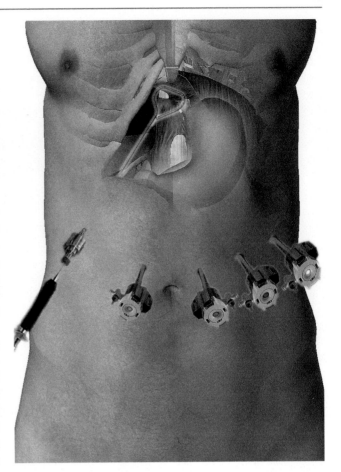

Fig. 5.1 Trocar positioning

the anterior esophagus are incised superficially in order to prevent any injuries to the esophagus or anterior vagus. This incision is extended to the left crus, and the esophagus is peeled off the right crus providing access to the mediastinum. The posterior vagus is identified and preserved, and the dissection is extended circumferentially and in a clockwise fashion within the mediastinum. The esophageal hiatus is fully dissected, and the esophagogastric junction is reduced in to the abdomen. For this, intra-abdominal esophagus is mobilized anteriorly and posteriorly from the right and the left crus. The dissection should be extended as proximally as possible to ensure an adequate part of movable esophagus at least 4 cm of esophagus should be able to move below the diaphragm without any tension. Grasping the esophagus should be avoided at all times during the procedure. Complete excision of the sac should be performed. It is important to control any minor bleeding by using the robotic bipolar forceps rather than by using monopolar for hemostasis, to prevent delayed perforations.

In order to achieve mobilization of the fundus, a point along the upper third of the gastric fundus (approximately 10–15 cm from the angle of His) is selected to begin ligating the short gastric vessels with a robotic ultrasonic scissors (or Vessel Sealer). Alternatively, short gastric vessels are divided

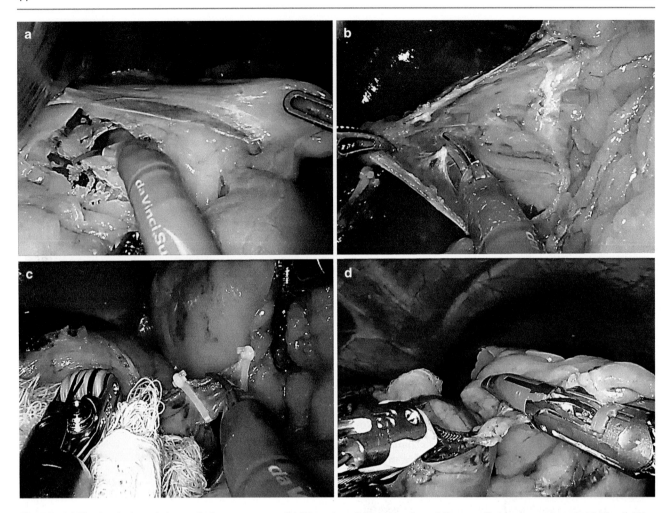

Fig. 5.2 (**a**) The developing window at the lesser omentum. (**b**) Dissection of phrenoesophageal ligament (Laimer's membrane). (**c**) The dividing of short gastric vessels between two Hem-o-Lok clips. (**d**) The ligating the short gastric vessels with a robotic Vessel Sealer

between two Hem-o-Lok clips (Fig. 5.2c, d). The ligation is continued up to the level of the left crus. Additional attention is needed during fundus dissection because the spleen is so near and can be injured easily. If there is minor hemorrhage, it can be controlled by prepositioned sponge in order to identify the bleeding source immediately. If needed, adhesions of the posterior gastric wall to the pancreas are divided.

After full mobilization of the fundus and esophagus, robotic fenestrated forceps is passed slowly around the esophagus and grasps a previously placed Penrose drain. With the aid of Penrose drain, which is wrapped and looped around distal esophagus, the stomach is pulled laterally and superiorly in order to expose lower junction of the crura (Fig. 5.3a–c). The robotic instruments are switched to needle drivers, and the hiatus is closed using nonabsorbable (0) sutures in a horizontal mattress fashion (Fig. 5.3d). Usually 2–3 interrupted sutures are applied, with thick bites including the peritoneum to strengthen it. The use of pledged is also advisable to avoid tearing diaphragmatic crura muscles, especially in large defects. It is suggested that a Nr. 52 bougie

be in place while closing the crural defect to prevent postoperative dysphagia and it also stays in esophageal lumen during fundoplication.

Subsequently, the fundus is pushed partly toward the posterior window, and then the robotic forceps is used to pull the fundus behind the esophagus. The fundus should be held by a larger bite. And then the rest of the fundus is pulled to bring it in front of the esophagus. Tension of the wrap by gently pulling and pushing the fundus around the esophagus can be assessed at this point, called shoeshine maneuver (Fig. 5.4). It can be determined if the mobilization is adequate or not with this maneuver. If your mobilization is adequate, the wrap should stay around the esophagus, or else it may return at its initial position, outside the posterior window, which denotes that further posterior dissection may be necessary. The anterior surface of the stomach is assessed in order to anchor the wrap properly.

The two sides of the fundus are sutured together with permanent 2-0 sutures. The stitches should pass through all gastric wall layers, and part of the anterior esophagus should be

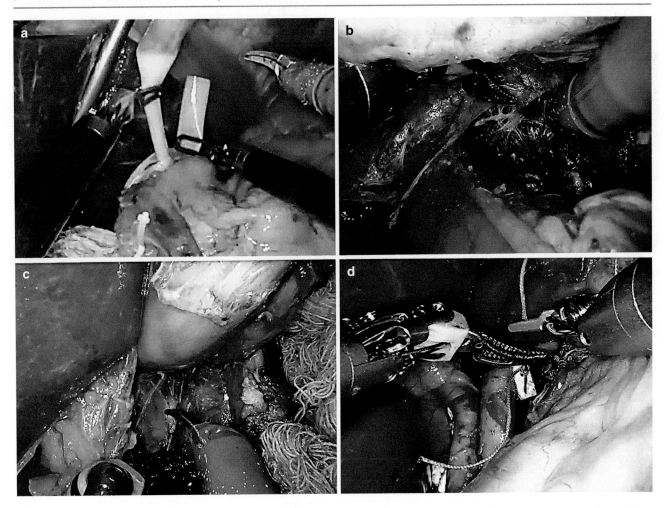

Fig. 5.3 (**a**) The looping of a Penrose drain around distal esophagus. (**b**) The anterior mobilization of distal esophagus. (**c**) The posterior mobilization of distal esophagus. (**d**) The closure of crura with pledged nonabsorbable suture in horizontal mattress fashion

included with partial thickness bites. Some surgeons suggest securing the wrap to the diaphragm using two coronal sutures (left and right). The wrap faces the patient's right side in its final position. The first suture is mostly cephalad and is placed up on the esophagus at least 2–3 cm above the gastroesophageal junction. The next suture incorporates a small bite of the esophagus and is placed 1 cm distal. The third suture only incorporates the fundus and is placed another centimeter distal (Fig. 5.5). Irrigation and suction are not needed if no bleeding occurred during procedure. All instruments under direct vision are removed. After injection of local anesthetic trocar sites, all incisions are closed by using monofilament absorbable suture in subcutaneous fashion.

Postoperative Care

Following the completion of the procedure, the patient is transferred to the postanesthesia recovery unit and afterward is getting admitted to the surgical floor. A clear liquid diet may be initiated when postanesthesia nausea has

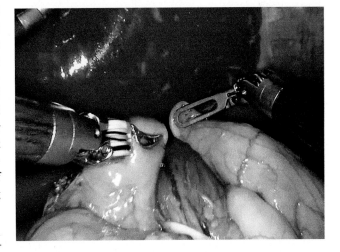

Fig. 5.4 The assessment of tension of the wrap by "shoeshine" maneuver

resolved. A soft mechanical diet is usually started on postoperative day 1, and the patient is maintained on that diet for 2–3 weeks after the operation. If no significant dyspha-

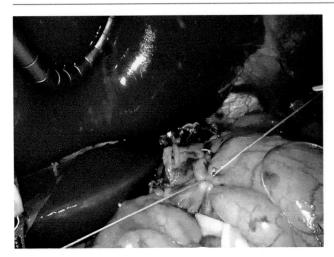

Fig. 5.5 The suturing of the fundus wrap

gia is encountered, then a regular diet can be instituted. Initial pain management is achieved with IV narcotics and a patient-controlled analgesia technique. Transition to oral narcotics pain medications is usually accomplished within 24 h after the procedure, and most of the patients are getting discharged home on postoperative day 1 on pain control medications and antiemetics.

References

1. Berselli M, Livraghi L, Latham L, Farassino L, Rota Bacchetta GL, Pasqua N, et al. Laparoscopic repair of voluminous symptomatic hiatal hernia using absorbable synthetic mesh. Minim Invasive Ther Allied Technol. 2015;24(6):372–6.
2. Dean C, Etienne D, Carpentier B, Gielecki J, Tubbs RS, Loukas M. Hiatal hernias. Surg Radiol Anat. 2012;34(4):291–9.
3. Kohn GP, Price RR, DeMeester SR, Zehetner J, Muensterer OJ, Awad Z, et al. Guidelines for the management of hiatal hernia. Surg Endosc. 2013;27(12):4409–28.
4. Roman S, Kahrilas PJ. Mechanisms of Barrett's oesophagus (clinical): LOS dysfunction, hiatal hernia, peristaltic defects. Best Pract Res Clin Gastroenterol. 2015;29(1):17–28.
5. van Herwaarden MA, Samsom M, Smout AJ. The role of hiatus hernia in gastro-oesophageal reflux disease. Eur J Gastroenterol Hepatol. 2004;16(9):831–5.
6. Velanovich V, Karmy-Jones R. Surgical management of paraesophageal hernias: outcome and quality of life analysis. Dig Surg. 2001;18(6):432–7; discussion 7-8.
7. Nissen R. A simple operation for control of reflux esophagitis. Schweiz Med Wochenschr. 1956;86(Suppl 20):590–2.
8. Goksoy E. Rudolf Nissen: his activities at the Cerrahpasa Surgical Clinic and his contributions to Turkish surgery. Turk J Surg. 2006;22(2):85–91.
9. Read RC. The contribution of Allison and Nissen to the evolution of hiatus herniorrhaphy. Hernia. 2001;5(4):200–3.
10. Galvani CA, Loebl H, Osuchukwu O, Samame J, Apel ME, Ghaderi I. Robotic-assisted paraesophageal hernia repair: initial experience at a single institution. J Laparoendosc Adv Surg Tech A. 2016;26(4):290–5.
11. Gehrig T, Mehrabi A, Fischer L, Kenngott H, Hinz U, Gutt CN, et al. Robotic-assisted paraesophageal hernia repair – a case-control study. Langenbeck's Arch Surg. 2013;398(5):691–6.
12. Brenkman HJ, Parry K, van Hillegersberg R, Ruurda JP. Robot-assisted laparoscopic hiatal hernia repair: promising anatomical and functional results. J Laparoendosc Adv Surg Tech A. 2016;26(6):465–9.
13. Owen B, Simorov A, Siref A, Shostrom V, Oleynikov D. How does robotic anti-reflux surgery compare with traditional open and laparoscopic techniques: a cost and outcomes analysis. Surg Endosc. 2014;28(5):1686–90.
14. Melvin WS, Needleman BJ, Krause KR, Schneider C, Ellison EC. Computer-enhanced vs. standard laparoscopic antireflux surgery. J Gastrointest Surg. 2002;6(1):11–5; discussion 5-6.
15. Muller-Stich BP, Reiter MA, Wente MN, Bintintan VV, Koninger J, Buchler MW, et al. Robot-assisted versus conventional laparoscopic fundoplication: short-term outcome of a pilot randomized controlled trial. Surg Endosc. 2007;21(10):1800–5.
16. Draaisma WA, Ruurda JP, Scheffer RC, Simmermacher RK, Gooszen HG, Rijnhart-de Jong HG, et al. Randomized clinical trial of standard laparoscopic versus robot-assisted laparoscopic Nissen fundoplication for gastro-oesophageal reflux disease. Br J Surg. 2006;93(11):1351–9.
17. Morino M, Pellegrino L, Giaccone C, Garrone C, Rebecchi F. Randomized clinical trial of robot-assisted versus laparoscopic Nissen fundoplication. Br J Surg. 2006;93(5):553–8.
18. Nakadi IE, Melot C, Closset J, DeMoor V, Betroune K, Feron P, et al. Evaluation of da Vinci Nissen fundoplication clinical results and cost minimization. World J Surg. 2006;30(6):1050–4.
19. Wang Z, Zheng Q, Jin Z. Meta-analysis of robot-assisted versus conventional laparoscopic Nissen fundoplication for gastro-oesophageal reflux disease. ANZ J Surg. 2012;82(3):112–7.
20. Mi J, Kang Y, Chen X, Wang B, Wang Z. Whether robot-assisted laparoscopic fundoplication is better for gastroesophageal reflux disease in adults: a systematic review and meta-analysis. Surg Endosc. 2010;24(8):1803–14.
21. Yao G, Liu K, Fan Y. Robotic Nissen fundoplication for gastroesophageal reflux disease: a meta-analysis of prospective randomized controlled trials. Surg Today. 2014;44(8):1415–23.
22. DeMeester TR, Johnson LF. The evaluation of objective measurements of gastroesophageal reflux and their contribution to patient management. Surg Clin North Am. 1976;56(1):39–53.
23. Peters JH. Modern imaging for the assessment of gastroesophageal reflux disease begins with the barium esophagram. J Gastrointest Surg. 2000;4(4):346–7.
24. Oelschlager BK, Quiroga E, Parra JD, Cahill M, Polissar N, Pellegrini CA. Long-term outcomes after laparoscopic antireflux surgery. Am J Gastroenterol. 2008;103(2):280–7; quiz 8.
25. Morgenthal CB, Lin E, Shane MD, Hunter JG, Smith CD. Who will fail laparoscopic Nissen fundoplication? Preoperative prediction of long-term outcomes. Surg Endosc. 2007;21(11):1978–84.
26. M. A. Outcomes of Antireflux Surgery. Antireflux surgery [Internet]. New York: Springer; 2015. p. 229–39.
27. D'Alessio MJ, Arnaoutakis D, Giarelli N, Villadolid DV, Rosemurgy AS. Obesity is not a contraindication to laparoscopic Nissen fundoplication. J Gastrointest Surg. 2005;9(7):949–54.

Robotic Heller Myotomy

6

Sharona B. Ross, Darrell Downs, Iswanto Sucandy,
and Alexander S. Rosemurgy

Introduction

Achalasia is a rare esophageal motility disorder that affects approximately 1 in 100,000 persons, often resulting in very debilitating symptoms [1]. It is an esophageal dysmotility disorder caused by haphazard or loss of esophageal peristalsis and an uncoordinated hypertensive lower esophageal sphincter mechanism, which can lead to a dilated and/or tortuous esophagus. Chronic dilation may lead to aperistalsis or vigorous uncoordinated contractions of the esophageal body. Patients are often plagued with choking sensations, inability to pass food boluses, and chest pain. Thereby, patients frequently avoid certain foods to help prevent exacerbation of their condition.

Endoscopic therapies, such as pneumatic balloon dilation and Botox® injections, have provided a nonoperative approach to alleviate symptoms but have not produced the same long-term success as operative interventions [2]. Pneumatic dilation has been shown to have a 5% perforation risk that many patients are not willing to take, and Botox® related palliation is transient at best. In recent years, surgical intervention has presented a more promising alternative than these therapies. POEM is the newest endoscopic therapy, but POEM is not widely available, and experience is lacking [3].

Over the last 30 years, the management options of achalasia have evolved and progressively promoted salutary benefit. From thoracotomy/celiotomy to minimally invasive techniques via thoracoscopy or laparoscopy, results of Heller myotomy improved, which manifested in shorter hospital stays and earlier returns to normal activities [4–13]. Because of associated morbidity, it was not until the 1990s, with the advent of laparoscopy, that the operative approach for the treatment of achalasia became the preferred approach over endoscopic therapies [4]. Thereafter, laparoscopic Heller myotomy became the favored approach, and thoracoscopy generally lost its place in the armamentarium treating achalasia. Over the last few decades, a partial fundoplication has been added to buttress the myotomy site and help prevent postoperative gastroesophageal reflux (GER), after a randomized trial supported its use [14, 15]. Most recently, in 2007, the advent of laparo-endoscopic single-site (LESS) surgery moved Heller myotomy with anterior fundoplication further along the path of minimally invasive surgery. Compared to conventional laparoscopy, LESS Heller myotomy with anterior fundoplication is as safe and efficacious, while allowing for better cosmesis, less postoperative pain, and quicker return to daily functional activities [5, 16].

In the last several years, advancement in surgical technology has introduced a robotic platform as a viable alternative approach for Heller myotomy. Robotic Heller myotomy was first reported in 2001 by Melvin et al. as an alternative technique to laparoscopic Heller myotomy [17]. The safety and efficacy, as measured by symptom resolution, have been reported to be similar between the robotic and laparoscopic approach, with a suggested lower rate of esophagotomy with the robotic platform [18]. Overall, the Heller myotomy has progressed through a variety of innovations that ultimately allow for better symptom amelioration and patient satisfaction [19]. Herein, we discuss our approach in treatment of achalasia using robotic technology.

Preoperative Preparation

Preoperative assessment and diagnosis of achalasia are often impacted by patient presentation and are obtained through a combination of studies including radiographic imaging, esophageal manometry, and upper endoscopy. Prior to surgical intervention, patients routinely undergo a timed barium swallow (Cohen test) to evaluate esophageal appearance, motility, and emptying, as well as to evaluate the gastroesophageal junction, looking for the classic "bird's beak" appearance of the gastroesophageal junction (i.e., a dilated

S. B. Ross (✉) · I. Sucandy · A. S. Rosemurgy
Department of Surgery, Florida Hospital Tampa, Tampa, FL, USA

D. Downs
Surgical Surgery, Florida Hospital Tampa, Tampa, FL, USA

© Springer Nature Switzerland AG 2019
S. Tsuda, O. Y. Kudsi (eds.), *Robotic-Assisted Minimally Invasive Surgery*, https://doi.org/10.1007/978-3-319-96866-7_6

proximal esophagus with distal tapering). Esophageal manometry is utilized to evaluate esophageal function along the length of the esophagus and through the gastroesophageal junction. Esophageal manometry is not undertaken routinely because the highly tortuous esophagus of most patients often limits its application; an esophageal diverticulum as well dissuades endoscopists from applying manometry to diagnostic testing. Upper endoscopy is necessary preoperatively to assess the distal esophageal mucosa and to rule out other causes of dysphagia (i.e., esophageal stricture, malignancy, or infectious etiology). Typical endoscopic findings are dilated proximal-mid esophagus with a narrowed distal esophagus that fails to relax (i.e., open) with air insufflation; the endoscope should be able to pass though the gastroesophageal junction with careful guidance but without force, unlike when a peptic stricture is present. If a stricture of unknown etiology or a mass is noted during endoscopy, then further investigation with dilation, pH testing, and endoscopic ultrasound (EUS) is warranted. In patients with long-standing achalasia, a highly serpiginous esophagus may be encountered.

Surgical Technique

Patient Positioning

Even though the laparoscopic approach is the "gold standard" for definitive therapy for achalasia, robotic technology offers inherent advantages over laparoscopy. The robot offers optimal visualization, adequate retraction and exposure, and the "fine" motor skills required for an uncomplicated and adequate Heller myotomy. Utilization of the robotic system allows and obviates the need for advanced laparoscopic skills. In sum, the robotic system provides a safe and effective approach for undertaking to Heller myotomy and anterior fundoplication.

The patient is placed in the supine position on the operating table. Compression stockings and sequential compression devices (SCDs) are used in all patients to prevent deep vein thrombosis (DVT). After general endotracheal anesthesia is established, both arms are extended, and all pressure points are padded. The patient's abdomen is widely prepped with alcohol, and a betadine-impregnated plastic drape is applied. The surgical table is then positioned in modest reverse Trendelenburg position with a slight left lateral tilt. The da Vinci Xi® (Intuitive Surgical, Sunnyvale, CA) robotic system is docked with the boom coming over the patient's right shoulder. The assistant surgeon stands on the patient's left, and the "scrub tech" stands to the patient's right. This arrangement enables easy access to the robotic arms for instrument exchange. Two surgeon consoles are placed in such a way that the surgeon at the console has a direct visu-

alization of the patient; we utilize dual consoles for the education and training of fellows and residents (see Fig. 6.1).

Port Placement

Prior to making any incision, approximately 5-8 cc of 0.25% Marcaine™ (AstraZeneca, Wilmington, DE) with epinephrine (1:1000) is injected into the umbilicus and all robotic port sites for local anesthesia. We believe this aids with decreasing postoperative pain. The abdomen is entered via 8 mm incision in the umbilicus, and pneumoperitoneum is established (up to 15 mmHg). The da Vinci Xi® is docked from over the patient's right shoulder.

After placement of the umbilical port, an 8 mm ports are placed along the left and right midclavicular line, cephalad to the umbilicus. A third 8 mm port is placed along the left anterior axillary line, cephalad to the umbilicus. A 5 mm AirSeal® Access Port (ConMed Inc., Utica, NY) is placed in the right upper quadrant along the right anterior axillary line for placement of a laparoscopic liver retractor. This port is very helpful in maintaining insufflation; this port is a particularly good adjunct for complex abdominal operations. The left lobe of the liver is retracted anteriorly, which provides exposure to the epigastric area (gastroesophageal junction and stomach). Only robotic arms 2, 3 (camera), and 4 are used. A fenestrated bipolar is placed in Arm 2, and a hook cautery is placed in Arm 4. The left midclavicular line port is used by the bedside assistant for suctioning or retraction (see Fig. 6.2).

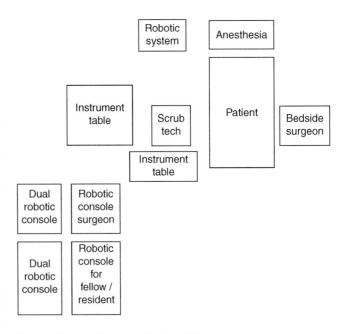

Fig. 6.1 Step 1 – Patient positioning/OR setup

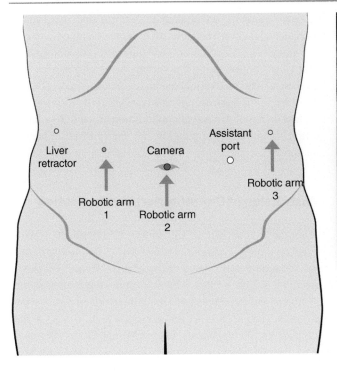

Fig. 6.2 Step 2 – Port placement

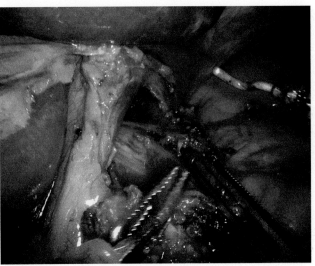

Fig. 6.3 Step 3 – Exposure of distal esophagus

Exposure of Distal Esophagus

The dissection begins with opening the gastrohepatic omentum in a stellate fashion using the robotic fenestrated bipolar instrument, a bowel grasper, and hook cautery. An accessory or replaced left hepatic artery must be anticipated in this location, and it should be preserved when the diameter is significant. The dissection is then carried toward the right crus, up and down the right crus, and into the mediastinum. Attention must be paid not to enter either pleural cavity. The dissection is continued anteriorly and cephalad to expose the anterior surface of the distal esophagus and gastroesophageal junction; care is undertaken to preserve the vagal trunks. The upper portion of the left crus then comes into view. The vagal nerve bundle is identified and preserved, and the gastroesophageal fat pad is excised (see Fig. 6.3).

Mobilization of Gastric Fundus

With the stomach retracted to the patient's right, the short gastric vessels are divided in a caudal to cephalad direction using the robotic vessel sealer sufficiently to reduce the gastroesophageal junction (GEJ) into the peritoneal cavity. The GEJ and the distal esophagus are mobilized only to expose the GEJ and reduce any hiatal hernia. Unnecessary dissection is to be avoided. As needed, the dissection is carried to the left crus, up and down the left crus, and into the mediastinum; any remaining hiatal hernia is fully reduced. The esophagus needs not be circumferentially mobilized. Our goal was to have 8 cm of esophagus in the peritoneal cavity.

Heller Myotomy

The myotomy starts on the esophageal side of the GEJ, approximately 1–2 cm superior to the gastroesophageal junction. Identifying the GEJ can be difficult, and the benefits of esophagoscopy/gastroscopy cannot be overstated. Carrying the myotomy unnecessarily cephalad is counterproductive; this carries risk without benefit and myotomized esophagus not covered by anterior fundoplication notably bulges over time. Utilizing robotic hook cautery, and while avoiding the anterior vagus nerve, the longitudinal muscle fibers are divided, which exposes the underlying circular muscle fibers (see Fig. 6.4). The plane exterior to the submucosa is divided carefully with hook cautery. The division of circular muscle fibers is carried out initially in a cephalad direction using robotic hook cautery (see Fig. 6.5). Then the myotomy is carried in a cephalad-to-caudad direction as the myotomy is carried along the anterior aspect of proximal stomach. The muscle edges are teased off the submucosa until about 50% of the esophageal circumference is freed of overlying muscle.

The goal is to defunctionalize the LES mechanism; the robotic 3D camera and stable platform facilitate a precise myotomy. The myotomy must defunctionalize the LES mechanism, nothing more. It is not productive, and is, in fact, counterproductive, to carry the myotomy unnecessarily "high" on the esophagus and unnecessarily "far" onto the stomach. Endoscopically, the myotomy must be carried across the Z-line; that is the goal. A bit more cephalad and caudad is OK, but excessive dissection is risk without benefit.

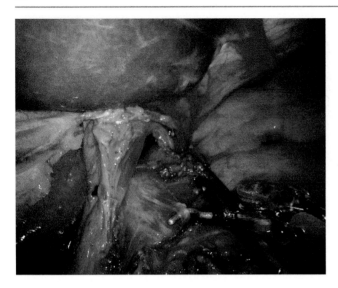

Fig. 6.4 Step 4 – Heller myotomy (dividing the *longitudinal* muscle fibers)

It is important to free submucosa from overlying muscle to free about 50% of the esophagus of "hypertensive" "uncoordinated" muscle. Blood loss should not be an issue, and most bleeding can be easily controlled with the application of direct pressure. Electrocautery should be used very judiciously to avoid thermal injury to the esophageal and gastric submucosal layers.

Intraoperative Esophagogastroscopy

Once the myotomy extends well above and below the gastroesophageal junction, intraoperative esophagogastroscopy

(EGD) is routinely undertaken to confirm that the gastroesophageal junction (i.e., the myotomized segment) opens with gentle CO_2 insufflation (see Fig. 6.6). The endoscopy should also confirm that the myotomy is "clean" enough and that there are no inadvertent esophagotomies and/or gastrotomies. Next, the gastroscope is advanced to the distal stomach, and an anterior fundoplication is constructed in order to prevent inadvertent angulation at the gastroesophageal junction.

Construction of Dor (Anterior) Fundoplication

We routinely construct a Dor (anterior) fundoplication with Heller myotomy. The fundus is brought "over" to the myotomy and completely covers the myotomy. We use 3–4 interrupted 3.0 V-Loc sutures. The first brings the fundus to the left side of the esophagus, proximal (on the esophagus) to the myotomy (see Fig. 6.7a). The second brings the fundus to the right side of the esophagus, also proximal to the myotomy (see Fig. 6.7b). The third brings the fundus to the right side of the esophagus but caudal to the previous suture (see Fig. 6.7c). With these three sutures, the myotomized segment is completely covered. The fundus is anchored to the esophagus and right crus to remove tension on the wrap and twisting of the esophagus (see Fig. 6.7d).

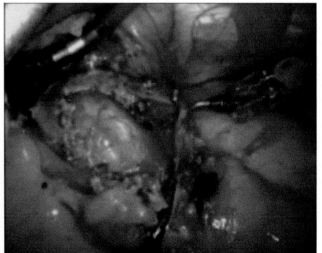

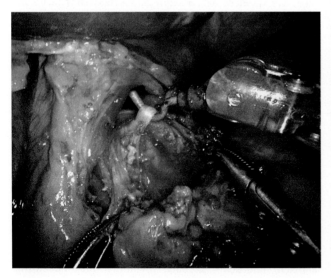

Fig. 6.5 Step 4 – Heller myotomy (dividing the *transverse* muscle fibers)

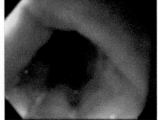

Fig. 6.6 Step 5 – Intraoperative EGD

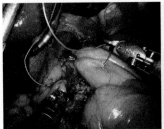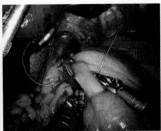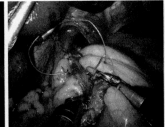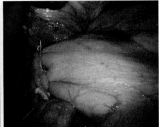

Fig. 6.7 Step 6 – Construction of Dor fundoplication

Closure

To decrease postoperative shoulder pain, the diaphragm is irrigated bilaterally and liberally with a solution of 7.5 mL of 0.25% Marcaine™ in 250 mL of normal saline. The fascial incisions are closed with 0-gauge monofilament absorbable sutures. The skin is approximated with interrupted 4-0 absorbable sutures. A sterile 1.5 × 6 silver dressing (Therabond® 3D, Alliqua Biomedical, Langhorne, PA) is applied to all incisions followed by sterile dry dressing with 2 × 2 gauze; it is covered with a Tegaderm™ (Tegaderm transparent dressing, 3M™, St Paul, MN) dressing. This watertight dressing allows the patients to shower at home. The dressing is removed at 7–8 days postoperatively in the office.

Postoperative Management

Esophagography (gastrografin followed by thin barium) is obtained upon discharge from the recovery room to evaluate integrity of the distal esophagus (i.e., evaluate for esophageal leak) and to document prompt emptying of the esophagus. In the absence of leak and delayed emptying, patients are started on a clear liquid diet. Pain is controlled and nausea is treated with anti-nausea medication. Retching and emesis must be avoided to prevent disruption of the myotomy and the fundoplication in the early postoperative phase. Patients are generally advanced to a full liquid diet the next morning, and they are discharged to home that day. Dietary instructions are provided to the patients and family prior to hospital discharge.

If the postoperative esophagogram indicates poor esophageal emptying, it is usually related to self-limited postoperative edema that resolves within 24–48 h [20]; if this is occurs, we just wait to start liquids until the next morning. We have never had the esophagogram detect an occult or unexpected esophagotomy. After discharge, patients are seen in the office in about 1–2 weeks postoperatively, and their diets are advanced to a more textured diet. Intermediate follow-up occurs in 2–6 months. Long-term follow-up occurs annually or semiannually thereafter in person, through mail, or by phone.

Possible Complications

1. Esophagotomy and/or gastrotomy can occur during myotomy, especially in patients with prior history of pneumatic balloon dilation and/or botulinum toxin injections. Primary treatment: primary repair and buttress with Dor (anterior) fundoplication.
2. Capnothorax rarely occurs during reduction of hiatal hernia, when the pleural space may be violated. Treatment: Placement of a pneumothorax catheter or a small tube thoracotomy intraoperatively to evacuate the carbon dioxide.
3. Postoperative dysphagia can occur due to swelling at the gastroesophageal junction. This is usually self-limited.

Outcomes After Robotic Heller Myotomy

Early in the application of robotic surgery, Galvani et al. reported a series of robotic Heller myotomy in 54 patients [21]. There were no intraoperative complications, and only two patients developed postoperative complications (i.e., incarcerated port site hernia and a delayed thermal injury to the transverse colon requiring a colon resection). Melvin reported another series of 104 patients undergoing robotic Heller myotomy [22]. There were no intraoperative esophagotomies, which suggests that the application of computer-enhanced operative techniques provide superior outcomes when compared with standard laparoscopic techniques. Conversion to "open" operations was needed for two patients because of bleeding and robotic system computer failure. Perry et al. reported similar results in a series of 56 patients which compared robotic Heller myotomy to laparoscopic Heller myotomy [23]. No esophagotomies occurred with the robotic approach, while 16% of patients had esophagotomies with the laparoscopic approach ($p = 0.01$). Finally, the lower rate of esophagotomy with the robotic platform was confirmed in a meta-analysis by Maeso et al. [24]. A large multicenter study reported by Shaligram confirmed a low morbidity of robotic Heller myotomy (149 patients), when compared with laparoscopic (2116 patients) and "open" (418 patients) myotomy; the morbidity after robotic Heller myotomy is like that seen with laparoscopic Heller myotomy (4% versus 5%) [25].

Resolution of dysphagia after robotic Heller myotomy is excellent and like that after laparoscopic myotomy. Horgan et al. demonstrated comparable dysphagia resolution after both robotic and laparoscopic Heller myotomy (92% versus 90%, $p = 0.5$) [26]. Perry et al. reported long-term outcomes following robotic and laparoscopic Heller myotomy [18, 23]. Their study has 9-year median follow-up, and all patients reported adequate relief of dysphagia; 84% of patients who underwent robotic Heller myotomy had enduring relief of dysphagia without needing further intervention compared to 70% of patients who underwent laparoscopic Heller myotomy.

There is currently a great degree of debate on the role of robotics in American Surgery. Surgeons, patients, healthcare payers, and hospital institutions are among the many stakeholders in this debate. A multitude of factors, therefore, determine when robotic surgical systems should be used in patient care. These factors include, but are not limited to, robot availability, surgeon aptitude, nature and scope of the planned operation, costs of care, and institutional goals and direction. One of the major concerns about robotic surgery is the cost of purchasing and maintaining a robotic surgical system. Short hospital stays deriving from minimally invasive procedures do not necessarily translate into cost savings for healthcare institutions; whether the robotic platform is overall cost-effective is difficult to evaluate. However, we have reported that costs can be manageable and cost-effective if the robotic systems are used to their maximum potential (i.e., in high-volume centers) [27]. The robotic platform will eventually become more affordable, and institutions with the latest technologies may hold a competitive edge for patients.

In conclusion, robotic Heller myotomy is a safe and efficacious alternative for Heller myotomy. The robotic platform offers several advantages to the surgeon while providing similar benefits of laparoscopic Heller myotomy.

References

1. Podas T, Eaden J, Mayberry M, Mayberry J. Achalasia: a critical review of epidemiological studies. Am J Gastroenterol. 1998;93(12):2345–7.
2. Gockel I, Junginger T, Bernhard G, Eckardt V. Heller myotomy for failed pneumatic dilation in achalasia: how effective is it? Ann Surg. 2004;239:371–7.
3. Schlottmann F, Luckett DJ, Fine J, Shaheen NJ, Patti MG. Laparoscopic Heller myotomy versus peroral endoscopic myotomy (POEM) for achalasia: a systematic review and meta-analysis. Ann Surg. 2017; https://doi.org/10.1097/SLA.0000000000002311.
4. Sharp K, Khaitan L, Schotz S, Holzman M, Richards W. 100 consecutive minimally invasive Heller myotomies: lessons learned. Ann Surg. 2002;235:631–9.
5. Rosemurgy AS, Morton CA, Rosas M, Albrink M, Ross SB. A single institution's experience with more than 500 laparoscopic Heller myotomies for achalasia. J Am Coll Surg. 2010;210(5):637–45. 645-7.
6. Finley R, Clifton J, Stewart K, et al. Laparoscopic Heller myotomy improves esophageal emptying and the symptoms of achalasia. Arch Surg. 2001;136:892–6.
7. Bloomston M, Boyce W, Mamel J, et al. Videoscopic Heller myotomy for achalasia: results beyond short term follow-up. J Surg Res. 2000;92:150–6.
8. Zaninotto G, Costantini M, Rizzetto C, et al. Four hundred laparoscopic myotomies for esophageal achalasia: a single centre experience. Ann Surg. 2008;248:986–93.
9. Bloomston M, Serafini F, Rosemurgy A. Videoscopic Heller myotomy as first-line therapy for severe achalasia. Am Surg. 2001;67:1105–9.
10. Zaninotto G, Costantini M, Molena D, et al. Minimally invasive surgery for esophageal achalasia. J Laparoendosc Adv Surg Tech A. 2001;11:351–9.
11. Bloomston M, Brady P, Rosemurgy A. Videoscopic Heller myotomy with intraoperative endoscopy promotes optimal outcomes. JSLS. 2002;6:133–8.
12. Ramacciato G, Mercantini P, Amodio PM, et al. Minimally invasive surgical treatment of esophageal achalasia. JSLS. 2003;7:219–25.
13. Bloomston M, Serafini F, Boyce HW, et al. The "learning curve" in videoscopic Heller myotomy. JSLS. 2002;6:41–7.
14. Richards W, Torquati A, Holzman M, et al. Heller myotomy versus Heller myotomy with Dor fundoplication for achalasia. Ann Surg. 2004;240:405–12.
15. Bloomston M, Rosemurgy A. Selective application of fundoplication during laparoscopic Heller myotomy. Surg Laparosc Endosc Percutan Tech. 2002;12:309–15.
16. Ross SB, Luberice K, Kurian TJ, Paul H, Rosemurgy AS. Defining the learning curve of laparoendoscopic single-site Heller myotomy. Am Surg. 2013;79(8):837–44.
17. Melvin WS, Needleman BJ, Krause KR, Wolf RK, Michler RE, Ellison EC. Computer-assisted robotic heller myotomy: initial case report. J Laparoendosc Adv Surg Tech A. 2001 Aug;11(4):251–3.
18. Afaneh C, Finnerty B, Abelson JS, Zarnegar R. Robotic-assisted Heller myotomy: a modern technique and review of outcomes. J Robot Surg. 2015 Jun;9(2):101–8.
19. Rosemurgy AS, Downs DJ, Jadick G, Swaid F, Luberice K, Ryan J, Ross SB. Dissatisfaction after laparoscopic heller myotomy: The truth is easy to swallow. Am J Surg. 2017. pii: S0002-9610(16)30692-4.
20. Cowgill SM, Villadolid D, Boyle R, Al-Saadi S, Ross S, Rosemurgy AS. Laparoscopic Heller myotomy for achalasia: results after 10 years. Surg Endosc. 2009;23(12):2644–9.
21. Galvani C, Gorodner MV, Moser F, Baptista M, Donahue P, Horgan S. Laparoscopic Heller myotomy for achalasia facilitated by robotic assistance. Surg Endosc. 2006;20(7):1105–12. Epub 2006 May 13.
22. Melvin WS, Dundon JM, Talamini M, Horgan S. Computer-enhanced robotic telesurgery minimizes esophageal perforation during Heller myotomy. Surgery. 2005;138(4):553–8; discussion 558-9.
23. Perry KA, Kanji A, Drosdeck JM, Linn JG, Chan A, Muscarella P, et al. Efficacy and durability of robotic Heller myotomy for achalasia: patient symptoms and satisfaction at long-term follow-up. Surg Endosc. 2014;28(11):3162–7. https://doi.org/10.1007/s00464-014-3576-9. Epub 2014 May 31.
24. Maeso S, Reza M, Mayol JA, Blasco JA, Guerra M, Andradas E, et al. Efficacy of the Da Vinci surgical system in abdominal surgery compared with that of laparoscopy: a systematic review

and meta-analysis. Ann Surg. 2010;252(2):254–62. https://doi.org/10.1097/SLA.0b013e3181e6239e.

25. Shaligram A, Unnirevi J, Simorov A, Kothari VM, Oleynikov D. How does the robot affect outcomes? A retrospective review of open, laparoscopic, and robotic Heller myotomy for achalasia. Surg Endosc. 2012;26(4):1047–50. https://doi.org/10.1007/s00464-011-1994-5. Epub 2011 Oct 25

26. Horgan S, Galvani C, Gorodner MV, Omelanczuck P, Elli F, Moser F, et al. Robotic-assisted Heller myotomy versus laparoscopic Heller myotomy for the treatment of esophageal achalasia: multicenter study. J Gastrointest Surg. 2005;9(8):1020–9; discussion 1029-30.

27. Ross SB, Downs D, Saeed SM, Dolce JK, Rosemurgy AS. Robotics in surgery: is a robot necessary? For what? Minerva Chirurgica. 2017;72(1):61–70. https://doi.org/10.23736/S0026-4733.16.07235-7.

Robotic Sleeve Gastrectomy

7

Brian Minh Nguyen and Benjamin E. Schneider

Introduction

The sleeve gastrectomy is a weight loss procedure that has rapidly replaced Roux-en-Y gastric bypass as the most common weight loss procedure performed in the United States (see Fig. 7.1). By reducing the stomach volume by 70–80%, there are obvious restrictive properties that promote weight loss. In addition to having restrictive properties, it is also postulated that the sleeve gastrectomy causes weight loss by promoting gastric emptying and inhibiting the release of ghrelin, a hormone that acts on the brain to stimulate appetite. Over 90% of the bodies circulating ghrelin is released from the stomach and duodenum. Significant reduction in stomach volume produced by the sleeve gastrectomy, in turn, reduces the amount of circulating levels of ghrelin, which results in suppression of appetite. It is likely the combination of these mechanisms that lead to the weight loss seen in this patient population.

	2011	2012	2013	2014	2015	2016
Total	158,000	173,000	179,000	193,000	196,000	216,000
RNY	36.7%	37.5%	34.2%	26.8%	23.1%	18.7%
Band	35.4%	20.2%	14%	9.5%	5.7%	3.4%
Sleeve	17.8%	33%	42.1%	51.7%	53.8%	58.1%
BPD/DS	0.9%	1%	1%	0.4%	0.6%	0.6%
Revisions	6%	6%	6%	11.5%	13.6%	13.9%
Other	3.2%	2.3%	2.7%	0.1%	3.2%	2.6%
Balloons					.03%	2.7%

Fig. 7.1 MBSAQIP bariatric surgery procedures. (Reprinted with permission of American Society for Metabolic and Bariatric Surgery, Copyright 2015, all rights reserved)

B. M. Nguyen
San Diego, CA, USA

B. E. Schneider (✉)
Minimally Invasive and Bariatric Surgery, Department of Surgery,
University of Texas Southwestern, Dallas, TX, USA
e-mail: Benjamin.Schneider@UTSouthwestern.edu

© Springer Nature Switzerland AG 2019
S. Tsuda, O. Y. Kudsi (eds.), *Robotic-Assisted Minimally Invasive Surgery*, https://doi.org/10.1007/978-3-319-96866-7_7

History

The idea for the sleeve gastrectomy originated in 1976, when Lawrence Tretbar noticed that patients undergoing an extended fundoplication for reflux also had significant weight loss as a side effect. The extended fundoplication effectively reduced the stomach volume to restrict food intake, which led to weight loss in addition to treating the patients' reflux [1]. This idea was incorporated by Doug Hess a decade later, although instead of an extended gastric plication, he created a vertical gastrectomy as a way to reduce the stomach volume. He first performed this as part of a duodenal switch procedure in 1988 [2].

With the advent of minimally invasive surgery, some bariatric surgeons began performing laparoscopic duodenal switches. One of the barriers to widespread adoption of the laparoscopic duodenal switch was a high complication rate associated with high body mass index (BMI) patients. As a way of mitigating this risk, some surgeons began staging the procedure by first performing the vertical gastrectomy portion of the procedure. This allowed for interval weight loss prior to completing the second stage of the procedure months later. This staged approach was found to have lower complication rates in patients with high BMI, when compared to a single-staged procedure [3].

Soon, others realized that weight loss associated with the vertical gastrectomy alone was sufficient in morbidly obese patients with lower BMI. The sleeve gastrectomy, as it is known today, is now recognized as a primary bariatric surgery procedure by the American Society of Metabolic and Bariatric Surgery and is the most commonly performed weight loss operation in the United States.

Robot-assisted sleeve gastrectomy has grown in popularity as the platform continues to evolve and surgeons continue to embrace the technology.

Literature Review

Along with the Roux-en-Y gastric bypass and the adjustable gastric band, sleeve gastrectomy is one of the most common weight loss surgeries performed in the world and has been gaining popularity in recent years. According to the Metabolic and Bariatric Surgery Accreditation and Quality Improvement Program (MBSAQIP) database, sleeve gastrectomy has overtaken gastric bypass as the most commonly performed weight loss procedure in the United States.

A meta-analysis comparing outcomes between gastric bypass and sleeve gastrectomy showed that gastric bypass is associated with a slightly better long-term weight loss but is similar to sleeve gastrectomy in terms of resolution of weight-related comorbidities, including type 2 diabetes mellitus, hypertension, hyperlipidemia, and hypertriglyceridemia [4].

In another meta-analysis, sleeve gastrectomy was associated with a lower postoperative complication rate when compared to gastric bypass (3.9% vs 11.6%, $p < 0.001$) [5].

When comparing robot-assisted sleeve gastrectomy to laparoscopic sleeve gastrectomy, operative times were slightly longer in the robot-assisted cases. One author attributed this to routine oversewing of the staple line during robot-assisted sleeve gastrectomy which is not routinely done laparoscopically [6]. Another author attributed this to robot docking times, which took an average of 16 min [7].

Patient outcomes have been shown to be similar between the two groups. After accounting for the learning curve associated with robotic surgery, hospital length of stay was shown to be slightly longer in the robotic group (1.7 ± 1.8 days vs. 1.2 ± 0.5 days, $p < 0.01$) but only on the magnitude of half a day, on average. The authors showed no difference in terms of readmission (2.4% vs 2.2%, $p = 0.88$), reoperation (1.2% vs. 0.7%, $p = 0.60$), and leak rate (1.9% vs 3.2%, $p = 0.28$) [8].

Preoperative Planning

In order for patients to be considered for weight loss surgery, they must meet certain criteria. These criteria were first outlined by the National Institute of Health (NIH) in 1991 and modified by the American Society of Bariatric Surgery in 2004.

Candidates for weight loss surgery include patients with a BMI greater than 40 kg/m^2 (or body weight greater than 100 pounds above ideal body weight) or a BMI of 35 to 39.9 kg/m^2 (or body weight greater than 80 pounds above ideal body weight) with at least one serious weight-related comorbidity, such as obstructive sleep apnea, type 2 diabetes, hyperlipidemia, heart disease, degenerative arthritis/chronic lower back pain, or hypertension. Patients should also demonstrate failure of nonsurgical weight loss attempts in the past.

Contraindications to weight loss surgery include no prior attempt at medical weight loss, life-threatening disease, prohibitive operative risk, uncontrolled psychiatric illness, active substance abuse, inability to follow up, and lack of social support.

Relative contraindications to the sleeve gastrectomy include patients with Barrett's esophagus or severe gastroesophageal reflux, as the surgery may exacerbate this condition.

Preoperative Assessment

When considering any weight loss procedure, patients routinely undergo an extensive psychological, medical, and anesthetic risk assessment. In preparation for a sleeve gastrectomy, patients with documented upper gastrointestinal symptoms such as reflux or dysphagia should undergo evaluation to exclude ulcers, polyps, dysplastic changes, and hiatal hernia. This step is important because patients with severe gastroesophageal reflux or Barrett's esophagus may have their conditions worsened with a sleeve gastrectomy and may be better suited for another weight loss procedure, such as gastric bypass. An unrecognized hiatal hernia may also worsen symptoms postoperatively and, if identified, should be repaired at the time of sleeve gastrectomy.

Patients should be encouraged to lose weight in the weeks leading up to surgery, as this can significantly reduce liver size and the amount of visceral fat, makes surgery easier to perform. Patients should also confirm that all of their home medications can be either crushed or obtained in liquid form, as pill swallowing may be difficult for a few weeks after surgery due to postoperative inflammation. Extended release medications should be converted to immediate release because they typically cannot be crushed. Patients should have nothing to eat or drink starting midnight prior to surgery and avoid taking pills on the day of surgery to avoid retained pills within the stomach during surgery.

Setup

Sequential compression stockings and subcutaneous heparin should be administered to reduce the risk of deep vein thrombosis. Preoperative antibiotics targeting upper gastrointestinal flora should be administered in case of perforation or spillage of gastric contents. A urinary catheter is not routinely needed but can be placed if a prolonged procedure is anticipated or for patients at high risk of urinary retention. An orogastric tube should be inserted into the stomach and placed on suction to remove excess fluid and air from the stomach prior to beginning the dissection.

The patient is positioned supine on the operating room table. The patient's arms do not need to be tucked as the patient cart is docked over the patient's left shoulder. Because the patient cart will be stationed above the patient's head, it is important that the anesthesia provider makes arrangements for easy airway and intravenous access. Circulating nurses and scrub techs should be familiar with the setup and use of the robot.

Procedure

A robot-assisted sleeve gastrectomy involves performing a vertically oriented partial gastrectomy that removes 70–80% of the stomach along the greater curve. The following procedure will be described using a 4-armed da Vinci SI High-Definition Surgical System.

For this procedure, the patient cart is docked above the head of the patient over the left shoulder. A Veress needle is used to insufflate the abdomen and is inserted in the left upper quadrant, below the costal margin. When planning port placement for robotic surgery procedures, it is important to note that the camera port should be oriented approximately 20 cm from the target anatomy and each additional port should be at least 8–10 cm away from any adjacent robotic port. Because the target anatomy for a sleeve gastrectomy is the stomach, located slightly above the xiphoid, the camera port is placed 15–20 cm below the xiphoid, above the umbilicus in the midline. A 12-mm extra-long trocar is used as the camera port. Robotic arm port 1 should be placed in the left midclavicular line, about 10 cm lateral to the camera port. Robotic arm port 2 should be placed in the right midclavicular line, 10 cm lateral to the camera port on the opposite side. Robotic arm port 3 should be placed in the left flank, 8–10 cm lateral to robotic arm 1. Lastly, a 15-mm assistant port is placed in the right lower quadrant at the level of the umbilicus to assist in suctioning and stapling of the stomach (see Fig. 7.2).

To begin the operation, the Veress needle is inserted in the left upper quadrant below the costal margin. To confirm placement within the peritoneal cavity, an aspiration test is performed to confirm that no intestinal contents or blood is aspirated, followed by a saline drop test. Once intraperitoneal placement is confirmed, the abdomen is insufflated to 15 mmHg. The camera port is then inserted under direct visualization using an optical trocar. A laparoscopic camera is then inserted into the abdomen to evaluate for adhesions or other findings that may alter port placement or operative planning. A Nathanson liver retractor is then placed to the left of the epigastrium to retract the liver away from the stomach. Then, the three 8-mm trocars are placed under

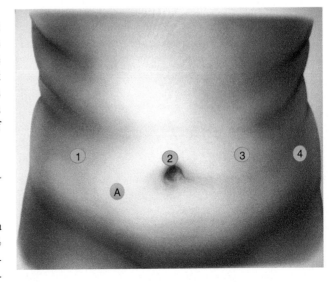

Fig. 7.2 Port placement

direct visualization in the aforementioned locations, followed by the assistant port trocar. Long cannulas should be used as high BMI patients tend to have a thicker abdominal wall. The bed should then be placed in reverse Trendelenburg.

The patient cart is then brought into the surgical field, positioned above the patient's left shoulder, and the robotic arms are attached to the trocars. The bed may need to be turned to facilitate this. Make sure that the elbow of the camera port is on the opposite side of robotic arm 3 to allow for maximal range of motion. A 30-degree camera is then inserted through the camera port in the down position. The camera port, target anatomy, and patient cart should be oriented in a straight line. Also, make sure that the blue arrow on the camera arm joint falls within the boundaries of the blue line, the so-called sweet spot.

The instruments are then inserted under direct visualization to avoid unintentional injury from blind insertion. Atraumatic forceps, such as a fenestrated bipolar forceps or Cadiere forceps, are inserted into ports 2 and 3. A vessel sealer is inserted into port 1. The accessory port can be used to suction or for extra retraction.

Dissection begins by separating the greater omentum from the greater curve of the stomach. A relatively avascular region is selected within gastrocolic ligament approximately 6 cm from the pylorus and a dissection begins using the vessel sealer (Fig. 7.3). This will open a window into the lesser sac, and the dissection should continue cephalad toward the spleen along the lateral border of the greater curve. To aid in this dissection, the stomach and omentum should be retracted with the forceps in opposite directions to create tension and adequate visualization. It is helpful to keep the line of dissection relatively close to the stomach, and it is important to avoid injuring the underlying colon. The dissection is further carried up toward the angle of His, dividing the short gastric vessels in the process. Extra care should be taken when approaching this dissection because of its proximity to the spleen (Fig. 7.4). There may be additional adhesions on the posterior wall of the stomach to the underlying pancreas, and

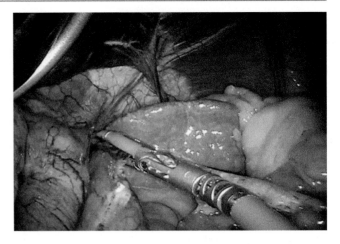

Fig. 7.4 Dissection of the short gastric vessels

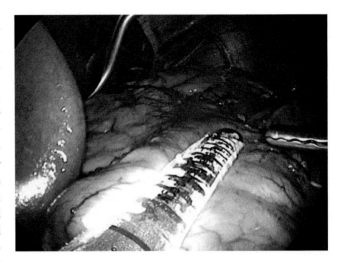

Fig. 7.5 Gastric division with bougie in place

these should be divided with a vessel sealer. Occasionally, additional dissection toward the pylorus may be necessary.

The orogastric tube should then be removed and replaced with a 36 Fr bougie tube. Starting 6 cm from the pylorus, 60-cm, linear cutting stapler should be inserted through the accessory port, and a horizontally angled firing of the stapling devise should be performed adjacent to the bougie (Fig. 7.5). Care should be taken to avoid narrowing the level of the incisura, which can lead to stricture. The remaining staple loads should be oriented vertically toward the angle of His, along the edge of the bougie. It is important to retract the fundus laterally to prevent corkscrewing of the staple line or leaving a redundant "neo-fundus" (Fig. 7.6). The thicker fungus may require a taller staple height, particularly for the first several staple loads. Some surgeons routinely oversew the staple line or use buttressing material to reinforce the staple line, although controversy exists regarding its benefits. If the staple line is

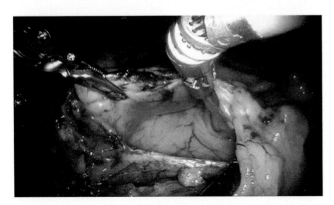

Fig. 7.3 Opening the gastrocolic ligament

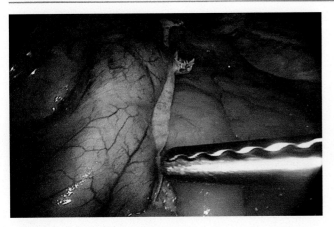

Fig. 7.6 Lateral retraction of the fungus

oversewn, it is imperative to keep the bougie in place to prevent narrowing of the lumen.

Once the stapling is complete, the bougie should be removed and replaced with a orogastric tube. To test for leaks, 120 ml of methylene blue is injected into the stomach via the orogastric tube to distend the stomach. Alternatively, endoscopy may be used in order to test the staple line.

Once hemostasis is achieved, the specimen is grasped through the accessory port with a locking forceps, the robot is undocked, and the specimen is removed. A 15-mm retrieval bag can also be used to facilitate removal of the specimen. The assistant port and cameral port need to be closed to prevent incisional hernia. This can be done using either an open or laparoscopic technique. The 8-mm port site fascia does not need to be re-approximated. The skin is then closed with and absorbable monofilament subcuticular suture.

Postoperative Care

Subcutaneous heparin and sequential compression stockings should be continued postoperatively. Patients can begin a clear liquid diet soon after surgery and are advanced to protein shakes as tolerated. Liquid should be taken in small boluses of no more than 15 mL at a time to account for the small stomach reservoir and swelling that occurs postoperatively. Maintenance IV fluids should be given until the patient is tolerating enough liquids to prevent dehydration. Patients are typically discharged on postoperative day 1 or 2 once they meet their discharge criteria. Patients should be seen 2 weeks after discharge for a postoperative check and be seen by the dietician to advance their diet as tolerated, based on symptoms. Patient surveillance is done at the 6-month and 1-year mark, then yearly from then on out.

Outcomes

Patients undergoing sleeve gastrectomy can expect to lose over 60% of their excess body weight. These results are slightly less than that of the gastric bypass [9].

Patient comorbidities, such as diabetes, hypertension, sleep apnea, and hyperlipidemia, also improve to varying degrees. Studies are conflicting regarding improvement of gastroesophageal reflux symptoms.

Complications

Although complications are rare, they can be serious. Acutely, complications include hemorrhage and leak. The rate of postoperative hemorrhage varies and can occur within the stomach lumen, at the trocar sites, or intra-abdominally. Most commonly, intra-abdominal bleeding occurs along the staple line as a result of the long staple line and well-vascularized stomach. Prior to finishing surgery, the staple line should be carefully examined to exclude potential sites of bleeding. Some surgeons routinely use buttressing material or oversew the staple line to prevent this potential complication.

Leaks can occur at any part of the long staple line and can be difficult to heal spontaneously because of increased intraluminal pressure keeping the perforation open. Evaluation of leaks can be done by injecting methylene blue or air through an orogastric tube. Other surgeons routinely perform endoscopy to detect leaks. Signs and symptoms of leaks include fever, tachycardia, respiratory distress, or worsening abdominal pain. Unstable patients require immediate reoperation. In patients with unexplained fever and tachycardia, surgeons should have a low threshold for re-exploration to rule out leak. Endo-luminal stenting has been shown to be effective treatment option. Other options include oversewing the leak with a bougie to prevent stricture or conversion to Roux-en-Y gastric bypass.

Strictures may occur over time, and patients typically present with symptoms that mimic gastroesophageal reflux. Endoscopy and balloon dilation can be used for short-segment strictures, but long-segment strictures may require conversion to Roux-en-Y gastric bypass.

Portal vein thrombosis is a rare but potentially serious complication that has been seen in sleeve gastrectomy patients and occurs in about 1% of patients undergoing laparoscopic sleeve gastrectomy [10]. Symptomatic patients will typically present with epigastric pain. Anticoagulation is the standard for asymptomatic patients with nonocclusive disease, but patients with occlusive disease may require thrombectomy in addition to anticoagulation.

References

1. Tretbar LL, Taylor TL, Sifer EC. Weight reduction. Gastric placation for morbid obesity. J Kans Med Soc. 1976;77(11):488–90.

2. Hess DS, Hess DW. Biliopancreatic diversion with a duodenal switch. Obes Surg. 1998;8(3):267–82.

3. Kim WW, Gagner M, Kini S, Inabnet WB, Quinn T, Herron D, Pomp A. Laparoscopic vs. open biliopancreatic diversion with a duodenal switch: a comparative study. J Gastrointest Surg. 2003;7(4):552–7.

4. Shoar S, Saber AA. Long-term and midterm outcomes of laparoscopic sleeve gastrectomy versus Roux-en-Y gastric bypass: a systematic review and meta-analysis of comparative studies. Surg Obes Relat Dis. 2017;13(2):170–80.

5. Rondelli F, Bugiantella W, Vedovati MC, Mariani E, Balzarotti Canger RC, Federici S, Guerra A, Boni M. Laparoscopic gastric bypass versus laparoscopic sleeve gastrectomy: a retrospective multicenter comparison between early and long-term post-operative outcomes. Int J Surg. 2017;37:36–41.

6. Ayloo S, Buchs NC, Addeo P, Bianco FM, Giulianotti PC. Robot-assisted sleeve gastrectomy for super-morbidly obese patients. J Laparoendosc Adv Surg Tech A. 2011;21(4):295–9.

7. Diamantis T, Alexandrou A, Nikiteas N, Giannopoulos A, Papalambros E. Initial experience with robotic sleeve gastrectomy for morbid obesity. Obes Surg. 2011;21:1172–9.

8. Moon RC, Stephenson D, Royall NA, Teixeira AF, Jawad MA. Robot-assisted versus laparoscopic sleeve gastrectomy: learning curve, perioperative, and short-term outcomes. Obes Surg. 2016;26(10):2463–8.

9. Garg H, Priyadarshini P, Aggarwal S, Agarwal S, Chaudhary R. Comparative study of outcomes following laparoscopic Roux-en-Y gastric bypass and sleeve gastrectomy in morbidly obese patients: a case control study. World J Gastrointest Endosc. 2017;16(4):162–70.

10. Salinas J, Barros D, Salgado N, Viscido G, Funke R, Pérez G, Pimentel F, Boza C. Portomesenteric vein thrombosis after laparoscopic sleeve gastrectomy. Surg Endosc. 2014;28(4):1083–9.

Robotic Gastric Bypass/Duodenal Switch

Keri Seymour and Ranjan Sudan

Introduction

Bariatric surgery incorporated the robotic surgical system into their surgical armamentarium with advanced hand-sewn techniques and improved outcomes. In 2000, the Food and Drug Administration approved the use of the da Vinci robot in general surgery, and the first robotic Roux-en-Y gastric bypass (RARYGB) and robotic-assisted biliary pancreatic diversion with duodenal switch (RABPD/DS) were performed the same year [1, 2].

Patients undergoing bariatric surgery often have a thick abdominal wall with substantial subcutaneous fat. These factors place significant torque on the straight laparoscopic instruments and may be physically demanding on the surgeon. Additionally, the significant visceral fat frequently reduces operating space. The robotic platform incorporates more durable instruments, additional arms for retraction, and enhanced ergonomics for the surgeon. Some surgeons prefer to use the robot for these reasons, especially in patients with higher body mass index (BMI) or technically challenging anatomy.

Literature Review

Robotic systems can offset many of the limitations of conventional laparoscopy including optics, ergonomics, and retraction. The earliest version of the robotic surgical system incorporated three robotic arms that were controlled from a remote console. The addition of a third arm created an opportunity for additional retraction or operating radius. The optical imaging was more advanced than standard laparoscopy and included binocular vision and a stable, 3D camera. The instruments introduced seven degrees of movement, two more than the standard laparoscopy. The "wristed" instruments allowed for precise actions and were frequently used for creating a hand-sewn anastomosis [3, 4]. In addition, the robotic system dampened unnecessary movements and tremors.

Himpens performed the first robotic-assisted adjustable gastric band in 1998 in Belgium [5]. By 2003, only 11 surgeons in the United States were publishing results on robotic bariatric surgery [6]. Initial implementation by six surgeons utilized a hybrid technique that reserved the robot for the gastrojejunostomy (GJ) or duodenoileostomy (DI) anastomosis [2, 3]. Even though the wristed instruments allowed hand-sewn anastomosis in complex surgeries like RABPD/DS, operating in multiple areas required additional setups and extended operating time. With experience and improvements in technology, docking times improved and totally RARYGB and totally RABPD/DS were developed [7, 8].

The first-generation robotic platform had three arms and a limited selection of instruments. Since then technology steadily developed, and the latest generation of the robot includes a fourth robotic arm, electrocautery, and stapler and is capable of multi-quadrant operations. Furthermore, updated instruments are longer, are more suited to gently handle bowel, and have increased range of motion.

With the development of the field of robotic bariatric surgery, the learning curve for surgeons has also been reported. Operative time for fellows performing the RARYGB was 154 min after the first 10 cases and decreased to 99 min after 20 cases [3]. Additionally, complications decreased after 50 RABPD/DS cases [9]. Overall, the surgeons experience reflected reduced operative times and low complication rates. The technical advances, along with surgeon proficiency, shorter operative time, and fewer complications, have promoted robotic-assisted bariatric surgery.

K. Seymour
Department of Surgery, Duke University Medical Center, Durham, NC, USA
e-mail: Keri.Seymour@duke.edu

R. Sudan (✉)
Department of Surgery, Duke University Health System, Duke University Medical Center, Durham, NC, USA
e-mail: Ranjan.sudan@duke.edu

© Springer Nature Switzerland AG 2019
S. Tsuda, O. Y. Kudsi (eds.), *Robotic-Assisted Minimally Invasive Surgery*, https://doi.org/10.1007/978-3-319-96866-7_8

RYGB

Initially, utilization of the robot was hindered by a complicated setup and technical inexperience. The first RARYGB was performed in 2000 [1], and studies that compared laparoscopic RYGB (LRYGB) to RARYGB reported mixed results [7, 10–12]. An interesting analysis comparing RARYGB to eight different LRYGB techniques demonstrated that the mean operative time for the RARYGB was 201 min, while the operative time for the various LRYGB procedures ranged from 60 to 260 min. The RARYGB fell within an acceptable range of operative times and included a mean time of 19.3 min to perform a hand-sewn GJ anastomosis [10]. Another study compared outcomes after RARYGB to the same surgeon's previous LRYGB outcomes [11]. The mean operative length for this single surgeon's LRYGB was 127 min while the first 15 RARYGB cases was completed in 212 min and included 30 min to dock and set up the robot. However, after 35 RARYGB cases, this surgeon's operative time reduced to a mean of 136 min [11]. This demonstrated the surgeon's and operative room staff's learning curve in mastering robotic technology.

Another study also reported decreased setup and operating time with increasing number of cases. Initial robotic setup time decreased by over 50% from an average of 17.3 min for the first 20 RARYGB patients to 7.7 min for the last 20 cases. Additionally, the average operative time decreased from 312.6 min during the first 20 RARYGB cases to a mean of 201.6 min for the last 20 patients [4]. Similarly, a case series demonstrated the mean operative time for the initial 40 RARYGB cases was 200 min while the final 100 RARYGB cases was 90 min [13].

Although the RARYGB requires training on the robotic system and technical expertise with the operation itself, the learning curve appears to be shorter than that of the LRYGB. While the learning curve of the LRYGB is 75–100 cases [14], the RARYGB is reported at 14–35 cases [3, 11, 14, 15].

BMI per minute is used as a surrogate to standardize procedure difficulty related to ergonomic challenges from torque and central visceral adiposity while acknowledging operative efficiency. When controlling for BMI, the operating time (mean minute per BMI) was faster for RARYGB than for LRYGB [3, 7]. The study also suggested BMI >43 kg/m^2 did not affect RARYGB time and the skill of the surgeon was more influential in operative length [3]. This was further supported when additional studies described mean operative minutes per BMI diminished with operative proficiency [7, 14, 15].

Overall complications for RARYGB were comparable to laparoscopy. The overall complication rate was 14% and mortality was 0% [3, 10, 12, 13, 16]. A GJ leak occurred in up to 0.09% [6, 10, 13, 16, 17]. Additionally, rates were low for deep venous thrombosis (DVT) (0.27%), pulmonary embolus (1%), bleeding events (0%), marginal ulcers (0.55%), and trocar site hernia (1%) [6, 10, 13, 16]. The postoperative course had 2% reoperations [16]. A GJ stricture was more common than a leak when the hand-sewn technique was incorporated in the robotic surgeries. A GJ stricture rate up to 4.4% occurred after RARYGB compared to 5.3% during hand-sewn LRYGB anastomosis [6, 10, 12, 13, 15–17]. No nutritional deficiencies were reported at 12 months after RARYGB [10], again proving that RARYGB was safe and comparable to LRYGB.

Weight loss was similar to LRYGB. One month after RARYGB, patients achieved 21% EWL [10]. This ranged from 38% to 48% EWL at 3 months and 57% to 64% EWL at 6 months [10, 15]. Weight loss was similar at 1 year for LRYGB (61.9% EWL) and RARYGB (61% EWL) [10, 12].

Cost analysis of robotic surgery is limited in direct comparison of open and laparoscopic surgery. The purchasing cost for the da Vinci robot platform (Intuitive Surgical, Sunnyvale, CA) is now close to $2 million and excludes the additional 10% cost for annual maintenance [3, 4, 10, 18]. When the cost per case includes analysis of instruments designated for robotic surgery or supplemental instruments, the material costs were highest for the RARYGB (US $5427) and LRYGB (US $5494) compared to open RYGB (US $2251) [18]. Some suggest the minimal difference is the result of fewer staple loads and the lower cost of suture, since the improved dexterity of the wristed instruments allows for hand-sewn anastomosis [3, 4]. The cost increased when comparing the robotic stapling system (US $2212.2) to laparoscopic staple loads (US $1787.4) [19]. Of note, the cumulative cost including postoperative care and cost of complications claimed RARYGB (US $19,363) to be the most cost-effective compared to LRYGB (US $21,697) and open RYGB (US $23,000) [18].

BPD/DS

The first RABPD/DS was performed by Sudan et al. [2] in 2000 and reported similar advantages and challenges with implementation as RARYGB.

The RABPD/DS is especially demanding since the surgery potentially progresses through all four abdominal quadrants. The right lower quadrant is accessed to measure the bowel from the terminal ileum. The sleeve gastrectomy and dissection of angle of His occur in the left upper quadrant (LUQ). The DI anastomosis is created in the right upper quadrant, and the ileoileostomy (II) occurs in the periumbilical region. The left lower quadrant may also need to be accessed if there are lower abdominal adhesions. Another impediment involves the increased torque on instruments from the thick abdominal wall of patients with a higher BMI. The mean BMI for the RABPD/DS was 56 kg/m² with a range of 40–85 kg/m². While 34% (20 patients) had a BMI of 60 kg/m², the procedure has been successful up to the highest weight of 505 lbs. (229.5 kg) [8].

The learning curve for RABPD/DS was established at 50 cases [9]. The median operative time was 514 min for 47 patients, but this declined to 379 min for the last 10 RABPD/DS. Conversion to open surgery occurred in only 2% of the patients during the learning curve and was related to difficult anatomy, iatrogenic injury, or bleeding. Initially, blood loss was an average of 179 ml per patient. Conversion decreased to 0% with surgeon experience and improved robotic technology [2, 8, 9].

Similar to RARYGB, the robotic technique did not significantly adversely impact outcomes. The hybrid technique for the RABPD/DS reported a mean operative duration of 366.6 min. Modifications to a totally robotic technique resulted in reduced operative time by 60 min, to an average of 306 min for the totally RABPD/DS [8]. Further analysis found female gender decreased complication risks but increased mean operative minute per BMI [9]. Few complications were reported after RABPD/DS. There were no perioperative deaths in the studies [2, 8, 9], and the average length of stay (LOS) for RABPD/DS was 4.6 days [8]. Conversion to open surgery was performed in 6.4% to 1.7% of cases [2, 8, 9]. Similarly, leaks occurred at the DI in 4 patients (8%) and decreased to 0% with operative experience [2, 8]. No DVT or bleed that required transfusion occurred after RABPD/DS [8]. Weight loss after RABPD/DS was not reported [2, 8, 9].

Preoperative Planning

The preoperative planning for robotic surgery is consistent with other bariatric procedures. This includes evaluation by a dietician, psychologist, and vitamin and nutrition panel, imaging studies or upper endoscopy, and appropriate risk stratification by cardiology, pulmonology, or other specialists as determined by the surgeon. The robotic assistance may be particularly useful when performing surgery on patients with a BMI ≥ 65 [6]. Some advocate a liver shrinking diet for up to 2 weeks prior to surgery to improve operative space when performing the GJ or DI anastomosis [9]. There are no absolute or relative contradictions for robotic surgery that are different than laparoscopic surgery.

Setup

Successful organization of the robotic platform involves appropriate docking, placement of the robotic arms, patient position, trocar use, instruments, and beside assistance. Both the RARYGB and RABPD/DS require operating in two or more areas of the abdomen. To overcome this, surgeons may perform a hybrid procedure that maximizes the precision of the robot by performing a hand-sewn anastomosis and includes laparoscopy to operate in multiple abdominal quadrants. However, with experience many surgeons perform a totally robotic operation with a single dock of the robot.

In order to utilize the robot, the patient must be appropriately positioned at the time of docking. With experience, arranging the robot becomes easier and may ultimately decrease operative time by 20 min or more [4]. Some studies suggest including two scrub nurses to reduce setup time, one nurse for the robot and one for the patient. This is ideal, but may not be realistic at some institutions. The robot can be docked at the head of the patient or 15–30° left of midline with the left arm tucked for RARYGB [7, 11, 13] or over the patient's right shoulder with outstretched arms for RABPD/DS [2].

Appropriate port placement is critical to improved technique. Ports should not be placed in folds of the abdominal wall because it limits instrument reach and places unnecessary torque on the instruments. The robot is docked at the head of the patient for the RARYGB, and a sample operating room configuration is demonstrated in Fig. 8.1. For the RABPD/DS, the robot is docked over the patient's right shoulder; the robotic arm and operating room setup is shown in Fig. 8.2 [8]. The robotic arms should be well spaced from each other to prevent collision and allow for smooth movement and full range of motion of the arms and instruments [3]. At least five to six ports, and a liver retractor, will be needed for both the RARYGB and RABPD/DS [6]. The camera is often placed in the periumbilical region [6, 7]. For the RARYGB, the robot instrument arm 2 is in the right midclavicular line (MCL). The accessory port for the assistant is between the MCL and the camera port. The port for the instrument arm 1 is placed in the left MCL, and the port for the instrument arm 3 is in the left subcostal area of the anterior axillary line (Fig. 8.3) [7, 13]. There are proponents of using 12 mm ports, so the 8 mm robotic port can be interchangeably used (port-in-port technique) and thus more easily transitions between two working areas of the abdomen [7].

The surgeon should develop technical proficiency in the use of instrumentation, including energy and stapling devices on the robotic platform. The Cadiere forceps, needle driver, and hook cautery were introduced early on by Intuitive Surgical (Sunnyvale, CA) [2, 7, 10]. Although the introduc-

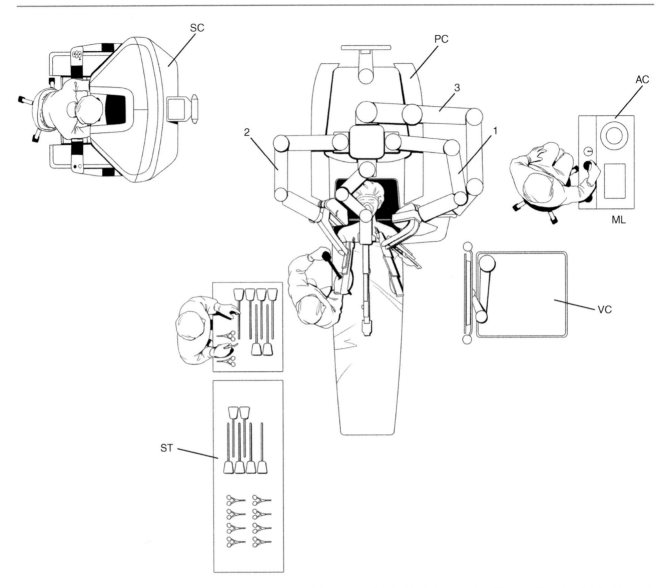

Fig. 8.1 Operating room setup for RARYGB. The patient cart (PC) is docked at the head of the patient. The surgeon console (SC), sterile Table (ST), and surgical assistant are positioned on the right side of the patient. The anesthesia cart (AC) and vision cart (VC) are on the patient's left side. Robot arm 1 and 3 are on the patient's left side, while robot arm 2 is on the patient's right side. (Illustration by Megan Llewellyn)

tion of the robotic stapler, upgraded instruments, and a fourth arm has provided the console surgeon with more sophisticated adjuncts, the bedside assistant is utilized to perform conventional laparoscopic stapling and pass suture through an accessory port. In the RABPD/DS, the bedside assistant is positioned on the patient's left side for the majority of the case and uses a 12 mm port placed in the left anterior axillary line to staple the duodenum [6, 7]. However, the sleeve gastrectomy portion of the case is performed from the patient's right side using a 12–15 mm port in the right mid-clavicular line. This port is also used robotically using the port-in-port technique.

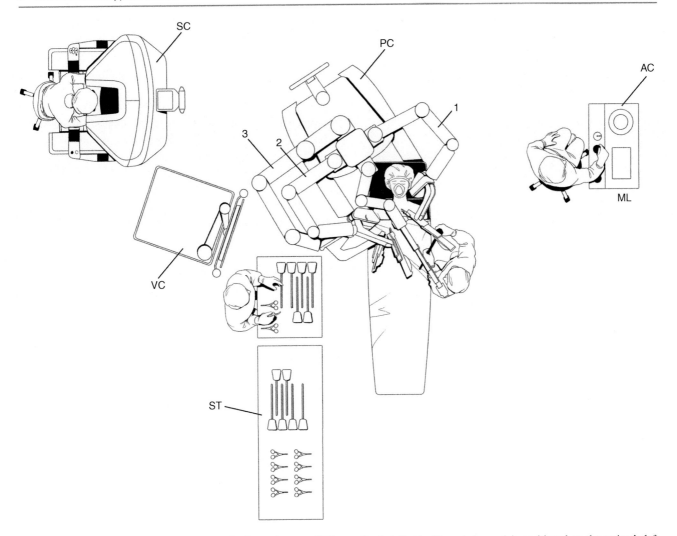

Fig. 8.2 Operating room setup for RABPD/DS. The patient cart (PC) is docked over the patient's right shoulder. The surgeon console (SC), sterile Table (ST), and vision cart (VC) are positioned on the right side of the patient. The anesthesia cart (AC) and surgical assistant are on the patient's left side. The robot arm 1 is positioned on the patient's left side, while robot arm 2 and robot arm 3 are on the patient's right side. (Illustration by Megan Llewellyn)

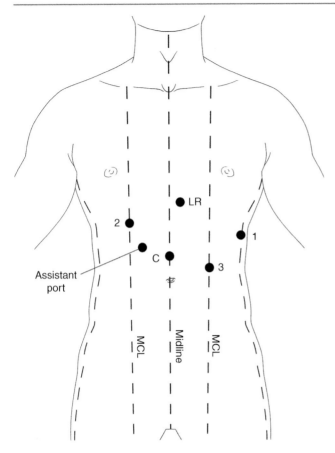

Fig. 8.3 Port placement for RARYGB. The camera port (C) is placed in the periumbilical region, while the liver retractor (LR) is placed in the epigastric region. The port for the first arm of the robot (1) is in the subcostal area of the left anterior axillary line, while the port for the third arm (3) is in the left midclavicular line (MCL). The port for the second arm of the robot (2) is placed in the MCL, and the assistant (assistant port) is between the right MCL and midline. (Illustration by Megan Llewellyn)

Procedure

RARYGB Steps

For the RARYGB, the patient is positioned supine and general anesthesia is induced. Appropriate DVT prophylaxis, perioperative antibiotics, Foley catheter, and OGT may be placed. The robot is docked at the patient's head or slightly to the left of the head [6, 7, 11].

The sequence of the case varies depending on surgeon preference. Some surgeons will begin with the jejunojejunostomy (JJ) anastomosis, either laparoscopically [1, 6, 10] or robotically [3, 7, 11, 16]. The omentum is lifted and tucked under the liver, and the transverse mesocolon is retracted superiorly to expose the ligament of Treitz. The proximal jejunum is transected 50 cm to create the biliopan-

creatic limb. The small bowel is run another 100–150 cm to create an alimentary limb. The JJ is performed with a unidirectional or bidirectional technique, and the suture or stapler closes the enterotomy. The mesenteric defect is closed with permanent suture [6, 16].

Next, the patient is placed in moderate reverse Trendelenburg and the robot is docked. The ports are placed as described above (Fig. 8.3). The lesser sac is entered using a perigastric or gastrohepatic dissection, and a 15–30 ml pouch is created with staple loads to completely divide the stomach. The GJ is performed using a hand-sewn two-layer anastomosis with the robotic platform [6, 7, 11, 13, 16, 18]. A leak test is performed with methylene blue or carbon dioxide insufflation [7, 10].

Our preference is to perform a totally robotic technique using an Omega loop. The bowel is first measured 50 cm from the ligament of Treitz and anchored to the anterior stomach wall laparoscopically with two orienting sutures. The robot is then docked, and the 15–30 ml stomach pouch is created using a vagal-sparing approach. Next, the bowel anchored to the stomach is anastomosed to the stomach pouch using a two-layer hand-sewn technique with barbed absorbable 3–0 sutures. The bowel is oriented such that the biliary limb will be toward the patient's left side and the alimentary limb will be to the patient's right side (Fig. 8.4a). Next, the Roux limb is measured to 150 cm, and a stapled JJ anastomosis is created while the biliary limb is still anchored in the LUQ by the GJ anastomosis. The biliary limb is divided using a 60 mm stapler to separate it from the GJ anastomosis, either prior to or after creating the JJ anastomosis depending on the ease with which the bowel can be manipulated while performing the JJ anastomosis. The enterotomy for the JJ is closed with absorbable 3-0 barbed suture (Fig. 8.4b). The mesenteric defects are closed with nonabsorbable 3-0 barbed suture.

RABPD/DS Steps

In the RABPD/DS, the pylorus is preserved, and a sleeve gastrectomy is performed to create a 150 ml stomach pouch, along with a 150 cm alimentary limb, and 100 cm common channel [8, 9]. Analogous to the RARYGB, the bedside assistant is utilized to perform the stapling during a RABPD/DS.

The patient is similarly placed supine, general anesthesia is induced, DVT and antibiotic prophylaxis are given, and OGT or Foley catheters are placed. Optical entry is performed with a 0° camera and 12 mm port in the supraumbilical region. Two additional 12 mm ports are placed, along with the Nathanson liver retractor as previously described [2, 8].

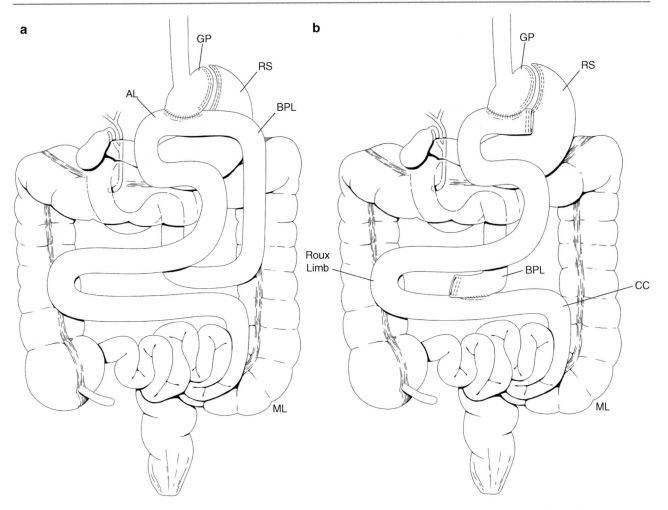

Fig. 8.4 (**a**) Omega loop configuration for the RARYGB. The bowel is measured at 50 cm from the ligament of Treitz and anchored to the abdominal wall in the left upper quadrant. The robot is docked, and the gastric pouch (GP) is separated from the remnant stomach (RS). The Omega loop orients the biliopancreatic limb (BPL) toward the patient's left side and the alimentary limb (AL) to the patient's right side. A hand-sewn gastrojejunostomy is sewn in a two-layer fashion. (Illustration by Megan Llewellyn). (**b**) Final configuration of RARYGB. The Roux limb is measured at 150 cm from the gastric pouch (GP). The stapled JJ anastomosis is performed over the remnant stomach (RS). This creates continuity with the biliopancreatic limb (BPL) and common channel (CC). The enterotomy is closed with a single-layer hand-sewn technique. Then the BPL is divided to separate it from the GJ anastomosis to create the final RYGB configuration. (Illustration by Megan Llewellyn)

For the totally RABPD/DS, the small bowel is measured from the ileocecal valve and marked at 100 cm and then anchored to the anterior abdominal wall at 250 cm, laparoscopically. The robot is then docked, and the patient is placed in moderate reverse Trendelenburg position. The robotic instrument arms 1 and 2 are placed in the left and right MCL, respectively, and the accessory arm (arm 3) is placed in the right anterior axillary line (Fig. 8.5). This allows the entire operation to be completed robotically using the Si model.

It is our preference to first perform a routine cholecystectomy, though some surgeons prefer to preform cholecystectomy selectively. Next, the stomach is mobilized to about 4 cm distal to the pylorus, and the duodenum is divided where the gastroduodenal artery lies posterior to the first portion of the duodenum. The rest of the stomach is then completely mobilized to the angle of His and the sleeve gastrectomy performed starting 5 cm proximal to the pylorus with the intention of creating a 150–200 cc pouch. The bedside assistant uses the right midclavicular port to provide stapling, and the staple line is reinforced with either buttress material or is oversewn by the console surgeon [2, 8, 9].

Thereafter, the console surgeon performs a hand-sewn antecolic or retrocolic two-layer DI anastomosis [2]. Our preference is to now to perform an antecolic anastomosis. The ileum at the 250 cm mark is sutured to the transected duodenum in two layers in an end-to-side fashion, using 3-0,

Fig. 8.5 Port placement for RABPD/DS [8]. The trocar for the camera (C) is in the periumbilical area, while the liver retractor (LR) is placed in the epigastric region. The robot is docked, and the first robotic arm (1) is placed in the left midclavicular line (MCL), and the assistant port is placed in the subcostal region of the left anterior axillary line. The trocar for arm 2 (2) is placed in the right MCL, and the trocar for arm 3 (3) is placed in the subcostal region of the right anterior axillary line. (Illustration by Megan Llewellyn)

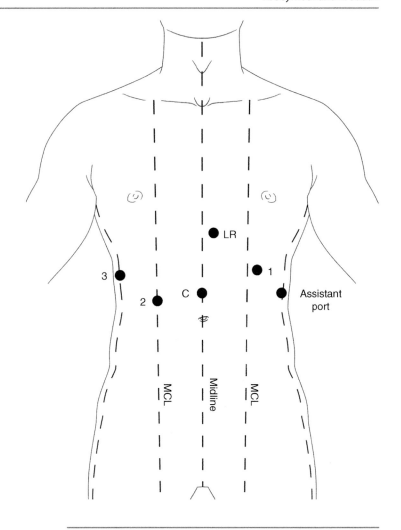

6 inch barbed suture. The bowel is positioned in Omega loop fashion to allow the totally robotic technique and prevent redocking [8] (Fig. 8.6a). Methylene blue is then placed in the stomach to perform a leak test while the II is being constructed.

Next, the II is performed between the biliary limb and the common channel at the 100 cm mark. The assistant through the left anterior axillary port uses a 60 mm stapler, and the enterotomy for the stapler is closed using a running 3-0 absorbable barbed suture. Finally, the biliary limb is separated from the DI anastomosis using a 60 mm stapler (Fig. 8.6b). The mesenteric defects between the common channel and the BPD limb, along with the alimentary limb and the transverse mesocolon, are closed with permanent 3-0 barbed suture [2, 8].

Postoperative Care

Postoperative care follows the same pathway as for laparoscopic bariatric surgery. Patients follow an enhanced recovery pathway that includes intraoperative removal of the Foley catheter, a liquid diet, and limited narcotics. Imaging studies are performed if there is concern for a complication. During the learning curve, conversion to open surgery occurred in 11% of RARYGB cases and conversion to laparoscopy in 9%. Iatrogenic bowel injury or bleeding was often a cause for conversion [11, 16]. Experienced surgeons report a much lower conversion rate of 0% for RARYGB and 1.7% for RABPD/DS [8, 13, 17]. The mean LOS was 2–3 days [1, 3, 6, 12, 16] with 6.1% readmissions [13].

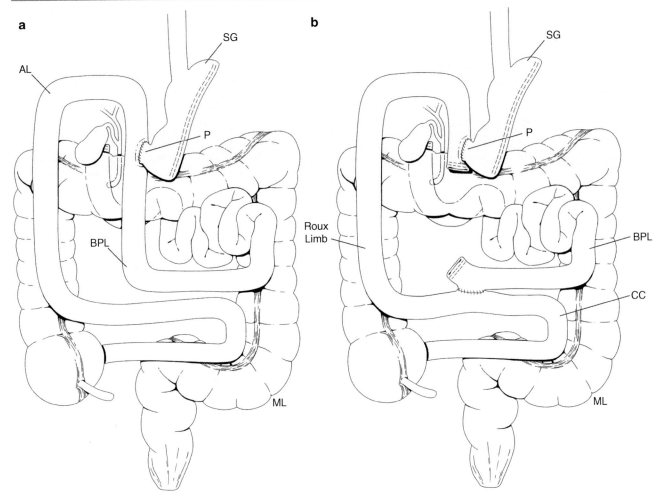

Fig. 8.6 (**a**) Omega loop configuration for RABPD/DS. The RABPDS begins by marking the alimentary limb (AL) at 100 cm and 250 cm. The sleeve gastrectomy (SG) is performed, along with the pylorus-preserving (P) duodenal transection. The duodenoileostomy is created in Omega loop configuration. The single-loop anastomosis at the 250 cm mark creates a very long biliopancreatic limb (BPL). (Illustration by Megan Llewellyn). (**b**) Final anatomy RABPD/DS [8]. The ileoile-ostomy is performed at the 100 cm mark. Then the bowel is divided between the duodenoileostomy and the ileoileostomy to separate the pylorus-preserving (P) sleeve gastrectomy (SG). The final BPDDS anatomy is a 150 cm alimentary limb (AL), 100 cm common channel (CC), and very long biliopancreatic limb (BPL). (Illustration by Megan Llewellyn)

Acknowledgment With gratitude to Megan Llewellyn for the illustrations.

Disclosure Statement The authors Keri Seymour and Ranjan Sudan have nothing to disclose.

References

1. Horgan S, Vanuno D. Robots in laparoscopic surgery. J Laparoendosc Adv Surg Tech A. 2001;11(6):415–9.
2. Sudan R, Puri V, Sudan D. Robotically assisted biliary pancreatic diversion with a duodenal switch: a new technique. Surg Endosc. 2007;21(5):729–33.
3. Sanchez BR, Mohr CJ, Morton JM, Safadi BY, Alami RS, Curet MJ. Comparison of totally robotic laparoscopic Roux-en-Y gastric bypass and traditional laparoscopic Roux-en-Y gastric bypass. Surg Obes Relat Dis. 2005;1(6):549–54.
4. Jacobsen G, Berger R, Horgan S. The role of robotic surgery in morbid obesity. J Laparoendosc Adv Surg Tech A. 2003;13(4):279–83.
5. Cadiere GB, Himpens J, Vertruyen M, Favretti F. The world's first obesity surgery performed by a surgeon at a distance. Obes Surg. 1999;9(2):206–9.
6. Moser F, Horgan S. Robotically assisted bariatric surgery. Am J Surg. 2004;188(4A Suppl):38S–44S.
7. Mohr CJ, Nadzam GS, Curet MJ. Totally robotic Roux-en-Y gastric bypass. Arch Surg. 2005;140(8):779–86.
8. Sudan R, Podolsky E. Totally robot-assisted biliary pancreatic diversion with duodenal switch: single dock technique and technical outcomes. Surg Endosc. 2015;29(1):55–60.

9. Sudan R, Bennett KM, Jacobs DO, Sudan DL. Multifactorial analysis of the learning curve for robot-assisted laparoscopic biliopancreatic diversion with duodenal switch. Ann Surg. 2012;255(5):940–5.

10. Parini U, Fabozzi M, Brachet Contul R, Millo P, Loffredo A, Allieta R, et al. Laparoscopic gastric bypass performed with the Da Vinci Intuitive Robotic System: preliminary experience. Surg Endosc. 2006;20(12):1851–7.

11. Hubens G, Balliu L, Ruppert M, Gypen B, Van Tu T, Vaneerdeweg W. Roux-en-Y gastric bypass procedure performed with the da Vinci robot system: is it worth it? Surg Endosc. 2008;22(7):1690–6.

12. Park CW, Lam EC, Walsh TM, Karimoto M, Ma AT, Koo M, et al. Robotic-assisted Roux-en-Y gastric bypass performed in a community hospital setting: the future of bariatric surgery? Surg Endosc. 2011;25(10):3312–21.

13. Tieu K, Allison N, Snyder B, Wilson T, Toder M, Wilson E. Robotic-assisted Roux-en-Y gastric bypass: update from 2 high-volume centers. Surg Obes Relat Dis. 2013;9(2):284–8.

14. Buchs NC, Pugin F, Bucher P, Hagen ME, Chassot G, Koutny-Fong P, et al. Learning curve for robot-assisted Roux-en-Y gastric bypass. Surg Endosc. 2012;26(4):1116–21.

15. Mohr CJ, Nadzam GS, Alami RS, Sanchez BR, Curet MJ. Totally robotic laparoscopic Roux-en-Y gastric bypass: results from 75 patients. Obes Surg. 2006;16(6):690–6.

16. Yu SC, Clapp BL, Lee MJ, Albrecht WC, Scarborough TK, Wilson EB. Robotic assistance provides excellent outcomes during the learning curve for laparoscopic Roux-en-Y gastric bypass: results from 100 robotic-assisted gastric bypasses. Am J Surg. 2006;192(6):746–9.

17. Stefanidis D, Bailey SB, Kuwada T, Simms C, Gersin K. Robotic gastric bypass may lead to fewer complications compared with laparoscopy. Surg Endosc. 2017;32(2):610–6.

18. Hagen ME, Pugin F, Chassot G, Huber O, Buchs N, Iranmanesh P, et al. Reducing cost of surgery by avoiding complications: the model of robotic Roux-en-Y gastric bypass. Obes Surg. 2012;22(1):52–61.

19. Hagen ME, Jung MK, Fakhro J, Buchs NC, Buehler L, Mendoza JM, et al. Robotic versus laparoscopic stapling during robotic Roux-en-Y gastric bypass surgery: a case-matched analysis of costs and clinical outcomes. Surg Endosc. 2017;32(1):472–7.

Robotic Total Gastrectomy with Lymphadenectomy

9

Yanghee Woo and Jared Rocky Funston

Introduction

Robotic gastrectomy has become an integral tool for surgeons treating gastric cancer worldwide. Since 2002 and 2003 when surgeons from Japan [1] and the United States [2] independently reported the initial safety and feasibility of robotic gastrectomy, adoption of the robotic approach has outpaced that of laparoscopy for gastric cancer operations. Studies have demonstrated the application of robotic technology in gastric cancer procedures to be safe and feasible, to allow adherence to oncologic principles, and to show improved patient outcomes compared to open operations and comparable outcomes to laparoscopic sur-

gery [3–6]. Moreover, robotic approach has been suggested to decrease the steep learning curve for laparoscopic radical gastrectomies [7, 8] opening the potential to achieve optimum minimally invasive surgical outcomes with less number of operations. In the United States where gastric cancer incidence and case volumes are generally low and patients present with more advanced disease state, robotic approach for a technically demanding total gastrectomy procedure is an appealing minimally invasive option for our gastric cancer patients.

To date, most studies in robotic gastrectomy combine both robotic total and distal gastrectomies (Table 9.1). In comparison to open procedures, laparoscopic and robotic

Table 9.1 Studies comparing robotic, laparoscopic, and/or open radical gastrectomies, which include total gastrectomy

Author	Year	# of RTG included	Operating time (min)	Blood loss (mL)	Lymph nodes retrieved	Hospital LOS (days)	Morbidity/mortality rate (%)
Patriti et al. [9]	2008	4	287	103	28.1	11	8
Song et al. [10]	2009	33	231	128	36.7	8	13
D'Annibale et al. [11]	2011	11	268	30	28	6	8
Woo et al. [4]	2011	64	220	92	39	8	11
Caruso et al. [12]	2011	12	290	198	28	10	41
Isogaki et al. [13]	2011	14	520	150	43	13	5
Yoon et al. [14]	2012	36	305	NA	42.8	9	17
Huang et al. [15]	2012	7	430	50	32.0	7	15
Kang et al. [16]	2012	16	202	93	NA	10	14
Kim et al. [6]	2012	109	226	85	40.2	8	10
Liu et al. [17]	2013	54	273	81	23.1	6	12
Hyun et al. [18]	2013	9	234	131	32.8	11	13
Junfeng et al. [19]	2014	26	235	118	34.6	8	6
Shen et al. [20]	2015	23	257	177	33	9	10
Kim et al. [21]	2016	43	226	50	33	6	1

Notes: *LOS* length of stay, *RTG* robotic total gastrectomy

Y. Woo (✉)
Department of Surgery, City of Hope National Medical Center, Duarte, CA, USA
e-mail: ywoo@coh.org

J. R. Funston
Department of Surgery, Huntington Hospital, Pasadena, CA, USA

© Springer Nature Switzerland AG 2019
S. Tsuda, O. Y. Kudsi (eds.), *Robotic-Assisted Minimally Invasive Surgery*, https://doi.org/10.1007/978-3-319-96866-7_9

Table 9.2 Case series of robotic total gastrectomies

Author	Year	RTG	Operating time (min)	Blood loss (mL)	Lymph nodes retrieved	Hospital LOS (days)	Morbidity/mortality rate (%)
Son et al. [22]	2014	51	264.1	163.4	47.2	8.6	15.7/NA
Parisi et al. [23]	2015	22	270	200	19.2	5.5	0/0
Jiang et al. [24]	2015	65	245	75	NA	5.4	1.5/0

Notes: *LOS* length of stay, *RTG* robotic total gastrectomy, *NA* not available. Operating time, blood loss, and hospital length of stay are all averages

surgeries have been found to decrease hospital length of stay, improve cosmesis, and decrease postoperative pain over open operations without compromising oncologic outcomes. A single prospective trial comparing robotic and laparoscopic subtotal distal gastrectomy for clinically stage 1 disease that demonstrated postoperative complication severity and frequency was comparable to standard technique [21]. However, the greatest disadvantage to robotic surgery has been the consistently longer operative times when compared to laparoscopic and open operations.

Direct comparison of robotic total gastrectomy to laparoscopic surgery has largely been retrospective (Table 9.2). In these studies, robotic total gastrectomy has been found to have a complication rate of 10.4% and mortality rate of 0.4% in a large meta-analysis [25]. The learning curve of the robotic total gastrectomy has been reported to be lower than for the laparoscopic approach with stabilization of operative times at between 95 and 127 cases compared to 262 and 270 cases [7]. A prospective study comparing robotic versus laparoscopic total gastrectomy is currently ongoing in South Korea. Over a decade of robotic surgery application for gastric cancer treatment informs us that robotic total gastrectomy with lymphadenectomy for curative resections remains a complex minimally invasive procedure which offers significant advantages to the patient and the surgeon when properly adopted.

Patient Selection and Preoperative Planning

The decision for robotic total gastrectomy depends on several factors including the patient's clinical condition and disease state and the surgeon's experience and expertise. Patient selection should consider the patient's comorbidities with special consideration given to patient's ability to tolerate pneumoperitoneum and prolonged operative time.

All patients being evaluated for total robotic gastrectomy should have pathologically confirmed diagnosis as well as proper staging of the disease:

- Upper endoscopy with biopsy to locate the tumor and confirm biological diagnosis
- Endoscopic ultrasound to evaluate tumor invasion and nodal status

- CT scan of the abdomen and pelvis to determine invasion depth, nodal status, and distant metastasis
- PET scan as indicated

Recognition of the tumor location within the stomach and clinically suspected nodal stations as well as aberrant vascular anatomy is of particular importance in the preoperative planning for robotic total gastrectomy. Localization of the lesion by endoscopy is critical with robotic surgery where intraoperative palpation or direct visualization of tumor is not possible. Careful planning will allow the surgeon to avoid unnecessary manipulation of the area of the tumor during surgery. In addition, CT evaluation of aberrant anatomy will aid the robotic surgeon in surgical decision-making during the nodal dissection along the vessels and to maintain vascular control.

The recommended indications for robotic total gastrectomy for gastric adenocarcinoma are equivalent to that of laparoscopic total gastrectomy and include:

- Early gastric cancer as defined by cT1abNxM0 by the 8th AJCC TNM classification
- Locally advanced disease as defined by cT2NxM0 disease
  - Mucosal and submucosal tumors not eligible for endoscopic resection
  - Failed endoscopic mucosal resection or endoscopic submucosal dissection

Minimally invasive surgery for more advanced disease states involving the serosa or having significant gross nodal disease remains controversial, and the decision for robotic surgery for these patients should be carefully considered. The robotic approach can also be considered for patients with CDH-1 mutations at risk for hereditary diffuse gastric cancer, gastrointestinal stromal tumors, and carcinoids who require total gastrectomies.

Another consideration in the perioperative planning for patients undergoing robotic total gastrectomy is the implementation of enhanced recovery after surgery (ERAS) protocols for gastric cancer. Several studies along with the recommended consensus guidelines by the European ERAS Society include the use of minimally invasive surgery and several key components of patient management that demonstrate improved short-term perioperative patient outcomes [26–29].

Setup

The setup of the operation begins with positioning of the patient in the supine position with both arms tucked at the patient's side. Standard practice of inserting an orogastric or nasogastric tube for gastric decompression is used but not routinely left in place after surgery. In addition, bilateral lower extremity sequential compression devices (SCDs) and urinary catheter are placed. The abdomen is prepped from the nipple line to the suprapubic region and draped in a standard sterile fashion. During the draping, the position of the endotracheal tube under the drapes is carefully noted to avoid clash with the robotic arms when docking.

Four robotic ports and one assistant port are used in the procedure of robotic total gastrectomy. A periumbilical camera port is either placed infraumbilically or supraumbilically depending on the distance from the xiphoid (~16 cm to 18 cm), and the patient's body habitus is placed either by cut down or direct entry at the preference of the surgeon. After the placement of the initial periumbilical port, the robotic camera is inserted, and the patient is placed in 15–30° reverse Trendelenburg position. The remaining ports are placed under direct vision as shown in Fig. 9.1. The placement of the 15 mm assist port should be in the left midaxillary line just inferior to the camera port.

Tips: The assist port should be slightly caudal to camera port to improve assistant access to the port. Also, the intra-abdominal distance from the assist port site to the esophageal hiatus should be considered as it pertains to the reach of laparoscopic instruments used by the bedside assist especially the staplers.

Once the trocars are in place, the robot is docked followed by instrument placement in the appropriate arms. Several options for instrument selection exist but ultimately are the surgeon's choice. The preferred instruments in each arm are

Table 9.3 Instrument selection

Arm (Si/Xi)	Primary instrument	Alternate	Purpose
1/1	Cadiere forceps	Tip-up	Grasper for retraction Suturing
2/2	Harmonic ultrasound	Vessel sealer Hem-o-Lok clips	Vascular control and division of tissue
	Needle holder	Large-suture cut needle holder	Suturing
3/camera	Camera (30° down)	Camera (30° down)	Visualization
4/3	Maryland bipolar	Maryland bipolar	Dissection and vascular control
	Needle holder	Large-suture cut needle holder	Large-suture cut needle holder

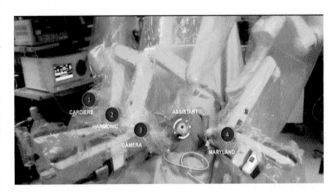

Fig. 9.2 Docking of the robotic system from the patient's left side. Arm #3 is docked on the periumbilical port for camera placement. Then, Cadiere forceps, ultrasonic shears (vessel sealer or monopolar shears), and Maryland Bipolar instruments are placed in Arms #1, #2, and #4, respectively

listed in Table 9.3. The setup differs slightly depending on whether a da Vinci Si or Xi system is utilized. A docked da Vinci Xi surgical system with selected instruments in each of the robotic arms is shown in Fig. 9.2.

Prior to beginning your dissection, create an adequate upper abdominal exposure using a self-sustaining liver retractor as per surgeon choice. Proper liver retraction must provide constant and adequate exposure of the lesser curvature of the stomach and easy access to esophageal hiatus.

Steps of the Procedure

The robotic total gastrectomy with D2 lymphadenectomy can be performed en bloc, and in summary, key steps include:

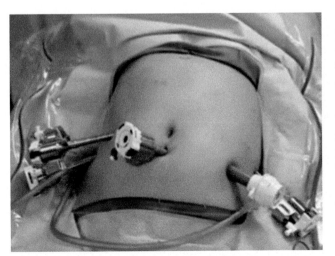

Fig. 9.1 Port placement for robotic total gastrectomy using da Vinci Xi Surgical System

1. Left-side dissection: division of the gastrocolic ligament, the left gastroepiploic vessels, and the short gastric vessels (LN stations 4sb, 4d, and 2)

2. Right-side dissection: division of the distal gastrocolic, the duodenocolic ligaments, and the right gastroepiploic vessels, clearance of the soft tissue along the head of pancreas (LN station 6), and transection of the duodenum

3. Hepatoduodenal and suprapancreatic dissection: clearance of LN stations 8a, 5, 12a, and 9

4. Left gastric and splenic vessel approach: clearance of LN stations 7, 11p, and 11d

5. Lesser curve and left-sided proximal dissection: clearance of LN stations 1 and 3

6. Roux-en-Y esophagojejunal reconstruction

Each of these steps is discussed below in detail.

Step 1: Left-Side Dissection

A robotic total gastrectomy begins with a partial omentectomy. Grasp the soft tissue along the edge of the greater curvature of the stomach near the distal body, and retract cephalad to create a draping of the lesser omentum between the stomach and transverse colon (Fig. 9.3a). This allows for efficient division of the gastrocolic ligament and entrance into the lesser sac. It also provides visualization of the posterior stomach and retention of LN station #4sb and #4d nodes along the specimen side of the dissection (Fig. 9.3b).

Start the division near the mid-transverse colon 4 cm from the greater curvature to enter the lesser sac, and divide the omentum toward the spleen; ensure that you are sufficiently

away from the gastroepiploic arcade to collect the nodal stations.

Next, identify, clip, and divide the left gastroepiploic vessels at their roots and continue superiorly along the greater curvature until the short gastric vessels are encountered (Fig. 9.3c). Identify and ligate the short gastric vessels close to the splenic hilum, taking care not to injure the spleen or the hilar vasculature. Continue to grasp more proximally along the stomach using the grasper in arm #1, and retract medially to create tension between the stomach and spleen, to exposure the gastrophrenic ligament, and to divide the short gastric vessels.

Tips: At this point, make sure that the posterior stomach is free of attachments and ensure ready medial mobility of the stomach. Once the greater curvature of the stomach is detached, the fundus of the stomach becomes floppy and can interfere with the exposure during the proximal dissection. Positioning the shaft and elbow of the grasper skillfully underneath the stomach during the retraction can be of great assistance in the proper exposure of this area. Ensure that all attachments of the fundus and the cardia on the left side and posteriorly are divided to free the proximal portion of the stomach to expose the left side of the diaphragmatic crux.

Step 2: Right-Side Dissection

During the second step of the surgery, mobilize the distal stomach, identify the right gastroepiploic vessels, and clear the soft tissues from the head of the pancreas with removal of the LN station #6 nodes. Release any remaining posterior

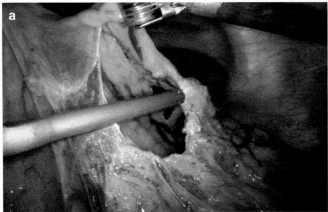
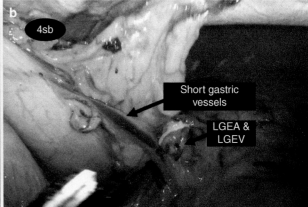

Fig. 9.3 Step 1, left-side dissection. (**a**) Left-side dissection with division of the gastrocolic ligament. Retraction of the greater curvature of the stomach creates a draping of the gastrocolic ligament and provides exposure between the stomach and the transverse colon. (**b**) Identification of the short gastric vessels. After ligation of the left gas-

troepiploic vessels, the dissection continues with identification and ligation of the short gastric vessels and retrieval of the soft tissue containing 4sb lymph nodes (LN) along the proximal greater curvature until all gastrophrenic attachments are divided

attachments of the distal stomach from the anterior pancreas. Divide the duodenocolic ligament until the inferior first portion of the duodenum is identified. Free any attachments of the duodenum to the gallbladder.

Dissect the soft tissue off the head of the pancreas, and identify the right gastroepiploic vein (RGEV) and anterior superior pancreaticoduodenal vein (ASPDV) (Fig. 9.4a, b). The RGEV is then ligated at the junction with the ASPDV. The LN station #6 nodes are within the confines of the middle colic vein, the anterior superior pancreaticoduodenal vein, and the right gastroepiploic vein. Then identify, ligate, and divide the right gastroepiploic artery at the level of its origin at the gastroduodenal artery (GDA).

Follow the dissection anterior to the GDA, and release the posterior attachments of the first portion of the duodenum before freeing the supraduodenal area (Fig. 9.4c) for duodenal transection. Either a robotic liner stapler or laparoscopic linear stapler can be used to transect the duodenum 2 cm distal to the pylorus.

Step 3: Hepatoduodenal and Suprapancreatic Dissection

After the duodenal transection, retract the stomach caudally and to the left side of the abdomen using the left-side robotic arm to expose the pars flaccida. Divide the pars flaccida proximally from the left side of the right gastric artery to the right side of the diaphragmatic crux. This is followed by meticulously continuing the dissection along the anterior aspect of the GDA to clear the soft tissue along the common

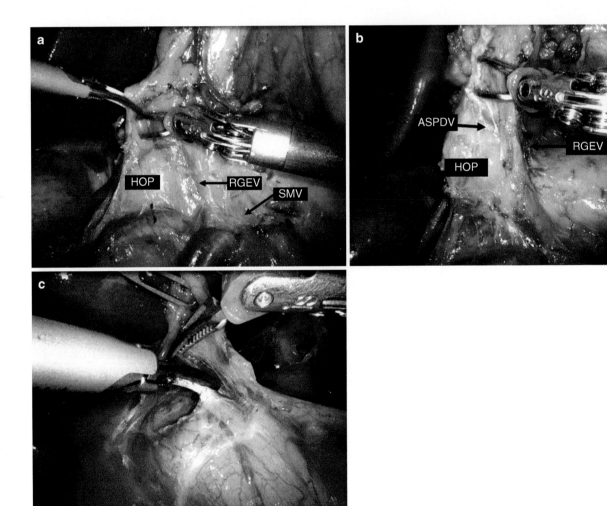

Fig. 9.4 Step 2, right-side dissection. (**a**) Dissection along the infrapyloric artery on the head of pancreas to identify the right gastroepiploic vein (RGEV) and right gastroepiploic artery (RGEA) and clear the soft tissue containing LN station 6. (**b**) The borders of LN station 6 are the anterior superior pancreaticoduodenal vein (ASPDV), the middle colic vein, and the RGEV. (**c**) Supraduodenal dissection. After exposure of the intraduodenal border for at least 3 cm distal to the pylorus, the window for duodenal transection is completed by dividing the supraduodenal attachments just distal to the insertion site of the right gastric vessels

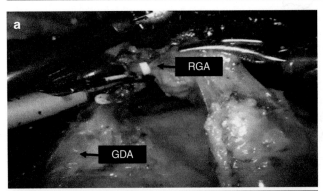

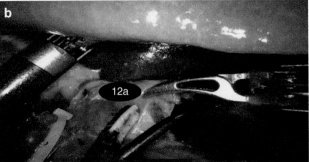

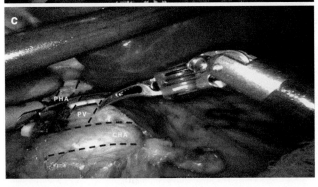

Fig. 9.5 Step 3, hepatoduodenal and suprapancreatic dissection. (**a**) Ligation of the right gastric artery (RGA) and retrieval of LN station 5. Retraction of the stomach using the right gastric vessels allows for exposure to its attachment to the proper hepatic artery. The root of the RGA is identified by clearing the soft tissue anterior to the GDA and the proper hepatic artery and ligated to release the distal stomach and retrieve LN station 5. (**b**) Dissection of the porta hepatis for removal of LN station 12a. The soft tissue along the anteromedial side of the proper hepatic artery (PHA) anterior to the portal vein is carefully removed. (**c**) Anatomic exposure after clearance of the soft tissue in the hepatoduodenal and proximal suprapancreatic region. The soft tissue containing LN stations 5, 12a, and 8 has been retrieved exposing the vasculature underneath

hepatic artery and proper hepatic artery with identification and ligation of the right gastric artery at its root (Fig. 9.5a). This allows collection of LN station #5. In order to complete the removal of the station #12a LN, grasp, pull up on the soft tissue anterior and medial to the proper hepatic artery and medial to the portal vein, and dissect along the portal vein to retrieve the LN in this region (Fig. 9.5b). Then continue the en bloc dissection of these nodes along the common hepatic artery for retrieval of LN station #8a (Fig. 9.5c). Next, identify and ligate the left gastric vein at its insertion into the portal vein. *Tips: Remember that left gastric vein at times drains into the splenic vein and must be ligated and divided anterior to the splenic artery.* Continue to trace and dissect the soft tissue on the common hepatic artery toward its origin at the celiac axis. Dissect free the soft tissue around the celiac axis to collect LN station #9. *Tips: The assistant may need to retract the pancreas inferiorly to improve visualization of suprapancreatic dissection plane.*

Step 4: Left Gastric and Splenic Vessel Approach

The dissection along the left gastric artery, celiac artery, and splenic vessels is critical in collecting LN stations #7, #9, and #11p, respectively. To begin dissection in the area, firmly grasps the lesser curvature of the stomach proximal to the incisura to straighten out the left gastric vessels for vertical exposure. Identify the origin of the left gastric artery, and clear the soft tissue along its base and the celiac artery.

Once the base of the left gastric artery is identified, ligate with Hem-o-Lok clips and divide it leaving two or three clips on the patient side (Fig. 9.6a). Then, move the stomach to the left upper quadrant in order to fully visualize the anterior aspect of the pancreas. Skeletonize the anterior surface of the splenic artery in order to collect the entirety of LN stations #11p and #11d (Fig. 9.6b).

Hilar lymphadenectomy for retrieval of #10 LN station is reserved for grossly positive disease and should only be performed by advanced robotic gastric cancer surgeons. If splenic hilar lymphadenectomy is required, a

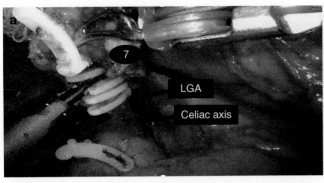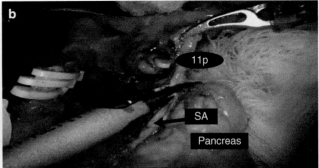

Fig. 9.6 Step 4, left gastric and splenic vessel approach. (**a**) Ligation of the left gastric artery and retrieval of the LN station 7. A vertical view of the left gastric artery perpendicular to the celiac artery is created by retraction of the lesser curvature of the stomach upward to facilitate dissection around the LGA and ligation at its root. (**b**) Distal suprapancreatic dissection along the splenic artery. The soft tissue along the proximal and distal splenic artery is dissected to retrieve soft tissues containing LN stations 11p and 11d

splenectomy incorporating this nodal station is recommended.

Step 5: Lesser Curve and Proximal Dissection

Return to the dissection of the retroperitoneal attachments of the proximal stomach, and continue it to the level of the esophageal crus. Contrary to previous reports, the posterior gastric artery branching from the mid- to distal splenic artery and inserting into the stomach is commonly encountered and must be ligated to free the stomach. The soft tissues along the intra-abdominal esophagus and the cardia are dissected until the esophagogastric junction is clearly identified (Fig. 9.7a). As dissection continues to free the distal esophagus from the crux, the anterior and posterior vagal trunks should be readily identifiable and transected. Perform a transhiatal dissection of the distal esophagus by dividing its surrounding attachments to mobilize about 5 cm of the intrathoracic esophagus into the abdominal cavity (Fig. 9.7b).

Next, place two 2-0 Vicryl on the right and left sides of the esophagus to mark the proximal resection and provide retraction of the distal esophagus during the reconstruction. The assist trocar is used to insert the linear stapler for the esophageal transection (Fig. 9.7c). Place the specimen into an Endo Catch bag and put it aside.

Tips: Options to check the frozen sections on the proximal margin prior to reconstruction include removing the robotic instruments and extending the assist port for specimen extraction or taking additional donut of the esophagus for pathologic evaluation without removing or undocking the robot.

Step 6: Reconstruction

Several methods for intracorporeal Roux-en-Y esophagojejunal reconstruction and restoration of continuity have been well-described, including the use of circular and linear staplers. To start creating the Roux-en-Y, identify a segment of the jejunum roughly 40 cm distal to the ligament of Treitz. Bring it up to the level of the esophageal hiatus in an antecolic fashion. Check the reach of the mesentery of the selected segment for tension-free anastomosis.

Circular Stapler Reconstruction

If you plan to use the circular stapling method (EEA 25 mm), instead of using a linear stapler to transect the esophagus, pull the distal esophagus into the abdominal cavity prior to transection, and place a heavy bulldog just proximal to the resection margin, and divide the esophagus using ultrasonic sheers. Using heavy suture such as 0-prolene or 0-PDS, place a running purse string at the open end of the cut esophagus. To insert the anvil into the abdominal cavity, remove the assist port trocar, slightly extend the incision, and insert the anvil and replace the trocar. *Tips: This may cause leaking of CO_2 and loss of intra-abdominal pressure and may require temporary skin closure of the extraincisional opening.*

Using two of the robotic instruments in the right lateral and left arms and the assistant, retract open the distal esophagus and remove the bulldog. Using the Cadiere forceps in the right medial robotic arm, insert the anvil into the distal esophagus, and tie the purse string to keep the anvil in place (Fig. 9.8a). Open the staple line of the alimentary limb of the jejunum, and confirm the correct orientation of the limb and mesentery. Using the assist port site, insert the shaft of the

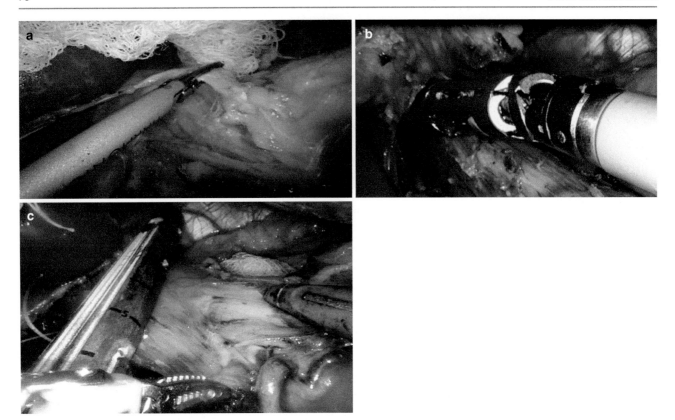

Fig. 9.7 Step 5, lesser curvature and proximal dissection. (**a**) The identification of esophagogastric junction (EGJ). The dissection along the anterior surface of the left esophageal crux proximally leads to the hiatus where EGJ is identified and dissected free from its surrounding structures. (**b**) Transhiatal mobilization of the distal esophagus. Firm traction of the stomach is seen, and a vessel sealer is being used to dissect free the attachments to the distal esophagus through the esophageal hiatus for sufficient mobilization into the abdominal cavity. (**c**) Transection of the esophagus. A linear stapler is used to transect the esophagus

EEA, and intubate shaft into the open end of the jejunal limb until about 6 cm of the shaft is firmly inserted (Fig. 9.8b).

Open the spike on the shaft of the EEA, and carefully bring the tip of the shaft along with the small bowel toward the anvil mate. As you approximate the two ends, pay close attention that the small bowel will not twist and no other tissue gets in between the mating of the anvil and the shaft. Once the stapler has been fired, remove the instrument and check that both the esophageal and jejunal donuts are intact. Examine the esophagojejunal (EJ) staple line. *Tips: If there is an incomplete donut or concern for anastomotic disruption, place simple interrupted sutures using 2-0 Vicryl or other dissoluble sutures.*

Linear Stapler Reconstruction

For the option of using the linear stapler for reconstruction of the EJ anastomosis, transect the distal esophagus using a linear stapler. Bring the alimentary limb antecolic to the distal esophagus, and using a 2-0 Vicryl, stitch the jejunal limb secured to the esophagus. The corners of the esophageal and jejunal limb staple lines are then removed, and a side-to-side esophagojejunostomy is created using a linear stapler (Fig. 9.9). The common enterotomy is closed with another

linear stapler. As with open and laparoscopic procedures, care must be taken to ensure the correct orientation of the bowel loops and the lack of tension on the small bowel mesentery.

Finally, create a side-to-side jejunojejunostomy (JJ). Measure another 40–60 cm from the EJ anastomosis, and bring it next to a correctly oriented biliary limb. Using two simple stitches about 4 cm apart, keep the two limbs together and stretched out while creating an enterotomy on each of the small bowel segments. Insert the linear stapler through the assist port and position the small bowel away from the abdominal wall to gain space for manipulation of the stapler, insert a jaw of the linear stapler into each of the jejunal limb, and complete the anastomosis (Fig. 9.10). The common enterotomy can be closed with another linear stapler or by robotically suturing it closed with continuous running stitches.

At the end of the operation, reexamine the duodenal stump, the esophagojejunal anastomosis, and the clips on the patient side of named vessels that were ligated. Check for hemostasis. Remove all instruments and undock the robot. Move to the bedside, and using laparoscopic instruments (robotic camera), place a drain (Jackson-Pratt) posterior to

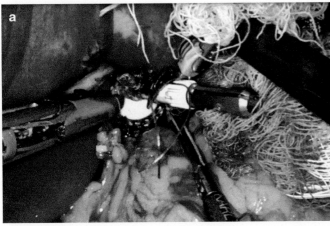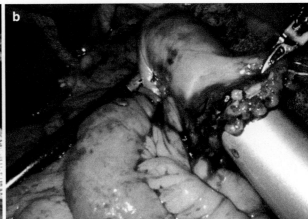

Fig. 9.8 Step 6, reconstruction. (**a**) Placement of the anvil into the distal esophagus. After a purse string is placed on the cut opening of the distal esophagus, the anvil is inserted and secured in place. (**b**) The

small bowel intubation of the shaft of the circular stapler. After extension of the assistant's port site and insertion of the shaft of the stapler into abdominal cavity, the jejunum has been intubated

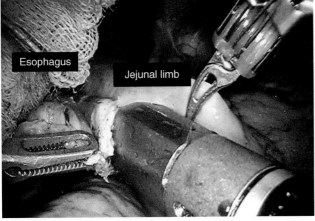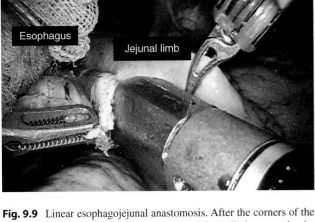

Fig. 9.9 Linear esophagojejunal anastomosis. After the corners of the staple line for both the distal esophagus and Roux limb are made, the jaws of the linear staple have been securely inserted and esophagojejunal anastomosis is created

Fig. 9.10 Jejunojejunal anastomosis. Approximately 40 cm distal to the esophagojejunostomy, a side-to-side jejunojejunostomy is created using a linear stapler

the EJ anastomosis and exteriorize it through the left lateral port site and suture in place.

Remove the specimen in the Endo Catch bag via the extended assistant's trocar site. May need to extend the incision to at least 3–4 cm (alternatively, extend the periumbilical incision for specimen extraction). This completes robotic total gastrectomy with lymphadenectomy and Roux-en-Y esophagojejunal anastomosis.

Postoperative Care and Potential Complications

Management of patients following robotic total gastrectomy does not deviate from that of patients who have undergone open and laparoscopic gastrectomies. Following robotic gastrectomy, the patient is at risk of several potential complications, including:

- Intra-abdominal fluid collections/abscesses
- Intraluminal and intra-abdominal bleeding
- Pancreatitis/pancreatic leak/pancreatic fistula
- Anastomotic leak/stricture
- Gastroparesis or ileus
- Obstruction

An ERAS protocol for gastrectomy patients for early recovery includes the standard careful monitoring for potential postoperative complications, pain, return of gastrointestinal function with timely initiation of DVT prophylaxis, pain control regiment that includes patient-controlled analgesics (morphine or Dilaudid), nonsteroidal anti-inflammatories (e.g., acetaminophen), and advancement of diet. Typically, patients are ambulating on postoperative day (POD) 1 and will tolerate sips of water on POD 2 with diet advanced through clear liquids to soft/regular foods by POD 5 to 7. Corresponding oral pain control can be achieved as soon as soft/regular food is tolerated. Median hospital length of stay following gastrectomy is 7 days. Without evidence of EJ anastomotic leaks or intra-abdominal collections, the JP drain can be removed prior to discharge.

In conclusion, robotic total gastrectomy is technically feasible and safe and provides minimally invasive benefits to patients undergoing surgery for gastric cancer. Understanding the key steps to performing this complex robotic procedure will allow for ready adoption of the robotic technology in a surgeon's practice in treating patients with gastric cancer. After performing a robotic total gastrectomy, the potential surgical advantages of the sophisticated robotic surgical platform and instrumentation may become more clearly evident, and experience will provide the foundation for individualized procedure improvements. As no long-term oncologic outcome of robotic total gastrectomy confirming the equivalence of minimally invasive total gastrectomy to open operations for advanced gastric cancer exists, caution must be taken in patient selection with consideration of the patient's disease state and the surgeon's experience and expertise in both gastric cancer and robotic surgery.

References

1. Hashizume M, Shimada M, Tomikawa M, Ikeda Y, Takahashi I, Abe R, Koga F, Gotoh N, Konishi K, Maehara S, Sugimachi K. Early experiences of endoscopic procedures in general surgery assisted by a computer-enhanced surgical system. Surg Endosc. 2002;16(8):1187–91. https://doi.org/10.1007/s004640080154.
2. Giulianotti PC, Coratti A, Angelini M, Sbrana F, Cecconi S, Balestracci T, Caravaglios G. Robotics in general surgery: personal experience in a large community hospital. Arch Surg (Chicago, IL: 1960). 2003;138(7):777–84. https://doi.org/10.1001/archsurg.138.7.777.
3. Tokunaga M, Makuuchi R, Miki Y, Tanizawa Y, Bando E, Kawamura T, Terashima M. Late phase II study of robot-assisted gastrectomy with nodal dissection for clinical stage I gastric cancer. Surg Endosc. 2016;30(8):3362–7. https://doi.org/10.1007/s00464-015-4613-z.
4. Woo Y, Hyung WJ, Pak KH, Inaba K, Obama K, Choi SH, Noh SH. Robotic gastrectomy as an oncologically sound alternative to laparoscopic resections for the treatment of early-stage gastric cancers. Arch Surg (Chicago, IL: 1960). 2011;146(9):1086–92. https://doi.org/10.1001/archsurg.2011.114.
5. Chen K, Pan Y, Zhang B, Maher H, Wang XF, Cai XJ. Robotic versus laparoscopic gastrectomy for gastric cancer: a systematic review and updated meta-analysis. BMC Surg. 2017;17(1):93. https://doi.org/10.1186/s12893-017-0290-2.
6. Kim KM, An JY, Kim HI, Cheong JH, Hyung WJ, Noh SH. Major early complications following open, laparoscopic and robotic gastrectomy. Br J Surg. 2012;99(12):1681–7. https://doi.org/10.1002/bjs.8924.
7. Kim HI, Park MS, Song KJ, Woo Y, Hyung WJ. Rapid and safe learning of robotic gastrectomy for gastric cancer: multidimensional analysis in a comparison with laparoscopic gastrectomy. Eur J Surg Oncol J Eur Soc Surg Oncol Br Assoc Surg Oncol. 2014;40(10):1346–54. https://doi.org/10.1016/j.ejso.2013.09.011.
8. Huang KH, Lan YT, Fang WL, Chen JH, Lo SS, Li AF, Chiou SH, Wu CW, Shyr YM. Comparison of the operative outcomes and learning curves between laparoscopic and robotic gastrectomy for gastric cancer. PLoS One. 2014;9(10):e111499. https://doi.org/10.1371/journal.pone.0111499.
9. Patriti A, Ceccarelli G, Bellochi R, Bartoli A, Spaziani A, Di Zitti L, Casciola L. Robot-assisted laparoscopic total and partial gastric resection with D2 lymph node dissection for adenocarcinoma. Surg Endosc. 2008;22(12):2753–60. https://doi.org/10.1007/s00464-008-0129-0.
10. Song J, Kang WH, Oh SJ, Hyung WJ, Choi SH, Noh SH. Role of robotic gastrectomy using da Vinci system compared with laparoscopic gastrectomy: initial experience of 20 consecutive cases. Surg Endosc. 2009;23(6):1204–11. https://doi.org/10.1007/s00464-009-0351-4.
11. D'Annibale A, Pende V, Pernazza G, Monsellato I, Mazzocchi P, Lucandri G, Morpurgo E, Contardo T, Sovernigo G. Full robotic gastrectomy with extended (D2) lymphadenectomy for gastric cancer: surgical technique and preliminary results. J Surg Res. 2011;166(2):e113–20. https://doi.org/10.1016/j.jss.2010.11.881.
12. Caruso S, Patriti A, Marrelli D, Ceccarelli G, Ceribelli C, Roviello F, Casciola L. Open vs robot-assisted laparoscopic gastric resection with D2 lymph node dissection for adenocarcinoma: a case-control study. Int J Med Robot Comput Assist Surg MRCAS. 2011;7(4):452–8. https://doi.org/10.1002/rcs.416.
13. Isogaki J, Haruta S, Man IM, Suda K, Kawamura Y, Yoshimura F, Kawabata T, Inaba K, Ishikawa K, Ishida Y, Taniguchi K, Sato S, Kanaya S, Uyama I. Robot-assisted surgery for gastric cancer: experience at our institute. Pathobiol J Immunopathol Mol Cell Biol. 2011;78(6):328–33. https://doi.org/10.1159/000330172.
14. Yoon HM, Kim YW, Lee JH, Ryu KW, Eom BW, Park JY, Choi IJ, Kim CG, Lee JY, Cho SJ, Rho JY. Robot-assisted total gastrectomy is comparable with laparoscopically assisted total gastrectomy for early gastric cancer. Surg Endosc. 2012;26(5):1377–81. https://doi.org/10.1007/s00464-011-2043-0.
15. Huang KH, Lan YT, Fang WL, Chen JH, Lo SS, Hsieh MC, Li AF, Chiou SH, Wu CW. Initial experience of robotic gastrectomy and comparison with open and laparoscopic gastrectomy for gastric cancer. J Gastrointest Surg Off J Soc Surg Aliment Tract. 2012;16(7):1303–10. https://doi.org/10.1007/s11605-012-1874-x.
16. Kang BH, Xuan Y, Hur H, Ahn CW, Cho YK, Han SU. Comparison of surgical outcomes between robotic and laparoscopic gastrectomy for gastric cancer: the learning curve of robotic surgery. J Gastric Cancer. 2012;12(3):156–63. https://doi.org/10.5230/jgc.2012.12.3.156.
17. Liu XX, Jiang ZW, Chen P, Zhao Y, Pan HF, Li JS. Full robot-assisted gastrectomy with intracorporeal robot-sewn anastomosis produces satisfying outcomes. World J Gastroenterol. 2013;19(38):6427–37. https://doi.org/10.3748/wjg.v19.i38.6427.
18. Hyun MH, Lee CH, Kwon YJ, Cho SI, Jang YJ, Kim DH, Kim JH, Park SH, Mok YJ, Park SS. Robot versus laparoscopic gastrectomy for cancer by an experienced surgeon: comparisons of surgery, complications, and surgical stress. Ann Surg Oncol. 2013;20(4):1258–65. https://doi.org/10.1245/s10434-012-2679-6.
19. Junfeng Z, Yan S, Bo T, Yingxue H, Dongzhu Z, Yongliang Z, Feng Q, Peiwu Y. Robotic gastrectomy versus laparoscopic gastrectomy for gastric cancer: comparison of surgical performance and short-term outcomes. Surg Endosc. 2014;28(6):1779–87. https://doi.org/10.1007/s00464-013-3385-6.
20. Shen W, Xi H, Wei B, Cui J, Bian S, Zhang K, Wang N, Huang X, Chen L. Robotic versus laparoscopic gastrectomy for gastric cancer: comparison of short-term surgical outcomes. Surg Endosc. 2016;30(2):574–80. https://doi.org/10.1007/s00464-015-4241-7.
21. Kim HI, Han SU, Yang HK, Kim YW, Lee HJ, Ryu KW, Park JM, An JY, Kim MC, Park S, Song KY, Oh SJ, Kong SH, Suh BJ, Yang DH, Ha TK, Kim YN, Hyung WJ. Multicenter prospective

comparative study of robotic versus laparoscopic gastrectomy for gastric adenocarcinoma. Ann Surg. 2016;263(1):103–9. https://doi.org/10.1097/sla.0000000000001249.

22. Son T, Lee JH, Kim YM, Kim HI, Noh SH, Hyung WJ. Robotic spleen-preserving total gastrectomy for gastric cancer: comparison with conventional laparoscopic procedure. Surg Endosc. 2014;28(9):2606–15. https://doi.org/10.1007/s00464-014-3511-0.

23. Parisi A, Ricci F, Trastulli S, Cirocchi R, Gemini A, Grassi V, Corsi A, Renzi C, De Santis F, Petrina A, Pironi D, D'Andrea V, Santoro A, Desiderio J. Robotic total gastrectomy with intracorporeal robot-sewn anastomosis: a novel approach adopting the double-loop reconstruction method. Medicine. 2015;94(49):e1922. https://doi.org/10.1097/md.0000000000001922.

24. Jiang ZW, Liu J, Wang G, Zhao K, Zhang S, Li N, Li JS. Esophagojejunostomy reconstruction using a robot-sewing technique during totally robotic total gastrectomy for gastric cancer. Hepato-Gastroenterology. 2015;62(138):323–6.

25. Haverkamp L, Weijs TJ, van der Sluis PC, van der Tweel I, Ruurda JP, van Hillegersberg R. Laparoscopic total gastrectomy versus open total gastrectomy for cancer: a systematic review and meta-analysis. Surg Endosc. 2013;27(5):1509–20. https://doi.org/10.1007/s00464-012-2661-1.

26. Mortensen K, Nilsson M, Slim K, Schafer M, Mariette C, Braga M, Carli F, Demartines N, Griffin SM, Lassen K. Consensus guidelines for enhanced recovery after gastrectomy: enhanced recovery after surgery (ERAS(R)) society recommendations. Br J Surg. 2014;101(10):1209–29. https://doi.org/10.1002/bjs.9582.

27. Yamada T, Hayashi T, Aoyama T, Shirai J, Fujikawa H, Cho H, Yoshikawa T, Rino Y, Masuda M, Taniguchi H, Fukushima R, Tsuburaya A. Feasibility of enhanced recovery after surgery in gastric surgery: a retrospective study. BMC Surg. 2014;14:41. https://doi.org/10.1186/1471-2482-14-41.

28. Sugisawa N, Tokunaga M, Makuuchi R, Miki Y, Tanizawa Y, Bando E, Kawamura T, Terashima M. A phase II study of an enhanced recovery after surgery protocol in gastric cancer surgery. Gastric Cancer Off J Int Gastric Cancer Assoc Japanese Gastric Cancer Assoc. 2016;19(3):961–7. https://doi.org/10.1007/s10120-015-0528-6.

29. Pedziwiatr M, Matlok M, Kisialeuski M, Migaczewski M, Major P, Winiarski M, Budzynski P, Zub-Pokrowiecka A, Budzynski A. Short hospital stays after laparoscopic gastric surgery under an enhanced recovery after surgery (ERAS) pathway: experience at a single center. Eur Surg ACA Acta Chirurgica Austriaca. 2014;46:128–32. https://doi.org/10.1007/s10353-014-0264-x.

Robotic Cholecystectomy

10

Thomas Swope

Cholecystectomy is one of the most common general surgery procedures performed each year. Laparoscopic cholecystectomy remains the standard of care for symptomatic gallbladder disease and has replaced open cholecystectomy for the vast majority of cases. Robotic surgical technology continues to advance, and robotics has become an attractive alternative to laparoscopic surgery for many surgeons. Robotic cholecystectomy, either multiport or single site, is an operation that is gaining traction. Robotic cholecystectomy keeps the advantage of a minimally invasive procedure but adds wristed instruments, a 3D immersive experience, fluorescence imaging, and greater surgeon comfort. Robotic surgery may potentially decrease the 5–10% open conversion rate that has been reported in the literature [1]. Situations that make surgery more difficult and can lead to open conversion include acute inflammation (infection or gangrene), scarring from previous surgery or infection, significant bleeding, advanced age, male gender, or injury to bile ducts or bowel. Lee et al. found a lower complication rate (3.8% vs 20.4%) and open conversion rate (0.0% vs 1.9%) in a study comparing robotic to laparoscopic cholecystectomy [2]. Other studies have not demonstrated a difference in clinical outcomes between robotic and laparoscopic cholecystectomy [3, 4]. A retrospective analysis comparing laparoscopic to robotic cholecystectomy found a lower conversion rate to open cholecystectomy with robotic cholecystectomy but with a slightly longer operative times and cost [5]. I am personally happy to accept a longer operative time on a difficult gallbladder and not have to convert to an open procedure. The patient benefit to me is worth the added time and effort in the operating room. The complications from an open subcostal incision include more pain, increased wound morbidity, longer recovery, and a higher hernia rate vs the smaller trocar incisions. The robot enables the ability to suture ligature, clip, or tie off the cystic duct. The suction irrigator is a wristed instrument that allows both suction and dissection which is very helpful in situations when there is an inflamed gallbladder with adhesions. When these enhanced abilities are combined with fluorescence imaging, the need for open conversion has decreased in my experience.

Multiport Cholecystectomy

Cholecystectomy was the introductory procedure for me into robotic surgery. Multiport cholecystectomy provides 3D immersion, wristed instrumentation, and fluorescence imaging. Once I worked past the loss of haptics on my initial cases and gained visual haptics, my technique greatly improved. Early in my experience, there was a tendency to pull too hard on the gallbladder with my robotic retracting instrument (i.e., my left hand) which led to gallbladder tearing and bile leakage in my first couple of cases. At first I was using the ProGrasp to retract the gallbladder because it had the greatest grip strength. As I quickly learned, unless you are very careful in the beginning stage with the ProGrasp, you will tear gallbladders. I quickly switched to the Caudier instrument to retract the gallbladder with my left hand, and the issues resolved immediately. There are three different grasping strengths among the graspers, with the ProGrasp having the strongest grip strength, the Caudier the weakest, and the bipolar grasper in between. My point is that there is a learning curve with every operation. Be patient and slow down in the beginning to be safe. My mantra with robotics is "get good, get fast, and then get cheap." In the early part of your learning curve you will be slower, have little patience for instrument exchanges, and have to learn to depend on your first assist more than you did laparoscopically. With experience not only you will become faster, but so will your team. They are learning a new system and your preferences. Only with repetition will consistency and speed be achieved.

T. Swope
Center for Minimally Invasive Surgery, Mercy Medical Center, Baltimore, MD, USA
e-mail: tswope@mdmercy.com

© Springer Nature Switzerland AG 2019
S. Tsuda, O. Y. Kudsi (eds.), *Robotic-Assisted Minimally Invasive Surgery*, https://doi.org/10.1007/978-3-319-96866-7_10

Multiport Setup

My preference is to use two robotic operative arms and the camera for a cholecystectomy. Some surgeons prefer the fourth arm for retraction using another robotic instrument to hold the gallbladder anteriorly and superiorly. I substitute a disposable 5 mm port laterally on the right abdominal wall and use a laparoscopic grasper to retract the gallbladder to save on cost. The patient is positioned in 10–15° of reverse Trendelenburg. Arms are usually tucked at the sides, but the left arm can be left out for anesthesia access if desired.

Si System

On the Si system, I dock the camera arm to a 12 mm disposable port at the umbilicus. That is where I remove the specimen later. I place an 8.5 mm port in the left upper abdominal wall and another in the right mid-abdomen (Fig. 10.1). Alternatively a fifth port can be placed to assist with retraction as seen in Fig. 10.2.

I place the left upper quadrant port lateral to the falciform ligament. This is different than the laparoscopic upper midline epigastric port placement. Other than that, my port placement is the same as a laparoscopic case on

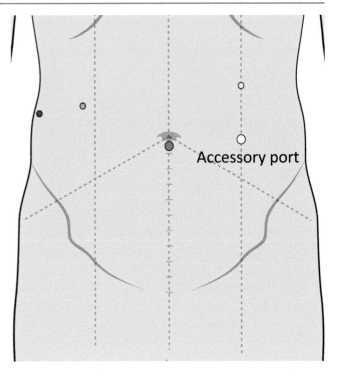

Fig. 10.2 Alternative Si port placement. (©2018 Intuitive Surgical, Inc. Used with permission)

the Si. The disposable 5 mm port is placed far laterally in the right upper quadrant through which the gallbladder is retracted.

Xi System

The port placement on the Xi is different than the SI. On the Xi, the ports are all aligned in a row parallel to your working area, in this case the right upper quadrant. I use three 8.5 mm ports (Fig. 10.3). I prefer to go in optically using a 5 mm laparoscope inside an 8.5 mm trocar with an optical obturator in place. Alternatively you could place a disposable 12 mm trocar at the umbilicus and then piggyback an 8.5 mm port through that as the camera port. The camera arm will only dock to an 8.5 mm port and not a 12 mm disposable port as it does on the Si system. Your method of establishing pneumoperitoneum laparoscopically should not change with the robot. Whether you prefer an optical entry, a Veress needle, or an open Hasson technique, your approach should remain the same and be something with which you are comfortable. Lastly, I place a disposable 5 mm port in the right lateral abdominal wall similar to my Si setup for retraction, but another robotic port and use of a third robotic arm for retraction are alternatives.

Instrumentation varies based on surgeon preference as it does laparoscopically. I prefer to use a Caudier and a hook to do the dissection. Others use a scissor or a Maryland dissector instead of a hook. Still others will use a bipolar instrument to

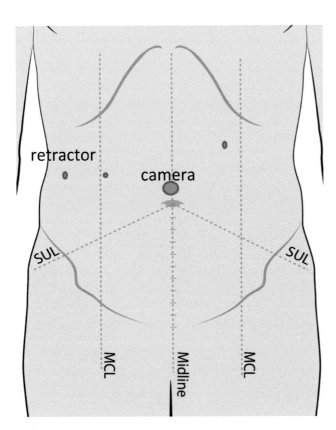

Fig. 10.1 Si port placement. (©2018 Intuitive Surgical, Inc. Used with permission)

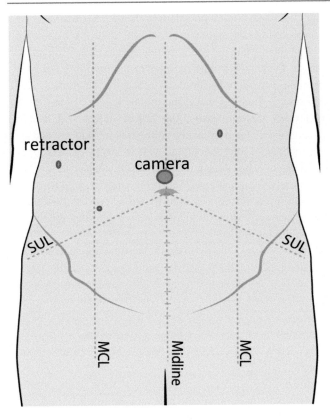

Fig. 10.3 Xi port placement. (©2018 Intuitive Surgical, Inc. Used with permission)

retract and for additional hemostasis. The bottom line starting out is to use similar instruments that you are already comfortable using to perform the case laparoscopically and modify from there if needed as your experience increases.

Single Site

I performed a lot of single-site laparoscopic surgery (SILS), and this approach is actually what initially drew me into robotics. I was exploring all technology related to single-incision minimally invasive surgery. I felt that the single-site robotic platform would solve some of the difficulties I experienced with SILS, namely, the sword fighting and lack of triangulation. By providing curved cannulas, the robotic platform gave back the triangulation that was missing with SILS. The triangulation isn't quite as good as multiport laparoscopy in my opinion, but it is adequate to operate safely and much better than traditional SILS. However, no wrist motion is provided on the single-site instruments. A prospective, multicenter, randomized controlled trial comparing robotic single-site cholecystectomy (RSSC) to multiport laparoscopic cholecystectomy (MPLC) found no difference in quality of life or complication rates between the techniques [6]. Operative times were longer for RSSC (61 min) vs MPLC (44 min). However, RSSC demonstrated signifi-

cant superiority in cosmetic satisfaction and body image perception with no difference in quality of life.

The single-site port is soft with an hourglass shape. It has an air insufflation channel, a camera port channel, two operative port channels, and an assist port channel (Fig. 10.4). Insertion is generally performed at the umbilicus. An incision can be made splitting the umbilicus vertically or horizontally (Fig. 10.5). Alternatively a curvilinear incision can be made beneath the umbilical fold preserving the umbilical stalk (Fig. 10.6). The advantage of the curvilinear incision is the preservation of the umbilical stalk. When the umbilical stalk is split, there is a higher incidence of wound complications in my experience. When drainage occurs, it will typically begin at about 2–3 weeks after surgery. Usually it is serosanguinous and resolves with time, but occasionally

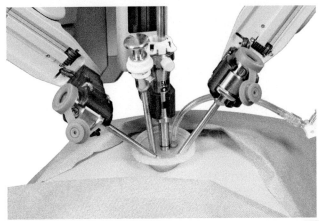

Fig. 10.4 Single-site port. (©2018 Intuitive Surgical, Inc. Used with permission)

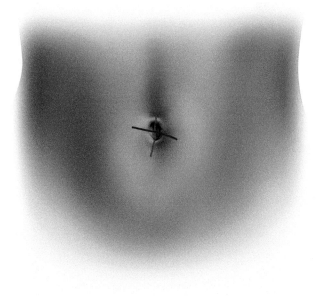

Fig. 10.5 Splitting the umbilical stalk. (©2018 Intuitive Surgical, Inc. Used with permission)

wound infections arise requiring drainage and antibiotics. To avoid that problem, I began preserving the umbilical stalk and switched to the curvilinear incision beneath the umbilical fold. There may a slight cosmetic advantage to splitting the umbilicus, but the trade-off is more frequent drainage and the resultant post-op visits and phone calls. This is not an issue in thinner patients where I continue to split the umbili-

cus. The issue is more prevalent in the obese patient population as you would expect.

The skin incision needs to be approximately 3 cm in length. Dissection is carried down to the fascia. A 2–2.5 cm opening is made in the fascia and the peritoneum is opened. My rule of thumb is that if the middle knuckle of my index finger fits through easily, the fascial defect will usually accommodate the port nicely. A finger is introduced, and the peritoneum of the abdominal wall is swept to make sure there are no adhesions in the area which would interfere and potentially complicate port insertion. Once assured there are no adhesions in the area, the insertion process continues. Next an Army Navy retractor is placed into the abdominal cavity. To insert the port I, place a large Kelly clamp about ¾ of the way across the port paralleling the internal skirt leaving about 2 cm of the port distal to the tip of my clamp. Using abdominal lift with the Army Navy retractor in my non-dominant hand, the port is then placed by applying pressure downward and toward the head to avoid the bowel with my dominant hand (Fig. 10.7). Once it is seated nicely, insufflation tubing is connected and pneumoperitoneum is established. The orientation arrow on the port is aimed at the area of the gallbladder. The camera trocar is then gently inserted lining up the marking on the port with the level of the fascia. The peritoneal cavity is then inspected using the robotic camera in a handheld fashion. I then place the curved operative trocars under vision. There are short (250 mm) and long (300 mm) versions of the operative trocars. I prefer the lon-

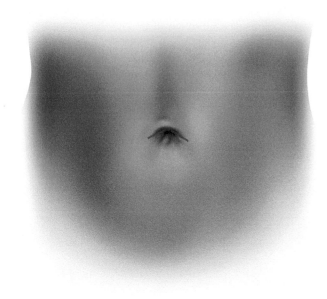

Fig. 10.6 Preserving umbilical stalk. (©2018 Intuitive Surgical, Inc. Used with permission)

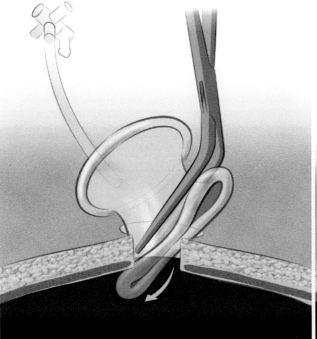
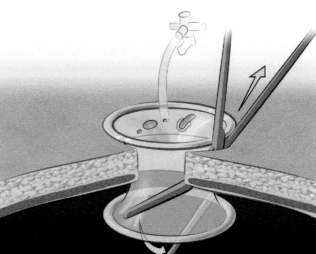

Fig. 10.7 Placing the single-site port. (©2018 Intuitive Surgical, Inc. Used with permission)

ger trocars as I feel they provide a greater arc inside of which I can move the camera without collisions. Others prefer the shorter trocars, especially if the umbilicus is close to the right upper quadrant. My advice is to try both and see which works better for you. The robot is then docked. Intuitive surgical training has you docking the robot to the camera first and then placing the operative ports after camera docking. I found it faster to place the curved trocars under visualization before docking to the camera trocar, using the robotic camera in a handheld fashion. On the Xi, there is a grounding cable that needs to be connected to the camera port. The patient is placed in 10–15° of reverse Trendelenburg. At this stage, I bring the robot in and dock. Docking all occurs from a lateral approach on the Xi since the boom is able to rotate into any position. On the Si, however, I like to turn the patient table after induction and before the patient is prepped. I turn the head of the OR table toward the direction of the robot to allow the robot to come in over the right shoulder at about a 45-degree angle (Fig. 10.8). I only want the nurse driving the robot in and out from the patient in a straight line for simplicity, repetition, and speed. On the Si, the elbows of the robotic arms need to face outward to minimize collisions. After docking I place the accessory trocar last. Through the accessory port, I place a laparoscopic grasper to hold the gallbladder anteriorly and superiorly. If the gallbladder needs to be decompressed, that can also be done through the accessory port using a laparoscopic needle aspiration instrument. Zero-degree and 30-degree camera both work. I prefer the zero-degree camera, keeping the retracting instrument superior to the camera. Others prefer a 30-degree scope either looking upward or downward. After docking sometimes the port is too close or too far away from the gallbladder. In that situation, the port complex can be moved slightly toward or away

from the gallbladder by burping all three arms simultaneously with your first assist helping. The port complex can also be lowered or more likely elevated to get the view and working distance that is needed. Alternatively the longer or shorter operative ports can be exchanged depending on how close the umbilicus is to the gallbladder.

Single site can be challenging in the obese patient. Early in your learning curve I would approach these patients in a multiport fashion. However, with experience they can be performed with single site as well. There is likely a higher hernia rate in the obese patient population with single site. If the port is too short to bridge the distance from inside the abdominal cavity to the skin surface, you have a couple of options. You can simply seat the port nicely in the fascia and have the upper surface in the subcutaneous space. Some surgeons will suture the skin down to the fascia to allow the port to seat nicely. The alternative that also works here is to use a small wound protector and then seat the single-site port inside of that. The last alternative is to use a gel port (GelPOINT). The gel port is placed, and then the single-site trocars are placed through the gel port in a similar configuration to the single-site port followed by docking. This does increase cost but is always effective.

Once the dissection is done and the critical view of safety has been obtained and verified using fluorescence imaging, the cystic duct and artery are clipped and divided. Critical view of safety entails seeing two structures (the cystic duct and artery) going to the gallbladder with the cystic plate exposed in the background (Fig. 10.9). This is obtained after clearing the hepatocystic triangle and freeing the lower third of the gallbladder off of the liver bed. Once critical view of safety is obtained, the cystic duct and artery are clipped and divided depending on your preferred method.

To save time, I single clip the artery and divide it with the hook cautery toward the gallbladder in coagulation mode. The remaining gallbladder is then freed from the gallbladder

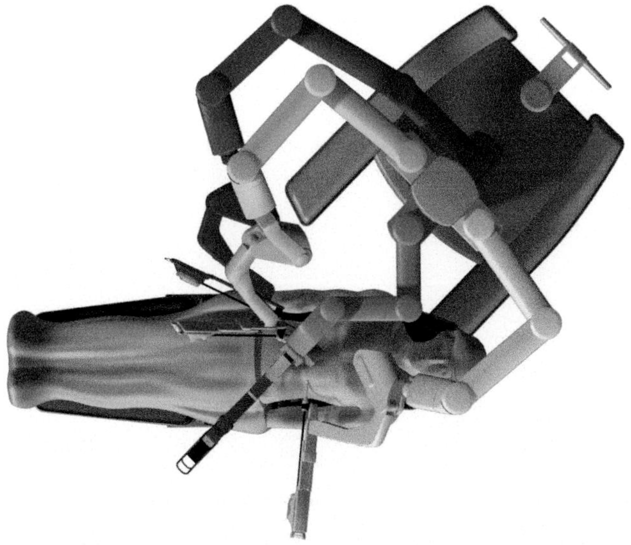

Fig. 10.8 Si Single-site robot position. (©2018 Intuitive Surgical, Inc. Used with permission)

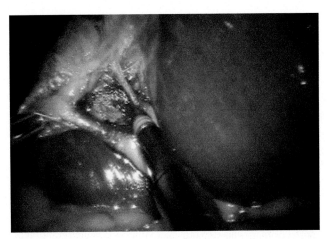

Fig. 10.9 Critical view of safety. (©2018 Intuitive Surgical, Inc. Used with permission)

fossa using hook cautery or your instrument of choice. Once the gallbladder is freed from the liver, the robot is undocked, the camera trocar and operative trocars are removed, and the port is removed through the umbilicus with the gallbladder attached to the grasper. Alternatively a 5 mm specimen bag can be used placing the gallbladder in the bag prior to removal.

Attention is then turned toward closing the fascia. I initially used 0-Vicryl figure-of-eight sutures to close the fascia but noticed a few hernias early in my SILS experience. I quickly switched to PDS, and the hernias dropped off quickly. I now close the fascia with 2–0 PDS taking 0.5 cm bites spaced 0.5 cm apart in a running fashion. The dermis is then reapproximated with absorbable deep dermal sutures. If the umbilicus was split, the base of the umbilicus is sutured to the fascia to reconstruct the umbilicus. Dermabond or Steri-Strips can be applied. I like to use a vacuum dressing for these cases. A 2 × 2 inch gauze is scrunched up and pushed inside the umbilicus and covered by a flat piece of 2 × 2 gauze. That is then covered with a large clear adhesive dressing. A 25-gauge needle is inserted laterally into the gauze in the center of the dressing, and air is aspirated out creating a vacuum dressing. I have my patients remove the dressing once the vacuum seal is gone. Postoperatively the only physical limitations are patient comfort levels. Patients can drive as soon as they are off pain medication and can comfortably drive without putting themselves or someone else at risk.

Fluorescence Cholangiography Utilizing Indocyanine Green (ICG)

ICG is a tricarbocynanine dye that has been used clinically for over 50 years for hepatic clearance, cardiovascular function testing, and retinal angiography on the basis of its dark green color, typically administered at concentrations of 2.5 mg/ml at typical total doses of 25 mg in adults [7]. It binds to albumin in the bloodstream and is selectively excreted through the biliary system. It fluoresces at near-infrared light making it very useful for identification of the biliary anatomy. It is not useful for identifying common bile duct stones and, therefore, is not a substitute for traditional intraoperative cholangiography for this purpose with the possible exception of an obstructing common bile duct stone blocking passage of the ICG. In terms of its safety profile, the incidence of mild adverse reactions was 0.05% and 0.05% for severe adverse reactions, with no deaths after 1923 procedures [7]. In a study of 2820 patients who underwent ICG angiography, the incidence rate of adverse events was 0.07% [8]. In comparison, the incidence rate reported for isosulfan blue dye in SLN identification was 1.1% [9].

The primary cause of bile duct injury is misinterpretation of the biliary anatomy which occurs in 71–97% of all cases [10]. According to Dip et al., the cystic duct was identified by intra-operative fluorescence cholangiography (IOFC) in 44 out of 45 patients (97.77%) [11]. Individual median cost of performing IOFC was cheaper than intraoperative cholangiography (IOC) (13.97 ± 4.3 vs 778.43 ± 0.4 USD) per patient ($p = 0.0001$). IOFC was faster than IOC (0.71 ± 0.26 vs 7.15 ± 3.76 min, $p < 0.0001$). Firefly imaging allows visualization of accessory ducts and superficial gallbladder bed ducts which in my experience occurs in approximately 2% of cholecystectomy cases. Schnelldorfer et al. in a systemic review identified a 4% incidence of accessory ducts [12]. Images of aberrant anatomy can be seen in Figs. 10.10 and 10.11. In Fig. 10.10, an accessory duct can be seen communicating between the common hepatic duct and the cystic duct/gallbladder junction. Fig. 10.11 demonstrates an aberrant duct between the right hepatic duct and the gallbladder. This patient also had the cystic duct inserting at the junction of the left and right hepatic ducts, all of which was easily identified using fluorescence imaging.

With ICG fluorescence, imaging of the bile ducts occurs in real time during the dissection and can be achieved without cutting any biliary structures to complete the imaging vs

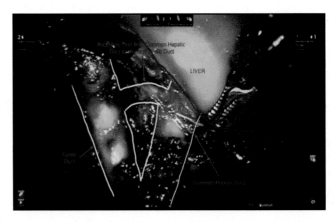

Fig. 10.10 Accessory duct from common hepatic duct to cystic duct

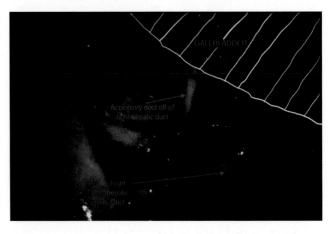

Fig. 10.11 Accessory duct from right hepatic duct to gallbladder

traditional cholangiography. It also eliminates radiation exposure to the patient and the OR staff that occurs with traditional cholangiography. In addition to being more easily able to identify aberrant anatomy, fluorescence imaging more easily allows identification of the anatomy on difficult cases. This in turn can allow a lower rate of open conversion in challenging cholecystectomy cases [13]. The intensity of the fluorescence can be adjusted using the brightness control on the console as well as by how close you are to the target tissue. Greater camera proximity to the target tissue gives a more robust fluorescence response.

The ICG needs to be injected IV at least 30 min before fluorescence imaging is utilized. At my institution, I have the anesthesia team give it in the pre-op area as they are evaluating the patient. That allows the ICG to circulate and be present in the liver and biliary tree during the operation. The usual dose is 2.5 mg (1 ml). If the patient is obese, I increase the dose to 5 mg (2 ml). That is my own protocol and is based on my clinical experience.

Traditional Cholangiography

Traditional cholangiography can also be performed during robotic cholecystectomy. A cholangiogram catheter is introduced through an angiocatheter in the right upper quadrant. The cholangiogram catheter is then introduced into the cystic duct as is done traditionally after clipping the proximal duct and opening the duct toward the common duct. Once inserted, the catheter can be held in position by placing a clip across the catheter and cystic duct securing the catheter in place. The clip will not prevent the ability to inject contrast. Alternatively the Reddick cholangiogram catheter curved introducer sheath can be passed through the accessory port and the balloon tipped catheter introduced into the cystic duct using the clip applier or Maryland grasper. The groove at the end of the clip applier is well suited for grasping and manipulating the catheter into the duct prior to clipping. To use the C-arm, the number 1 arm is undocked and moved out of the way. The C-arm is then rotated slightly clockwise to allow it to pass under the patient and not contact to the other robotic arms (Fig. 10.12). Once in position, the cholangiogram catheter is injected and fluoroscopic images are obtained. Once completed, the catheter is removed, and another clip can be placed on the cystic duct before complete division of the duct is performed.

Postoperative Care

Robotic cholecystectomy is an outpatient procedure for the majority of patients unless there are underlying comorbidities. Diet is initiated as tolerated as is postoperative activity and return to work.

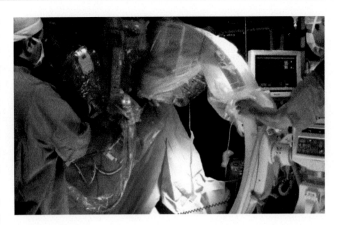

Fig. 10.12 Using the C-arm. (©2018 Intuitive Surgical, Inc. Used with permission)

References

1. Sakpal SV, Bindra SS, Chamberlain RS. Laparoscopic cholecystectomy conversion rates two decades later. JSLS. 2010;14(4):476–83.
2. Li YP, Wang SN, Lee KT. Robotic versus conventional laparoscopic cholecystectomy: a comparative study of medical resource utilization and clinical outcomes. Kaohsiung J Med Sci. 2017;33(4):201–6. https://doi.org/10.1016/j.kjms.2017.01.010. Epub 2017 Feb 28
3. Huang Y, Chua TC, Maddern GJ, Samra JS. Robotic cholecystectomy versus conventional laparoscopic cholecystectomy: a meta-analysis. Surgery. 2017;161(3):628–36. https://doi.org/10.1016/j.surg.2016.08.061. Epub 2016 Dec 20
4. Strosberg DS, Nguyen MC, Muscarella P, Narula VK. A retrospective comparison of robotic cholecystectomy versus laparoscopic cholecystectomy: operative outcomes and cost analysis. Surg Endosc. 2017;31(3):1436–41. https://doi.org/10.1007/s00464-016-5134-0. Epub 2016 Aug 5
5. Ayloo S, Roh Y, Choudhury N. Laparoscopic versus robot-assisted cholecystectomy: a retrospective cohort study. Int J Surg. 2014;12(10):1077–81. https://doi.org/10.1016/j.ijsu.2014.08.405. Epub 2014 Sep 9.
6. Kudsi OY, Castellanos A, Kaza S, McCarty J, Dickens E, Martin D, Tiesenga FM, Konstantinidis K, Hirides P, Mehendale S, Gonzalez A. Cosmesis, patient satisfaction, and quality of life after da Vinci Single-Site cholecystectomy and multiport laparoscopic cholecystectomy: short-term results from a prospective, multicenter, randomized, controlled trial. Surg Endosc. 2016;31:3242.
7. Hope-Ross M, Yannuzzi LA, Gragoudas ES, Guyer DR, Slakter JS, Sorenson JA, et al. Adverse reactions due to indocyanine green. Obana A, Miki T, Hayashi K, et al. Survey of complications of indocyanine green angiography in Japan. Am J Ophthalmol. 1994;118(6):749–53.en. Ophthalmology. 1994;101(3):529–33.
8. Obana A, Miki T, Hayashi K, et al. Survey of complications of indocyanine green angiography in Japan. Am J Ophthalmol. 1994;118(6):749–53.
9. Albo D, Wayne JD, Hunt KK, et al. Anaphylactic reactions to isosulfan blue dye during sentinel lymph node biopsy for breast cancer. Am J Surg. 182(4):393–8. 200. Albo D, Wayne JD, Hunt KK, et al. Anaphylactic reactions to isosulfan blue dye during sentinel lymph node biopsy for breast cancer. Am J Surg. 182(4):393–8. 200.
10. Way LW, Stewart L, Gantert W, Liu K, Lee CM, Whang K, Hunter JG. Causes and prevention of laparoscopic bile duct injuries: analy-

sis of 252 cases from a human factors and cognitive psychology perspective. Ann Surg. 2003;237:460–9.

11. Dip F, Roy M, Lo Menzo E, Simpfendorfer C, Szomstein S, Rosenthal RJ. Routine use of fluorescent incisionless cholangiography as a new imaging modality during laparoscopic cholecystectomy. Surg Endosc. 2015;29(6):1621–6. https://doi.org/10.1007/s00464-014-3853-7. Epub 2014 Oct 3.

12. Schnelldorfer T, Jenkins RL, Birkett DH, Georgakoudi I. From shadow to light: visualization of extrahepatic bile ducts using image-enhanced laparoscopy. Surg Innov. 2015;22(2):194–200. https://doi.org/10.1177/1553350614531661. Epub 2014 Apr 30.

13. Gangemi A, Danilkowicz R, Elli FE, Bianco F, Masrur M, Giulianotti PC. Could ICG-aided robotic cholecystectomy reduce the rate of open conversion reported with laparoscopic approach? A head to head comparison of the largest single institution studies. J Robot Surg. 2017;11(1):77–82. https://doi.org/10.1007/s11701-016-0624-6. Epub 2016 Jul 19.

Robotic Liver Resection

11

Charles R. St. Hill, Christopher Francis McNicoll, and Daniel M. Kirgan

Introduction

Liver surgery has been performed for decades and was initially fraught with high morbidity and mortality and poor overall survival [1]. The indications for resection have broadened with improved outcomes following liver surgery, due to advancements in critical care, surgical technique, and hemostatic devices. Minimally invasive surgery has further improved perioperative outcomes with decreased blood loss, decreased postoperative morbidity, and decreased length of hospital stay. Despite these advantages, laparoscopic surgery has certain limitations as to which liver segments can be easily accessed and safely removed. This is a result of instruments and laparoscopes that have limited articulation and have not been well adapted to the specific challenges of parenchymal-sparing hepatectomy. This may limit the indications of minimally invasive liver resection and therefore the potential benefit to patients. A relevant example of this are the right posterolateral liver segments (segments 7,8) which have been approached laparoscopically but with mixed perioperative outcomes and are not widely performed.

The advent of robotic instrumentation shows promise in extending the indications for minimally invasive surgery while still retaining the benefits of laparoscopic surgery, specifically robotic surgery for right posterior segments. There may also be a future role for robotic surgery in central hepatectomy. Wristed instruments and more degrees of freedom provide improved articulation. Improved optics due to the steady camera and from the binocular vision provides better depth perception [2]. These technical advantages may allow

for more confident suturing, vessel isolation, and control of hemorrhage.

Although new technology brings the promise of expanding the role and advantages of minimally invasive surgery, there are some disadvantages of robotic surgery that should be considered. Disconnect from the tissue in terms of distance and loss of haptic feedback, increased time required to convert to an open approach in case of catastrophic or audible hemorrhage. Finally, the difficulty to utilize a hybrid technique (i.e., laparoscopic hand-assisted) with robotic surgery may limit early adoption by surgeons.

Additional barriers to adoption of robotic surgery include access to the robotic system, a dedicated and well-trained operative team, institutional experience, as well as the surgeon's technical learning curve. Liver surgeries are often performed by highly specialized surgeons. They may not have access to low-risk, high-volume cases, like cholecystectomies and ventral or inguinal hernia repairs. This may make the transition from laparoscopic to robotic liver resection less intuitive due to technical nuances of the robotic system. In earlier iterations of the robotic system, the arms were docked over the patient's head, which limited access to the head and thorax for the anesthesiologist. This potentially puts the patient at higher risk of complications, during these high-risk procedures. There has also been a lack of empiric evidence proving similar oncologic outcomes between laparoscopic and robotic surgery.

The current chapter will discuss relevant evidence regarding the indications, efficacy, outcomes, and cost of robotic liver resection. We will also outline the procedure including room setup, technical steps of the procedure, as well as perioperative considerations.

When deciding to delve into robot liver resection, as with any new procedure, several issues should be carefully considered. Your own expertise in liver surgery is clearly paramount. However, the system that you work in should also be taken into account. A liver resection as we know has high potential for morbidity and even mortality implications for technical mistakes. Given this issue, we recommend that sur-

C. R. St. Hill (✉) · D. M. Kirgan
Department of Surgery, Division of Surgical Oncology, UNLV School of Medicine, Las Vegas, NV, USA
e-mail: charles.sthill@unlv.edu

C. F. McNicoll
Department of Surgery, University of Nevada, Las Vegas School of Medicine, Las Vegas, NV, USA

© Springer Nature Switzerland AG 2019
S. Tsuda, O. Y. Kudsi (eds.), *Robotic-Assisted Minimally Invasive Surgery*, https://doi.org/10.1007/978-3-319-96866-7_11

geons be familiar with the robotic system prior to delving into this procedure. Familiarity with your operating room staff and environment may also minimize some of the issues associated with starting a procedure using a new technique. Despite these challenges, these authors believe that the robotic system has several advantages to standard laparoscopy that are worth the effort required to start a robotic liver resection program.

Literature Review

As with any new tool or technique introduced in surgery, robot-assisted laparoscopic liver resection deserves critical appraisal before being recommended as a mainstream option for patients. We will examine the somewhat limited but salient studies performed to date.

It is accepted that compared to open liver resection, laparoscopic as a minimally invasive technique has the advantage of decreased blood loss, decreased perioperative morbidity, and decreased length of hospital stay. For example, the OSLO-COMET randomized controlled trial shows improved perioperative outcomes in laparoscopic versus open liver resection for colorectal liver metastasis. The authors of this trial report a significant decrease in postoperative complications 19 vs 31% (95% confidence interval 1.67–21.8; $P = 0.021$) and length of hospital stay. Improved quality of life scores were also noted. There were no differences in blood loss, operation time, or rate of positive resection margins. The reported mortality at 90 days did not differ significantly from the laparoscopic group (0 subjects) to the open group (1 subject) [3].

Improvements in these areas are potentially obtained with a trade-off of higher operative cost that is generally recovered by the decreased length of hospital stay mentioned above. Our literature review sought to explore whether the same could be said of robot-assisted laparoscopic liver resection. Further, attributes of robot assistance could extend the indications for laparoscopic resection, offering benefits of minimally invasive resection to a much larger proportion of patients requiring resection.

A summary table of prospective clinical trials is included (Table 11.1 [4]), several of which we will discuss later in this

Table 11.1 Perioperative surgical outcomes

Authors (number of subjects)	Operating time (min)	Blood loss (mL)	Conversion rate n(%)	LOS (days)	Positive surgical margins	Transection method	Patients with ≥1 complication n(%)	Mortality
Giulianotti et al. (70)	270 (90–660)	260 (20–2000)	4 (6)	7 (2–26)	0/42	Harmonic device and bipolar forceps	15 (21)	0
Tsung et al. (57)	255 (62–597)	200 (30–3600)	4 (7)	4 (1–31)	2/42	NR	11 (19)	0
Wu et al. (38)	380 ± 165 SD	325 ± 480	2	8 ± 5	NR	NR	3	0
Lai et al. (41)	230 ± 85 SD	415 (10–3500)	2	6 ± 4	3/42	NR	3	0
Toisi et al. (40)	270 ± 100 SD	330 ± 300	8	6 ± 3	3/28	Straight line: Harmonic scalpel Curved and angulated section lines: Kelly clamp crushing technique using endo-wristed bipolar precise forceps	5	0
Choi et al. (30)	510 (120–815)	345 (95–1500)	2	12 (5–46)	0/13	Harmonic curved shears and Maryland bipolar forceps	13	0
Spampinato et al. (25)	430 (240–725)	250 (100–1900)	1	8 (4–22)	0/17	NR	4	0
Felli et al. (20)	140 (100–200)	50 (0–200)	0	6 (4–14)	2/17	Combination of Kelly crushing technique, bipolar forceps, monopolar crochet, and harmonic scalpel	2	0
Ji et al. (13)	340 (150–720)	280	0	7	0/8	Harmonic curved shears and bipolar electrocautery	1	NR
Yu et al. (13)	290 ± 85 SD	390 ± 65	0	8 ± 2	0/12	Harmonic scalpel	0	0
Berber et al. (9)	260 ± 30 SD	135 ± 60	1	NR	0/9	Harmonic scalpel, clips, scissors, or stapler	1	NR
Kandil et al. (7)	60 ± 30 SD	100 (10–200)	0	2 (1–5)	NR	Harmonic scalpel	2	0

From Nota et al. [4] with permission of Elsevier

text. It is apparent that there is a paucity of definitive prospective clinical trials designed to answer the pertinent questions clinicians have regarding this topic. However, there are some important questions that have been addressed with these studies.

First we will discuss some of the potential advantages of the robotic platform. Milone et al. published an article describing the state of the art in hepatobiliary surgery and suggest several potential advantages that the robotic platform could provide. They propose that it could be utilized to overcome the limitations of the laparoscopic approach to hepatectomy. The increased range of motion could be used to suture bleeding vessels. Additionally, improved visualization with three-dimensional stereoscopic view could improve dissection of critical structures [5]. Kitisin and colleagues expand on this idea when discussing the da Vinci © S and newer iterations of their robotic platform. These systems assist in overcoming the limitations of two-dimensional imaging, tremor amplification, and fulcrum effect suffered by laparoscopic instrumentation. They also address the limited degrees of freedom and awkward ergonomics often experienced by laparoscopic surgeons. This is accomplished by the three-dimensional imaging that adds depth perception, improved dexterity with endo-wristed instruments, and integrated filtration of surgeon tremor for precise tissue dissection [6].

The learning curve becomes important in deciding if these potential advantages will be worth taking the time to acquire the new skill in your particular practice. Choi and his colleagues sought to assess their learning curve by recording the operative time in ten consecutive patients who underwent left hepatectomy. Interestingly, they found a clear cutoff point by the seventh case, where the total operating and console time began to gradually decrease [2]. In 2003, Giulianotti et al. addressed this topic while describing a decreased mean operative time from 96.5 to 66.4 min, following a series of 20 robotic cholecystectomies. In their article describing their personal experience with a large variety of abdominal procedures, they stated that the learning curve at the console was relatively short, even for an inexperienced surgeon. They found that when using robotic cholecystectomy as a basic training model, 20 operations were necessary to complete the learning phase, after which the operative time was similar to that for traditional laparoscopy. Of importance, the authors also noted that in order to perform advanced procedures, full training in open and laparoscopic surgery was mandatory [7]. This learning phase can also be used as an important starting point for training of the operating room nursing staff. Nelson et al. also reported a significant decrease in robot setup time from 30.6 min in the first 16 cases to 18.3 min in the last 16 cases. They determined that robotic cholecystectomy was an excellent procedure for teaching the basics of robotic surgery [8].

We explored relevant literature to address potential benefits and shortcomings of robot-assisted laparoscopic liver resection. Compared to open resection, laparoscopic techniques have shown improved or equivalent perioperative outcomes including blood loss, operative time, morbidity, and mortality with an acceptable conversion rate. A study by Yoon et al. points out the weakness of laparoscopic liver resection compared to open resection for hepatocellular carcinoma in the posterosuperior segments. They report longer operative times as well as increased length of hospital stay and intraoperative blood loss [9].

Several reports show decreased or equivalent intraoperative blood loss compared to open or laparoscopic resection. Ji et al. report a series of their initial experience in China containing 13 consecutive patients. They had a significantly lower mean blood loss in the robotic group, 280 versus 350 ml for laparoscopic procedures and 470 mL for the open group [10]. In another study, Lai et al. analyzed short-term outcomes after liver resection for hepatocellular carcinoma (HCC). They included 42 consecutive robot liver resections. In the subgroup analysis of minor liver resection, when compared with the conventional laparoscopic approach, the robotic group had similar blood loss (mean, 373.4 mL vs 347.7 mL) [11]. Matched patients undergoing robotic and open liver resections displayed no significant differences in postoperative outcomes as measured by blood loss [12]. Another study including matched patients by Montalti et al. displayed no significant differences in postoperative outcomes as measured by blood loss [13]. Sham et al. found approximately half the blood loss and two-thirds less chance of transfusion in robot versus open resections [14]. A case series of 16 patients underwent robot-assisted laparoscopic liver resection at the University Medical Center Utrecht. Fifteen robot-assisted laparoscopic liver resections were completed in a minimally invasive manner. Mean blood loss was 245 mL; transfusion was required in only 2 cases (8.6%) [15].

Spampinato and his Italian colleagues address the issue of intraoperative blood loss in a report including a total of 50 major hepatectomies, inclusive of 25 robotic and 25 laparoscopic cases. The two groups had comparable demographic and tumor characteristics aside from more frequent use of neoadjuvant chemotherapy in the laparoscopic resection group. Regarding operative technique, the only difference between groups regards the use of intermittent pedicle clamping, which was employed in one-third of laparoscopic major hepatectomy (LMH) and in none of the robot assisted major hepatectomy (RMH). The cumulative rate of blood transfusions was higher after RMH (44%) than that after LMH (16%) ($p = 0.031$). However, these rates include autologous blood transfusions, which were given to five patients undergoing RMH because of symptomatic giant hemangioma. The rate of allogeneic blood transfusion was not different between the two groups (24 vs 16%) although still slightly higher after RMH. Median estimated blood loss, indeed, was similar after RMH (250 mL; range 100–1900) and LMH (400 mL; range 50–1200) [16]. Overall, blood loss and transfusion appear to be comparable between robotic and laparoscopic liver resection techniques and less than that required for open approaches.

Operative time, however, is consistently longer in robotic vs open or laparoscopic approaches. A single-institution, retrospective cohort study was performed that included robotic and open liver resections performed for benign and malignant pathologies. Clinical and cost outcomes were analyzed using adjusted generalized linear regression models. Clinical and cost data for 71 robotic and 88 open hepatectomies were analyzed. Operative time was significantly longer in the robotic group (303 vs 253 min; $p = 0.004$) [14]. Patriti et al. matched patients undergoing robotic or open liver resections, they reported significantly longer operative time in the robot group (mean, 303 vs 233 min) [17]. In the analysis of short-term outcomes after liver resection for HCC by Lai et al., they included 42 consecutive robot liver resections, and when compared with the conventional laparoscopic approach, the robotic group had a significantly longer operative time (202.7 min vs 133.4 min) [11].

Troisi's group performed a comparative analysis involving two institutions that sheds more light on the intraoperative blood loss issue as noted above but also analyzed their conversion rates. They concluded that despite higher conversion rates and blood loss, robot-assisted surgery may allow the resection of more liver lesions, especially those located in the posterosuperior segments, therefore facilitating parenchymal-sparing surgery with a comparable complication rate with respect to laparoscopic resection. Their major hepatectomy rate was significantly higher in laparoscopic hepatectomy (16.6% vs 0%, $p = 0.011$), while a parenchymal-preserving approach was favored in robot-assisted resection (55% vs 34.1%, $p = 0.019$). More nodules were resected in the robotic group (1.971.4 vs 1.571.1, $p = 0.04$). Overall conversion rate was 8/40 (20%) in the robotic and 17/223 (7.6%) in the laparoscopic group ($p = 0.034$) [18]. Pelletier et al. examined 170 procedures in a systematic review of 8 studies in order to determine the safety and oncologic efficacy of robotic liver resection. They found a low average conversion rate of 6.6% [13].

Perhaps the most important outcomes relating to care of our patients are morbidity and mortality. In Pelletier's systematic review discussed above, they found low average morbidity (11.6%) and no mortality [13]. Ji et al.report a series of their initial experience in China containing 13 consecutive patients. The morbidity rate was lower in the robotic group in this series. Additionally, they reported postoperative morbidity was lower than either the laparoscopic or open groups, 7.8 versus 10 and 12.5%, respectively [10]. Lai et al. analyzed 104

consecutive patients undergoing liver resection. They included total laparoscopic ($n = 17$), hand-assisted laparoscopic ($n = 55$), and robot-assisted laparoscopic liver resection ($n = 32$). Their study looked specifically at surgical complications, postoperative course, disease-free survival, and overall survival for malignant pathologies. Conversion from laparoscopic to open approach and from laparoscopic to hand-assisted approach occurred in 1.9 and 1% of the cases, respectively. Overall mortality was 0%, and morbidity was 17.3% [9]. In another study by Lai et al., they analyzed short-term outcomes after liver resection for HCC. They included 42 consecutive robot liver resection. The hospital mortality and morbidity rates were 0% and 7.1%, respectively. In the subgroup analysis of minor liver resection, when compared with the conventional laparoscopic approach, the robotic group had similar blood loss (mean, 373.4 mL vs 347.7 mL), morbidity rate (3% vs 9%), and mortality rate (0% vs 0%) [11].

Before extending this technique to include malignant pathologies, studies evaluating oncologic outcomes should also be considered. Pelletier et al. examined 170 procedures in a systematic review of 8 studies in order to determine the safety and oncologic efficacy of robotic liver resection. Their negative margins ranged from 11 to 18 mm, with R0 resection in 14/15 and R1 resection in 1/15 patients [13]. Lai et al. analyzed short-term outcomes after liver resection for HCC. They included 42 consecutive robot liver resection. Five resections (11.9%) were carried out for recurrent HCC, and 23.8% were hemihepatectomy procedures. The R0 resection rate was 93%. The 2-year overall and disease-free survival rates were 94% and 74%, respectively. In the subgroup analysis of minor liver resection, when compared with the conventional laparoscopic approach, the robotic group had similar R0 resection rate (90.9% vs 90.9%). However, the robotic group had a significantly longer operative time (202.7 min vs 133.4 min). These authors also confirm feasibility, safety, and favorable short-term HCC outcomes following robot liver resection [11].

A study by Montalti evaluated the overall survival (OS) in patients with colorectal liver metastases which was 92.3, 64.6, and 40.4% versus 96.4, 70.8, and 62.9% ($p = 0.24$) at 1, 3, and 5 years in robotic versus laparoscopic groups, respectively. Accordingly, recurrence-free survival (RFS) was 73.3, 46.2, and 46.2% versus 63.7, 37.1, and 32.5% ($p = 0.56$) in the robotic versus laparoscopic groups, respectively. These results show no difference in OS or RFS between robot and laparoscopic resections [13]. In 2012 Lai et al. analyzed 104 consecutive patients undergoing liver resection. They included total laparoscopic ($n = 17$), hand-assisted laparoscopic ($n = 55$), and robot-assisted laparoscopic liver resection ($n = 32$). Their study looked specifically at surgical complications, postoperative course, disease-free survival, and overall survival for malignant pathologies. Overall mortality was 0%, and morbidity was 17.3%. The median follow-up period was 24 months, the 5-year overall survival for hepatocellular carcinoma (HCC) was 52%, and the 3-year overall survival for colorectal liver metastasis was 88% [9]. Consistent with other literature reviewed, this illustrates low morbidity and acceptable oncologic outcome for both primary and secondary metastatic disease.

Cost is another important consideration for deciding to adopt new techniques or technology. It is also remarkably difficult to analyze. Most studies evaluate charges, direct costs, and length of hospital stay as a surrogate for the actual cost. To complicate this further, robotic systems have high upfront costs shouldered by the hospital, and the procedure codes used to charge payers are often identical to the open or laparoscopic procedure.

Other laparoscopic procedures afford decreased length of hospital stay and more than make up for the increased equipment costs. Ji et al. report a series of their initial experience in China containing 13 consecutive patients. In terms of hospital stay, they reported 5.2 days for the laparoscopic group, 6.7 days for the robotic group, and 9.6 days for the open group. Thus, while the robotic group resulted in higher operative costs, as compared to the other two groups, the authors suggest that this can be counterbalanced by the shorter hospital stay, particularly when comparing overall cost for open resection [10]. Yoon et al. point out the weakness of laparoscopic liver resection for hepatocellular carcinoma in the posterosuperior segments. They report longer operative times as well as increased length of hospital stay and intraoperative blood loss. Additionally, a higher conversion to open rate was noted. Only 38% of their study patients with lesions in posterosuperior segments received minimally invasive resection [12]. It is intuitive that each of these factors would lead to increased costs to hospitals and decreased or negative case margins at the hospital level. Pelletier's systematic review found average direct cost of robot-assisted resection of $12,046, open $10,548, and laparoscopic $7618 [13]. However, a single-institution, retrospective cohort study was performed that included robotic and open liver resections for benign and malignant pathologies. Clinical and cost outcomes were analyzed using adjusted generalized linear regression models. Clinical and cost data for 71 robotic and 88 open hepatectomies were analyzed. Operative time was significantly longer in the robotic group (303 vs 253 min, $p = 0.004$). Length of hospital stay was more than 2 days shorter in the robotic group (4.2 vs 6.5 days, $p = 0.001$). Predictably, perioperative costs were higher in the robot resection group ($6026 vs $5479, $p = 0.047$). However, postoperative costs were significantly lower, resulting in lower total hospital direct costs compared with open hepatectomy controls ($14,754 vs $18,998, $p = 0.001$). Similar to previous studies comparing laparoscopic to open surgery, the robotic approach increased perioperative costs, but overall robotic

direct costs were not greater than open resection approach [14].

As we alluded to earlier, resection of the right posterolateral segments (segments 7, 8, 4a, and 1) can be challenging using laparoscopic techniques. Two centers reviewed their outcomes using robot versus open resection for lesions in the right posterior section between January 2007 and June 2012. A 1:3 matched analysis was performed by individually matching patients in the robotic cohort to patients in the open cohort on the basis of demographics, comorbidities, performance status, tumor stage, and location. They showed that matched patients undergoing robotic and open liver resections displayed no significant differences in postoperative outcomes as measured by blood loss, transfusion rate, hospital stay, overall complication rate (15.8% vs 13%), R0 negative margin rate, and mortality. Patients undergoing robotic liver surgery had significantly longer operative time (mean, 303 vs 233 min) and inflow occlusion time (mean, 75 vs 29 min) compared with their open counterparts. These authors concluded that robotic and open liver resections in the right posterior section display similar safety and feasibility [17]. In another study, 36 patients were included who underwent robot-assisted liver resection and matched with 72 patients undergoing laparoscopic liver resection. Matched patients displayed no significant differences in postoperative outcomes as measured by blood loss, hospital stay, R0 negative margin rate, and mortality. The overall morbidity according to the comprehensive compilation index was also similar (34.6 ± 33 vs 18.4 ± 11.3, respectively, for robotic and laparoscopic approach, $p = 0.11$). Patients undergoing robotic liver surgery had significantly longer inflow occlusion time (77 vs 25 min, $p = 0.001$) as compared with their laparoscopic counterparts. Although the number and severity of complications in the robotic group appear to be higher, robotic and laparoscopic parenchymal-preserving liver resections in the posterosuperior segments display similar safety and feasibility [18]. So although more work needs to be done in this area, it appears to be safe to conclude that posterosuperior segmentectomies can be approached robotically when preoperative imaging suggests difficult access by standard laparoscopy.

In summary, initial reports suggest similar results of robot-assisted laparoscopic liver resection to standard laparoscopy. These include intraoperative outcomes such as blood loss and transfusion rate, although inflow occlusion time is consistently longer in robotic cohorts. Short-term postoperative morbidity and mortality are similar. Oncologic outcomes including R0 resection rate and short-term overall survival are also comparable. Cost is generally less with laparoscopy, although maturing data may prove more patients are able to reap the benefits of minimally invasive resection using robotic assistance.

Preoperative Planning

Preoperative planning should be focused on the correct indication for the procedure, evaluation of the patient's operative risk based on comorbidities, and optimization of these to minimize perioperative morbidity. Assessment of the patient's cardiac risk should be no different when considering robot-assisted resection compared to any other liver resection access. This remains a high-risk surgery, and adequate preoperative risk assessment and appropriate medical optimization are very important. Additionally, we know that many of these patients are being treated for cancer and do not have the luxury of a prolonged period of cardiac optimization or intervention.

According to the Louisville consensus statement, indications for laparoscopic liver resection are patients with solitary lesions, 5 cm or less, located in liver segments 2–6 [15]. Over time this has evolved to a definition of resectability for colorectal liver metastases requiring removal of all metastases with negative microscopic margins. Adequate future liver remnant is preserved by retaining at least two consecutive liver segments with adequate vascular inflow, outflow, and biliary drainage and demonstrating regenerative capability [19]. Recent, high-quality imaging such as contrast-enhanced CT, MRI, or PET/CT should be used to assess resectability, future liver remnant, and vascular invasion.

With regard to pathologic considerations, there are no indications specific to robotic resection as compared to standard open or laparoscopic techniques. They include HCC, colorectal liver metastases, hepatic cysts, symptomatic hemangioma, intrahepatic cholangiocarcinoma, and possibly gallbladder cancer. Practitioners should use appropriate clinical judgment when planning a robotic liver resection.

Assessment of liver function or extent of liver dysfunction through preoperative laboratory testing is important in determining appropriate candidates for surgical resection. Calculating Child-Pugh-Turcotte [20] and/or MELD [21] scores may assist in guiding the limits of safe resection to avoid liver insufficiency, failure, or even mortality following resection.

There are no absolute contraindications to robotic surgery, though relative contraindications mimic those of laparoscopic surgery and include physiologic and anatomic conditions that limit prolonged tolerance of increased intra-abdominal pressure and CO_2 peritoneum such as COPD [22]. If the patient has relative contraindications, closely assess the patient's pulmonary and hemodynamic status during the initial laparoscopic portion of the procedure. If the patient is tolerating this well, then it is reasonable to continue to the robotic portion of the procedure based on clinical judgment of the surgeon and anesthesiologist.

Setup

The robotic approach should be standardized with a team experienced in assisting with robot procedures. Having the ability to convert quickly to either laparoscopic or open approaches is essential. Early in one's experience, utilizing a two-attending method or an experienced surgical first assistant is as well beneficial. A skilled assistant is necessary to place an ablation probe and provide suction or retraction throughout the case. As one's experience grows, modifications to these recommendations can be tailored to the needs of the individual surgeon.

Vascular access with two large-bore intravenous catheters or a central line and arterial line placement to monitor pulse pressure versus noninvasive measurements should routinely be employed. We prefer using low central venous pressure or pulse pressure monitoring during parenchymal transection to further reduce blood loss.

The patient and table positioning should allow the robot to appropriately access the target segments. Please refer to Fig. 11.1 for an example of the operating room setup.

Intraoperative ultrasound is essential and requires a 12 mm assist port to place the ultrasound device. Robotic graspers then position and manipulate the drop-in probe or robotic arm attachment for the ultrasound.

Precoagulation is achieved using an ablation device, either microwave or radiofrequency, prior to parenchymal transection. The probe(s) may be placed directly through the

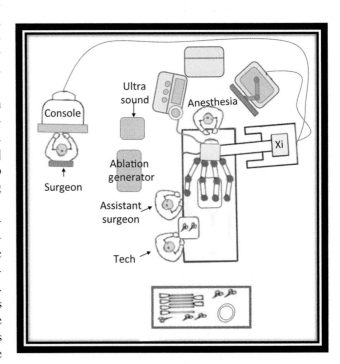

Fig. 11.1 Robotic-assisted laparoscopic hepatectomy room layout. (Illustration by Alouette Vera)

abdominal wall through a small stab incision. Parenchymal transection is started with advanced bipolar device or harmonic scalpel. Deep parenchymal transection including large vessels is completed with endoscopic vascular staplers.

Procedure

Port placement – For clarity of terminology, this text will use the Brisbane 2000 terminology of liver anatomy and resection in the description of procedures [23]. We strongly recommend, when considering port placement, the review of preoperative imaging to plan for the target segment(s). We will start by describing a robot-assisted laparoscopic right hepatectomy and then describing modifications needed for resection of other areas. For resection of right or right anterior segments, ports are placed in a similar position to a robot-assisted cholecystectomy (see Fig. 11.2). This configuration is used for parenchymal-sparing segmentectomies including lesions in segments 5 and 6 and superficial aspects of segment 8 as well. An infraumbilical port is placed for the camera, right midaxillary port at the level of the umbilicus is placed for retraction or dissection, a right lateral subcostal port is placed for retraction or dissection, and the final robotic port is placed at the left midaxillary line. This port may be placed more cephalad for lesions located in segment 4b or 8 to allow for adequate instrument reach. A 12 mm assistant port is added for placement of the ultrasound probe and for

suctioning by the surgical assistant (see Fig. 11.1 for alternate assistant port sites). The operating room table should then be placed in 8–12° of reverse Trendelenburg.

Exploration – After initial port placement, the peritoneal cavity is inspected carefully for peritoneal carcinomatosis or extrahepatic spread which may preclude resection for curative intent. Any suspicious masses should be sampled and sent for intraoperative pathologic evaluation to assist in decision-making based on the respective disease. For example, extrahepatic disease in hepatocellular carcinoma would preclude resection. However, with neuroendocrine carcinoma, where cytoreductive techniques may be advantageous to patients, one may continue with resection based on overall risk and benefit assessment.

Mobilization – The falciform ligament is transected using an energy device followed by mobilization of the right triangular and coronary ligaments. A careful and systematic evaluation of the entire liver parenchyma using high-resolution intraoperative ultrasound is of paramount importance as occult metastases may be found using this modality. This often changes the planned approach as proximity to vessels or occult masses missed on other preoperative imaging modalities are revealed [24]. For example, new bilobar lesions may be amenable to ablation rather than resection. If high-volume, diffuse metastases are encountered, then you may elect to obtain pathologic confirmation with ultrasound-guided biopsy and abort the procedure at this time.

Ultrasound evaluation – In addition, ultrasound guidance can be utilized to obtain the desired gross resection margins.

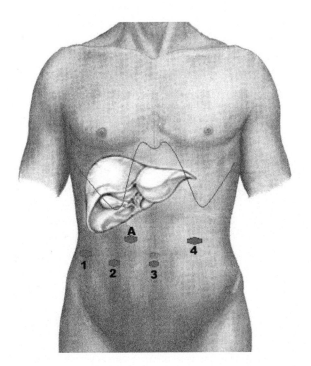

1. Prograsp/ tip up fenestrated grasper

2. Fenestrated bipolar

3. Camera

4. Monopolar scissors/ vessel sealer

A. 12 mm assistant port

Fig. 11.2 Robotic-assisted laparoscopic right hepatectomy. (Illustration by Alouette Vera)

The transaction lines are marked at the liver surface using electrocautery with the monopolar scissors or hook device. If your technique includes vascular isolation of the respective pedicle, this is performed at this time. Vascular isolation of the inflow is achieved by encircling the hepatic artery and right portal vein separately with ligation using a vascular stapler, suture ligature, or hemolock clips and sharp transection with endoshears. Alternatively, the entire portal triad may be encircled for intermittent vascular inflow occlusion via application of the Pringle maneuver during the procedure. The outflow may be controlled by isolating and ligating the right and middle hepatic veins.

Parenchymal transection – We have adopted a parenchymal transection technique using precoagulation of the transection line using microwave thermal ablation. This has the advantage of limiting hemorrhage during parenchymal transection as well as extending the effective margin on the remnant liver side; in most cases, we avoid the need for vascular inflow occlusion (Pringle maneuver). Transection is started with the vessel-sealing device by the operating surgeon at the console. Other options include the surgical assistant using an advanced bipolar or harmonic device, although the latter does not take advantage of the increased degrees of freedom gained with the robot system instruments. Intraoperative ultrasound is used periodically to ensure adequate margins are obtained and that larger vessels are avoided or completely controlled. When the bottom third of the parenchyma is reached, we use an endoscopic vascular stapler controlled by the surgical assistant to complete the transection. The robotic stapler may also be utilized for this crucial portion of the case.

We cauterize the transected parenchymal surface using Argon beam coagulation through the assistant port. Next the surface is carefully inspected and sprayed with absorbable hemostatic polysaccharide as it assists with hemostasis and remains true to its color, facilitating identification of bile leaks. If none are noted, we spray with procoagulant tissue sealant as well.

Specimen extraction – Our group favors extension of the periumbilical port as the extraction site. Other options include a Pfannenstiel incision or extension of the 12 mm port site. A wound protector or laparoscopic retrieval bag should be used to decrease postoperative extraction site infection and theoretical risk of port site tumor seeding.

Specific procedure modifications – For left hepatectomy or left lateral segmentectomy, the port placement is reversed (see Fig. 11.3). For optimal access of the endostapler, the assist port should be placed in line with the parenchymal transection plane through the gallbladder fossa for formal left hepatectomy. For parenchymal-sparing segmentectomy, the placement should be adjusted accordingly. During the mobilization phase, the left triangular and coronary ligaments are incised, and if vascular isolation is desired, the left hepatic artery, portal vein, and hepatic veins would then be carefully dissected. The remainder of the steps in the procedure have been described above.

Right posterior or posterolateral sectionectomy – segments 7 and 8. Segments 4a and 1 may also be accessible using this port placement strategy. Setup for right posterior segments by placing the patient in the supine position with the surgical table in 10–12° of reverse Trendelenburg and rotating the patient's right side up 8–15°.

Alternatively, the patient may be placed in the left lateral decubitus position and ports placed more laterally. The left trocars are placed at the level of the right costal margin. The right trocar is inserted between the 10th and 11th intercostal space along the scapular line. Assistant port trocars can be

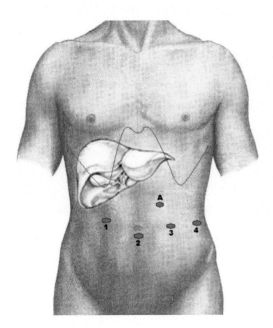

1. 8 mm fenestrated bipolar

2. Camera

3. Monopolar scissors/vessel sealer

4. Prograsp/tip-up fenestrated grasper

A. 12 mm assist port

Fig. 11.3 Robotic-assisted laparoscopic left hepatectomy. (Illustration by Alouette Vera)

placed along the midline or anterior axillary line. This configuration facilitates liver mobilization and inferior vena cava dissection [17, 25–27]. Patriti et al. describe an extracorporeal Pringle maneuver which should be considered as access to inflow for emergent conversion may be more challenging with the patient in the lateral position [25].

Postoperative Care

There is nothing unique to the postoperative care of robotic patients as compared to laparoscopic patients. As with laparoscopic surgery, one must be aware of CO_2 embolism, pneumothorax, bleeding, bile leak, hepatic insufficiency, and the other common complications. Postoperative patients may require intensive care unit (ICU) stay; however, that is not determined by the nature of the surgical technique but rather dictated by the comorbidities of the patient or other intraoperative factors. Thus, patients may be placed in appropriate floor status, ICU, an intermediate care, or standard postoperative surgical unit, based on the patient's medical status and the nature of the procedure.

There appears to be lower intraoperative intravenous fluid requirements for robotic procedures. This is likely due to a decrease of blood loss as well as insensible fluid loss during robotic liver surgery. Thus, the postoperative labs expected to be required for a given patient should not be impacted negatively by the use of the robotic approach. In fact there is a potentially positive impact of robotic surgery on overall hospital stay.

In summary, robot-assisted laparoscopic surgery is a viable technique that can be employed to extend the benefits of minimally invasive surgery to parenchymal-sparing liver resection in all segments. The literature supporting this is growing, and practitioners should tailor specific indications and improved techniques as it matures.

References

1. Yim SY, Seo YS, Jung CH, Kim TH, Lee JM, Kim ES, et al. The management and prognosis of patients with hepatocellular carcinoma: what has changed in 20 years? Liver Int. 2016;36(3):445–53.
2. Choi SB, Park JS, Kim JK, Hyung WJ, Kim KS, Yoon DS, et al. Early experiences of robotic-assisted laparoscopic liver resection. Yonsei Med J. 2008;49(4):632–8.
3. Fretland ÅA, Kazaryan AM, Bjørnbeth BA, Flatmark K, Andersen MH, Tønnessen TI, et al. Open versus laparoscopic liver resection for colorectal liver metastases (the Oslo-CoMet Study): study protocol for a randomized controlled trial. Trials. 2015;16(1):73.
4. Nota CL, Rinkes IHB, Molenaar IQ, van Santvoort HC, Fong Y, Hagendoorn J. Robot-assisted laparoscopic liver resection: a systematic review and pooled analysis of minor and major hepatectomies. HPB Off J Int Hepato Pancreato Biliary Assoc. 2016;18(2):113–20.
5. Milone L, Daskalaki D, Fernandes E, Damoli I, Giulianotti P. State of the art in robotic hepatobiliary surgery. World J Surg. 2013;37(12):2747–55.
6. Kitisin K, Packiam V, Bartlett DL, Tsung A. A current update on the evolution of robotic liver surgery. Minerva Chir. 2011;66(4):281–93.
7. Giulianotti PC, Coratti A, Angelini M, Sbrana F, Cecconi S, Balestracci T, et al. Robotics in general surgery: personal experience in a large community hospital. Arch Surg. 2003;138(7):777–84.
8. Nelson EC, Gottlieb AH, Muller HG, Smith W, Ali MR, Vidovszky TJ. Robotic cholecystectomy and resident education: the UC Davis experience. Int J Med Robot. 2014;10(2):218–22.
9. Lai E, Tang C, Li M. Conventional laparoscopic and robot-assisted laparoscopic liver resection for benign and malignant pathologies: a cohort study. J Robot Surg. 2012;6(4):295–300.
10. Ji W, Wang H, Zhao Z, Duan W, Lu F, Dong J. Robotic-assisted laparoscopic anatomic hepatectomy in China: initial experience. Ann Surg. 2011;253(2):342–8.
11. Lai ECH, Yang GPC, Tang CN. Robot-assisted laparoscopic liver resection for hepatocellular carcinoma: short-term outcome. Am J Surg. 2013;205(6):697.
12. Yoon YS, Han HS, Cho JY, Ahn KS. Total laparoscopic liver resection for hepatocellular carcinoma located in all segments of the liver. Surg Endosc. 2010;24(7):1630–7.
13. Pelletier J, Gill RS, Shi X, Birch DW, Karmali S. Robotic-assisted hepatic resection: a systematic review. Int J Med Robot Comput Assist Surg. 2013;9(3):262–7.
14. Sham J, Richards M, Seo Y, Pillarisetty V, Yeung R, Park J. Efficacy and cost of robotic hepatectomy: is the robot cost-prohibitive? J Robot Surg. 2016;10(4):307–13.
15. Buell JF, Cherqui D, Geller DA, O'Rourke N, Iannitti D, Dagher I, et al. The international position on laparoscopic liver surgery: the Louisville statement, 2008. Ann Surg. 2009;250(5):825–30.
16. Spampinato M, Coratti A, Bianco L, Caniglia F, Laurenzi A, Puleo F, et al. Perioperative outcomes of laparoscopic and robot-assisted major hepatectomies: an Italian multi-institutional comparative study. Surg Endosc. 2014;28(10):2973–9.
17. Patriti A, Cipriani F, Ratti F, Bartoli A, Ceccarelli G, Casciola L, et al. Robot-assisted versus open liver resection in the right posterior section. JSLS J Soc Laparoendosc Surg Soc Laparoendos Surg. 2014;18(3):e2014.00040.
18. Troisi RI, Patriti A, Montalti R, Casciola L. Robot assistance in liver surgery: a real advantage over a fully laparoscopic approach? Results of a comparative bi-institutional analysis. Int J Med Robot Comput Assist Surg. 2013;9(2):160–6.
19. Adams RB, Aloia TA, Loyer E, Pawlik TM, Taouli B, Vauthey JN, et al. Selection for hepatic resection of colorectal liver metastases: expert consensus statement. HPB (Oxford). 2013;15(2):91–103.
20. Child CG, Turcotte JG. The liver and portal hypertension. Major Probl Clin Surg. 1964;1:1–85.
21. Kamath PS, Wiesner RH, Malinchoc M, Kremers W, Therneau TM, Kosberg CL, et al. A model to predict survival in patients with end-stage liver disease. Hepatology. 2001;33(2):464–70.
22. Arkell H. Introduction. London: Helen Arkell Dyslexia Centre; 1977.
23. Pang YY. The Brisbane 2000 terminology of liver anatomy and resections. HPB. 2000;2:333–9. HPB (Oxford) 2002;4(2):100.
24. Parker GA, Lawrence W, Horsley JS, Neifeld JP, Cook D, Walsh J, et al. Intraoperative ultrasound of the liver affects operative decision making. Ann Surg. 1989;209(5):7.
25. Patriti A, Ceccarelli G, Bartoli A, Casciola L. Extracorporeal Pringle maneuver in robot-assisted liver surgery. Surg Laparosc Endosc Percutan Tech. 2011;21(5):e244.
26. Montalti R, Scuderi V, Patriti A, Vivarelli M, Troisi R. Robotic versus laparoscopic resections of posterosuperior segments of the liver: a propensity score-matched comparison. Surg Endosc. 2016;30(3):1004–13.
27. Casciola L, Patriti A, Ceccarelli G, Bartoli A, Ceribelli C, Spaziani A. Robot-assisted parenchymal-sparing liver surgery including lesions located in the posterosuperior segments. Surg Endosc. 2011;25(12):3815–24.

Robotic Total Pancreatectomy

12

Anusak Yiengpruksawan

Introduction

Since total pancreatectomy (TP) was first reported in the 1940s [1], it has always been under close scrutiny by the surgical community. Initially TP was greeted with enthusiasm because it would, by definition, completely eliminate the potential source of cancer and dreaded pancreatic fistula [2]. However, such enthusiasm gradually waned as the postoperative long-term metabolic effects including death due to hypoglycemia and high readmission rates for glycemic control [3] became apparent. As such, after an initial rise in the 1970s, TP became a less performed procedure in the following decades.

In the recent years, we have again seen resurgence of TP due to several factors. First and foremost was the improvement in diabetes mellitus management [4], especially for pancreatogenic diabetes after pancreatic resection. Secondly, better understanding of the tumor biology of pancreatic neoplasms such as IPMN and PNET [5], and pathophysiology of chronic pancreatitis, helps to justify expanding indications for TP. Lastly, innovation in surgical technique and technology [6–8], particularly in the areas of minimally invasive surgery and autologous islet transplantation, has brought about improved surgical outcomes and quality of life for patients with TP. The latest addition of robotic surgical technology to the MIS armamentarium may bring about new surgical paradigm where all digital information can be integrated into the system that further enhances safety, precision, and accuracy.

Historical Evolution of Robotic Total Pancreatectomy (RTP)

Giulianotti et al. [9] reported the first series of robotic pancreatic surgeries in 2010. Initially this was met with skepticism due to the early primitive design of the dVSS and the difficulty inherent to pancreatic surgery. However, over time, as both the technology for the newer dVSS improved and robotic surgery became an accepted minimally invasive approach, there has been renewed interest and increased participation by non-MIS pancreatic surgeons in robotic pancreatic surgery, as evidenced from the rise in published reports. Challenging and complex pancreatic procedures have also increasingly been performed with dVSS by high-volume pancreatic surgeons [10]. Of all robotic pancreatic procedures, TP presents the most challenging strategic and tactical considerations at both preoperative and intraoperative stages. RTP was first reported by Giulianotti et al. [11] and followed subsequently by others [12–14]. Short-term outcomes for RTP were reportedly acceptable in all series (see Table 12.1). Two groups reported successful RTP with simultaneous autologous islet transplantation. Because of the high complexity of the procedure, these reports were all generated from few high-volume pancreatic centers and by highly experienced pancreatic surgeons. Since RTP is still in its early development stage, there has not yet been an established standard approach. Each center had its own strategy not only in the technical aspect but also in the setup of the dVSS. As such, the technical approach described as follows should be considered as just one of the optional techniques that has been developed and is proven to be safe and feasible by the author.

A. Yiengpruksawan
The Valley Minimally Invasive and Robotic Surgery Center, The Valley Hospital, Ridgewood, NJ, USA

Minimally Invasive Surgery Unit, Department of Surgery, Faculty of Medicine, Siriraj Hospital, Mahidol University, Bangkok, Thailand

© Springer Nature Switzerland AG 2019
S. Tsuda, O. Y. Kudsi (eds.), *Robotic-Assisted Minimally Invasive Surgery*, https://doi.org/10.1007/978-3-319-96866-7_12

Table 12.1 Comparison of published robotic total pancreatectomy series and current series

Column 1	Giulianotti	Galvani	Zureikat	Boggi
Year published	2011	2014	2015	2015
N	5	6	10	11
Age (years)	N/A	41 (22–58)	58 (20–76)	61.8 (50–74)
BMI (kg/m^2)	N/A	23.2 (18.5–30.1)	28.2 (24.5–29.75)	24.8 (18.4–35.0)
Diagnosis	PC 2, IPMN 1, PNET 1, CP1	CP 6 (+AIT)	PC 1, IPMN 6, CP 3(+1AIT)	PC 2, IPMN 8, PNET 1
OR time (min)	480 (300–560)	712 (612–835)	560 (461–592)	600 (400–800)
EBL (ml)	300 (50–650)	630 (500–800)	650 (400–1000)	220 (100–450)
LOS (days)	7 (5–10)	12.6 (11–14)	10 (7–10)	27 (12–88)
SP	2 (40%)	4 (66.6%)	2 (20%)	3 (27.2%)
PP	N/A	6(100%)	0	10(90.9%)
LGV	N/A	N/A	N/A	11(100%)

N/A information not available, *BMI* body mass index, *EBL* estimated blood loss, *LOS* length of stay, *SP* spleen preservation, *PP* pylorus preservation, *PC* pancreatic cancer, *IPMN* intraductal papillary mucinous neoplasm, *PNET* pancreatic neuroendocrine tumor, *CP* chronic pancreatitis, *AIT* autologous islet cell transplantation

Indications for RTP

The most common indications for RTP are as follows:

Diffuse IPMN with potential malignant changes
Pancreatic cancer involving the body of the pancreas with extension into either the head or the tail
Multifocal PNET
Pancreas with diffuse high-grade dysplasia (panIN3) with or without hereditary pancreatic cancer
Chronic pancreatitis with intractable pain

Preoperative Planning

RTP, a biquadrant procedure, demands careful preoperative planning starting with proper positioning of the patient, surgical cart (robot), and trocars. This step is crucial, specifically with the da Vinci Si that is still in use in many facilities globally. The system does not permit repositioning of the camera into a different trocar unless instruments on each side are also moved together. Furthermore, in a multi-quadrant procedure, it is necessary to undock and reposition the surgical cart each time the procedure is changed to the different quadrant thus increasing time and reducing efficiency. However, with the new dVSS Xi system, some of these issues have been solved. The smaller camera can now be placed in any 8 mm trocar with instant position recognition by the system computer. With robotic arms installed on the rotatable boom, the surgical cart can now be parked at one position while the boom rotated to accommodate positioning of the robotic arms for the corresponding quadrant using the automated "target positioning" function. The dedicated operating table is synched to the robotic surgical system via Bluetooth and, therefore, can be adjusted, while it is docked to the robot providing additional convenience and efficiency.

For most patients with average size, a single docking with standard setup for a Whipple's procedure (Fig. 12.1) can generally cover both quadrants. However, for those with wide and deep upper abdomen, repositioning of the cart for distal pancreatectomy may be required to allow for safe and efficient dissection. This principle applies for both the Si and Xi systems.

Since robotic surgery is essentially a visual-based (without haptic feedback) surgery, analysis of preoperative imaging studies is critical for strategic and tactical planning of a complex procedure such as RTP. If available, 3D rendering images of the regional anatomy based on CT or MRI should be obtained and studied prior to the surgery.

All patients undergoing RTP should be medically evaluated and optimized for blood sugar and albumin levels. Those with severe cardiopulmonary conditions are generally excluded. Smoking and/or alcohol usage is strictly prohibited at least 2 weeks preoperatively. Timing of discontinuing anticoagulation medication especially for a postcoronary stenting patient should be discussed with the primary cardiologist. Patients can take a minidose aspirin (81 mg) until the day of the surgery. For those with high risk for DVT, they may be admitted for preoperative heparin or its derivative treatment, which can be discontinued at an appropriate time preoperatively depending on its half-life.

Setup of the Robotic Cart and Port Placement

The patient is placed supine in a reverse Trendelenburg position with both arms tucked and protected with foam padding along the body. Pneumoperitoneum is established with a

Fig. 12.1 Port positions are shown in the circle. *Blue*, camera port, below the umbilicus; *green*, instrument arm 1; *yellow*, instrument arm 2; *red*, instrument arm 3; *black*, assistant ports

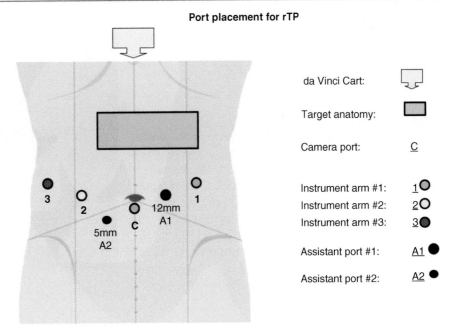

Fig. 12.2 Robot setup for total pancreatectomy. The patient is placed in 30° reverse Trendelenburg position. The surgical cart is brought in directly over the head

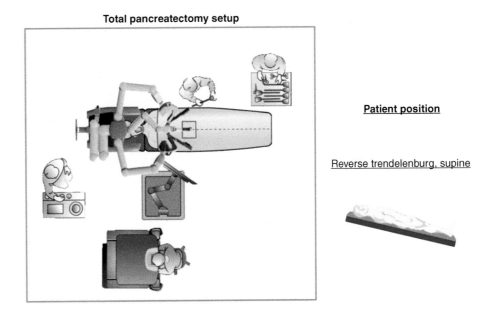

Veress needle inserted through a left subcostal stab incision or Hasson's technique if the patient has previous abdominal surgery. Four robotic ports and two accessory ports are placed as shown in Fig. 12.1.

Instrumentation

We use bipolar forceps in arm 2, hook or scissors in arm 1 (scissors have become the author's preferred instrument), and a grasper forceps in arm 3. The robotic cart (Si system) is brought directly over the head of the patient with arms 2

and 3 on the right lateral side of the table (Fig. 12.2). As the surgeon assumes his position at the robot console, the first assistant stands at the patient's right side.

Operative Details

In general, we like to start on the left side with distal pancreatic dissection and mobilization and then shift to the right for proximal pancreatic resection, once the distal pancreatectomy is completed. However, the sequence of steps can and should be flexible depending on the circumstance and on the type of procedure selected (see Table 12.2).

Left-Sided Pancreatic Dissection

Pancreatic Exposure

The dissection commences with the opening of the gastro-colic ligament along the gastroepiploic arcade from the pylorus to the level of the short gastric vessels. The stomach is then retracted anteriorly and to the right with arm 3 to expose the pancreas. To maximize utilization of arm 3, the stomach can also be sutured to the falciform ligament (Fig. 12.3). The pancreatogastric fold is divided at this stage for full pancreatic exposure. Care is taken to identify and preserve the left gastric vein during this dissection. The right gastroepiploic vein is then followed toward the pancreas until the Henle's trunk is identified and the root of the superior mesenteric vein (SMV) is seen (Fig. 12.4). Gentle dissection in the avascular plane between the anterior wall of the SMV and the neck of the pancreas creates a tunnel that leads to the upper border of the pancreas and the portosplenic junction.

Table 12.2 Abbreviations of procedure

S: Splenectomy
SP: Spleen plus splenic vessels preservation
WSP: Warshaw's type spleen minus splenic vessel preservation
TP: Total pancreatectomy
PPTP: Pyloric preserving total pancreatectomy
PPTP-S: PPTP with splenectomy
PPTP-SP: PPTP with SP
PPTP-WSP: PPTP with WSP
CTP: Classic (distal gastrectomy) total pancreatectomy
CTP-S-: CTP with splenectomy
CTP-SP: CTP with SP
CTP-WSP: CTP with WSP

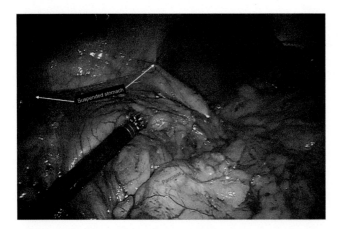

Fig. 12.3 Stomach was suspended to the diaphragm and falciform ligament to provide stability of the operative field and to maximize the utility of the instrument arm

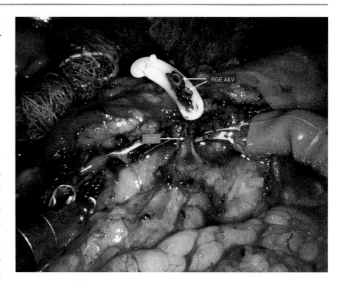

Fig. 12.4 Tributaries of the superior mesenteric vein below the pancreatic neck. RGE A&V right gastroepiploic artery and vein, GCT gastrocolic trunk, SMV superior mesenteric vein, MCV middle colic vein

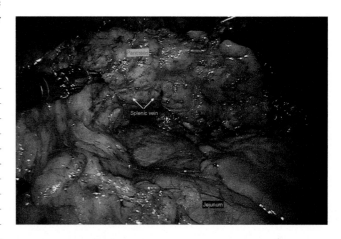

Fig. 12.5 Completion of posterior dissection of the pancreas showed embedded splenic vein

Dissection and Mobilization of the Pancreas and Spleen (Fig. 12.5)

From here, the dissection progresses leftward, along the splenic vein and posterior avascular plane of the pancreas, toward the pancreatic tail. The splenocolic and splenorenal ligaments may be divided at this stage, if splenectomy is planned. Otherwise, once the splenic hilum is reached, attention is turned to the upper pancreatic border.

Dissection of the Superior Pancreas and Splenic Vessels (Fig. 12.6)

Umbilical tape may be used to encircle the previously dissected PN for traction, at the surgeon's discretion. We routinely perform celiac lymph node dissection, irrespective of pathology, to expose the common hepatic artery (CHA), left gastric artery and vein, and the splenic artery (SA).

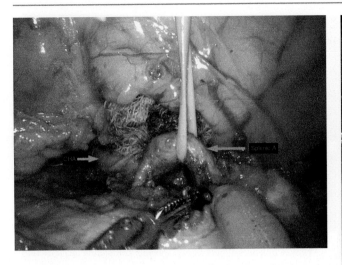

Fig. 12.6 Dissection of superior aspect of the pancreas with clearance of celiac lymph nodes and isolation of splenic artery. CHA common hepatic artery

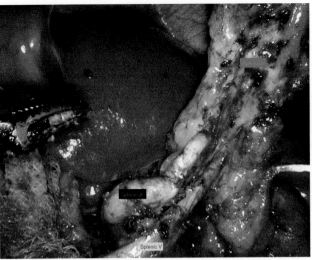

Fig. 12.7 Dissection of distal pancreas with preservation of splenic vessels. Transected pancreatic stump was lifted upward to show the dissected pancreas and exposed vessels

When splenectomy or WSP is planned, we perform early ligation of the splenic vessels near their origin. The PN is pulled cranially using the placed umbilical tape, and the splenic vein (SV) is then encircled with a vessel loop for traction control. Dissection moves superiorly, where the SA is dissected free from the pancreas, clipped at its root, or divided using a vascular cartridge linear stapler.

After the division of the SA, the vessel loop used to identify SV is pulled inward, and the vein is then clipped with Hem-o-Lok® and subsequently divided.

For an en bloc splenectomy case, short gastric vessels are cauterized with bipolar energy and divided. After this point, dissection continues as previously described [15, 16] until the entire pancreatic body, tail, and spleen are mobilized en bloc. Preservation of LGV is recommended for gastric venous drainage.

For WSP, meticulous dissection and preservation of LGV is crucial in order to ensure both splenic viability and gastric venous congestion, as it will become the only reliable splenic outflow channel once the main splenic vein is interrupted. After LGV is secured, splenic vessels can now be divided. Both short gastric vessels and splenocolic ligament, which contains the blood supply to the lower pole of the spleen, are also preserved in WSP. After the hilar vessels are ligated and the distal pancreas is disconnected from the spleen, the splenic viability test is performed. Two to four milliliter of indocyanine green (25 mg/vial, Patheon Italia S.p.A./HUB Pharmaceuticals LLC) is injected IV in the bolus. After 1–2 min, the dVSS scope illumination is switched to the near-infrared mode to assess the perfusion. Perfused spleen will illuminate green; otherwise it remains dark.

For SP, the dissection progresses in medial-to-lateral direction starting at the portosplenic junction. The pancreas is carefully retracted and stabilized with the third arm, while it is being dissected free from the vessels (Fig. 12.7). Small venous branches can be safely cauterized and divided if their dissected length is greater than 1 cm, while shorter veins and arterial branches are ligated or clipped. The dissection proceeds from the pancreatic neck toward the spleen until the distal pancreas is completely free from the vessels.

Right-Sided Pancreatic Dissection: A Caudad to Cephalad Approach [17]

A classic distal gastrectomy is performed at this stage if the decision is made not to preserve the pylorus. Otherwise dissection is carried out along the CHA toward the GDA, removing surrounding lymph nodes along the way. Once the GDA is encountered, it is dissected free and ligated. The right gastroepiploic vessels are next dissected and ligated. The duodenum can now be divided with a linear stapler just above the head of the pancreas. Next, the transverse mesocolon is carefully separated from the underlying uncinate process along the defined tissue plane until the infra-pancreatic SMV along with its tributaries is exposed. The gastrocolic trunk is carefully dissected toward the SMV and then ligated. This will facilitate safe retraction of the SMV during uncinate dissection. Hepatic flexure is next mobilized and extended Kocherization performed to free the pancreatic head, duodenum, and proximal jejunum. If the jejunum can be brought behind the mesentery to the right, it can now be divided. Alternatively, the jejunum can be located and brought up to the lesser sac directly by opening the mesocolon through the avascular portion on the left of the SMA. The proximal jejunum is then divided, demesenterized, and then brought behind the mesentery to the right subhepatic area. To avoid losing the distal jejunum, we routinely attach the proximal and distal stumps together with a long 2-0 silk suture.

We also place a stay suture between the stomach and the jejunal wall, 20 cm from the distal stump, to mark the site of the anastomosis. The duodenum is retracted to the right by the third arm to expose the uncinate process and its attachment to the superior mesenteric vessels. With the area exposed, detachment of the uncinate process from the vessels can now be carried out meticulously using a combination of monopolar and bipolar energy. The procedure is moved on to the hepatic hilum. The gallbladder is dissected in a retrograde fashion until the common bile duct is reached. The latter is then divided above the cystic duct junction. We then rotate the distal pancreas with or without spleen over to the right side of the SMV (Fig. 12.8). With the PV fully in view, we carefully dissect distal CBD together with surrounding soft tissue away from the vein toward the detached pancreas until the entire specimen is freed.

Reconstruction

The stapled distal jejunum stump is brought up to the hilum where an end-to-side hepaticojejunostomy is performed, using 5-0 PDS in continuous running fashion (Fig. 12.9). A biliary stent is used only for small bile duct with diameter less than 5 mm. Next, the previously marked loop of jejunum is brought into the lesser sac through the mesocolic window to anastomose to the duodenum (or gastric remnant) using 3-0 V-Loc sutures in a traditional two-layer continuous running fashion (Fig. 12.10). The anastomotic site, which is approximately 30 cm distal to the biliary anastomosis, is then pushed through the same window until it is resting under the mesocolon. Interrupted sutures are then placed between the edge of the window and the duodenum (or stomach) just above the anastomosis to seal the window and secure the anastomosis below the mesocolon. This trick prevents not only internal herniation but also potential bowel obstruction.

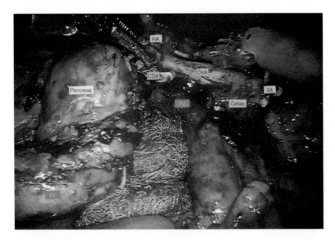

Fig. 12.8 Completely dissected distal pancreas and spleen were rotated to the right of the SMV to facilitate the last stage – dissection of uncinate process and pancreatic head

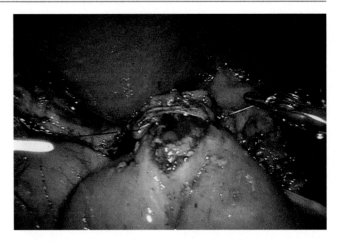

Fig. 12.9 Choledochojejunostomy showed completion of posterior wall

Specimen Extraction

The specimen is placed in a 15 mm bag and then extracted through a small Pfannenstiel incision or an enlarged camera port incision. We routinely place a 19 French Blake drain in the right subhepatic space adjacent to the biliary anastomosis and bring it out through the right lateral port incision.

Postoperative Care

A post RTP patient should be monitored in the ICU for at least 24 h by teamwork that consists of, at least, an intensivist and an endocrinologist. Blood sugar is meticulously monitored and titrated hourly with insulin drip. Pain management with intravenous opioid medication is quite straightforward during the first 24 h and may not be needed after that. A patient can get out of bed with assistance on the first postoperative day and is encouraged to ambulate on the second. NG tube is removed on the second postoperative day unless the output is greater than 200 ml/8 h shift. Clear liquid diet is generally started on the second postoperative day and can be advanced to diabetic diet as tolerated. JP drain is removed on the third or fourth operative day. Patient is generally discharged on the fifth day if stable. An endocrinologist who will also follow the patient in a long-term basis should do the order and adjustment of insulin dosage and formula prior to discharge. Predischarge comprehensive diabetic education is essential in order to prevent complications related to hypoglycemic event. As for pancreatic exocrine insufficiency, pancreatic enzyme replacement therapy should be initiated while inpatient and adjusted accordingly after discharge, preferably by a gastroenterologist, depending on the type of diet or character of stool (steatorrhea).

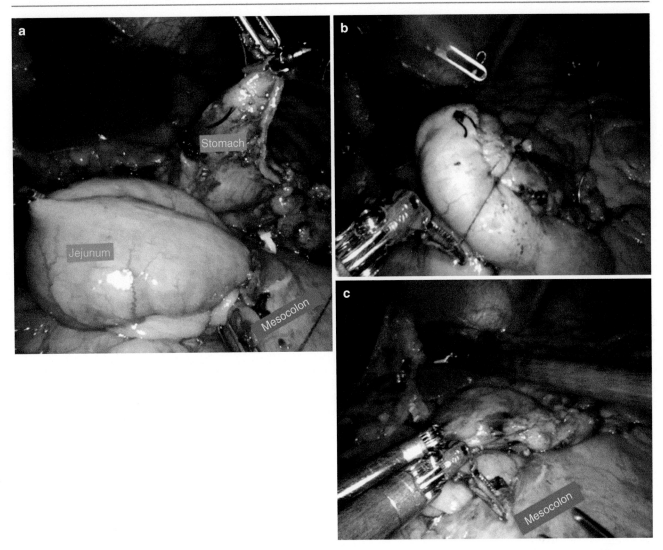

Fig. 12.10 Billroth II retrocolic gastrojejunostomy. (**a**) A loop of jejunum was brought up through the mesocolic defect to the upper abdomen. (**b**) Completion of anastomosis. (**c**) The anastomosis was pushed through the mesocolic defect and secured to the edge with 3-0 silk sutures

References

1. Rockey EW. Total pancreatectomy for carcinoma: a case report. Ann Surg. 1943;118(4):603–11.

2. Almond M, Roberts KJ, Hodson J, Sutcliffe R, Marudanayagam R, Isaac J, et al. Changing indications for a total pancreatectomy: perspectives over a quarter of a century. HPB. 2015;17(5):416–21.

3. Barbier L, Jamal W, Dokmak S, Aussilhou B, Corcos O, Ruszniewski P, et al. Impact of total pancreatectomy: short- and long-term assessment. HPB (Oxford). 2013;15:882–92.

4. Jethwa P, Sodergren M, Lala A, Webber J, Buckels JAC, Bramhall SR, et al. Diabetic control after total pancreatectomy. Dig Liver Dis. 2006;38(6):415–9.

5. Nathan H, Wolfgang CL, Edil BH, Choti MA, Herman JM, Schulick RD, et al. Peri-operative mortality and long-term survival after total pancreatectomy for pancreatic adenocarcinoma: a population-based perspective. J Surg Oncol. 2009;99(2):87–92.

6. Dallemagne B, De Oliveira ATT, Lacerda CF, D'Agostino J, Mercoli H, Marescaux J. Full laparoscopic total pancreatectomy with and without spleen and pylorus preservation: a feasibility report. J Hepatobiliary Pancreat Sci. 2013;20(6):647–53.

7. Kitasato A, Tajima Y, Kuroki T, Adachi T, Kanematsu T. Hand-assisted laparoscopic total pancreatectomy for a main duct intra-ductal papillary mucinous neoplasm of the pancreas. Surg Today. 2011;41(2):306–10.

8. Kim DH, Kang CM, Lee WJ. Laparoscopic-assisted spleen-preserving and pylorus-preserving total pancreatectomy for main duct type intraductal papillary mucinous tumors of the pancreas: a case report. Surg Laparosc Endosc Percutan Tech. 2011;21(4):e179–82.

9. Giulianotti PC, Sbrna F, Bianco FM, Elli EF, Shah G, Addeo P, Caravaglios G, Coratti A. Robot-assisted laparoscopic pancreatic surgery: single-surgeon experience. Surg Endosc. 2010;24(7):1646–57.

10. Zuirekat AH, Nguyen KT, Bartlett DL, Zeh HJ, Moser AJ. Robotic-assisted major pancreatic resection and reconstruction. Arch Surg. 2011;146(3):256–61.

11. Giulianotti PC, Addeo P, Buchs NC, Bianco FM, Ayloo SM. Early experience with robotic total pancreatectomy. Pancreas [Internet]. 2011;40(2):311–3.

12. Galvani CA, Rodriguez Rilo H, Samame J, Porubsky M, Rana A, Gruessner RWG. Fully robotic-assisted technique for total pancreatectomy with an autologous islet transplant in chronic pancreatitis patients: results of a first series. J Am Coll Surg. 2014;218(3):73–8.

13. Zureikat AH, Nguyen T, Boone BA, Wijkstrom M, Hogg ME, Humar A, et al. Robotic total pancreatectomy with or without autologous islet cell transplantation: replication of an open technique through a minimal access approach. Surg Endosc. 2015;29:176–83.

14. Boggi U, Palladino S, Massimetti G, Vistoli F, Caniglia F, De Lio N, et al. Laparoscopic robot-assisted versus open total pancreatectomy: a case-matched study. Surg Endosc Other Interv Tech [Internet]. 2015;29(6):1425–32. Springer US

15. Suman P, Rutledge J, Yiengpruksawan A. Robotic distal pancreatectomy. JSLS. 2013;17:627–35.

16. Yiengpruksawan A. Technique for laparobotic distal pancreatectomy with preservation of spleen. J Robot Surg. 2011;5(1):11–5.

17. Yiengpruksawan A, Carnevale N. Laparobotic pancreatoduodenectomy: caudad to cephalad approach. In: Asbun HJ, Fuchshuber PR, editors. ACS multimedia atlas of surgery, pancreas surgery volume. Chicago: American College of Surgeons; 2010. p. 347–60.

Robotic Adrenalectomy

13

Bora Kahramangil and Eren Berber

Introduction

Open adrenalectomy used to be the standard of care for adrenal tumors prior to the initial report of laparoscopic adrenalectomy (LA) by Gagner et al. in 1992 [1]. Over the following years, LA has been shown to be safe and efficacious and has become the treatment of choice for adrenal tumors [2, 3]. In 1999, Piazza et al. [4] and Hubens et al. [5] described robotic adrenalectomy (RA) for the first time. Studies have shown comparable outcomes with RA to LA, and RA is now accepted as a valid alternative to LA for the treatment of adrenal tumors [6].

Despite its safety and efficacy, laparoscopic technique has certain limitations including handheld unstable camera platform, two-dimensional view, and rigid instruments with limited motion. Robotic technique, on the other hand, has a stable camera platform that provides three-dimensional images, and the robotic arms allow seven degrees of freedom [7]. Given these advantages over LA, RA looks promising and will likely expand the limits of minimally invasive adrenal surgery in the future. This chapter reviews the progress made so far and also describes our surgical technique.

Literature Review

Robotic adrenalectomy was first described in 1999 by Piazza et al. [4] and Hubens et al. [5] using AESOP 2000 Surgical System (Computer Motion Inc., Goleta, CA). Piazza et al. performed a right adrenalectomy for Conn's syndrome, and Hubens et al. performed a left adrenalectomy for Cushing's syndrome. Both studies were from Europe. In the United States, the first RA experience was reported from the Cleveland Clinic in a preclinical study on pigs [8]. Following the FDA approval of the da Vinci Robotic System (Intuitive Surgical Inc., Sunnyvale, CA) for general surgical procedures, Horgan

et al. reported a series of 34 robotic general surgical procedures including one bilateral adrenalectomy [7]. In the following years, many other studies on RA have been published [9–19]. The perioperative parameters of studies with at least 30 patients were summarized (Table 13.1). Below is a chronological discussion of important studies in this field.

In 2004, Morino et al. [9] conducted a prospective randomized controlled trial to assess the benefits and disadvantages of RA. In this study of 20 patients, 10 patients were assigned each to laparoscopic adrenalectomy (LA) and RA. RA group was found to have a longer operative time (169.2 min vs 115.3 min, $p < 0.001$) and higher total cost ($3467 vs $2737, $p < 0.01$) than LA group. Length of postoperative stay was reported to be similar (5.7 vs 5.4 days, RA and LA, respectively, $p = $ NS).

Winter et al. [10] published a prospective study of 30 RAs in 2006. Mean operative time was 185 min, and operative time decreased by 3 min with each operation. Perioperative morbidity was 7%, and conversion to open adrenalectomy or laparoscopy was not required in any case. No significant difference in hospital charge was found between robotic, laparoscopic, and open adrenalectomy ($12,977, $11,599, and $14,600, respectively, $p = $ NS).

Brunaud et al. [11] studied the learning curve of RA in a prospective evaluation of 100 RAs in 2008. Mean operative time was reported to be 95 min and conversion rate 5%. Morbidity rate was 10% without any mortality. Mean operative time was found to decrease by 1 min for every 10 cases, and the improvement in operative time after the first 50 cases was greater in junior than senior surgeons ($p = 0.006$). The predictors of operative time were surgeon experience, first assistant training level, and tumor size.

In 2011, Nordenstrom et al. [13] reported their RA experience in a prospective study of 100 patients. Conversion rate was 7% and postoperative complication rate was 13%. Median operative time was reported to be 113 min and console time 88 min. The console time decreased as the number of patients operated increased, suggesting a learning curve ($r = 0.37, p < 0.001$).

B. Kahramangil · E. Berber (✉)
Department of Endocrine Surgery, Cleveland Clinic, Cleveland, OH, USA
e-mail: berbere@ccf.org

© Springer Nature Switzerland AG 2019
S. Tsuda, O. Y. Kudsi (eds.), *Robotic-Assisted Minimally Invasive Surgery*, https://doi.org/10.1007/978-3-319-96866-7_13

Table 13.1 Summary of perioperative parameters in studies with more than 30 patients undergoing robotic adrenalectomy

Study	Number of patients	Approach	Tumor size, cm (mean)	Conversion rate	Operating time, minutes (mean)	Complication rate	Hospital stay, days (mean)
Brunaud et al. [11]	100	LT	2.9 ± 1.9	5%	95 ± 27	10%	6.4 ± 3.0
Nordenstrom et al. [13]	100	LT	5.3 (median)	7%	113 (median)	13%	Not reported
Karabulut et al. [16]	50	LT, PR	3.9 ± 0.3	1%	166 ± 7	2%	1.1 ± 0.3
Giulianotti et al. [12]	42	LT	5.5 ± 2.5	0%	118 ± 46	4.8%	4 (median)
Aksoy et al. [17]	42	LT, PR	4.0 ± 0.4	0%	186.1 ± 12.1	4.8%	1.3 ± 0.1
Morelli et al. [20]	41	LT	4.9 ± 3.1	0%	177.2 ± 57.0	4.8%	3.3 ± 1.1
Agcaoglu et al. [14]	31	PR	3.1	0%	163.2	0%	1 (median)
Winter et al. [10]	30	LT	2.4 (median)	0%	185	7%	2 (median)
Pineda-Solis et al. [18]	30	Not reported	3.2 ± 2.1	0%	189.7 ± 32.7	0%	1.3 ± 0.5
Brandao et al., 2014 [19]	30	LT	3.0 (median)	0%	120 (median)	20%	2 (median)

LT lateral transabdominal, *PR* posterior retroperitoneal

Later same year, Giulianotti et al. [12] published the results of a single-surgeon 43-patient RA series. Mean lesion size was 5.5 cm, with tumors as large as 10 cm successfully removed robotically. Overall, morbidity and mortality rates were 2.4%, and there were no conversions. Mean operative time was reported to be 118 min and median hospital stay 4 days. Given good postoperative outcomes, the conclusion was RA would be a valid treatment option for adrenal tumors and would possibly expand the limits of minimally invasive adrenal surgery.

Our group compared the outcomes of RA with LA in 2012 [16]. Each group had 50 patients, 32 approached LT, and 18 approached PR. In LT approach, RA was found to have similar operative time to LA (168 vs 159 min, p = NS) despite larger tumor size (4.7 vs 3.8 cm, p = 0.05). In PR approach, both tumor size (2.7 vs 2.3, p = NS) and operative time (166 vs 170, p = NS) were similar. For both approaches, the docking time for robot was found to decrease by 50% by the second year of the study. Overall, RA resulted in shorter hospital stay (1.1 vs 1.5, p = 0.006) and similar complication rates (2% vs 10%, p = NS). Same year, we also reported a comparison of RA (n = 31) and LA (n = 31) in PR approach, specifically [14]. For all patients, operative times were similar (163.2 vs 165.7 min, p = NS). However, when the first 10 RA patients were excluded (i.e., after initial learning curve), RA had significantly shorter operative time (139.1 vs 166.9 min, p = 0.046). Also, PR RA resulted in less pain on postoperative day #1 (2.5 vs 4.2 mean pain score, p = 0.008) with similar pain of postoperative day #14 (p = NS).

D'Annibale et al. published a series of 30 unilateral transperitoneal RAs in 2012 [15]. Their results were comparable with the previous studies with a mean tumor size of 5.1 cm. 6.6% intraoperative complication rate and 10% hospital morbidity without mortality were reported. Rate of conversion to open adrenalectomy was 3.3%, and the mean hospital stay was 5.2 days. As with previous studies, reduction in operative time was noted with increasing number of operations.

In 2013, our group compared the outcomes of RA and LA in obese patients in a study of 99 patients with BMI ≥ 30 kg/

m² [17]. Forty-two patients that underwent RA and 57 that underwent LA were comparable in tumor properties and demographics except for slightly lower BMI in robotic group (35.4 vs 38.8 kg/m², p = 0.01). Perioperative parameters including operative time (186.1 vs 187.3 min, RA and LA, respectively, p = NS), estimated blood loss (50.3 vs 76.6 ml, p = NS), hospital stay (1.3 vs 1.6 days, p = 0.06), conversion rate (0% vs 5.2%, p = NS), and 30-day morbidity (4.8% vs 7%, p = NS) were found to be similar.

Again in 2013, Pineda-Solis et al. compared RA with LA in a prospective study of 60 patients [18]. Each group had 30 patients and were comparable in demographic and pathologic parameters except for more pheochromocytomas in LA group (43% vs 17%, p = 0.02). RA was found to have longer operative time than LA (190 vs 160 min, p = 0.003). A trend for less blood loss was noted in RA; however it did not reach statistical significance (30 vs 55 ml, p = 0.07). Morbidity and length of hospital stay were similar in RA and LA. No mortality was recorded. It was concluded that RA was feasible and safe given comparable outcomes to LA.

Brandao et al. reported a retrospective comparison of 30 RAs and 46 LAs in 2014 [19]. Groups were comparable except for smaller median tumor size in RA group (3 cm vs 4 cm, p = 0.02). Less intraoperative blood loss was noted in the RA group (50 vs 100 ml, p = 0.02). Other perioperative parameters including operative time (120 vs 120 min, RA and LA, respectively, p = NS), length of stay (2 vs 2.5 days, p = NS), rate of postoperative complication (20% vs 10.9%, p = NS), and conversion rate (0% vs 2.3%, p = NS) did not significantly differ between groups. Overall, good postoperative outcomes recapitulated the safety and efficacy of RA for the treatment of adrenal tumors.

Finally, in 2016, Morelli et al. [20] compared 41 RAs with 41 LAs in a case-control study. Groups were comparable in terms of demographics and pathology. RA group had shorter operative time than LA group (177.2 vs 207.1 min, p = 0.047). On subgroup analysis, RA was found to result in shorter operative time in patients with tumors larger than 6 cm (p = 0.002), BMI ≥ 30 kg/m² (p = 0.009), and previous

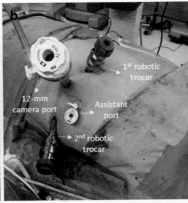
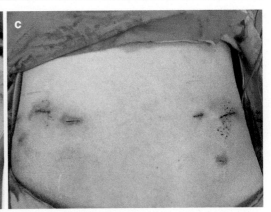

Fig. 13.1 Intraoperative photos demonstrating the placement of trocars for bilateral robotic adrenalectomy through posterior retroperitoneal approach. (**a**) Placement of trocars for right adrenalectomy. (**b**) Placement of trocars for left adrenalectomy. (**c**) Picture showing bilateral trocar placement sites after skin closure

history of abdominal operation ($p = 0.042$). Multiple regression model confirmed the decreased operative time with RA in patients with tumors larger than 6 cm ($p = 0.01$).

Preoperative Planning

Preoperatively, all patients undergo abdominal CT scan and a thorough hormonal workup for the adrenal mass. Patients with pheochromocytoma require 3 weeks of α-blockade with phenoxybenzamine preoperatively. In patients with primary hyperaldosteronism, lateralization of the disease may require adrenal venous sampling in select patients.

At our institution, selection between PR vs TL approach is made according to a laparoscopic selection algorithm we have previously reported [21]. This algorithm takes into consideration the preoperative CT as well as the preoperative examination. We prefer LT approach in patients with tumors larger than 6 cm. In patients with smaller tumors, PR approach is preferred if the measured distance on CT scan between the skin and Gerota's fascia is less than 7 cm and the 12th rib is rostral to the renal hilum. Meeting these criteria allows efficient movement of the robotic arms after docking. Also, PR approach is preferred in patients with bilateral tumors and with extensive adhesions from prior abdominal surgeries. When patients are selected appropriately, both approaches have comparable outcomes [16].

Setup

Robotic Posterior Retroperitoneal Adrenalectomy

The patient is placed on a Wilson frame in prone jackknife position after intubation and administration of anesthesia.

An incision is made below the 12th rib, and a 12 mm optical trocar is introduced (Fig. 13.1). After entering Gerota's space, the optical trocar is removed and a balloon trocar is inserted. With the help of the balloon trocar, a potential space is created under direct visualization. Then, the balloon trocar is removed, and the space is insufflated with CO_2 to a pressure of 15 mmHg. On medial and lateral sides of the first trocar, two more 5 or 8 mm trocars are placed. Depending on surgeon's preference, one more 5 or 8 mm trocar can be inserted for the first assistant. For docking, the robot is brought in from the head-side end of the table, in between the patient's shoulders. Fine adjustment is made depending on the location of the adrenal gland. When mandated by the patient's anatomy, the operating table may be rotated.

Robotic Lateral Transabdominal Adrenalectomy

The patient is intubated and anesthesia is administered. Then, the patient is placed on right or left lateral decubitus position on a beanbag, and the table is flexed at the flank. An incision is made midway in between the umbilicus and the costal margin, and a 12 mm optical trocar is introduced (Fig. 13.2). After the peritoneal space is entered, the abdomen is insufflated with CO_2 to a pressure of 15 mmHg. Following insufflation, two 8 mm and one 15 mm trocars are inserted below the costal margin in a configuration that would allow the first assistant to operate the suction/irrigation device and the clip applier when needed. Usually, the assistant port is the most medial one for right-sided and the most lateral one for left-sided tumors. In obese patients and in patients with short stature, the position of the first assistant trocar may be changed as needed. In obese patients, adequate retraction is critical. For right-sided tumors, retraction is maintained by a self-retain-

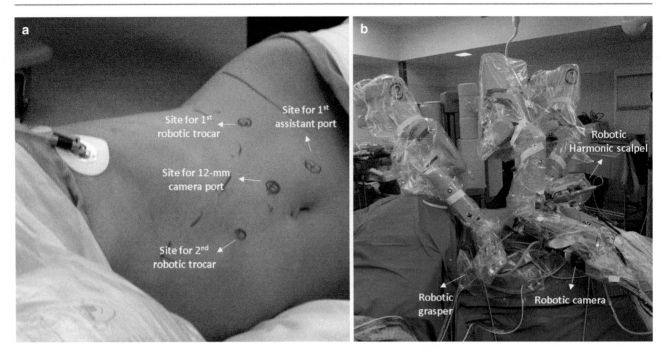

Fig. 13.2 Intraoperative pictures describing the placement of trocars for left robotic adrenalectomy through lateral transabdominal approach. For left adrenalectomy, the patient is placed in right lateral decubitus position. (**a**) Preoperative marking of trocar placement sites. (**b**) Photo demonstrating the surgical setup after completion of docking

ing laparoscopic liver retractor introduced through a 5 mm port. For left-sided tumors, the fourth robotic arm is used for retraction. For docking, the robot is brought in from above the ipsilateral shoulder. The operating table may be rotated depending on the patient's anatomy.

Procedure

Robotic Posterior Retroperitoneal Adrenalectomy

We use a hybrid laparoscopic-robotic technique (Fig. 13.3). In this hybrid technique, the exposure of the retroperitoneal space and the retrieval of the specimen after completion of dissection are done laparoscopically. The dissection of the adrenal gland is carried robotically.

Ports are positioned as described in the setup, and the retroperitoneal space is developed using laparoscopic instruments. Following adequate exposure, laparoscopic ultrasound is performed to help localize the adrenal gland. After completion of the ultrasound, the robot is docked. A robotic grasper is introduced from the lateral port and a robotic vessel sealer from the medial port. The instruments may be changed as needed. First, superior and lateral borders of the adrenal gland are dissected. Next, the inferior border is mobilized, and the medial border is dissected the last. The adrenal vein is

identified and divided depending on its size either with the vessel sealer or with 5 mm clips deployed by the first assistant. If clips are used, they can be introduced through the first assistant port. When a first assistant port is not present, the vessel sealer is removed temporarily and the medial port can be used for this purpose. When needed, suctioning can be done in a similar manner. After the completion of dissection, the robot is undocked, and the specimen is removed laparoscopically using a specimen retrieval bag. Tumors larger than 3 cm can be morcellated to help with removal. The fascial incision for the 12 mm port and all skin incisions are closed.

Robotic Lateral Transabdominal Adrenalectomy

As in PR approach, a hybrid laparoscopic-robotic technique is utilized. Initial hepatic/splenic mobilization and removal of the specimen after completion of dissection are done laparoscopically. The adrenal gland is dissected robotically.

Ports are positioned as described in the setup. For left-sided tumors, the splenocolic and splenorenal ligaments need to be divided to expose the adrenal gland. For right-sided tumors, the right triangular ligament is divided and the liver is mobilized. This initial exposure is performed laparoscopically. After adequate exposure, laparoscopic ultrasound is

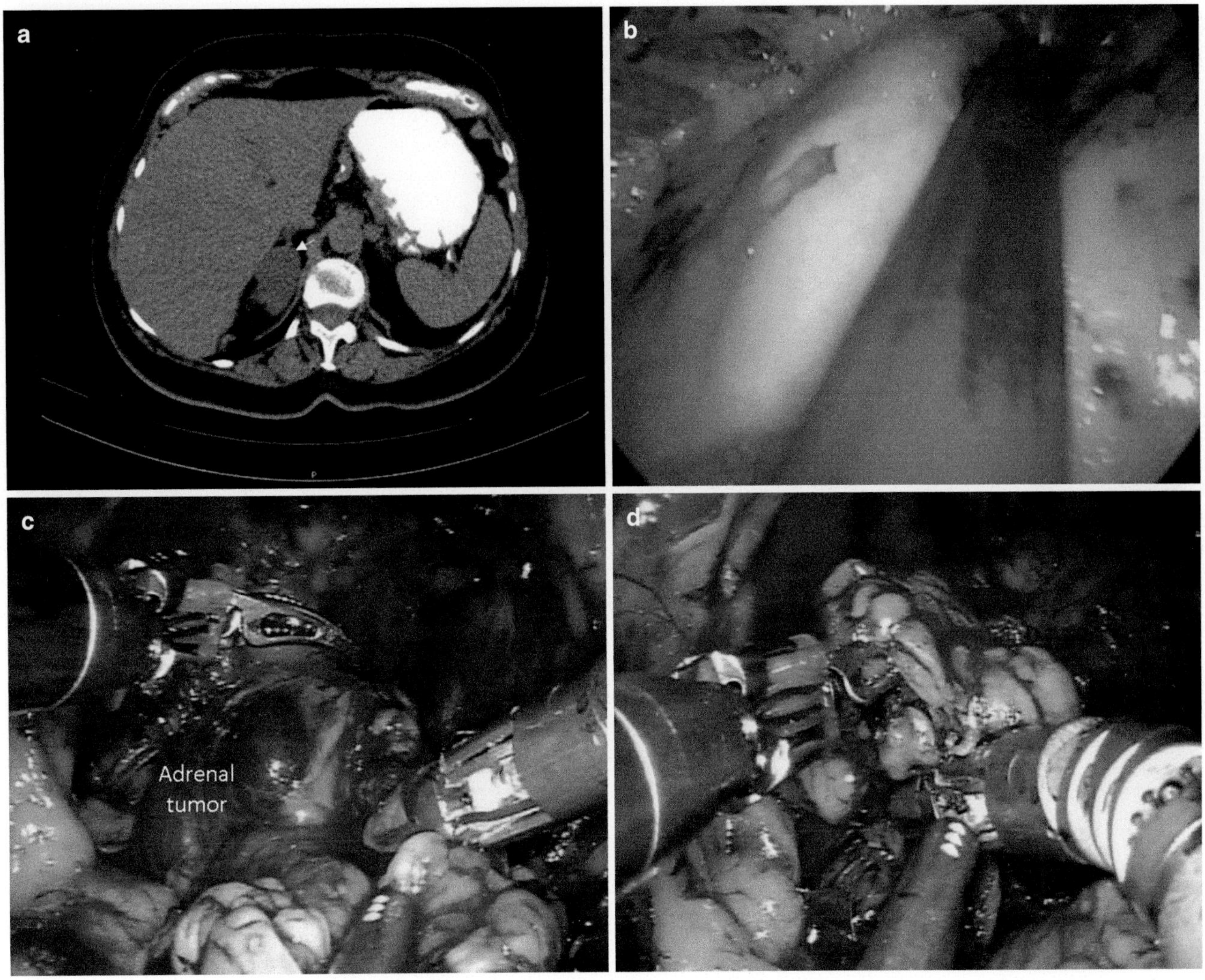

Fig. 13.3 Preoperative CT scan and intraoperative captures of a 4.6 cm right adrenal cyst removed robotically through posterior retroperitoneal approach. (**a**) Preoperative CT scan showing the right-sided adrenal cyst. Arrow points at the lesion. (**b**) Intraoperative laparoscopic ultrasound for the localization of the adrenal gland. (**c**) Dissection of the tumor with the help of a robotic grasper (on the left-hand side) and a robotic vessel sealer (right-hand side). Suction/irrigation device (at the bottom) is operated laparoscopically by the first assistant. (**d**) Division of the adrenal vein using the robotic vessel sealer

performed. The robot is docked after completion of the ultrasound. As in PR approach, the superior and lateral borders are dissected first, followed by the inferior, and finally the medial border (Fig. 13.4). The adrenal vein is divided either with the vessel sealer or by applying clips. After completion of adrenal dissection, the robot is undocked. The tumor is removed laparoscopically using a specimen retrieval bag. Twelve millimeter trocar fascial incisions and all skin incisions are closed.

Postoperative Care

Most patients require an overnight hospital stay. Diet is started in the recovery room, narcotics avoided, and ambulation encouraged. Next morning, a complete blood count and a basic metabolic panel are obtained. Patients with Cushing's syndrome are started on stress dose steroids and discharged home on oral hydrocortisone. Patients without evidence of Cushing's have their cortisol levels checked the next morning. If greater than 10 µg/dl, oral steroids are not required at discharge. If the patient exhibits signs of adrenal insufficiency or AM cortisol level is less than 10 µg/dl, the patient is placed on steroids and needs to follow up with endocrinology. Patients with primary hyperaldosteronism also have their aldosterone and renin levels checked the next morning. Catecholamine levels in patients with pheochromocytoma are checked in a month and then annually.

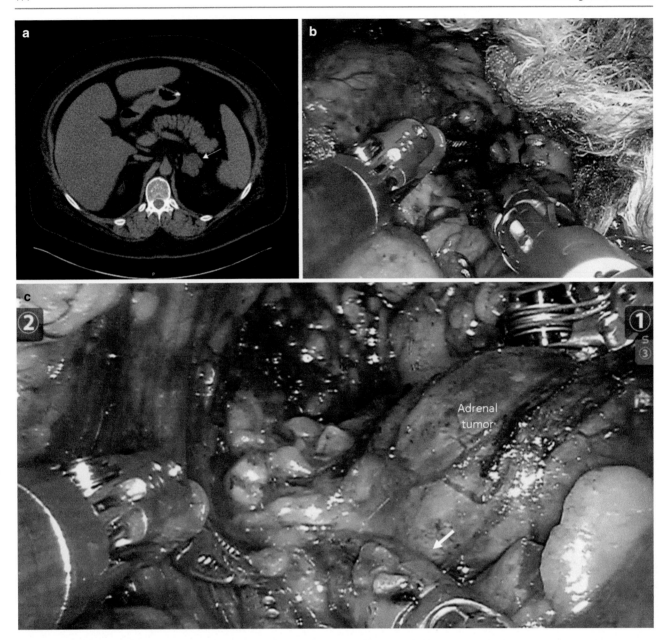

Fig. 13.4 Preoperative CT scan and intraoperative photos of a 3.6 cm left-sided adrenal tumor causing Cushing's syndrome. The tumor was removed robotically through lateral transabdominal approach. (**a**) 3.6 cm left adrenal tumor on CT scan. Arrow points at the tumor. (**b**) Intraoperative photo demonstrating the dissection of the tumor using a robotic grasper (left-hand side) and a robotic vessel sealer (right-hand side). (**c**) Division of the adrenal vein using a laparoscopic clip applier operated by the first assistant. Arrow points at the laparoscopic clip applier

References

1. Gagner M, Lacroix A, Bolte E. Laparoscopic adrenalectomy in Cushing's syndrome and pheochromocytoma. N Engl J Med. 1992;327(14):1033.
2. Sommerey S, Foroghi Y, Chiapponi C, Baumbach SF, Hallfeldt KK, Ladurner R, et al. Laparoscopic adrenalectomy – 10-year experience at a teaching hospital. Langenbeck's Arch Surg. 2015;400(3):341–7.
3. Eichhorn-Wharry LI, Talpos GB, Rubinfeld I. Laparoscopic versus open adrenalectomy: another look at outcome using the Clavien classification system. Surgery. 2012;152(6):1090–5.
4. Piazza L, Caragliano P, Scardilli M, Sgroi AV, Marino G, Giannone G. Laparoscopic robot-assisted right adrenalectomy and left ovariectomy (case reports). Chir Ital. 1999 Nov-Dec;51(6): 465–6.
5. Hubens G, Ysebaert D, Vaneerdeweg W, Chapelle T, Eyskens E. Laparoscopic adrenalectomy with the aid of the AESOP 2000 robot. Acta Chir Belg. 1999;99(3):125–7; discussion 127–9.
6. Brandao LF, Autorino R, Laydner H, Haber GP, Ouzaid I, De Sio M, et al. Robotic versus laparoscopic adrenalectomy: a systematic review and meta-analysis. Eur Urol. 2014;65(6):1154–61.
7. Horgan S, Vanuno D. Robots in laparoscopic surgery. J Laparoendosc Adv Surg Tech A. 2001;11(6):415–9.

8. Gill IS, Sung GT, Hsu TH, Meraney AM. Robotic remote laparoscopic nephrectomy and adrenalectomy: the initial experience. J Urol. 2000;164(6):2082–5.

9. Morino M, Beninca G, Giraudo G, Del Genio GM, Rebecchi F, Garrone C. Robot-assisted vs laparoscopic adrenalectomy: a prospective randomized controlled trial. Surg Endosc. 2004;18(12): 1742–6.

10. Winter JM, Talamini MA, Stanfield CL, Chang DC, Hundt JD, Dackiw AP, et al. Thirty robotic adrenalectomies: a single institution's experience. Surg Endosc. 2006;20(1):119–24.

11. Brunaud L, Ayav A, Zarnegar R, Rouers A, Klein M, Boissel P, et al. Prospective evaluation of 100 robotic-assisted unilateral adrenalectomies. Surgery. 2008;144(6):995–1001; discussion 1001.

12. Giulianotti PC, Buchs NC, Addeo P, Bianco FM, Ayloo SM, Caravaglios G, et al. Robot-assisted adrenalectomy: a technical option for the surgeon? Int J Med Robot. 2011;7(1):27–32.

13. Nordenstrom E, Westerdahl J, Hallgrimsson P, Bergenfelz A. A prospective study of 100 robotically assisted laparoscopic adrenalectomies. J Robot Surg. 2011;5(2):127–31.

14. Agcaoglu O, Aliyev S, Karabulut K, Siperstein A, Berber E. Robotic vs laparoscopic posterior retroperitoneal adrenalectomy. Arch Surg. 2012;147(3):272–5.

15. D'Annibale A, Lucandri G, Monsellato I, De Angelis M, Pernazza G, Alfano G, et al. Robotic adrenalectomy: technical aspects, early results and learning curve. Int J Med Robot. 2012;8(4):483–90.

16. Karabulut K, Agcaoglu O, Aliyev S, Siperstein A, Berber E. Comparison of intraoperative time use and perioperative outcomes for robotic versus laparoscopic adrenalectomy. Surgery. 2012;151(4):537–42.

17. Aksoy E, Taskin HE, Aliyev S, Mitchell J, Siperstein A, Berber E. Robotic versus laparoscopic adrenalectomy in obese patients. Surg Endosc. 2013;27(4):1233–6.

18. Pineda-Solis K, Medina-Franco H, Heslin MJ. Robotic versus laparoscopic adrenalectomy: a comparative study in a high-volume center. Surg Endosc. 2013;27(2):599–602.

19. Brandao LF, Autorino R, Zargar H, Krishnan J, Laydner H, Akca O, et al. Robot-assisted laparoscopic adrenalectomy: step-by-step technique and comparative outcomes. Eur Urol. 2014;66(5):898–905.

20. Morelli L, Tartaglia D, Bronzoni J, Palmeri M, Guadagni S, Di Franco G, et al. Robotic assisted versus pure laparoscopic surgery of the adrenal glands: a case-control study comparing surgical techniques. Langenbeck's Arch Surg. 2016;401(7):999–1006.

21. Agcaoglu O, Sahin DA, Siperstein A, Berber E. Selection algorithm for posterior versus lateral approach in laparoscopic adrenalectomy. Surgery. 2012;151(5):731–5.

Robotic Right and Left Colectomy

14

Sandeep S. Vijan

Introduction

Approximately 135,000 individuals in the United States are diagnosed with colorectal cancer every year [1]. Surgical colectomy is the centerpiece of care for most patients. Our role as surgeons is integral to battling this disease that claims 50,000 lives annually [1]. Our surgical principles teach us to provide a safe, oncologic operation, with a steadfast recovery and return to normal function. Today, we can all agree that a minimally invasive approach fulfills these criteria [2]. Robotic surgery aims to increase the penetrance of minimally invasive surgery. Enhanced 3D visualization and wristed instrumentation allow a 50% increase in manual dexterity and a 93% reduction in skills-based errors [3]. Despite these technological advancements, robotic surgery has been surrounded by a shroud of controversy. In colorectal surgery, multiple studies [4–6] have demonstrated safety, efficacy, and oncologic adequacy; however lack of improvement in clinical outcomes and apparent increased costs [7] have weighed on the practice. More recently, however, clinical improvements in terms of lower conversion rates, especially in obese, male patients, with low rectal cancers [8] and reductions in length of stay in complicated diverticulitis [9] have been documented. This seemingly parallels my personal clinical experience; and I propose that earlier studies have been limited by older generation machines and the lack of routine application of intracorporeal anastomotic techniques. Despite sequential years of controversy, robotic surgery today is more widely utilized than ever before. The newer robots (da Vinci Xi©, Intuitive Surgical, Sunnyvale, CA) are more efficient and agile and have extended range of motion. These features allow for single docking operations in multiple abdominal quadrants and the performance of a *routine intracorporeal anastomosis*. It is the feasibility of this internal anastomosis construct that has proven

reductions in length of hospital stay, postoperative narcotic use, accelerated gastrointestinal recovery, and lower wound morbidity [10–12]. Even more relevant in the longer term is the decreased incisional hernia risk with non-midline specimen extraction [13] or even natural orifice (trans-anal) extraction that is facilitated by a robotic approach. In the following chapter, I share the robotic surgical techniques for a true minimally invasive right and left hemicolectomy, with an completely intracorporeal anastomosis, so that your patients may benefit as much as mine.

Indications and Contraindications

The indications for a robotic colectomy in surgical practice are similar to traditional open or laparoscopic techniques. While malignant neoplasm is a common indication, benign adenomatous polyps often require a colectomy, especially those larger than 1 cm, sessile, or simply not amenable to endoscopic resection for anatomic or technical reasons. Benign polyps with suspicious pathologic features also warrant colectomy, due to the risk of occult malignancy. Diverticular disease, inflammatory bowel disease, and enteric duplication cysts round up the other common indications for surgical colectomy.

More importantly, however, are the contraindications to a minimally invasive colectomy. Most contraindications are *relative* but ultimately rest on accurate localization of disease, patient's comorbid conditions, and surgeon expertise. I usually refrain from robotic colectomy in cases of intestinal obstruction and multi-visceral organ involvement and for patients in whom prolonged pneumoperitoneum is deemed unsafe. Intestinal obstructions pose very specific surgical challenges. Namely, lack of operative domain due to dilated bowel and friability of bowel, resulting in increased risk of iatrogenic injury with minimal instrument manipulation. Multi-visceral resections are certainly selectively possible, robotically, but these are not the cases to initiate your practice. Lastly, patients at risk of intra-abdominal adhesive

S. S. Vijan
Sangre de Cristo Surgical Associates P.C.,
Parkview Medical Center, Pueblo, CO, USA
e-mail: sandeep_vijan@parkviewmc.com

© Springer Nature Switzerland AG 2019
S. Tsuda, O. Y. Kudsi (eds.), *Robotic-Assisted Minimally Invasive Surgery*, https://doi.org/10.1007/978-3-319-96866-7_14

disease, such as those whom have had multiple prior laparotomies, should be approached with caution and evaluated by diagnostic laparoscopy to judge the feasibility of a robotic procedure.

Surgical Planning

A thorough history and physical, basic blood work including a serum carcinoembryonic antigen and axial imaging are essential for all cancer patients. Of utmost importance in the era of robotic colectomy is localization of disease. There is little to no haptic feedback with current robotic instrumentation. The extent of resection in robotic colectomy must be determined well before any surgical incision is made. Polyps and smaller neoplasms must be accurately localized on colonoscopy, and I encourage my fellow gastroenterologists to routinely, and liberally, tattoo (with India ink) both the proximal and distal margin of any suspicious lesions. The tattoo marks usually stay in situ for several months after the index endoscopy. If there is any concern regarding the location of a lesion, then enhanced CT abdomen and pelvis with rectal contrast or a barium enema can be of immense value. As a last resort, certain patients will need a repeat colonoscopy *by the surgeon*, for surgical planning. Although this is uncomfortable and duplicative for our patients, it is often a necessary step to facilitate an oncologically appropriate, minimally invasive operation.

Bowel preparation in colorectal surgery has been the source of much debate over the last few decades. However, contemporary data from the National Surgical Quality Improvement Project has clearly demonstrated that the use of a mechanical bowel prep in conjunction with oral antibiotics reduces nearly by half the risks of surgical site infection, anastomotic leakage, and postoperative ileus [14]. Hence, as a routine, combination of mechanical and antimicrobial bowel preparation is recommended for all patients undergoing a robotic colectomy.

Robotic Instrumentation and Technology

Currently, the only FDA-approved surgical robots that are capable of intestinal surgery are the da Vinci Si© and Xi© machines (Intuitive Surgical, Sunnyvale, CA). The surgical techniques described in this chapter will revolve entirely around these machines and their many accouterments. The majority of the text is devoted to the Xi system, which is my robot of choice to facilitate an efficient colectomy. Before we continue, it is essential to devote some time to a discussion around the variety of instruments that are necessary for a robotic colectomy.

Grasping Forceps

Two graspers are necessary in a robotic colectomy. A Cadiere (Si) or Fenestrated Bipolar (Xi) grasper is usually my left-handed instrument. Both harness the power of bipolar energy and have similar short lengths (28 mm) and medium jaw closing strength. They are atraumatic to healthy bowel. My right-handed instrument is a large grasping forceps (Si) or Tip-Up fenestrated grasper (Xi). Both are devoid of energy, are longer, and have even lower jaw closing strength. These are also atraumatic to any bowel.

Energy Devices

Monopolar energy with a da Vinci Endowrist® scissor is used throughout a robotic colectomy, much like a laparoscopic scissor, however more versatile due to the addition of an articulating wrist. The da Vinci Endowrist® Vessel Sealer is a bipolar energy device, coupled with a knife. Similar in principle to the more familiar LigaSure™ (Covidien/Medtronic, Minneapolis, MN), it will coagulate vessels safely unto 7 mm diameter and then is able to divide the tissue. Key difference emerges with the articulated wrist that allows for 90° approaches to vascular pedicles. It operates much cooler than its contemporaries, and lateral thermal spread is very minimal. Of special note, I find the jaws to be essentially bulky, allowing for its use as a blunt dissector. It is my instrument of choice for the entire mesenteric ligation portion of the procedure.

Stapler

The da Vinci Endowrist® 45 mm stapler is a significant step forward in stapling technology.

Although shorter than traditional laparoscopic staplers, its greater articulation allows for reach in tight quarters such as the pelvis. In comparison to currently available laparoscopic staplers, using the robotic stapler is both cost-effective, and there is a clear *trend* in decreasing anastomotic leakage (not statistically significant) [15]. Central to this trend is SmartClamp® technology, which gives immediate feedback to the user regarding the adequacy of stapler sealing. This allows for real-time adjustments to the amount of tissue being stapled and the potential to upsize staple cartridge thickness if clinical necessary. Vascular (white, 1 mm closed staple height) and bowel (blue, 1.5 mm, and green, 2 mm, closed staple height) cartridges are available. This stapler provides two secure rows of staples on either side of transected tissue.

Needle Driver

There are two types of needle drivers available for robotic use. A Mega Needle driver has a small cutting knife in the proximal joint, whereas a Large Needle driver is bladeless. Both have articulating wrists and provide significant dexterity during intracorporeal suturing. A word of caution, these are traumatic instruments and should *never* be used to grab intestines or any vulnerable anatomic structure.

Firefly® Technology

Standard equipment on the Xi robot, and an add-on technology for the Si machine, is fluorescence angiography. Intravenous administration of 8 mg indocyanine green dye during colectomy will provide real-time information on adequacy of vascular perfusion. "Firefly mode" allows the surgeon to visualize mesenteric and intestinal perfusion, which will fluoresce bright green. Perfusion is obvious within 60 s of administration and valid for 2–3 min. Emerging data proposes that use of this new technology could decrease the risk of anastomotic leakage [16]. I use this technology routinely during colectomy both before staple transection and after construction of anastomosis.

Right Colectomy

Surgical Position and Setup

The patient is positioned supine and secured on the operating room table. Pressure points are padded. Arms are preferably tucked on both sides. Laparoscopic access can be obtained using a traditional cutdown technique or an optical trocar system. My preference is optical access in the left subcostal area; the disposable trocar can then be exchanged for a metal 12 mm robotic trocar. The operative table is then repositioned to 30° Trendelenburg and 30° of left tilt. A robotic colectomy is a four-arm procedure; hence four robotic trocars are necessary. Port positions and trocar sizes are depicted in Figs. 14.1 and 14.2, for Xi and Si systems, respectively. Three 8 mm trocars are routine, with a 12 mm trocar used for the robotic stapler. An optional 5 mm assistant trocar site is also demonstrated, to assist with retraction and suction. The versatile, boom-mounted, Xi robot can be docked from any angle, either from the left or right side of the patient. However, the Si robot must be docked over the right hip or right shoulder. Xi robotic instruments are inserted under laparoscopic visualization as follows: arm 1 holds a Fenestrated Bipolar grasper, arm 2 holds a 30° camera, and arm 3

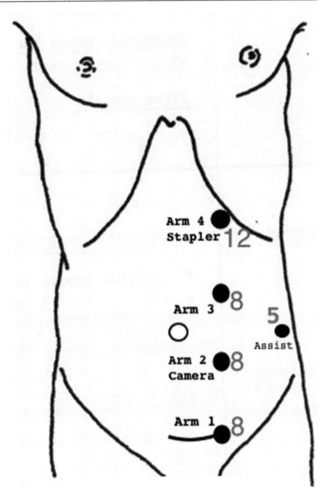

Fig. 14.1 Right colectomy trocar positions, Xi

sequentially holds the monopolar scissor, then the Vessel Sealer, and eventually a needle driver. Arm 4 holds a Tip-Up grasper, later exchanged with a robotic 45 mm blue load stapler. At this point, the surgeon commences the operation at the robotic console. The assistant remains as bedside, usually on the left side of the patient.

Initial Mobilization

The aforementioned setup allows the best visualization for a medial-to-lateral mobilization of the right colon. If the surgeon is more comfortable with a lateral-to-medial approach, this too is easily accomplished with an identical trocar setup. More often, a hybrid approach is necessary. The cecum is grasped with the Tip-Up grasper and retracted anteriorly. The small bowel is swept to into the left upper quadrant. This exposes the root of the cecal mesocolon, wherein the ileocolic pedicle is visualized. Using the

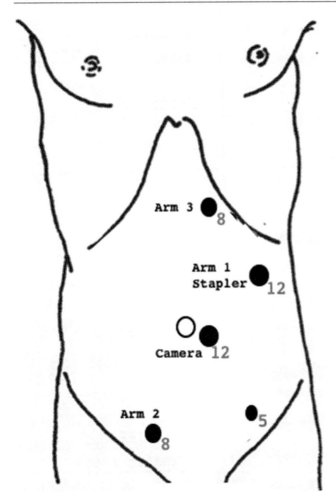

Fig. 14.2 Right colectomy trocar positions, Si

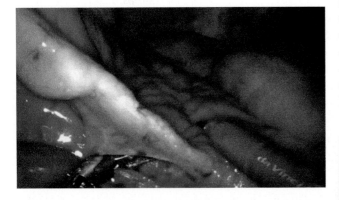

Fig. 14.3 Identification of ileocolic pedicle to begin mobilization

monopolar scissor, the peritoneum over the base of the ileocolic pedicle is incised (Fig. 14.3), extending caudally into the mesentery and cranially into naturally occurring clear space in the mesocolon. Using blunt dissection with the scissors as the right-handed instrument and the Fenestrated Bipolar grasper as the left-handed instrument, we can enter the space between the mesocolon and retro-

peritoneum. There mere presence of pneumoperitoneum facilitates this dissection. The correct plane is identified by wisps of tissue resembling a cobweb and the near absence of bleeding. At this point, the ileocolic pedicle can be divided at its base using the Vessel Sealer, or robotic clips, or even a vascular load robotic stapler, inserted into arm 4. The next step is to identify the *left ureter* and *duodenum* in this dissected plane. Great care must be taken to preserve both these structures in their entirety. Using the scissors or Vessel Sealer as a blunt instrument, the entire hemicolon can be mobilized from the terminal ileum to the hepatic flexure, until the white line of Toldt is completely divided. At this point, the hepatic flexure is retracted caudally with the Tip-Up grasper, and the lesser sac is entered through the gastrocolic omentum with the Vessel Sealer. Dissection is continued to divide the hepatocolic ligament and completely mobilize the hepatic flexure of the colon. Position change of the patient reverse Trendelenburg is not usually necessary given the minor degree of Trendelenburg used at the beginning of the case.

Mesocolic Vascular Ligation and Transection

Once mobilization is complete, the Vessel Sealer is used to divide the mesentery of the terminal ileum and ligate the right colic pedicle and associated mesocolon, proceeding to the right branch of the middle colic vessels (Fig. 14.4). Of note, mesentery of the terminal ileum should be taken 25 cm proximal to the ileocecal valve for an adequate lymphadenectomy. The robotic 45 mm stapler, blue load, is introduced into arm 4, after removing the Tip-Up grasper. Division of the proximal transverse colon requires two staple loads, and division of three terminal ileum requires an additional load. Sites of transection are guided by extent of mesenteric clearance and use of Firefly®. The divided and disconnected specimen can be left in situ or, if bulky, placed over the right lobe of the liver, for later extraction.

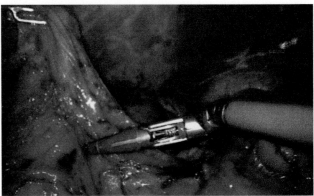

Fig. 14.4 Division of right branch of middle colic vessels

Intracorporeal Anastomosis

After ensuring that the terminal ileum is mobile, by dividing its retroperitoneal attachments, the anastomosis can be constructed. The ileum must be brought up to the right upper quadrant and placed in an isoperistaltic or antiperistaltic fashion, adjacent to the transverse colon. Using a robotic needle driver and a single 2-0 silk suture (cut to 15 cm), the anti-mesenteric surfaces must be approximated. This silk suture serves as an anchor to suspend the bowel loops anteriorly, with a Tip-Up grasper, typically in arm 3. Next, a monopolar scissor is inserted in arm 4, and a 1 cm enterotomy and colotomy are made, adjacent to each other, approximately 45 mm away from the anchoring silk. As long as the patient has received a bowel prep, the pneumoperitoneum (which is greater than intraluminal pressure) prevents enteric spillage. Another blue load of the robotic stapler is then inserted through arm 4, and a side-to-side ileocolic anastomosis is created (Fig. 14.5). The common channel or stapler access enterotomy then must be closed. My preference is to use an absorbable 3-0 V-Loc™ (Covidien, Minneapolis, MN), 9 inches long, with a robotic needle driver in arm 4, to close the defect (Fig. 14.6). A two-layered closure is recommended: the first layer approximates mucosa and submuco-

sal, and the second layer is a buttress of seromuscular Lembert. Alternatively, this can be closed with an additional blue stapler load. The mesenteric defect is not closed routinely. The anastomosis is wrapped in a tongue of omentum and allowed to anatomically retract into the right upper quadrant, where it is under least tension.

Specimen Extraction

Once the anastomosis is constructed, secure hemostasis is achieved; arm 1 is undocked, and the specimen is grasped by the assistant using a locking laparoscopic bowel grasper. The surgeon now scrubs back to the patient's bedside, the remaining robotic instruments are removed, and the robot is undocked and stowed. All trocars are removed. The trocar site of arm 1 is expanded medially using a Pfannenstiel technique. A wound protector is inserted, and the specimen is removed. The specimen is oriented for the pathologist and sent off for review in formalin. The fascia of the specimen extraction site is closed with running absorbable suture. The fascia of the left upper quadrant 12 mm trocar site must also be closed. Skin is closed, dressings are applied, and the operation is deemed complete.

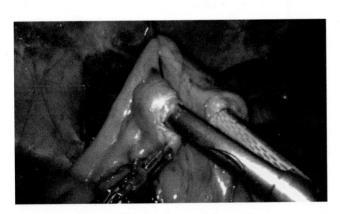

Fig. 14.5 Creation of a side-to-side isoperistaltic stapled ileocolic anastomosis

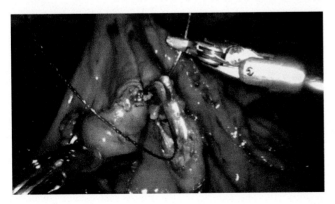

Fig. 14.6 Intracorporeal suture closure of common enterotomy

Left (Sigmoid) Colectomy

Surgical Position and Setup

After induction of general anesthesia, the patient is positioned in lithotomy using Allen stirrups, taking off the foot piece of the operating table. Arms are preferably tucked; pressure points must be padded. It is important to secure the patient to the operating table with a safety strap or nonslip padding. Port positions and trocar sizes are depicted in Figs. 14.7 and 14.8, for Xi and Si systems, respectively. With that schema in mind, I commence the operation in the right lower quadrant, with a transverse 3–4 cm skin incision over McBurney's point. A muscle-splitting approach is used, much like the approach to a traditional appendectomy. Once access to the abdomen is accomplished, an Alexis® wound retractor (Applied Medical, Rancho Santa Margarita, CA) with its cap cover is placed in this incision. This site is extremely multifunctional, as the initial camera port, stapler port, anvil introduction site, specimen extraction site, and ultimately a diverting loop ileostomy site if indicated. A 12 mm robotic trocar is inserted directly through the cap, and pneumoperitoneum is insufflated. At this point, I tend to use a little more Trendelenburg, 35°–40°, with 35° of right tilt in a left colectomy, than in right colectomy. Three additional 8 mm robotic trocars are placed, creating a gentle half-moon or oblique line, parallel to the sigmoid colon. An optional

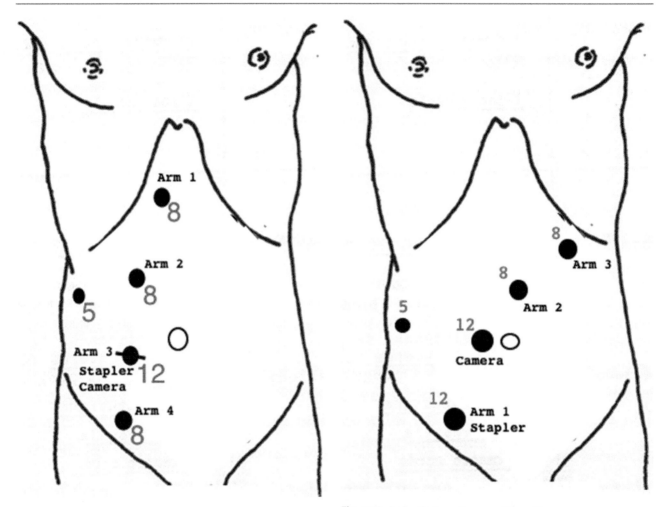

Fig. 14.7 Left colectomy trocar positions, Xi

Fig. 14.8 Left colectomy trocar positions, Si

5 mm assistant port is usually placed laterally in the right abdomen, behind the 12 mm trocar site. Once again, the Xi robot can be docked from either side, but the Si must be docked over the left hip. Xi robotic instruments are inserted under laparoscopic visualization as follows: arm 1 holds a Tip-Up grasper, arm 2 holds a Fenestrated Bipolar grasper, and arm 3 sequentially holds the 30° camera and then is replaced by a robotic 45 mm blue load stapler. Arm 4 holds a monopolar scissor, later exchanged with a Vessel Sealer. At this point, the surgeon retreats to the robotic console. The assistant remains as bedside, typically on the right side of the patient.

Initial Mobilization

The sigmoid colon is grasped with the Tip-Up grasper and retracted anteriorly; and the small bowel is swept into the right upper quadrant, clearing the pelvic brim. Using the monopoly scissor, the peritoneum over the root of the sigmoid mesocolon is incised. The inferior mesenteric artery

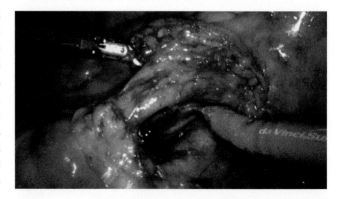

Fig. 14.9 Isolation of inferior mesenteric artery pedicle

pedicle is identified and dissected free, during the medial-to-lateral blunt dissection (Fig. 14.9). Here, the left ureter should be identified in the retroperitoneum (Fig. 14.10). As the cobweb tissue is blunt dissected, the mesocolon is retracted anteriorly, and the retroperitoneum is pushed posteriorly. The large jaws of the Vessel Sealer, inserted through arm 4, in lieu of the scissor, are perfect for this blunt

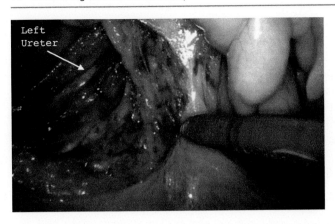

Fig. 14.10 Medial-to-lateral mobilization, identification of left ureter

dissection. As mobilization proceeds proximally to the splenic flexure, the Tip-Up grasper (arm 1) is used to retract the descending colon medially and caudally. The vessel sealer is used to divide the anterior abdominal wall adhesions of the splenic flexure and the spleno-colic ligament. Without table position change, even entry into the lesser sac is possible through the gastrocolic omentum. As the splenic flexure is mobilized and retracted medially, the inferior mesenteric vein comes into view. Given this anticipation of an intracorporeal anastomosis, extensive splenic flexure mobilization is rarely necessary, as the colon will not need to be exteriorized at all. Next, the scissor is reintroduced in arm 4, and the lateral sigmoid colon adhesions are divided, and mobilization is complete unto the white line of Toldt. Incising the peritoneum on either side of the upper rectum allows the pneumoperitoneum to expose the lateral upper rectal stalks which, based on surgical anatomy, may or may not need to be divided (Vessel Sealer). In cases of diverticular disease, mobilization of the upper rectum is essential to expose healthy, diverticula-free rectum for reanastomosis.

Mesocolic Vascular Ligation and Transection

I routinely use the Vessel Sealer to divide the skeletonized inferior mesenteric artery pedicle. Frequently, this is accomplished in more than one bite. I prefer a "Seal-Seal-Cut" approach to major vascular pedicles, in which the base of the pedicle is coagulated first and then coagulated again 5 mm distally before being cut. This allows two layers of thermal sealing on a vessel that has systolic blood pressure behind it. Alternatively, robotic clips or vascular load stapler can be used. The Vessel Sealer in arm 4 is used to divide the mesocolon proximally to the descending colon/sigmoid colon junction and distally to the rectosigmoid junction. This allows for a wide lymphadenectomy, both in cases of neoplasm, as well in those patients with a bulky mesenteric abscess from diverticulitis. Firefly® technology is critical in

assessment of perfusion of the margin artery and proximal colon. Once the mesocolon is completely divided, the camera is hopped to arm 2, removing the Fenestrated Bipolar grasper. The robotic stapler with a green load (1.5 mm closed staple height) is introduced into arm 3. The rectosigmoid junction is herein divided. At this point, the sigmoid colon is pushed into the pelvis, to judge adequacy of length of the proximal colon for construct of the anastomosis. If further mobilization of the splenic flexure is necessary, now is the time. The camera remains in arm 2 for the remainder of the operation.

Intracorporeal Anastomosis

Once satisfied with proximal colonic length, the anvil of an end-to-end anastomotic stapler (EEA) is introduced though the wound retractor in the right lower quadrant. Routinely, a 29 mm size is adequate for most patients, but one can upsize or downsize based on the diameter and flexibility of the colon. *Tip:* Fenestrated Bipolar grasper measures 28 mm from wrist to tip and is a useful measuring tool. The anvil requires a little preparation by the assistant who remains sterile. A dyed, 6-inch, 0-V-Loc™ (Covidien, Minneapolis, MN) is passed through the spike of the anvil and looped through the "eye" at the tail of the suture. The needle is cut off and the suture is left long. The anvil is introduced by the assistant and temporarily placed in the left lower quadrant. This requires removal of the robotic stapler and undocking of arm 3. Arm 3 can be re-docked, and monopolar scissor is inserted. A needle driver will need to be inserted in arm 4. Next, on the descending colon, a transverse 3 cm colotomy is made with the scissor on the anti-mesenteric border. The prepared anvil is inserted through the colotomy into the descending colon, such that only the 0-V-Loc is visible exiting the colon (Fig. 14.11). Use the Tip-Up grasper in arm 1 to hold the proximal descending colon anteriorly (to prevent

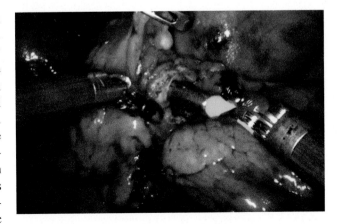

Fig. 14.11 Intracorporeal insertion of stapler anvil

excessive proximal anvil migration). The colotomy is then closed with a whip stitch of 3-0 V-Loc; the anvil suture should exit through the middle of the repair. The robotic stapler with a blue load (1.5 mm closed staple height) is reintroduced in arm 3. The proximal descending colon is amputated just proximal to the repaired colotomy. The anvil suture is usually cut by the stapler, but its dyed color is usually visible in the proximal staple line. That nub of suture can be grasped with the needle driver, and the anvil can be "popped" out through the descending colon staple line (Fig. 14.12). The spike of the anvil is then removed by holding the 0-V-Loc with a needle driver in the right hand and an open Tip-Up grasper at the anvil base in the left hand. The spike is then retrieved by the assistant.

My work flow is to remain at the console, while my trained assistant will insert the receptacle of the EEA stapler trans-anally. As I remain in robotic control, using the Tip-Up grasper, the anvil and receptacle are reconnected intracorporeally (Fig. 14.13). The EEA stapler is closed, fired, and removed. The assistant performs rigid proctoscopy with air insufflation, while the surgeon occludes the proximal descending colon with the atraumatic Tip-Up grasper. The

scrub tech can fill the pelvis with saline, using a laparoscopic suction irrigator. This completes the standard "air leak" test. If bubbling is seen from the anastomosis, I recommend circumferential reinforcement of the staple line with a 3-0 V-Loc suture, in a seromuscular Lembert fashion, placement of a pelvic drain, and creation of a diverting loop ileostomy.

Specimen Extraction

The specimen is grasped with a laparoscopic instrument; the robot is undocked and stowed. The surgeon scrubs back to the patient's bedside, and the specimen is extracted through the wound retractor in the right lower quadrant. The specimen and anastomotic donuts are sent off for pathologic review in formalin. A loop of ileum can be brought up at this point, if an ileostomy is necessary. Otherwise the fascia of the extraction site is closed with two layers of absorbable suture. The fascia of the 8 mm trocars is not routinely closed. The skin is closed, dressings are placed, and the operation is deemed complete.

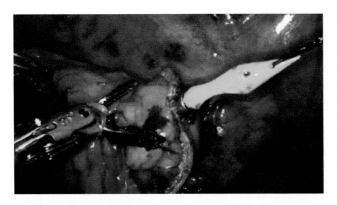

Fig. 14.12 Pulling of anvil through descending colonic staple line

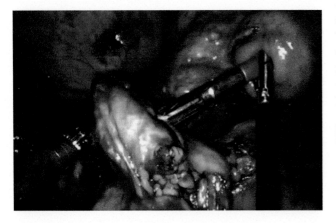

Fig. 14.13 Creation of end-to-end stapled anastomosis

Postoperative Care

The patient is allowed a liquid diet the night of surgery and a regular diet the next morning. An intravenous fluid restrictive strategy with an aggressive bowel regimen, early mobilization, and minimizing opioid analgesia is recommended. No protocol of minimally invasive colectomy is complete without an enhanced intestinal recovery pathway. In today's clinical practice, where patient satisfaction and quality metrics are measured in part by length of stay, current literature supports the use of the abovementioned strategies, to accelerate bowel recovery and shorten hospitalization [17]. Drugs such as Alvimopan (Entereg®, Merck & Co, Inc., Kenilworth, NJ) are opioid receptor antagonists at the intestinal level and are often included in such protocols, to improve postoperative bowel function in select patients [18]. After a robotic colectomy with an intracorporeal anastomosis, the vast majority of patients will pass flatus the day after surgery and will be ready for dismissal, after a bowel movement the following day.

Conclusion

With careful preoperative planning and due diligence in operative technique, a robotic colectomy is a safe, oncologic operation. Incorporating a routine intracorporeal anastomosis and adherence to an enhanced recovery pathway will shorten hospitalization and can improve short-term outcomes.

References

1. Surveillance Research Program, N.C.I. Surveillance epidemiology and end results—cancer statistics. April 11, 2013; Available from: http://seer.cancer.gov/statfacts/html/colorect.html.

2. Jayne DG, Thorpe HC, Copeland J, Quirke P, Brown JM, Guillou PJ. Five-year follow-up of the Medical Research Council CLASICC trial of laparoscopically assisted versus open surgery for colorectal cancer. Br J Surg [Internet]. 2010;97(11):1638–45.

3. Moorthy K, Munz Y, Dosis A, Hernandez J, Martin S, Bello F, et al. Dexterity enhancement with robotic surgery. Surg Endosc. 2004;18(5):790–5.

4. DeSouza AL, Prasad LM, Park JJ, Marecik SJ, Blumetti J, Abcarian H. Robotic assistance in right hemicolectomy: is there a role? Dis Colon Rectum. 2010;53(7):1000–6.

5. Luca F, Leal T, Valvo M, Cenciarelli S, Pozzi S, Radice D, Crosta C, Biffi R. Surgical and pathological outcomes after right hemicolectomy: case-matched study comparing robotic and open surgery. Int J Med Robot Comput Assist Surg. 2011;7:298–303.

6. Patel CB, Ragupathi M, Ramos-Valadez DI, Haas EM. A three-arm (laparoscopic, hand-assisted, and robotic) matched-case analysis of intraoperative and postoperative outcomes in minimally invasive colorectal surgery. Dis Colon Rectum. 2011;54:144–50.

7. Tyler JA, Fox JP, Desai MM, Perry WB, Glasgow SC. Outcomes and costs associated with robotic colectomy in the minimally invasive era. Dis Colon Rectum [Internet]. 2013;56(4):458–66.

8. Collinson FJ, Jayne DG, Pigazzi A, Tsang C, Barrie JM, Edlin R, et al. An international, multicentre, prospective, randomised, controlled, unblinded, parallel-group trial of robotic-assisted versus standard laparoscopic surgery for the curative treatment of rectal cancer. Int J Color Dis. 2012;27(2):233–41.

9. Ragupathi M, Ramos-Valadez DI, Patel CB, Haas EM. Robotic-assisted laparoscopic surgery for recurrent diverticulitis: experience in consecutive cases and a review of the literature. Surg Endosc [Internet]. 2011;25(1):199–206.

10. Trastulli S, Coratti A, Guarino S, Piagnerelli R, Annecchiarico M, Coratti F, et al. Robotic right colectomy with intracorporeal anastomosis compared with laparoscopic right colectomy with extracorporeal and intracorporeal anastomosis: a retrospective multicentre study. Surg Endosc Other Interv Tech. 2015;29(6):1512–21.

11. Morpurgo E, Contardo T, Molaro R, Zerbinati A, Orsini C, D'Annibale A. Robotic-assisted intracorporeal anastomosis versus extracorporeal anastomosis in laparoscopic right hemicolectomy for cancer: a case control study. J Laparoendosc Adv Surg Tech A [Internet]. 2013;23(5):414–7.

12. Grams J, Tong W, Greenstein AJ, Salky B. Comparison of intracorporeal versus extracorporeal anastomosis in laparoscopic-assisted hemicolectomy. Surg Endosc Other Interv Tech. 2010;24(8):1886–91.

13. Shapiro R, Keler U, Segev L, Sarna S, Hatib K, Hazzan D. Laparoscopic right hemicolectomy with intracorporeal anastomosis: short- and long-term benefits in comparison with extracorporeal anastomosis. Surg Endosc Other Interv Tech. 2016;30(9):3823–9.

14. Kiran RP, Murray ACA, Chiuzan C, Estrada D, Forde K. Combined preoperative mechanical bowel preparation with oral antibiotics significantly reduces surgical site infection, anastomotic leak, and ileus after colorectal surgery. Ann Surg [Internet]. 2015;262(3):416–25; discussion 423–5.

15. Jeremy L Holzmacher, Samuel Luka, Madiha Aziz, Richard L Amdur, Samir Agarwal, Vincent Obias. The use of robotic and laparoscopic surgical stapling devices during minimally invasive colon and rectal surgery – a comparison [Internet]. Dis Colon Rectum. 2015;58:e174.

16. Jafari MD, Lee KH, Halabi WJ, Mills SD, Carmichael JC, Stamos MJ, et al. The use of indocyanine green fluorescence to assess anastomotic perfusion during robotic assisted laparoscopic rectal surgery. Surg Endosc Other Interv Tech. 2013;27(8):3003–8.

17. Rawlinson A, Kang P, Evans J, Khanna A. A systematic review of enhanced recovery protocols in colorectal surgery. Ann R Coll Surg Engl. 2011;93:583–8.

18. Wang S, Shah N, Philip J, Caraccio T, Feuerman M, Malone B. Role of alvimopan (entereg) in gastrointestinal recovery and hospital length of stay after bowel resection. P T. 2012;37(9):518–25.

Robotic Total Mesorectal Excision for Rectal Cancer

Mark K. Soliman and Beth-Ann Shanker

Introduction

There are few operations that demand the same degree of technical precision and flawless execution like the total mesorectal excision (TME). The TME involves removing the fatty envelope – or mesorectum – surrounding the rectum itself. First described by Heald and Rydall, the TME proved critical in the surgical treatment of rectal cancer for decreasing local recurrence, reducing operative blood loss, and preserving genitourinary function.

Many techniques have been employed to perform a TME, such as open, laparoscopic, or robotic operative modalities. More recently transanal approaches have also been used. Prior to full adoption of minimally invasive approaches to the TME, oncologic outcomes were critically evaluated relative to open surgery. Non-inferiority was established through a number of studies including the CLASICC, COREAN, and COLOR II trial which primarily compared the oncologic outcomes between open and laparoscopic surgery for colorectal resections – as seen in the CLASICC trial – and rectal resections as investigated in the COREAN and COLOR II trials [1–4]. These studies showed open and laparoscopic surgery had similar oncologic outcomes; however outcomes were worse in patients who underwent a conversion from laparoscopic to open surgery. In the COLOR II trial, despite the expertise of the laparoscopic surgeons, there was a 16% conversion rate to open technique [4].

Since the short-term benefits of laparoscopic surgery have clearly been demonstrated – such as shorter hospital stay and earlier return of bowel function – and oncologic benefits are equivalent, one would expect more minimally invasive TME surgery to be performed. However, this has not been the case. The open approach to TME is still the most commonly performed method worldwide. As Bianchi et al. [1] noted in their review of the status of minimally invasive surgery and rectal cancer, the lack of widespread adoption of laparoscopic TME is because it requires high technical skill and a long learning curve.

The robotic approach is a newer technique to TME that overcomes some of the technical difficulties posed by open surgery or standard laparoscopy. The three-dimensional visual environment, wristed instrumentation, and decrease in surgeon fatigue are advantages of the robotic modality.

Compared to laparoscopy, robotic TME has a shorter learning curve, which has contributed to its adoption worldwide as a safe and feasible method for proctectomy. Kim et al. [5] reported on their robotic proctectomy learning curve. This was a single-surgeon retrospective study of 167 patients. The first 33 cases had significantly longer operative times and increased blood loss, but their documented conversions to open surgery were 1.2% (2 cases) and occurred only in their first 33 cases. A second decrease in overall operative time was seen again at 72 cases for this group. As noted previously, conversion rate for laparoscopic proctectomy is high. Moghadamyeghaneh et al. [6] used the National Inpatient Sample (NIS) database which is the largest all-payer inpatient database in the United States. They cited a 31.2% conversion rate from laparoscopic to open surgery for proctectomy. However, a meta-analysis by Sun et al. [7] reported on eight studies comparing laparoscopic and robotic low anterior resection for rectal cancers below the anterior reflection. They found a lower conversion rate to open surgery for robotic proctectomy.

More recently, a randomized prospective trial – Robotic vs Laparoscopic Resection for Rectal Cancer (ROLARR) [8] – compared laparoscopic and robotic proctectomy. Its primary endpoint was conversion to an open operation. The authors did not show a statistically significant difference in

M. K. Soliman (✉)
Colon and Rectal Surgery, Colon and Rectal Clinic of Orlando, Orlando, FL, USA
e-mail: mark.soliman@crcorlando.com

B.-A. Shanker
Department of Surgery, Saint Joseph's Mercy Hospital Ann Arbor, Ypsilanti, MI, USA

© Springer Nature Switzerland AG 2019
S. Tsuda, O. Y. Kudsi (eds.), *Robotic-Assisted Minimally Invasive Surgery*, https://doi.org/10.1007/978-3-319-96866-7_15

Fig. 15.1 Anatomy of the lower rectum

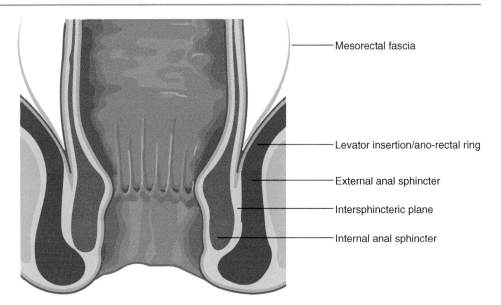

— Mesorectal fascia

— Levator insertion/ano-rectal ring

— External anal sphincter

— Intersphincteric plane

— Internal anal sphincter

conversion rate in the general study population; however a subset analysis demonstrated the obese male patient was less likely to undergo open conversion in the robotic group. The study did also show that less experienced robotic surgeons were able to achieve equal or better results than experienced laparoscopic surgeons with regard to conversion and all secondary endpoints.

As the benefits of minimally invasive surgery continue to be demonstrated, as well as the negative consequences of conversion on patient outcomes, learning a robotic TME – a modality with a shorter learning curve and low conversion rate – becomes of more interest. This chapter will review relevant anatomy to performing a robotic TME, go over the appropriate evaluation for clinical staging of rectal cancer, discuss key features of surgical planning, and review the robotic operative approach.

Anatomy for the Robotic TME

Rectum

For the purposes of operative planning and therapeutic management, the rectum is divided into lower, middle, and upper sections based on distance from the anal verge, rectal valves, and the peritoneal reflection. The anterior and lateral portions of the upper and mid rectum are peritonealized. The anterior peritoneal reflection marks the change between low and mid rectum, as the low rectum is not peritonealized. Understanding which part of the rectum a neoplasm is located in is paramount to both operative planning and deciding on possible neoadjuvant therapy [9].

Puborectalis Muscle (PRM)

The PRM is an important component to identify in devising a surgical plan. A mass above the puborectalis is likely to have a sphincter-sparing operation. The origin of the PRM is at the symphysis pubis and forms a sling which can be palpated as the anorectal ring on exam. Magnetic resonance imaging (MRI) should identify and report the relationship of a low rectal mass to this anatomical structure (Fig. 15.1) [10].

Fascial Planes

Understanding the fascial relationships of the rectum is important for a successful oncologic procedure and to minimize complications [9].

The mesorectum is the fascial envelope of the rectum which contains the terminal branches of the inferior mesenteric artery and lymph nodes. When performing a TME, this mesorectal envelope should not be violated due increased likelihood of locoregional recurrence. Morphologically, the mesorectum is larger in men and in obese individuals, which can affect the success of a high-quality surgical dissection [5].

The presacral fascia is a thickened part of the parietal endopelvic fascia. It covers the sacrum and coccyx, and dorsal to this fascia are the middle sacral artery and presacral veins. The presacral veins communicate with the internal vertebral venous system through the basivertebral veins. There are two lateral sacral veins and a middle sacral vein. The adventitia of the basivertebral veins is quite adherent to the sacral periosteum at the S3-S4 sacral foramina [11].

A dissection too deep into this fascia can lacerate these veins and cause life-threatening venous sacral hemorrhaging due both to retraction of the vessel through the sacral foramina and the elevated hydrostatic pressure of this system while the patient is in lithotomy. Bleeding rates to be as high as 1 liter/minute [11]. Awareness of this anatomy is critical during a posterior rectal mobilization.

Denonvilliers' fascia is a structure between the prostate or vagina and the anterior rectum that is often described as a peritoneal fusion of fascia. The anterior dissection plane for a TME and whether or not Denonvilliers' fascia should be included in the TME resection remain controversial. Some cadaveric studies indicate that Denonvilliers' fascia is not part of the rectal fascia itself and therefore does not have to be removed with the rectum during TME. Zhang et al. [12] performed cadaveric studies confirming that there are two layers of this fascia and advocated that the rectal mobilization should be between these layers to avoid injury to the pelvic autonomic nerves.

From a clinical standpoint, Wei et al. [13] evaluated the effect of sparing Denonvilliers' fascia in men with stage 1 mid to low rectal cancer undergoing a complete TME. They found sparing the fascia resulted in improved urogenital function. However, patients with advanced rectal cancer were not studied, as it is still unclear at this time if leaving the fascia will result in higher locoregional rectal cancer recurrence.

Denonvilliers' fascia should be resected if there is a concern that the circumferential resection margin (CRM) will be compromised. Anterior-based tumors can also include this fascia in the resected specimen. If the rectal neoplasm has a posterior or lateral location, leaving the anterior fascia may be considered. Other difficulties in identifying the fascial plane include patients who received radiation, a narrow pelvis, or a bulky mass [12].

Nerve Innervation

Sympathetic nerve fibers of the superior hypogastric plexus arise from L1 to L3 and synapse in the preaortic plexus. The nerves descend along the sacral promontory and bifurcate into bilateral hypogastric nerves which are medial to the ureters and common iliac arteries [13, 14].

As noted by Chew et al. [15], there are several potential points where the superior hypogastric plexus may be injured. Essential surgical techniques to protect the nerves include (1) ligating the IMA approximately 2 cm distal to its aortic origin to avoid nerve fibers ventral to the aorta; (2) preserving Gerota's fascia, as this contains the superior hypogastric nerve fibers; and (3) maintaining a posterior mesorectal plane of dissection immediately posterior to superior rectal artery, which preserves the parietal presacral fascia and the nerves it invests.

Right and left hypogastric nerves extend to the lateral pelvic sidewall and join the inferior hypogastric plexus adjacent to the lateral stalks. This plexus is formed from parasympathetic nerve fibers from S2 to S5. The existence of the lateral stalks as a distinct anatomical structure is of some debate. Surgical techniques to avoid injury include dividing the lateral stalks after posterior and anterior rectal mobilization has been performed as caudal as possible and gently teasing adherent nerves off the lateral mesorectum [15, 16].

As a branch of the pelvic plexus, the periprostatic plexus is located anterior to the rectum at the location of Denonvilliers' fascia. This will supply the prostate gland, seminal vesicles, corpora cavernosa, vas deferens, ejaculatory ducts, and bulbourethral glands. Neurovascular bundles run at the lateral aspects of the seminal vesicles in the 2 and 10 o'clock positions. In women the pelvic plexus lies just above the uterosacral ligament. Nerves extend lateral to the cervix and vaginal fornix. Injury at this location of the TME will cause urogenital dysfunction. Damage to these nerve bundles occurs both when dissecting outside the appropriate fascial planes and when excessive traction is applied to the rectum [14–16].

Arterial Supply

Blood supply to the rectum comes from both mesenteric and iliac supply. The IMA arises several centimeters proximal to the bifurcation of the aorta and is relatively short in nature. The IMA bifurcates into two branches: the left colic artery, which courses acutely cephalad toward the splenic flexure, and a descending branch that gives off the sigmoidal arteries and the superior rectal artery. The sigmoidal arteries vary in number and orientation. The superior rectal artery forms a rectosigmoid branch and then divides into right and left terminal branches, which extend to the level of the levator ani muscles [9].

The marginal artery is a series of arterial arcades along the mesenteric border of the colon starting at the ileocolic branches. The watershed area is at the splenic flexure. The arc of Riolan is found in 7% of the population and is collateral circulation between the left branch of the middle colic artery and the IMA. This is critical in an individual with a diseased SMA or IMA in providing adequate perfusion during rectal resection.

The pudendal artery gives rise to the middle rectal artery. The internal iliac artery gives rise to the inferior gluteal artery. The inferior rectal arteries, which are also from the pudendal artery, supply the anal canal and external anal sphincter muscle [9].

Evaluating Rectal Cancer

Standardizing Care

Before discussing the individual component of a rectal cancer workup, it is important to address the evolution of the multidisciplinary approach which is leading to the National Accreditation Program from Rectal Cancer (NAPRC).

As noted in the start of this chapter, over the past several decades, advances in our management of rectal cancer have grown tremendously. Surgically, it has been demonstrated that a quality TME results in decreased local recurrence as well as negative circumferential margins [17, 18]. Determining clinical staging and appropriate treatment has been advanced by MRI protocols, which utilize high-resolution oblique T2-weighted imaging cut in 3 mm slices perpendicular to the tumor axis in the sagittal view. The preoperative clinical staging determines whether or not neoadjuvant therapy is indicated. Studies from multiple countries have demonstrated that the implementation of national standards including staging, surgical technique, and centralized care results in improved 5-year survival [19].

In the United States, a group of 14 centers was organized to standardize management and improve rectal cancer outcomes. This group is called the consortium for Optimizing Surgical Treatment of rectal cancer (OSTRich). Data compiled from OSTRich has been used to implement a National Accreditation Program for Rectal Cancer (NAPRC). NAPRC is currently being trialed at a number of centers, but it is the expectation that improvements in outcomes will be seen through standardization of care and a multidisciplinary approach to rectal cancer [20].

Patient History

A complete history will give the surgeon an indication of more advanced disease, hereditary syndromes, the potential need for a permanent ostomy, and comorbidities that can and cannot be optimized prior to intervention [21–23].

Weight loss, tenesmus, anal pain, and fecal incontinence may indicate more advanced disease.

A complete family history will determine the potential for hereditary cancer that may require genetic counseling and other treatment paths.

History of anorectal surgery, urogenital surgery, or trauma may predict problems with postoperative incontinence of stool. If there is suspicion that anal sphincter control is suboptimal, then prior to any neoadjuvant or surgical treatment begins, further testing such as anal manometry may prudent to consider. Testing can help define the degree of impairment before adjuvant therapy and surgery take place. Helping the patient understand their current function will guide discussions on what to expect with regard to fecal continence in the postoperative setting, since those with poor anorectal function may consider a permanent ostomy.

Previous cancer treatments such as radiation for gynecologic cancers will impact neoadjuvant options and may indicate a hostile pelvis. Significant vascular disease may also represent a potential obstacle in creating a low anastomosis and maintaining adequate blood supply. Knowledge of these issues will help guide recommendations with the patient and family.

Medical comorbidities should be assessed to determine which patient factors may be optimized prior to surgery. Congestive heart failure, previous myocardial infarction, advanced age, and diabetes have correlations with cardiac complications. Patient with unintentional loss of >10% of their body weight and serum albumin <3.0 g/dL should be evaluated for perioperative nutritional support [21].

Physical Examination

A complete physical examination focusing on the abdomen and rectum is necessary for successful operative planning. Previous surgical scars and the patient's body habitus should be noted.

Rectal examination should assess the distance of the neoplasm from the anal verge and its circumference. Documentation of the relationship of the tumor to the puborectalis muscle (i.e., anorectal ring), degree of fixation and circumferential involvement, as well as orientation are all critical. Involvement of the anal sphincters, prostate or vagina, and sacrum may indicate the need for an abdominoperineal resection or en bloc resection of other organs with a multidisciplinary surgical team [20].

Colonoscopy

A complete colonoscopy will find a synchronous malignancy in 1–3% of patients and a synchronous polyp in 20–30% of all patients. If the mass is partially obstructing and a colonoscopy cannot be completed, a CT colonography or a barium enema should be performed. If the patient is symptomatic from a partial obstruction and the surgery is more urgent, a complete colonoscopy can either be performed at the time of surgery or within 6 months postoperatively [22].

Imaging and Laboratory Work

To evaluate for metastatic disease, a computerized tomographic (CT) scan of the chest, abdomen, and pelvis is performed with oral and intravenous contrast. Carcinoembryonic antigen levels

(CEA) should also be obtained. CEA levels >15 mg/mL should prompt a positron emission tomography (PET-CT) if CT imaging does not show distant disease [24, 25].

Local staging should be performed by rectal cancer protocol MRI over a transrectal ultrasound, which is in accordance with the NAPRC standards. Findings on MRI should be reported using standardized synoptic reporting system such as the Cancer Care Ontario reporting system [26]. Features to be reported include tumor depth of invasion, circumferential resection margin (CRM), spiculations, relationship to the puborectalis, mesorectal fascial involvement, extramural vascular invasion, and mesorectal lymph nodes. Malignant lymph node characteristics include mixed signal intensity, irregular contours, and size 8 mm or greater. Sensitivity and specificity are 77% and 71% for MRI detecting nodal involvement [26].

Neoadjuvant Management

After the workup is completed, the patient should be presented at a multidisciplinary conference for individualized treatment planning [27, 28]. Treatment should begin within 60 days of presentation per NAPRC standards.

Patients found to have a threatened resection margin, either distal resection margin (DRM) or CRM, or those found to have malignant lymphadenopathy typically require neoadjuvant treatment. However, treatment modalities are still an area of controversy. Short-course radiation is the standard of care in Northern Europe, and long-course radiation is the standard in Northern America. Our institutions typically utilize long-course radiation, which involves external beam radiation given as 45–50 Gy in a 25–28 fractionated conformational fashion [29]. This is given with a chemo-sensitizing agent. Surgery is performed 8–12 weeks after completing this treatment. There are current investigations that are looking at giving chemotherapy +/− radiation therapy prior to surgical resection for locally advanced stage II/III rectal cancers [30].

Operative Planning for Robotic TME

Operative planning starts with patient education. The patient and family should be educated on the overall plan as well as risks of the procedure including bowel and genitourinary dysfunction. Qin et al. [31] looked at functional impairment in 142 patients who either had chemotherapy or chemotherapy plus radiation prior to curative TME. They used a validated low anterior resection syndrome (LARS) score for assessment and preoperative MRI imaging to evaluate anatomical features that may predict dysfunction. They reported 71.1% of patients reported some dysfunction, and 44.4% of

patients experienced major LARS. Most common symptoms included clustering of bowel movements, urgency, incontinence to gas, and incontinence to liquid stool. Those with tumors in the lower 1/3 of the rectum and neoadjuvant chemoradiation were at increased risks of developing major LARS [31]. It is imperative that the patient understands the potential posttreatment issues regarding bowel function. Those with poor pre-treatment bowel control, or certain jobs not allowing frequent access to the bathroom, may choose an end colostomy as mentioned previously.

Patients should be sent to an enterostomal therapist for stoma marking and diet education. This is important for both an end colostomy and diverting loop ileostomy if planned. Preoperative marking and education are recommended by the American Society of Colon and Rectal Surgeons, the Wound, Ostomy and Continence Nurses Society, and the American Urological Association prior to any procedure. Stomal counseling and assessment have been shown to improve functional and lifestyle outcomes [32, 33].

Staging MRI should have already informed the decision of primary anastomosis versus APR for low rectal cancers. However, low-lying tumors located at or below the puborectalis benefit from repeat MRI and a flexible sigmoidoscope after neoadjuvant treatment is complete to determine if a sphincter-sparing operation is possible.

As part of an enhanced recovery pathway, patients are extensively counseled in the preoperative setting and are given documentation of their expectations after surgery (e.g., ambulation 5 times per day, incentive spirometer use, etc.).

The day prior to surgery, our patients undergo both mechanical and antibiotic bowel preparation (neomycin and metronidazole). Patients will also carbohydrate-load the evening before and 2 h prior to surgery with a maltodextrin-containing drink. This drink contains complex carbohydrates and a mixture of electrolytes, minerals, and vitamins, all of which reduce nausea, emesis, and hunger and accelerate gastrointestinal recovery postoperatively.

In the preoperative area, our patients typically receive a transversus abdominis plane (TAP) peripheral nerve block or epidural. Patients are also given gabapentin, alvimopan, acetaminophen, methocarbamol, and ondansetron.

The Setup

Once general anesthesia is established, the patient is carefully positioned. Proper positioning cannot be overemphasized, as nerve injuries can occur as a result of poor setup. The incidence of permanent nerve damage ranges from 0.03% to 1.4%. Specific patient factors increase risk of nerve injury including thin and obese body habitus, vascular disease, diabetes, and tobacco use. However, the most important risk factor for peripheral nerve injury is the surgery itself [34].

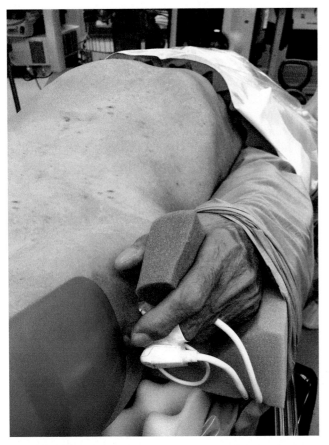

Fig. 15.2 Protecting the upper extremity with liberal foam padding placement of the hand in the neutral anatomic position

Proper positioning includes making certain the patient is secured to the table, all limbs are placed in their natural position without stretch, and all pressure points are carefully padded. Avoiding pronation of the upper extremity will reduce ulnar injury through the cubital tunnel. Arms are padded and tucked to prevent neuropraxia (Fig. 15.2).

The patient is placed in lithotomy positioning which can cause obturator, sciatic, or femoral nerve injury depending on the degree of stretch. The common peroneal nerve is also at risk for compression injury. If while in the lithotomy position the calf is compressed, this may result in the development of a deep vein thrombosis or even a catastrophic compartment syndrome. Compartment syndrome results from decreased perfusion and elevation of the limb above the level of the heart. Procedures requiring lithotomy positioning for more than 5 h increase the risk of these complications. Appropriately padding and positioning the lower extremities as well as limiting the degree of Trendelenburg positioning is helpful [34, 35].

Surgeons may choose to place ureteral stents at this time. If ureteral stents are placed, an open 5 French stent may be used where the author will instill 3 mL of indocyanine green and connect the stents to ureteral drainage bags. This will enable fluorescence imaging identification of the ureters

during the operation if such technology exists on the platform being used. Stents can be reinjected if needed, but this does not typically occur.

The abdomen is prepped and draped, and then abdominal entry is gained by whatever method the surgeon is most comfortable with. It is the preference of the author to gain intra-abdominal access via optical entry technique using a 5 mm laparoscope via the assistant trocar in the right upper quadrant. If the patient had previous surgery, we may enter with a 5 mm port in the left upper quadrant. This right upper quadrant port then becomes our bedside assist port. Robotic port placement commences based on surgeon preference, robotic system being used, and patient-specific considerations (Figs. 15.3, 15.4, and 15.5). Strategic port placement is critical for operative success, most notably to allow frustration-free case progression and to eliminate external and internal arm collisions. An optional second assist port may be place at the discretion of the surgeon. It is the preference of the author to place this second assist port. This has been found to be of high value in deep pelvic dissections, since it gives the assistant two working instruments – one to grasp and retract the rectum cephalad and the other to use for suctioning smoke and fluid that liberally collects in the dependent portions of the pelvis.

Operative Steps

Once the ports are placed, the patient is then positioned in the Trendelenburg position, just enough to clear and expose the pelvis, sacral promontory, and IMA. The patient is tilted with the left side up to obtain exposure additional exposure. Laparoscopic instruments may be used to assist in gaining this exposure, which ideally should be done prior to robotic arm docking.

The robot is docked, and instruments include a medium strength grasper (such as Tip-Up grasper), the fenestrated bipolar, and a monopolar dissecting instrument such as hook cautery or scissors. Other instruments to be used include the vessel sealer and robotic or laparoscopic stapling device.

We begin with a medial to lateral dissection. Our medium strength grasper is used to elevate the sigmoid colon toward the anterior abdominal wall. For a sigmoid colon with significant fatty epiploica, we may introduce an Endoloop transabdominally and place this around an epiploica to help elevate it toward the anterior abdominal wall.

Once the sigmoid colon is on stretch, we identify the inferior mesenteric artery. Distal to the IMA, the peritoneum is scored at the juncture of the mesentery and the retroperitoneum (Fig. 15.6). This is identified by a subtle color change from the bright yellow associated with the colon mesentery to a pinkish opaque color over the retroperitoneal structures. The peritoneum is scored, and dissection begins in this avascular plane.

Fig. 15.3 Robotic sigmoid or low anterior resection for da Vinci Si port placement

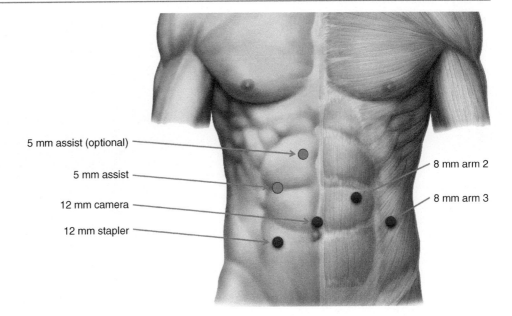

5 mm assist (optional)

5 mm assist

12 mm camera

12 mm stapler

8 mm arm 2

8 mm arm 3

Fig. 15.4 Robotic or low anterior resection for the da Vinci Xi port placement

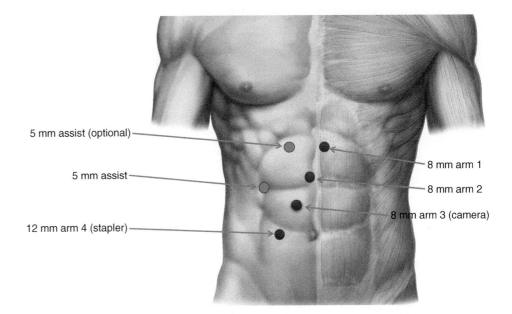

5 mm assist (optional)

5 mm assist

12 mm arm 4 (stapler)

8 mm arm 1

8 mm arm 2

8 mm arm 3 (camera)

The superior hemorrhoidal artery is identified and carefully swept anteriorly with the colon. The ureter can be identified in this window and swept downward (Fig. 15.7).

Next the window proximal to the IMA is developed. This is performed by incising the peritoneum between the IMA and IMV to unequivocally identify the two structures.

The left ureter is again identified and swept out of the way prior to ligation of the arterial vascular pedicle (Fig. 15.8). Once the vessel is isolated from the ureter, it is divided 1.5–2 cm from its origin off of the aorta to prevent injury to the superior hypogastric plexus. Typically, the robotic vessel dealing device suffices. A Hem-o-Lok clip can also be placed at the base of the IMA if the surgeon so chooses.

Alternatively, larger vessels may be divided with a vascular stapler load (e.g., white load). Bleeding from a ligated or stapled pedicle may be managed with any number of methods, including suture ligature, Endoloop application, or Hem-o-Lok clip placement.

Mobilization of Splenic Flexure

Once the pedicle is ligated, a medial dissection can continue up toward the splenic flexure. The inferior mesenteric vein needs to be divided at the inferior border of the pancreas. Separation of the mesentery from the retroperitoneum continues, staying

Fig. 15.5 Robotic low anterior resection Xi – alternative port placement

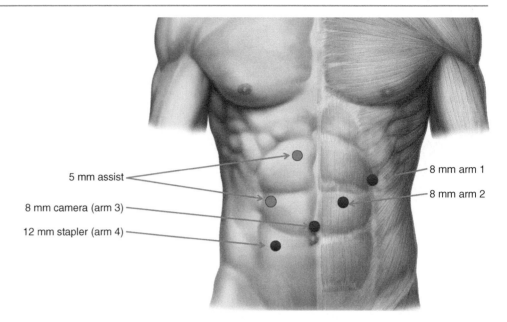

5 mm assist

8 mm camera (arm 3)

12 mm stapler (arm 4)

8 mm arm 1

8 mm arm 2

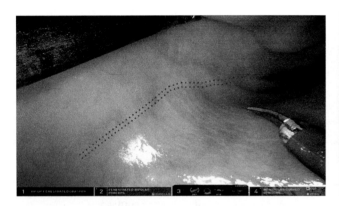

Fig. 15.6 Image of sacral promontory showing border of the retroperitoneum and mesentery

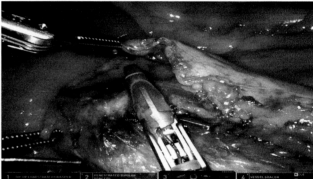

Fig. 15.8 Isolation of the IMA through medial dissection

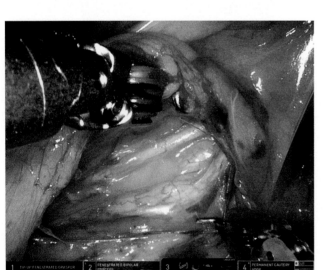

Fig. 15.7 Image after scoring of the peritoneum with resultant exposure of the left ureter and left gonadal vessel

anterior the pancreas. This allows anterior separation of the transverse mesocolon off of the retroperitoneum by entering into the lesser sac (Fig. 15.9). Once this medial dissection is completed, we turn our attention to lateral mobilization.

The sigmoid colon is gently grasped medially, and the white line of Toldt is identified. The peritoneum is scored just medial to this line. The lateral descending colonic mobilization continues cephalad, dividing the lienocolic ligament, ometocolic attachments, and gastrocolic ligaments from the spleen, omentum, and greater curve of the stomach, respectively. More often than not, full splenic flexure mobilization may be attained in the Trendelenburg position; however, if needed, the bed may be repositioned to complete this task.

Mobilization of Sigmoid Colon

With the proximal sigmoid colon on stretch, the white line of Toldt is again identified, and the lateral attachments are divided

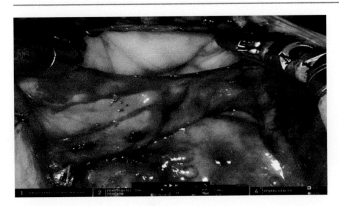

Fig. 15.9 Image shows medial dissection to the level of the lesser sac, with the pancreas posterior to the window and the transverse mesocolon anterior to the window

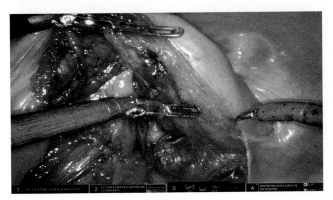

Fig. 15.10 Image shows rectum being tented anteriorly to facilitate posterior mesorectal dissection

to the level of the peritoneal reflection. As the mobilization continues caudad, identify the left ureter at the level of the sigmoid fossa. Once the sigmoid colon has been freed from its lateral attachments, we begin with the rectal mobilization.

Posterior Rectal Mobilization

Mobilization begins posteriorly (Fig. 15.10). The rectum is positioned again by having the third arm with the medium strength grasper elevate the sigmoid colon toward the anterior abdominal wall. Using the fenestrated bipolar device also on the left hand, anterior traction is provided on the posterior side of the proximal rectum, exposing the thin areolar tissue plane. This is the plane between the fascia propria of the rectum and the presacral fascia. Hypogastric nerves should be identified coming down both the right and left side of the sacral promontory and the should be preserved. Tension and counter tension will allow for visualization and to guide an avascular dissection. It is important to note that the mesorectum curves anterior at the level of the coccyx. Not being aware of this curvature may result in entry into the presacral fascia and sacral bleeding.

Once the distal-most aspect of the posterior dissection is accomplished, attention is then turned anteriorly.

Anterior Rectal Mobilization

Electrocautery is used to score the anterior peritoneal reflection to create a full-thickness peritoneal incision (Fig. 15.11). This incision is matured, and the third arm-fixed retractor is used to elevate the anterior pelvic structures, thus exposing the areolar tissue of the rectovaginal septum in the female patient or the prostate gland and seminal vesicles in the male patient. This retraction is best obtained by fanning out the fixed retractor and the bedside assist pulling the rectum of the pelvis. Denonvilliers' fascia may be incised at this point, and the anterior rectal dissection is carried down to the level of the distal rectum/proximal anal canal. Denonvilliers' fascia is often referred to as a thick fusion of peritoneum that can be divided into two layers and contains the prostatic plexus. Leaving behind or taking this fascia is controversial with concerns for increased local recurrence versus urogenital dysfunction.

Frequently, in the female patient, a gloved finger or vaginal dilator is placed transvaginally to assist in the proper identification of this anterior plane.

Lateral Rectal Mobilization

With the assistant applying contralateral tension on the rectum, the so-called lateral stalks are attended to next. This is a best performed by cephalad retraction of the rectum of the pelvis. The author begins with the left lateral stalk dissection, thereby having the assistant pull the rectosigmoid to the right upper quadrant.

This dissection is performed using electrocautery with the third arm applying traction on the left anterolateral pelvis, and the fenestrated bipolar continues to place countertraction on the medial aspect of the left lateral stalk. This dissection continues to the level of the distal rectum/proximal anal canal and is repeated on the right side in a mirrored fashion.

Rectal Division

Mobilization for a TME occurs down to the level of the anorectal ring. A perineal assistant may need to confirm the distal extent of the dissection as well as sufficient distance from the tumor. Once the distal aspect of the dissection has been identified and the bare area of the rectum encountered (i.e., the point at which the mesorectum tapers off), a robotic stapler is then introduced and used to divide the rectum distally (Fig. 15.12).

Fig. 15.11 Anterior mobilization of the rectum off of the anterior-based structures (labeled)

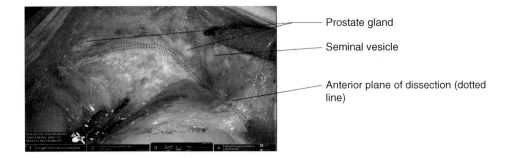

Prostate gland

Seminal vesicle

Anterior plane of dissection (dotted line)

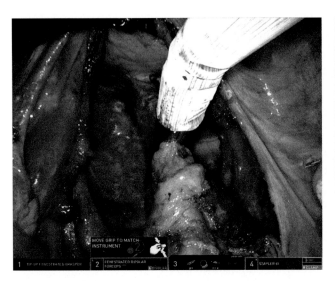

Fig. 15.12 Distal rectal division with robotic stapler

Coloproctostomy

At this time with the rectum divided, attention is turned to fashioning a suitable anastomotic surface. This can either be done in an intracorporeal or extracorporeal fashion.

The IMA pedicle is again identified and tented to the right lower quadrant of the patient. Using the vessel-sealing device, the mesentery is divided to the level of the mesenteric border of the descending/sigmoid junction, which will be the proximal dividing point (Fig. 15.13). At this time anesthesia administers indocyanine green to confirm the vascularity of the proximal portion of the colon that will be used for anastomosis.

If an intracorporeal anastomosis is chosen to be performed, a circular stapler anvil is introduced intra-abdominally. The author prefers placing the anvil through the 12 mm stapler port in the right lower quadrant.

If an end-to-end anastomosis is desired, the spike is affixed to the circular stapler anvil (Fig. 15.14). A 0-Vicryl suture is tied to this spike with two sets of air knots, as depicted in the diagram. On the specimen side, a colotomy is created large enough to accommodate the anvil. The anvil is

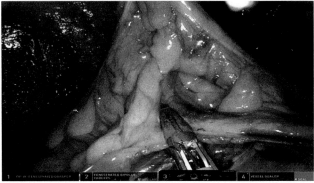

Fig. 15.13 Division of sigmoid mesentery to divide the proximal colon

then inserted with the spike just proximal to our intended transection site. Once the anvil is in place, the colotomy is sutured closed, and colon divided with a stapler. The ends of the Vicryl suture will be embedded within this newly fashioned staple line. The embedded end of the suture is then grasped and the suture pulled to guide the stem of the anvil through the linear staple line. The spike may be removed from the anvil by rotating it 90 degrees by pulling the suture with gentle but deliberate force.

If a Baker anastomosis is chosen, a site 2 cm from the proximal staple line is identified, and small colotomy is created on the anti-mesenteric side for which the stem of the anvil will exit the colon through (Fig. 15.15).

Next the colotomy is made using monopolar cautery. This colotomy is large enough to accommodate the base of the circular stapler anvil. Beginning with the stem first, the anvil is introduced into this colotomy and passed to the predesignated exit site that will be used in the coloproctostomy. If needed the anvil is secured with 2–0 Vicryl purse-string stitch. The colotomy on the specimen side, which the anvil was initially introduced, is closed with a running suture.

Once the anvil is in place, the colon is divided, and the specimen is then placed in the right upper or lower quadrant for extraction later.

Next an assistant introduces the circular stapler transanally to the level of the rectal staple line. Under direct visualization

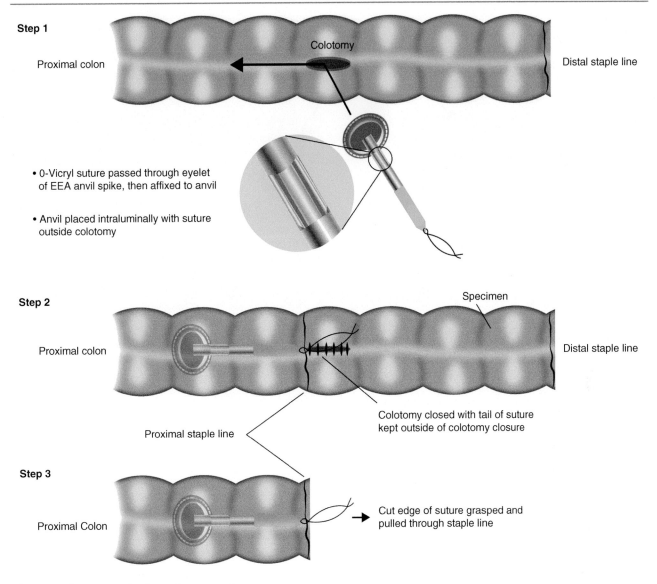

Step 1

Proximal colon

Colotomy

Distal staple line

- 0-Vicryl suture passed through eyelet of EEA anvil spike, then affixed to anvil

- Anvil placed intraluminally with suture outside colotomy

Step 2

Specimen

Proximal colon

Distal staple line

Proximal staple line

Colotomy closed with tail of suture kept outside of colotomy closure

Step 3

Proximal Colon

Cut edge of suture grasped and pulled through staple line

Fig. 15.14 Intracorporeal end-to-end anastomosis

the stapler is opened completely, the anvil connected to the stapler, and the stapler is then closed and deployed. Great care should be taken to assure the descending colonic conduit is correctly oriented and the mesentery remains on the posterior aspect of the anastomosis.

An alternative to this intracorporeal anastomosis is an extracorporeal anvil placement. For this, the mesentery is divided to the intended proximal transection site robotically. ICG is administered to confirm blood supply. The robot arms are undocked from the port sites, and the robot is backed away from the patient but kept sterile in case redocking is needed. A Pfannenstiel incision is made, and the abdomen is entered. The rectum is brought through this site, and a purse-string device is placed at the proximal site on the descending colon. The specimen is passed off, and the anvil is placed and secured. The colon and anvil are returned to the abdomen,

and the insufflation is re-established. We continue to use the robotic camera here. An assistant introduces a stapler into the rectum. This is opened and connected to the anvil. The alignment of the colon is checked to rule out any twisting of the mesentery, and finally the stapling unit is closed and deployed.

Anastomotic Leak Test

Regardless of how the anastomosis is created, we keep the robot draped in sterile in case there is a leak detected on pneumatic testing. If this is the case, then the surgeon may choose to revise the entire anastomosis or oversew the anastomosis and create a diverting ostomy. Both scenarios involve repeat pneumatic testing.

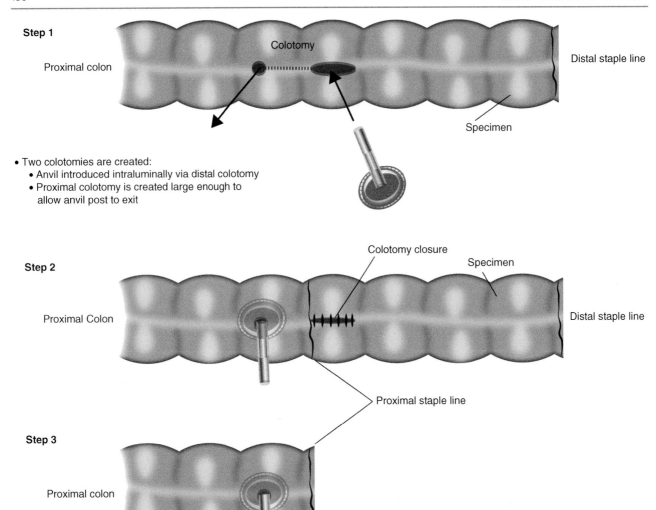

Step 1

Proximal colon

Colotomy

Distal staple line

Specimen

- Two colotomies are created:
  - Anvil introduced intraluminally via distal colotomy
  - Proximal colotomy is created large enough to allow anvil post to exit

Step 2

Colotomy closure

Specimen

Proximal Colon

Distal staple line

Proximal staple line

Step 3

Proximal colon

Fig. 15.15 Intracorporeal side-to-end anastomosis

To perform pneumatic testing, the pelvis is filled with irrigation in order to submerge the anastomosis. Proximal to the anastomosis, the colon is gently clamped off, while a sigmoidoscope (either rigid or flexible) is then introduced into the anal canal and advanced to the anastomosis. The anastomosis is identified and gently traversed. The appearance of bubbling in the pelvic irrigant indicates anastomotic disruption, which should immediately be examined and corrected. The endoscopy also allows the surgeon to check for bleeding at the staple line. Excessive bleeding may be managed with judicious use of cautery or an endoscopic clip.

Creation of a Diverting Loop Ostomy and Completion of the Operation

A loop of ileum is selected laparoscopically approximately 15 cm proximal to the ileocecal valve and brought out

through the previously marked ileostomy site. The remaining fascial and skin incisions are closed in a standard manner, and the operation is completed.

References

1. Bianchi PP, Petz W, Luca F, Biffi R, Spinoglio G, Montorsi M. Laparoscopic and robotic total mesorectal excision in the treatment of rectal cancer. Brief review and personal remarks. Front Oncol. 2014;4(98):1–6.
2. Green BI, Marshall HC, Collinson F, Quirke P, Guilou P, Jayne DG, Brown JM. Long-Term follow-up of the medical research council CLASICC trial of conventional cancer. Br J Surg. 2013;100:75–82.
3. Jeong S-Y, Park J-W, Nam BY, Kim S, Kang S-B, Lim S-B, Choi H-S, Kim D-W, Chang HJ, Kim DY, Jung KH, Kim T-Y, Kang GH, Chie EK, Kim SY, Sohn DK, Kim D-H, Kim J-S, Lee HS, Kim JH, Oh JH. Open versus laparoscopic surgery for mid-rectal or low-rectal cancer after neoadjuvant chemoradiotherapy (COREAN trial): survival outcomes of an open-label, non-inferiority, randomised controlled trial. Lancet Oncol. 2014;15:767–74.

4. Bonjer HJ, Deijen CL, Abis GA, Cuesta MA, Van der Pas MGH, Elly Klerk SM, Lacy AM, Bemelman WA, Andersson J, Angenete E, Rosenberg J, Fuerst A, Haglind E. A randomized trial of laparoscopic versus open surgery for rectal cancer. N Engl J Med. 2015;372:1324–32.

5. Kim HJ, Choi G-A, Park JS, Park SY. Multidimensional analysis of the learning curve for robotic total mesorectal excision for rectal cancer: lessons from a single surgeon's experience. Dis Colon Rectum. 2014;57(9):1066–74.

6. Moghadamyeghaneh Z, Masoomi H, Mills SD, Carmichael JC, Pigazzi A, Nguyen NT, Stamos MJ. Outcomes of conversion of laparoscopic colorectal surgery to open surgery. JSLS. 2014;18(4):1–10.

7. Sun Y, Xu H, Li Z, Han J, Song W, Wang J, Xu Z. Robotic versus laparoscopic low anterior resection for rectal cancer: a meta-analysis. World J Surg Oncol. 2016;14:61–9.

8. Jayne D, Pigazzi A, Marshall H, et al. Effect of robotic-assisted vs conventional laparoscopic surgery on risk of conversion to open laparotomy among patients undergoing resection for rectal cancer: the ROLARR randomized clinical trial. JAMA. 2017;318(16):1569–80.

9. Carmichael JC, Mills S. Anatomy and embryology of the colon, rectum, and anus. In: The ASCRS textbook of colon and rectal surgery. 3rd ed. Arlington Heights: Springer Publishing; 2016. p. 3–26.

10. Shihab OC, Moran BJ, Heald RJ, Quirke P, Brown G. MRI staging of low rectal cancer. Eur Radiol. 2009;19:643–50.

11. Harrison JL, Hooks VH, Pearl RK, Cheape JD, Lawrence MA, Orsay CP, Abcarian H. Muscle fragment welding for control of massive presacral bleeding during rectal mobilization: a review of eight cases. Dis Colon Rectum. 2003;46(8):1115–7.

12. Zhang C, Ding Z-H, Li G-X, Yu J, Wang Y-N, Hu Y-F. Perirectal fascia and spaces: annular distribution pattern around the mesorectum. Dis Colon Rectum. 2010;53(9):1315–22.

13. Wei HB, Fang JF, Zheng ZH, Wei B, Huang JL, Chen TF, Huang Y, Lei PR. Effect of preservation of Denonvilliers' fascia during laparoscopic resection for mid-low rectal cancer on protection of male urinary and sexual functions. Medicine (Baltimore). 2016;95(24):e3925. https://doi.org/10.1097/MD.0000000000003925.

14. Pappou EP, Weiser MR. Proctectomy. In: The ASCRS textbook of colon and rectal surgery. 3rd ed. Arlington Heights: Springer Publishing; 2016. p. 517–9.

15. Chew MH, Yeh YT, Lim E, Seow-Choen F. Pelvic autonomic nerve preservation in radical rectal cancer surgery: changes in the past 3 decades. Gastroenterol Rep (Oxf). 2016;4(3):173–85.

16. Açar HI, Kuzu MA. Perineal and pelvic anatomy of extralevator abdominoperineal excision for rectal cancer: cadaveric dissection. Dis Colon Rectum. 2011;54(9):1179–83.

17. Heald RJ, Moran BJ, Ryall RD, Sexton R, MacFarlane JK. Rectal cancer: The Basingstoke experience of total mesorectal excision, 1978–1997. Arch Surg. 1998;133(8):894–9.

18. Stelzner S, Koehler C, Stelzer J, Sims A, Witzigmann H. Extended abdominoperineal excision vs. standard abdominoperineal excision in rectal cancer—a systematic overview. Int J Colorectal Dis. 2011;26:1227.

19. Quirke P, Durdey P, Dixon MF, Williams NS. Local recurrence of rectal adenocarcinoma due to inadequate surgical resection. Histopathological study of lateral tumour spread and surgical excision. Lancet. 1986;2(8514):996–9.

20. Wexner SD, Berho ME. The rationale for and reality of the new national accreditation program for rectal cancer. Dis Colon Rectum. 2017;60(6):595–602.

21. Pickham DM, Hicks TC, Margolin DA. Preoperative preparation of the patient for colon and rectal surgery. In: Current therapy in colon and rectal surgery. Philadelphia: Elsevier, Inc; 2015. p. 167–73.

22. Marcet J. Rectal cancer: preoperative evaluation and staging. In: The ASCRS textbook of colon and rectal surgery. 3rd ed. Arlington Heights: Springer Publishing; 2016. p. 471–9.

23. Boutros M, Wexner SD. Preoperative evaluation of the patient with rectal cancer: staging and strategy. In: Current therapy in colon and rectal surgery. Philadelphia: Elsevier, Inc; 2015. p. 135–40.

24. Diamandis EP, Hoffman BR, Sturgeon CM. National Academy of Clinical Biochemistry laboratory medicine practice guidelines for use of tumor markers in testicular, prostate, colorectal, breast, and ovarian cancers. Clin Chem. 2008;54(12):1935–9.

25. Briggs RH, Chowdhury FU, Lodge JP, Scarsbrook AF. Clinical impact of FDG PET-CT in patients with potentially operable metastatic colorectal cancer. Clin Radiol. 2011;66(12):1167–74.

26. Al-Sukhni E, Milot L, Fruitman M, Brown G, Schmocker S, Kennedy E. User's guide for the synoptic MRI report for rectal cancer. 2015. Available from: www.http:www.cancercareontario.ca.

27. Snelgrove RC, Subendran J, Jhaveri K, Thipphavong S, Cummings B, Brierley J, Kirsch R, Kennedy ED. Effect of multidisciplinary cancer conference on treatment plan for patients with primary rectal cancer. Dis Colon Rectum. 2015;58(7):653–8.

28. Palmer G, Martling A, Cedermark B, Holm T. Preoperative tumour staging with multidisciplinary team assessment improves the outcome in locally advanced primary rectal cancer. Colorectal Dis. 2011;13(12):1361–9.

29. Cercek A, Garcia-Aguilar J-G. Rectal cancer: neoadjuvant therapy. In: The ASCRS textbook of colon and rectal surgery. 3rd ed. Arlington Heights: Springer Publishing; 2016. p. 481–94.

30. Cercek A, Goodman KA, Hajj C, Weisberger E, Segal NH, Reidy-Lagunes DL, Stadler ZK, Wu A, Weiser MR, Paty PB, Guillem JG, Nash GM, Temple LK, Garcia-Aguilar J, Leonard B, Saltz LB. Neoadjuvant chemotherapy first, followed by chemoradiation and then surgery, in the management of locally advanced rectal cancer. J Natl Compr Canc Netw. 2014;12(4):513–9.

31. Qin Q, Huang B, Cao W, Zhou J, Ma T, Zhou Z, Wang J, Wang L. Bowel dysfunction after low anterior resection with neoadjuvant chemoradiotherapy or chemotherapy alone for rectal cancer: a cross-sectional study from China. Dis Colon Rectum. 2017;60(7):697–705.

32. Berry K, Carmel J, Gutman N, et al. ASCRS and WOCN joint position statement on the value of preoperative stoma marking for patients undergoing fecal ostomy surgery. Mount Laurel: Wound, Ostomy, and Continence Nurses Society; 2007.

33. Hendren S, Hammond K, Glasgow SC, Perry BW, Buie DW, Steele SR, Rafferty J. Clinical practice guidelines for ostomy surgery. Dis Colon Rectum. 2015;58:375–87.

34. Knight D, Rahajan RP. Patient positioning in anaesthesia. Contin Educ Anaesth Crit Care Pain. 2004;4(5):160–3.

35. Seddon HJ. Surgical experiences with peripheral nerve injuries. Quarterly Bulletin of the Northwestern University Medical School. 1947;21(3):201–10.

Robotic Abdominoperineal Resection

Joshua MacDavid and Ovunc Bardakcioglu

Introduction

Numerous advances in robotic colorectal surgery have been made since the first robotic colectomy was performed in 2002 by Weber et al. [1]. New technologies such as haptic feedback, single-port systems, and eye-sensing camera technology are only some of a plethora of advancements that will be seen in the near future. Initial drawbacks to robotic surgery were steep learning curves, operative time, cost, and availability. Now, as robotic-assisted techniques have become more widespread, many of these initial limitations have been mitigated. Increasing evidence is showing robotic-assisted surgery to be superior to traditional laparoscopic, as in the case of rectal surgery, given the increased visibility and degrees of freedom afforded by robotic instruments. Given the narrow surgical field and proximity to major reproductive organs and autonomic centers, rectal dissections are challenging even for experienced surgeons. Herein we describe our technique of robotic-assisted cylindrical abdominoperineal resection, where the abdominal dissection is carried through the levator muscles, providing a complete total mesorectal excision with adequate circumferential resection margins (CRM) specifically at the level of the levator plate, while limiting open pelvic floor dissection from the perineum.

Background

The abdominoperineal resection (APR) is performed primarily for cancers in the lower third of the rectum where the sphincter complex cannot be salvaged. An APR includes total mesorectal excision along with resection of the sphincter complex and a portion of the pelvic floor musculature and perineum. The original total mesorectal excision, as described by Heald, drastically improved overall survival and local recurrence of rectal cancer [2]. The technique is considered standard of care in both the low anterior resection and the abdominoperineal resection and involves carrying sharp dissection in the avascular presacral plane anterolaterally until the entirety of the mesorectal envelope and its contents are excised. In APR, the dissection is continued through the levator musculature either via an abdominal approach or as a continuation of the perineal dissection.

Miles described the original APR in two phases. The first consisting of the abdominal mobilization of the rectum until the levator musculature, with the maturation of a colostomy and abdominal closure. The patient was then flipped over into the prone position where an extensive perineal dissection could be performed [3]. Miles advocated for taking the levators "as far outwards from their origin from the white line" [3, 4]. This wide resection of the levator musculature yields a cylindrical specimen. A recent retrospective study using morphometric data performed by West et al. showed that this traditional cylindrical approach yielded lower rates of positive circumferential resection margins (14.8% vs. 40.6%) and lower rates of intraoperative perforations (22.8% vs. 3.7%) [5]. Major drawbacks to this technique were increased operative time given that the two dissections could not be performed at the same time, and there was a tendency to perform a much wider excision of the perineum than what was necessary, taking the resection through to the origins of the levator muscles near the pelvic sidewall. This led to an increased size of the perineal defect and greater perineal morbidity [6]. If the perineal dissection was performed in a more conservative approach, there was a greater risk of tumor perforation given the paucity of mesorectum at the anorectal junction [7, 8].

The current technique for abdominoperineal resection involves carrying the dissection down the mesorectal

J. MacDavid
UNLV School of Medicine, Department of Surgery, University Medical Center, Las Vegas, NV, USA

O. Bardakcioglu (✉)
Department of Surgery, University of Nevada Las Vegas Medicine, Las Vegas, NV, USA
e-mail: Ovunc.Bardakcioglu@unlv.edu

© Springer Nature Switzerland AG 2019
S. Tsuda, O. Y. Kudsi (eds.), *Robotic-Assisted Minimally Invasive Surgery*, https://doi.org/10.1007/978-3-319-96866-7_16

envelope to the levators, where a second surgical team works on the perineal dissection, carrying the dissection through the levator muscles until met from above [9]. Given that the mesorectum tapers significantly as the levator muscles are approached and is nearly absent at the level of the anorectal junction, carrying out the above dissection will yield a conical, rather than cylindrical, specimen. The incompleteness of the total mesorectal excision will yield higher rates of circumferential resection margin positivity and local recurrence. The Dutch TME/TME and radiotherapy trial found that APR total mesorectal excisions were poorly excised, with only 34% showing complete excision, whereas 73% of anterior resections showed complete excision [9].

Given the numerous benefits of minimally invasive colorectal surgery, including shorter length of stay, earlier return of bowel function, and less analgesic requirements, it is becoming at minimum the standard of practice [10]. The debate is now between whether robotic surgery is superior to traditional laparoscopic. In their study of 113 patients, Baik et al. provided evidence for the superiority of the robotic low anterior resection over laparoscopic low anterior resection, with robotic resections achieving a significantly better mesorectal grade [11]. Additionally, the overall complication rate was nearly double in the laparoscopic group when compared to the robotic group, 19.3% vs. 10.7%, respectively. Given the technical challenge of laparoscopic rectal dissections, six of the patients in the laparoscopic group required conversion to open secondary to rectal perforation, hemorrhage from lateral pelvic wall, or severely compromised visualization from an anatomically narrow pelvis. Operative times were not significantly different between the two groups. In a similar study, Bedrili et al. showed the quality of TME specimens was superior in patients undergoing robotic resections [10].

The benefits of robotic surgery are numerous. Dissection of the rectum requires tremendous precision given the proximity to reproductive organs and major autonomic nerves [12, 13]. We would agree with deSouza et al. that the robot offers superior retraction, an enhanced three-dimensional field of view, and human anatomical articulation, all allowing for a more precise and superior dissection. These "7 degrees of freedom" and 90-degree articulation mimic human anatomy allowing the surgeon real-life ergonomic control [13].

Our approach, first described by Marecik et al., employs robotic transabdominal transection of the levator muscles with robotic dissection carried into the subcutaneous tissue [7]. This allows for an appropriate oncologic resection that limits the risk of tumor perforation and perineal morbidity while providing the benefits of minimally invasive surgery with the technical superiority of robotic surgery. Though large trials have yet to be performed specifically analyzing robotic transabdominal levator resection, our experience leads us to believe that it offers a tailored approach of dividing the levator muscles leading to adequate R0 resection and minimizing larger perineal defects and subsequent morbidity.

Preoperative Planning

Indications

The robotic abdominoperineal resection is primarily performed for adenocarcinoma in the lower third of the rectum where the sphincter complex cannot be spared and patients with preexisting fecal incontinence. Additional indications include recurrent anal squamous cell carcinoma.

Contraindications

Relative contraindications are extensive adhesive disease discovered during initial exploration.

Workup

All patients require a complete colonoscopy to evaluate for synchronous disease. Obtaining accurate information about the size and distance from the sphincter complex is necessary by digital rectal exam and proctoscopy. Staging includes a CT of the chest abdomen pelvis to evaluate for distant metastases, and a pelvic MRI should be performed not only for local staging but particularly in anterior tumors to rule out invasion into adjacent organs and need for exenteration. Patients will then undergo stage-dependent neoadjuvant therapy or immediate surgery.

Room Setup and Positioning

The best technique is to place the patient in the modified lithotomy position with both arms tucked. The lithotomy positioning allows for on-table colonoscopy to be performed. The robot will be docked from the left of the patient. It is important to secure the patient such that sliding will not occur, as the patient will need to be placed in steep Trendelenburg position to facilitate exposure. Some find the usage of a bean bag or a gelpad to be helpful. All extremities should be appropriately padded to prevent nerve injury.

Operative Steps

To facilitate easier reading, all technicalities are in reference to the da Vinci Xi system (Intuitive Surgical, Inc., Sunnyvale, CA).

Exploratory Laparoscopy, Port Placement, and Docking

Port placement will vary with patient body habitus; however it is important to have a general set of rules. The da Vinci Xi system requires a minimum of 8 cm distance between ports. The optimal distance from the camera to the area of interest is between 10 and 20 cm. If the camera is placed greater than 20 cm away, there will be difficulty obtaining appropriate reach with the instruments.

There are numerous ways to enter the abdomen and obtain capnoperitoneum. We prefer to place a 5 mm left upper quadrant laparoscopic port for using the OptiView technique, which is then exchanged to an 8 mm robotic port. The insufflation is then attached to this port (R4). A 12 mm staple port (R1) is then placed in the right lower quadrant either medial or lateral to the inferior epigastric ports depending on the patient's body habitus. The distance between these two ports is then measured, and the remaining two 8 mm robotic ports (R2, R3) are placed equidistant in this oblique line. An assistant 5 mm port is to be placed in the right upper quadrant. We prefer to use the AirSeal access port (CONMED, Utica, NY) (Fig. 16.1). An alternative port configuration can be used if reconstruction will be performed with a robotic rectus muscle flap (Fig. 16.2).

Exploratory laparoscopy with a thorough examination of the abdominal and pelvic cavity should be performed as the first step to rule out metastatic disease and determine the feasibility of a robotic approach. Both the surgeon and the assistant stand on the patient's right side, and the patient is placed in steep Trendelenburg with the left side up, approximately 15° to facilitate movement of small bowel and omentum out of the pelvis.

Initial setup includes fenestrated bipolar grasping forceps on R3 and a tip up grasping forceps on R4 to facilitate rectosigmoid retraction to the abdominal wall. The camera is used through the R2 port, while monopolar curved scissors are placed through R1.

Establishment of the Presacral Plane and Ligation of the IMA

Steep Trendelenburg is maintained with the left side up, the small bowel and omentum are retracted out of the pelvis, and the rectosigmoid is elevated to the abdominal wall.

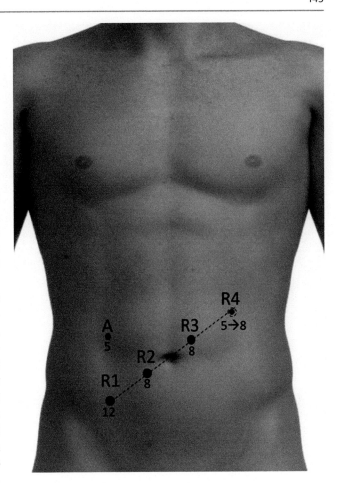

Fig. 16.1 Port configuration: R1, 12 mm staple port; R2, camera port; R3, fenestrated bipolar grasping forceps; R4, grasping forceps; A, assistant port. All numeric values in millimeters

Using monopolar shears through R1, the peritoneum is incised posterior to the inferior mesenteric vessels at the level of the sacral promontory, allowing entrance into the avascular presacral plane (Fig. 16.3). This "holy plane" is anterior to the presacral fascia, otherwise known as the endopelvic fascia. It is important not to violate this layer, as the pelvic and sacral splanchnic nerves as well as the inferior hypogastric plexus lie behind it. At this point the superior rectal artery should be identified along with the left ureter. The ureter can be found posterior to the inferior mesenteric artery (IMA), deep to the parietal peritoneum and medial to the gonadal vessels. It is important however to not perform deep dissection in order to facilitate ureter exposure as there are nearby autonomic centers and the iliac vessels. Occasionally, the ureter will be found on the posterior portion of the inferior mesenteric pedicle. The inferior mesenteric artery pedicle, including the inferior mesenteric vein, should be visualized at this point and taken with a robotic vessel sealer or stapler (Fig. 16.4).

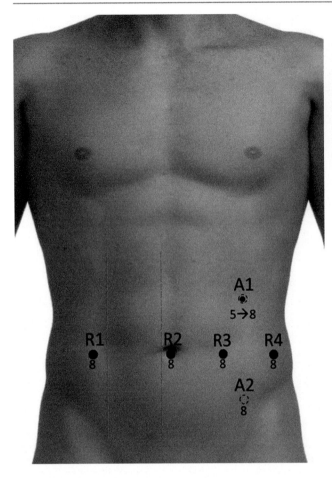

Fig. 16.2 Alternative port configuration for robotic rectus muscle flap. R1–R4, robotic arm configurations; A1, 5 mm assistant AirSeal port changed to 8 mm robotic port for flap; A2, 8 mm robotic port placed for flap. All numeric values in millimeters

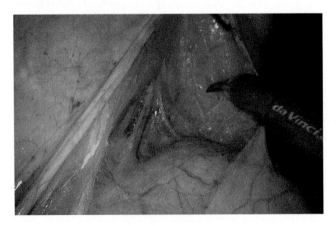

Fig. 16.3 Entry into the presacral space

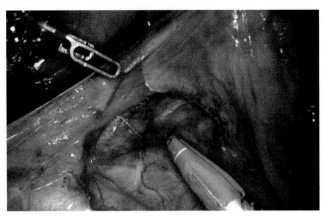

Fig. 16.4 Isolation of the IMA

Mobilization and Division of the Left Colon

Mobilization and division of the left colon proceed in a medial to lateral fashion. The left colon mesentery is divided using the vessel sealer in R1 or R3 cranially starting at the previously divided IMA pedicle toward the junction of sigmoid colon and descending colon. Dissection then proceeds laterally up the white line of Toldt. Mobilization of the splenic flexure is not usually required and dissection only needs to be carried out to obtain adequate reach of the descending colon to the abdominal wall. The colon is then divided with a 45 mm green load robotic stapler through the R1 port.

Dissection of the Mesorectum and Total Mesorectal Excision

The dissection of the mesorectum proceeds in the "holy plane" using Heald's technique, starting the dissection posteriorly and finishing in the anterior plane.

Posterior Dissection

Using R4, the rectosigmoid is elevated to the anterior abdominal wall. Dissection then proceeds in this presacral space using R1 and R3 that has previously been exposed. We prefer to use sharp dissection with monopolar scissors through R1 (Fig. 16.5). It is important to identify and preserve the fascia propria of the rectum. The dissection is continued down well above the anorectal junction through Waldeyer's fascia. It is crucial not to proceed to the anorectal junction as it would be in a low anterior resection in order to prevent coning of the specimen. Initial complete posterior dissection greatly facilitates further lateral and anterior dissection.

Lateral Dissection

The lateral pelvic space is exposed by applying medial and superior traction on the rectosigmoid and countertraction of the pelvic sidewall through R3 and R4. The hypogastric nerve and its branches can be seen directly posterolateral to the dissection plane, protected by the lateral pelvic wall fascia. It is very important to not violate the fascia as damage to the nerves may lead to autonomic dysfunction. Dissection starts on the patient's right side, taking down the lateral rectal stalk. The anterior reflection of the peritoneum is divided, and dissection of the left lateral stalk is performed in the same fashion (Fig. 16.6).

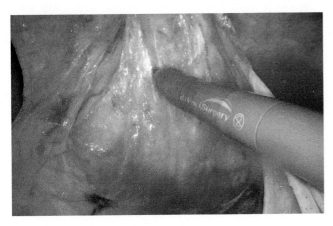

Fig. 16.5 Posterior TME dissection

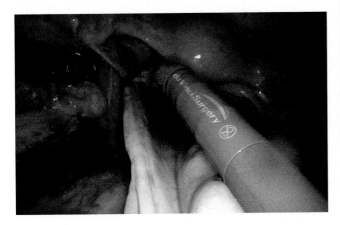

Fig. 16.6 Lateral TME dissection

Anterior Dissection

The location and stage of the rectal cancer will determine whether or not dissection will proceed either anterior or posterior to Denonvilliers' fascia. In males, the prostatic and vesicle plexus along with the seminal vesicles is located in the space just anterior to Denonvilliers' fascia. The risk of damage is much greater when dissection is to be performed anterior; however it may be necessary. The anterior peritoneal reflection is incised at the rectovesicular or rectouterine pouch. An assistant can facilitate anterior dissection by retracting the rectum out of the pelvis. R3 and R4 should be used to retract either the prostate and seminal vesicles in males or the vagina in females upward, while the R3 or R4 provides countertraction pulling the rectal wall out of the pelvis and downward (Fig. 16.7). It is helpful here to grasp the peritoneal reflection which was created with the initial incision within the Douglas pouch. Sharp dissection proceeds distally taking care to avoid excessive lateral dissection given the proximity of autonomic nerves as well as hypogastric veins and tributaries. Any remaining portions of the lateral rectal stalks are divided.

At this point, once all tissue has been dissected off close to the levator complex and it is circumferentially exposed, transection of the levators is performed using electrocautery as lateral as possible to allow a cylindrical excision. Based on preoperative MR imaging, this dissection can also be tailored to perform a wider excision on one side only. It is important to not carry the dissection between the levators and the rectal

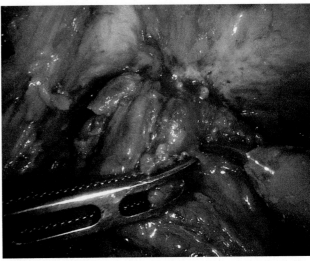

Fig. 16.7 Anterior TME dissection, tumor invasion into vaginal wall prior to perineal dissection

wall, as violation of the tumor plane may occur. Dissection is then carried into the ischiorectal fat, completing the robotic portion of the procedure. Of note when performing a proctectomy for benign disease, the levator is not transected, and dissection should continue between the levators and the rectal wall, as having the levators and external sphincter complex preserved will aid in closure of the perineum and potentially decrease perineal morbidity and hernia rates. Thus, a tailored robotic dissection of the levator muscles may allow an R0 excision and decreased morbidity.

Perineal Dissection

In a circumferential fashion, wide excision of the anus and perineal tissue is performed. The lateral margin should be about 1–2 cm from the anal verge. Dissection is carried into the ischiorectal fat until the previous robotic dissection is met. Once circumferential excision has been performed, the specimen is extracted from the perineal wound. If performed in an appropriate fashion, the specimen will be cylindrical in nature with intact fascia propria.

Port Site Closure and Colostomy Maturation

A colostomy is completed in a standard fashion according to surgeon preference. The 12 mm RLQ port is closed using an assisted closure device such as the Carter-Thomason (CooperSurgical, Trumbull, CT).

Perineal Closure and Reconstruction

Depending on the size of the perineal defect, closure may be performed primarily or with various pedicle flaps. If performing primary closure, the levators are imbricated with 2–0 Vicryl sutures with the subcutaneous and superficial tissues closed with 3–0 Vicryl. The skin is closed with interrupted 2–0 nylon sutures.

Preoperative radiation has been shown to greatly increase the odds of developing a perineal wound complication when primary closure is performed, with some authors quoting a 2–10-fold increase in complications [14]. Flap reconstruction provides volume as well as highly vascularized healthy tissue with the primary goal of maximizing healing and minimizing complications. However, flap reconstruction is not without substantial risks. Longer operative times, the risk of flap failure, and additional donor site morbidity are complications that can arise [14].

Reconstructive flaps can be separated into two main categories: fasciocutaneous flap and myocutaneous flaps. Common fasciocutaneous flaps include the anterolateral flap, the tensor fascia lata flap, and the V-to-Y advancement flaps. Pedicled myocutaneous flaps include the vertical rectus abdominus myocutaneous (VRAM) flap, the gracilis flap, and the gluteus maximus flap. A recent single-institution study by Scheckter et al. demonstrated that pedicled muscle flaps had overall lower rates of complications than local fasciocutaneous flaps, with the VRAM flap being superior to the gracilis flap [15]. In our institution we utilize a robotically harvested VRAM flap or gracilis flap.

The reconstructive technique for each of these flaps is beyond the scope of this text. Consultation with an experienced reconstructive surgeon should be initiated prior to resection.

References

1. Weber P, Stephen Merola MD, Annette Wasielewski RN, Ballantyne GH, M.D. Dis Colon Rectum. 2002;45:1689. https://doi.org/10.1007/s10350-004-7261-2.
2. Heald RJ. Recurrence and survival after total mesorectal excision for rectal cancer. Lancet. 1986;1(8496):1479.
3. Miles WE. A method of performing abdomino-perineal excision for carcinoma of the rectum and of the terminal portion of the pelvic colon. Lancet. 1908;2:1812–3.
4. Kim JC, Kwak JY, Yoon YS, et al. Int J Colorectal Dis. 2014;29:961. https://doi.org/10.1007/s00384-014-1916-9.
5. West NP, et al. Evidence of the oncologic superiority of cylindrical abdominoperineal excision for low rectal cancer. J Clin Oncol (0732-183X). 2008;26(21):3517.
6. West NP, Anderin C, Smith KJE, Holm T, Quirke P. Multicentre experience with extralevator abdominoperineal excision for low rectal cancer. Br J Surg. 2010;97:588–99. https://doi.org/10.1002/bjs.6916.
7. Marecik SJ, Zawadzki M, Desouza AL, Park JJ, Abcarian H, Prasad LM. Robotic cylindrical abdominoperineal resection with transabdominal levator transection. Dis Colon Rectum. 2011;54:1320–5.
8. Eriksen MT, Wibe A, Syse A, Haffner J, Wiig JN. Inadvertent perforation during rectal cancer resection in Norway. Br J Surg. 2004;91:210–6. https://doi.org/10.1002/bjs.439.
9. Marr R, Birbeck K, Garvican J, et al. The modern abdominoperineal excision: the next challenge after total mesorectal excision. Ann Surg. 2005;242:74–82.
10. Bedirli A, Salman B, Yuksel O. Robotic versus laparoscopic resection for mid and low rectal cancers. JSLS. 2016;20(1):e2015.00110. https://doi.org/10.4293/JSLS.2015.00110.
11. Baik SH, Kwon HY, Kim JS, et al. Ann Surg Oncol. 2009;16:1480. https://doi.org/10.1245/s10434-009-0435-3.
12. Weaver A and Steele S. Robotics in Colorectal Surgery [version 1; referees: 2 approved]. F1000Research 2016, 5(F1000 Faculty Rev):2373. https://doi.org/10.12688/f1000research.9389.1
13. de Souza AL, Prasad LM, Marecik SJ, et al. Total mesorectal excision for rectal cancer: the potential advantage of robotic assistance. Dis Colon Rectum. 2010;53:1611–7.
14. Nisar PJ, Scott HJ. Myocutaneous flap reconstruction of the pelvis after abdominoperineal excision. Colorectal Dis. 2009;11:806–16. https://doi.org/10.1111/j.1463-1318.2008.01743.x.
15. Sheckter CC, Shakir A, Vo H, Tsai J, Nazerali R, Lee GK. Reconstruction following abdominoperineal resection (APR): indications and complications from a single institution experience. J Plast Reconstr Aesthet Surg. November 1, 2016;69(11):1506–12. https://doi.org/10.1016/j.bjps.2016.06.024.

Robotic Inguinal Hernia

Peter Michael Santoro and Anthony R. Tascone

Introduction

Few procedures could be considered more "bread and butter general surgery" than the inguinal hernia repair. Inguinal hernia surgery is the most common general surgical technique performed in the United States with approximately 1 million procedures performed annually [1]. Herniation involving the groin region is a common ailment affecting both men and women, with lifetime risk of developing inguinal hernias estimated at 27% in men and 3% in women [2], while development of femoral hernia is more than twice as likely in women as compared to men.

Inguinal hernias are caused by a weakening of the abdominal wall fascia, leading to an opening through which peritoneum protrudes. Inguinal hernias are more common on the right side than on the left and are ten times more common in men than women. They can be divided into direct and indirect types, whereby a direct hernia protrudes medial to the inferior epigastric vessels traversing Hesselbach's triangle, while an indirect hernia represents a defect lateral to the vessels and traverses the inguinal canal traveling with the components of the spermatic cord. Indirect inguinal hernias are twice as common as direct hernias. Femoral hernia can be included in the discussion of groin hernias, and these occur medial to the femoral vessels through the femoral space.

The major risk factors for inguinal hernias are male sex, advanced age, and family history. Other risk factors include chronic obstructive pulmonary disease, smoking, high intra-abdominal pressure, collagen vascular disease, thoracic or abdominal aortic aneurysm, patent process vaginalis, history of open appendectomy, and peritoneal dialysis [3]. There is no conclusive evidence to show that heavy lifting is a risk factor.

Inguinal hernias are diagnosed by physical examination. A visible bulge may be present in the groin area, sometimes induced with straining. If no bulge is visible, a mass can be palpated protruding through the external inguinal ring with straining (asking the patient to cough) and Valsalva maneuver. Patients may endorse symptoms of pain, burning, or heaviness associated with the bulge. Patients with symptomatic inguinal hernias should be offered repair, although watchful waiting in patients with reducible hernias is also an acceptable strategy in certain patient populations [4].

Over the years the techniques utilized for inguinal hernia repair have evolved substantially. Early repairs were primarily completed by closing the defect using the patient's native tissue, as described in the various tissue repair techniques. However, due to closure of the hernia defect with excessive tension, these techniques were fraught with high recurrence rates [5]. Use of prosthetic mesh in inguinal hernia repairs was a major breakthrough, leading to a reduction in hernia recurrence by 50–75% and a lower risk of chronic groin pain compared to the primary tissue repairs [6]. Inguinal hernia repair continued to evolve with the advent of laparoscopy. Laparoscopic inguinal hernia repair techniques aim to utilize the preperitoneal space to place a piece of synthetic mesh over the entire myopectineal orifice. This space can be entered directly from the abdomen by incising the peritoneum (TAPP) or by gaining access to the preperitoneal space without entering the abdomen (TEP). Regardless of the specific method used, laparoscopic herniorrhaphy has been shown to result in less initial pain and an earlier return to normal activities compared to the open technique [7].

Current guidelines suggest that open or laparoscopic inguinal hernia repairs are comparably safe and effective in treating primary, unilateral inguinal hernias [8, 9]. The laparoscopic (or minimally invasive) approach, however, is the preferred method of repair for bilateral inguinal hernias and recurrent inguinal hernias previously repaired using an open approach [8, 9].

To date, there has been little published regarding the specific role of robotic surgery in the field of inguinal hernia repair. Regardless, the robotic platform, with its improved

P. M. Santoro (✉) · A. R. Tascone
Department of Surgery, Christiana Care Health System, Wilmington, DE, USA

© Springer Nature Switzerland AG 2019
S. Tsuda, O. Y. Kudsi (eds.), *Robotic-Assisted Minimally Invasive Surgery*, https://doi.org/10.1007/978-3-319-96866-7_17

dexterity and 3D visualization, serves as an excellent tool to aid the general surgeon in performing a minimally invasive inguinal hernia repair. The world of robotic hernia surgery has been rapidly evolving and expanding in the last several years. With the help of social media, closed Facebook groups including the International Hernia Collaboration (IHC) and the Robotic Surgery Collaboration (RSC) have allowed hernia surgeons around the world to collaborate and discuss new techniques with a common goal of providing excellent outcomes for patients undergoing hernia surgery. Inguinal hernia surgery is a commonly discussed topic as robotic inguinal hernia surgery has gained much notoriety and is quickly becoming a popular technique utilized by hernia surgeons for everything from unilateral primary inguinal hernias to complex recurrent hernias.

Preoperative Planning

Hernia involving the groin is a common pathology, affecting up to 5–7% of the general population, including the very young to the elderly. By far, the most common type of groin hernia is the indirect inguinal hernia, followed by direct and femoral hernias. Regardless of anatomic location, patients most frequently present to the surgeon for inguinal hernia due to the presence of a bulge in the groin. To a lesser extent, pain can be associated with groin hernia; however this type of hernia is not typically painful unless it has become either incarcerated or strangulated.

It is at least academically interesting to attempt to predict which type of herniation of the groin a patient has prior to taking them for surgical repair. The availability of computed tomography (CT) scanners in the present day eases this task. However, typically these hernias can be differentiated based on physical exam with some certainty. Examining a patient while standing and palpating the inguinal region frequently yields a diagnosis. A bulge originating at the external ring and pulsating down toward the scrotum on Valsalva maneuver is consistent with an indirect inguinal hernia, while a bulge medially thru the inguinal floor closer to the pubic tubercle frequently represents a direct hernia. A femoral hernia occurs through the femoral space and presents as a bulge on the lower abdomen or upper thigh, below the inguinal ligament. It is useful to get a sense of what type of hernia a patient has going in to surgery. However, regardless of which of these is present, either one or all of them, the surgical approach and technique in robotic inguinal hernia surgery are essentially the same, which will be discussed in a later section.

There are many considerations which one must take into account when planning on approaching a patient's inguinal hernia robotically. Some of these are common to most minimally invasive operations, but several are specific to this operation. Prior surgical history must be reviewed, and a careful history about this topic should be discussed with the patient. Types of abdominal operations in the past, surgical approach, etc. are very important pieces of information which can be used to risk stratify patients in regard to the presence of intra-abdominal adhesions and possibility of visceral injury on abdominal entry. Knowledge of history of prior hernia repairs is a must as well, including surgical approach for the previous repairs. A recurrent hernia previously repaired minimally invasively may warrant an anterior (open) approach in certain instances. In addition, history of pelvic surgery, particularly open or robotic prostatectomy in men, is vital information. In this situation, the preperitoneal dissection required for robotic inguinal hernia surgery will likely be more difficult, particularly medially, due to the dissection required to perform a prostatectomy. Pelvic irradiation further complicates the matter, and the surgeon should be well informed about this history prior to any attempt at robotic inguinal herniorrhaphy.

Not to be forgotten is the patient's ability to tolerate general anesthesia. Robotic surgery necessitates general anesthesia as paralysis is required, and in certain situations a patient may not be an ideal candidate for the physiologic stress of being placed under general anesthesia. These patients may be best suited with an anterior approach under either conscious sedation or local anesthesia.

Setup

Robotic inguinal hernia surgery is performed via a transabdominal approach typically utilizing three (3) 8 mm robotic trocars, although some surgeons elect to place an additional assistant port for passage of suture and mesh or to aid in retraction during the case. The operating room should be sufficiently sized to accommodate the *daVinci* patient cart and surgeon console. Typically to complete this operation, there is little to no need to move the operating room table. The patient is positioned in the supine or lithotomy position. The decision on patient positioning is based on where the patient cart will be placed relative to the patient and is at the discretion of the operating surgeon. There are many options for docking when planning robotic inguinal hernia surgery, including pelvic docking with patient in lithotomy position and several options for side docking. Other considerations in regard to patient preparation include the option to place a Foley catheter to decompress the urinary bladder, particularly when the dissection medially is anticipated to be difficult, and tucking the arms if leaving them out at a 90° angle relative to the patient presents difficulty for the bedside assistant. If the arms are tucked at the sides, care should be taken to pad the bony prominences to prevent nerve injury intraoperatively. The patient should be carefully and fully secured to the operating room table to prevent any slipping or shifting while positioning or during surgery.

If pelvic docking is preferred, the patient is placed in a lithotomy position with legs placed in adjustable stirrups, and the patient cart is guided toward the patient between the legs and adjusted accordingly. Parallel docking, or "side docking," is the preferred approach of the author (Fig. 17.1). In this setup, the patient cart is driven into the operative field from one side of the patient or the other. There are many variations on this type of docking technique. The robot can be placed in parallel to the patient on either side of the bed. Similarly, the cart can be placed at a 45° angle over the patient's hip. Docking in this fashion from either side facilitates access to either groin for either bilateral or unilateral repair.

There are several main considerations when docking utilizing this approach. It is important that all robotic arms be in line with the pelvis. Again, either side should be easily accessible with the patient cart docked on either side of the patient, i.e., a hernia on the right side can be approached with the patient cart docked on either the patient's left or right side. With the arms docked in line with the pelvis, both inguinal regions can be approached with ease. The patient will likely be placed in some degree of Trendelenburg position, and the

patient cart should be positioned high enough to clear the height of the patient's legs when placed in this position. Once docked, it is recommended that the spacing between instrument and camera arms be maximized to prevent intraoperative collisions.

Procedure

Technical aspects of the robotic transabdominal preperitoneal inguinal hernia repair will now be described. This is an operation that is rapidly gaining popularity due to relative technical ease, and patient benefits when compared to open surgery including less pain, faster recovery and return to normal activity, superior visualization, and decreased surgical site infections. It is estimated that approximately 20% of all inguinal hernia surgery in the United States currently is performed utilizing the *daVinci* robotic platform. This represents a tremendous surge in interest from the surgical community in minimally invasive hernia surgery, as the laparoscopic approach peaked around 15% nationally and has fallen off in recent years with the evolution of robotic hernia surgery. The critical principles of this operation when done robotically are nearly the same as those when completed laparoscopically, namely, establishment of the "critical view of the myopectineal orifice," popularized in text by Jorge Daes and Edward Felix described in a letter published in the *Annals of Surgery* in 2016. In this article, they report that "the objective of the critical view of the myopectineal orifice concept is to teach and standardize MIS inguinal hernia repair, facilitate evaluation of videos and live surgery transmissions, reduce recurrences, prevent complications, and ultimately improve patient care" [10].

With the patient positioned as described in the previous section, based on preoperative planning and surgeon preference, the abdomen is sterilely prepped and sterile draping applied. An 8 mm supraumbilical incision is made, and pneumoperitoneum is established to 15 mmHg with method of access being surgeon specific. Port placement is critical when doing any robotic surgery, and this holds true for robotic inguinal hernia surgery (Fig. 17.2). Once the supraumbilical port is placed, which will be the camera port, lateral ports should be placed at least 10 cm away laterally on either side of the abdomen to minimize instrument and camera collisions. The lateral ports should be high enough also to establish several centimeters of clearance from the patient's anterior superior iliac spine (ASIS) to facilitate work higher up on the abdominal wall. After appropriate port placement, the robot is driven in by operating room staff and docked to the trocars based on surgeon preference. The camera is inserted into the abdomen, and robotic instruments are passed thru the lateral trocars. Once these steps are complete, the surgeon scrubs out of the case to proceed to the console.

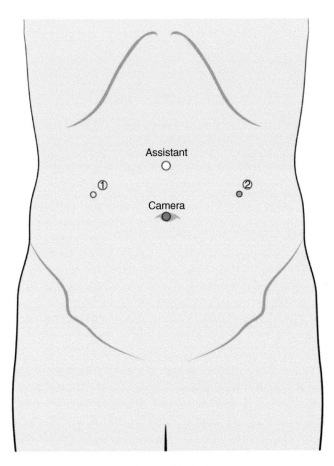

Fig. 17.1 Patient cart positioning, side dock

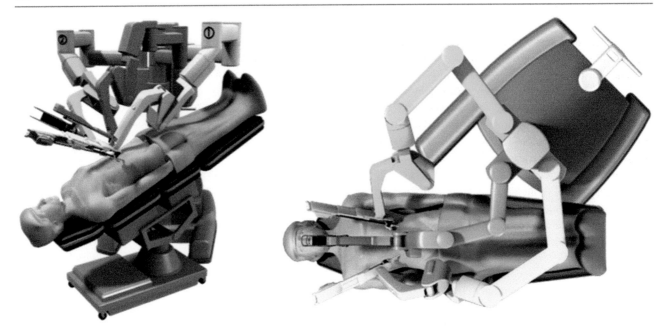

Fig. 17.2 Port positioning

Initial inspection proceeds to evaluate the contents of the hernia sac and type of hernia present whether it be indirect, direct, femoral, or a combination thereof. The choice of instruments is at the discretion of the operating surgeon but typically includes a grasping tool and an instrument that allows for electrocautery, either shears or a hook cautery device commonly. The dissection commences with the creation of a peritoneal flap to gain access to the preperitoneal space. It is suggested that this be made at least 5 cm above the uppermost aspect of the hernia defect to allow adequate space creation for wide overlap with prosthetic mesh. The flap extends from the ipsilateral median umbilical ligament to the ASIS. Care should be taken during this initial step to avoid injury to the inferior epigastric artery which courses vertically along the abdominal wall originating from the external iliac artery. Once the peritoneal flap is opened, dissection through the loose areolar tissue in the preperitoneal space ensues. Peritoneum should be followed carefully. Dissection is initially taken medially to identify and expose Cooper's ligament (Fig. 17.3). The dissection should extend medially at least to the pubic symphysis and, in the case of a large direct hernia, to the contralateral Cooper's ligament. During exposure of Cooper's ligament, the presence of a direct hernia will be evaluated, as the direct space is immediately superior to the ligament, within Hesselbach's triangle. If present, reduce herniated preperitoneal fat in the direct space. Once Cooper's ligament is identified, its dissection should continue laterally to the level of the external iliac vein. This step allows for evaluation of the femoral space and, if present, reduction of contents.

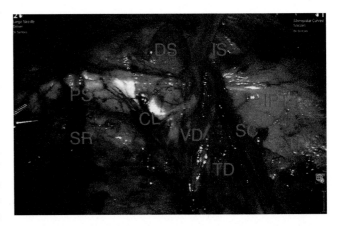

Fig. 17.3 Inguinal anatomy. *PS* pubic symphysis, *SR* space of Retzius, *CL* Cooper's ligament, *VD* vas deferens, *SC* spermatic cord (testicular vessels), *DS* direct space, *IS* indirect space (inguinal canal), *IPT* iliopubic tract, *TD* triangle of Doom, *TP* triangle of pain

After the medial dissection is completed, attention is turned laterally. Following the peritoneal flap, preperitoneal fat laterally is cleared back away from the peritoneum and spermatic cord structures. Dissection laterally proceeds carefully as to not injure or traumatize the peripheral nerves running in the triangle of pain below the iliopubic tract in this area. Lateral dissection should continue to the level of the lateral border of the psoas muscle. An indirect sac, if present, can now be dissected and reduced. The sac must be dissected off of the spermatic cord and mobilized sufficiently posteriorly. The spermatic cord elements must be parietalized adequately to avoid mesh disruption due to inadequate posterior dissection. This step is most frequently not completed appropriately and accounts for the majority of posterior repair failures. Care should be taken during this process, being aware that the iliac artery is directly deep to this area between the vas deferens and gonadal vessels, i.e., the triangle of doom (Fig. 17.3). Adequate dissection can be assured by pulling up on the peritoneal flap and then toward the camera. If the cord structures are not disrupted by this motion and continue to lie flat on the retroperitoneum without tenting upward, parietalization of the cord is complete. An effort should be made to try to identify and reduce cord lipomas, which typically run lateral to the cord elements and into the inguinal canal. These do not require resection, rather complete reduction, and once mesh is placed, the lipoma may be placed behind it. Once complete dissection of the MPO is accomplished, a synthetic mesh of the surgeon's choice may be deployed. If placing mesh that requires fixation with either sutures or tacks, care should be taken to avoid the so-called triangle of pain bounded by the iliopubic tract and the spermatic vessels, thereby avoiding injury to the peripheral nerves passing through this area. Robotic technology and instrumentation allow for easy suturing techniques and obviate the need for expensive tacking devices in most situations.

The mesh should lie flat without any creases, and there should be adequate clearance between the inferior border of the mesh and the posteriormost dissection of the parietalized cord and peritoneum. This prevents subsequent folding (so-called tacoing) of mesh due to inadequate posterior dissection as described above. In addition, there should be wide overlap of mesh to cover the defect, and an appropriately sized mesh should be chosen. Once the mesh is deployed and fixated, positioned appropriately, and hemostasis is evaluated and ensured, closure of the peritoneal flap is completed. This can be done in a variety of ways, typically with a running barbed suture thanks to the intuitive nature of robotic sewing.

Postoperative Care

Robotic inguinal hernia surgery is typically done as an outpatient procedure, either at an outpatient surgicenter or a hospital. The immediate postoperative management includes ensuring adequate pain control if necessary. Urinary retention can also be an issue in the immediate postop period, particularly for older men with prior history of retention or hesitancy related to prostatic hypertrophy. It is recommended

in these instances that patients remain at the facility where the procedure was performed until able to void.

Once the patient is home, instructions should be clear regarding activity restrictions. Typically it is recommended that the postoperative patient remain active. A heavy lifting and strenuous activity restriction is frequently recommended to allow healing and scarring of mesh to occur. At the follow-up appointment, physical exam is performed. The groin should be examined and early recurrence ruled out. The area of the inguinal canal should be examined for development of seroma. Seromas form more commonly after repair of large hernias, since reduction of a large hernia sac can result in leaving a potential space in which fluid can collect. It is uncommon that any intervention need be done for seromas in the inguinal region. They almost always resolve with time. Each surgeon makes recommendations to his/her patients in regard to duration of activity restriction. Typically the patient is able to resume normal activities in a matter of weeks. This approach to inguinal hernia repair is generally very well tolerated and results in excellent surgical outcomes.

References

1. Burcharth J, Pedersen M, Bisgaard T, et al. Nationwide prevalence of groin hernia repair. PLoS One. 2013;8(1):e54367.
2. Primatesta P, Goldacre MJ. Inguinal hernia repair: incidence of elective and emergency surgery, readmission and mortality. Int J Epidemiol. 1996;25:835–9.
3. Lau H, Fang C, Yuen WK, Patil NG. Risk factors for inguinal hernia in adult males: a case-control study. Surgery. 2007;141:262–6.
4. Fitzgibbons RJ Jr, Giobbie-Harder A, Gibbs JO, et al. Watchful waiting vs repair of inguinal hernia in minimally symptomatic men: a randomized clinical trial. JAMA. 2006;295:285–92.
5. Kux M, Fuchsjager N, Schemper M. Shouldice is superior to Bassini inguinal herniorrhaphy. Am J Surg. 1994;168:15–8.
6. Scott NW, McCormack K, Graham P, Go PM, Ross SJ, Grant AM. Open mesh versus non-mesh for repair of femoral and inguinal hernia. Cochrane Database Syst Rev. 2002;4:CD002197.
7. McCormack K, Scott NW, Go PM, Ross S, Grant AM. Laparoscopic techniques versus open techniques for inguinal hernia repair. Cochrane Database Syst Rev. 2003;1:CD001785.
8. Bittner R, Arregui ME, Bisgaard T, et al. Guidelines for laparoscopic (TAPP) and endoscopic (TEP) treatment of inguinal hernia [international Endohernia society (IEHS)]. Surg Endosc. 2011;25:2773–843.
9. Simons MP, Aufenacker T, Bay-Nielsen M, et al. European hernia society guidelines on the treatment of inguinal hernia in adult patients. Hernia. 2009;13:343–403.
10. Daes J, Felix E. Critical view of the Myopectineal orifice. Ann Surg. 2016;266:e1.

Robotic Transabdominal Preperitoneal Repair for Ventral/Incisional and Atypical Hernias

18

Anushi Shah and Conrad Ballecer

Introduction

Robotic transabdominal preperitoneal repair (rTAPP) for ventral hernias incorporates skills and techniques learned from both open and conventional laparoscopic ventral hernia repairs. The rTAPP hernia repair is borrowed from conventional laparoscopic transabdominal preperitoneal repair (TAPP) for the treatment of groin hernias [1]. This technique is built upon utilizing an uncoated mesh placed in a preperitoneal position [1, 2]. The robot allows for improved vision, ergonomics, and precision in separating and dissecting the individual layers of the abdominal wall. The preperitoneal approach allows for mesh to be placed in a position protected from the intra-abdominal content, thereby, reducing risk of visceral adhesions to mesh and perhaps eliminating the requirement of extensive mesh fixation [1–5]. This chapter introduces rTAPP for ventral and incisional hernias.

Anatomy

The key to rTAPP is to have adequate understanding of the individual layers of the abdominal wall. Initial dissection begins with incising the peritoneum to enter an avascular plane between the peritoneum and transversalis fascia or posterior sheath. Blunt and sharp dissection is used to carefully develop the preperitoneal plane following the principles of adequate 5 cm overlap circumferential to the hernia defect. The dissection is complete when the hernia sac is reduced and a large preperitoneal plane is developed to accommodate an adequately sized mesh. Mesh is placed for reinforcement and can be sutures or tacked to abdominal wall at cardinal points. The mesh is then covered with the dissected perito-

neal flap. This method is best suited for small- to medium-sized ventral hernias and atypical hernias such as subxiphoid, suprapubic, flank, and Spigelian defects.

Preoperative Considerations

A thorough history and physical exam are important in formulating a surgical plan for repair. Individual comorbidities such as BMI, smoking history, prior repairs, and immuno-compromised states can be determining factors for operative vs non-operative management.1 In patients with small primary hernias, a complete history and physical exam is usually sufficient in preoperative planning. However, abdominal/pelvis CT can be a useful adjunct especially in patients with recurrent and large incisional hernias.

Operative Steps

Umbilical Hernias

Positioning, Port Placement, Docking, and Instrumentation

Patient is placed in a supine position on the operating room table with bilateral arms tucked. Raising the kidney rest positioned at the level of the umbilicus can widen the space between the costal margin and the pelvic rim in order to place trocars with adequate separation. Flexing the bed can accomplish the same goal as well. Optional placement of Foley catheter can be considered if a prolonged case is expected.

A 5 mm OptiView trocar (with or without initial Veress insufflation) is used to achieve intra-abdominal access at Palmer's point in the left or right upper quadrant, and pneumoperitoneum is established to a pressure of 15 mmHg. Under direct visualization, a 12 mm robotic port is placed in the mid-lateral abdomen position at least 15 cm from the defect. Another 8 mm robotic port is placed in the left or

A. Shah
General Surgery, Maricopa Medical Center, Phoenix, AZ, USA

C. Ballecer (✉)
Department of Surgery, Abrazo Arrowhead Hospital, Peoria, AZ, USA
e-mail: cballecer1@mac.com

© Springer Nature Switzerland AG 2019
S. Tsuda, O. Y. Kudsi (eds.), *Robotic-Assisted Minimally Invasive Surgery*, https://doi.org/10.1007/978-3-319-96866-7_18

right lower quadrant. The 5 mm OptiView port is then replaced with an 8 mm robotic port (Fig. 18.1).

The robot is docked over the contralateral abdomen in line with the ports. A 30° up scope is used for initial dissection of the ipsilateral abdominal wall but can be adjusted to 0° or 30° down in order to facilitate contralateral preperitoneal dissection.

Preperitoneal Plane Dissection, Primary Repair of Defect, and Mesh Placement

Adhesions are carefully taken down to adequately visualize the hernia defect. The peritoneum is incised at least 5 cm from the closest (ipsilateral) edge of the hernia defect with monopolar scissors (Fig. 18.2). Blunt and sharp dissection is used to develop the preperitoneal avascular plane. While developing the peritoneal flap, cautery should be used judiciously to avoid peritoneal and posterior sheath rents. Blunt sweeping with adequate countertraction provides safe and easy dissection of the peritoneum off the posterior sheath. The hernia sac is defined by developing a preperitoneal plane cephalad and caudad to the hernia sac (Fig. 18.3, 18.4 and 18.5). The hernia sac is reduced meticulously to avoid peritoneal rents.

After reduction of the hernia sac, the peritoneal plane is developed on the contralateral abdomen. Minimum preperitoneal dissection is deemed complete when an adequately sized mesh with at least 5 cm overlaps in every direction. Creating a large flap is helpful to create a redundancy in the peritoneum, thereby facilitating its closure.

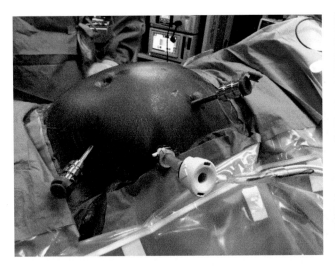

Fig. 18.1 Patient docking/trocar placement for umbilical/midline ventral hernia

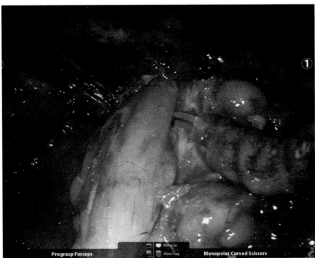

Fig. 18.3 Gentle reduction of hernia contents

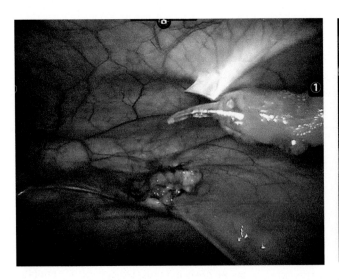

Fig. 18.2 Development of preperitoneal space at least 5 cm from hernia site

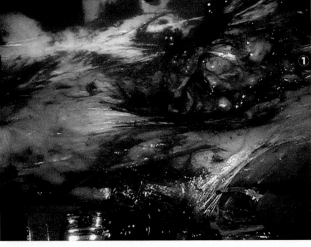

Fig. 18.4 Continuation of preperitoneal dissection past hernia defect with use of tension-countertension

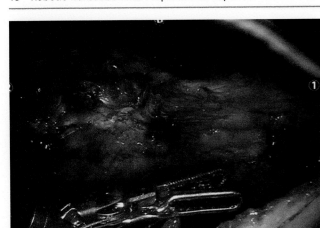

Fig. 18.5 Completed preperitoneal dissection with reduced hernia

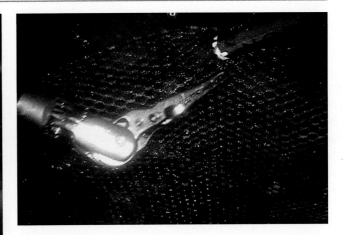

Fig. 18.7 Mesh fixation with tacker at cardinal points on anterior abdominal wall

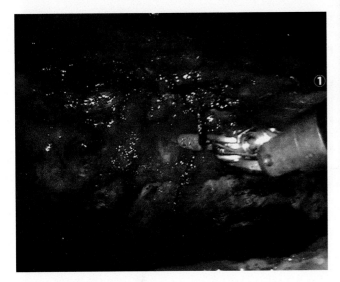

Fig. 18.6 Primary repair of suture defect with absorbable locking suture

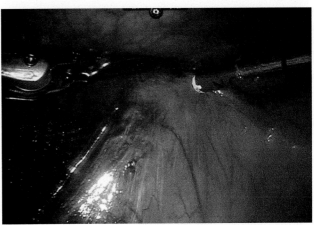

Fig. 18.8 Covering mesh with peritoneal flap with tacker

Subxiphoid Hernias

Positioning, Port Placement, Docking, and Instrumentation

After adequate preperitoneal dissection is completed, the hernia defect is primarily closed. This is usually performed with absorbable barbed suture in a continuous fashion (Fig. 18.6). The anterior dead space of the hernia defect can be obliterated by incorporating thin bites of subcutaneous skin which recreates an inverted umbilicus. Small peritoneal disruptions can be closed with absorbable suture.

An appropriately sized uncoated mesh can be introduced through the 8 mm trocar and situated in the preperitoneal space against the abdominal wall. The mesh is then fixated with tacks or sutures positioned at cardinal points (Fig. 18.7). The peritoneum is then re-approximated to cover the mesh with tacks or suture. The 12 mm port site is closed with absorbable suture (Fig. 18.8).

Atypical hernias such as those located in a subxiphoid location or Morgagni diaphragmatic defects are well suited to the rTAPP approach. By virtue of sandwiching the mesh within layers of the abdominal wall, the difficulty of lack of fixation points is overcome. Patient is placed in a supine position on the operating room table with bilateral arms tucked. Special consideration of the kidney rest at the level of the umbilicus or table flexion can be made if the patient has a short torso to allow for optimal space between trocars and separation from the site of the hernia. Optional placement of a Foley catheter can be considered if a prolonged case is expected.

A midline camera port situated at least 15 cm from the hernia defect is placed to obtain intra-abdominal access. Two 8 mm ports are subsequently placed under direct vision at or near the same level of the camera port. The robot is docked over the patient's left or right shoulder. A 30° up scope is used for adequate visualization of the anterior abdominal wall.

Preperitoneal Plane Dissection, Primary Repair of Defect, and Mesh Placement

Bowel and omental adhesions are carefully taken down to adequately visualize the abdominal wall anatomy and the hernia defect. Hernia content if any is reduced safely to avoid iatrogenic injury. The peritoneum is incised at least 5 cm from the edge of the hernia defect with scissors. Blunt and sharp dissection is used to develop a preperitoneal avascular plane in a caudal to cephalad direction. In developing the peritoneal flap, cautery should be used judiciously to avoid peritoneal and fascial defects. Blunt sweeping utilizing traction/countertraction principles provides safe and meticulous separation of the peritoneum from the posterior sheath. The hernia sac is reduced and preserved to become confluent with the peritoneal flap. The falciform ligament can be mobilized and dissected off the anterior abdominal wall to allow for better visualization and can subsequently be used to cover any peritoneal defects.

Once adequate dissection of at least 5 cm overlap is achieved in all directions surrounding the defect, the defect is primarily closed. This is usually performed with absorbable barbed suture in continuous fashion.

An appropriately sized uncoated mesh can be introduced through 8 mm trocar and situated in the preperitoneal space against the abdominal wall. The mesh is then fixated with tacks or sutured at cardinal points. The peritoneum is then re-approximated to cover the mesh with tacks or suture.

Suprapubic Hernias

Positioning, Port Placement, Docking, and Instrumentation

The rTAPP approach to atypical suprapubic hernias also exploits the enabling quality of the robotic instrument to develop a large preperitoneal space and ultimately hide the mesh from the visceral content once the peritoneal flap is re-approximated.

The patient is placed in a supine lithotomy position on the operating room table with bilateral arms tucked. The placement of Foley catheter is recommended as it can help with identification and possible reduction of the bladder from the hernia defect.

A midline camera port situated at least 15 cm from the hernia defect is placed to obtain intra-abdominal access. Two 8 mm ports are placed at bilateral lateral upper quadrants 10 cm apart from midline port (Fig. 18.9).

The patient is placed in a reverse Trendelenburg position, and the robot is docked in between the patient's legs

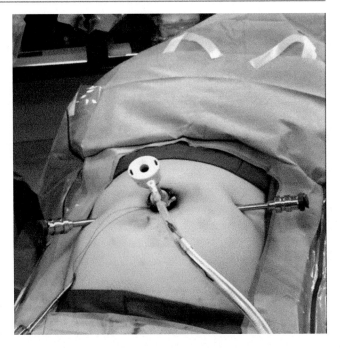

Fig. 18.9 Suprapubic hernia trocar placement and docking

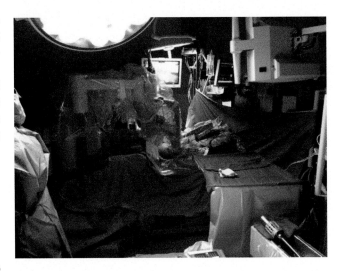

Fig. 18.10 Suprapubic hernia trocar placement and docking

(Fig. 18.10). Grasper and monopolar scissors are used for combination of blunt and sharp dissection. A 0 or 30° angled scope is used for abdominal wall visualization.

Preperitoneal Plane Dissection, Primary Repair of Defect, and Mesh Placement

Bowel and omental adhesions are carefully taken down to adequately visualize the abdominal wall anatomy and the hernia defect. The peritoneum is incised at least 5 cm from the edge of the hernia defect with scissors. Blunt and sharp dissection is used to develop a preperitoneal avascular plane in a cephalad to caudad direction encompassing bilateral medial umbilical ligaments at minimum. Wide retropubic and space of Retzius dissection is performed for this type of hernia in order to ensure adequate mesh coverage. Anatomical visualization and considerations to inguinal anatomy such as the retroinguinal space to expose Cooper's ligaments and bladder identification are important for repair of this hernia. In developing the peritoneal flap, cautery should be used judiciously to avoid peritoneal defects and potential injury to the bladder, cord elements, blood vessels, and nerves.

Once adequate dissection of at least 5 cm overlap circumferential to hernia defect is completed, the defect can be primarily repaired. This is usually performed with absorbable barbed suture in a continuous fashion. Desufflation of pneumoperitoneum to 6–10 mmHg may help in closing large suprapubic defects.

An appropriately sized uncoated mesh can be introduced through 8 mm trocar and situated in the preperitoneal space against the abdominal wall. The mesh is then fixated at cardinal points as well as Cooper's ligaments. It is important to avoid fixation in proximity to the bladder, triangles of doom, and pain. The peritoneum is then re-approximated to cover the mesh with tacks or suture. All port sites larger than 8 mm are closed with absorbable suture.

Conclusion

rTAPP for ventral/incisional and atypical hernias is an emerging surgical method vetted from well-established open and laparoscopic principles. The preperitoneal approach allows for protection of mesh from intra-abdominal contents and avoidance of full-thickness transfascial sutures. Inability to access preperitoneal plane limits the use of this repair, and other techniques may be utilized. However, this is a safe and versatile option for repair of abdominal wall hernias. The robot provides improved ergonomics, visualization, and precision with not only similar patient satisfaction compared to laparoscopic repair but also improved physician satisfaction and quality of life.

References

1. Prasad P, Tantia O, Patle NM, Khanna S, Sen B. Laparoscopic transabdominal preperitoneal repair of ventral hernia: a step towards physiological repair. Indian J Surg. 2011;73:403–8.
2. Gray SH, Vick CC, Graham LA, Finan KR, Neumayer LA, Hawn MT. Risk of complications from enterotomy or unplanned bowel resection during elective hernia repair. Arch Surg. 2008;143:582–6.
3. Halm JA, De Wall LL, Steyerberg EW, Jeekel J, Lange JF. Intraperitoneal polypropylene mesh hernia repair complicates subsequent abdominal surgery. World J Surg. 2007;31:423–9.
4. Colavita PD, Tsirline VB, Belyansky I, Walters AL, Lincourt AE, Sing RF, Heniford BT. Prospective, long-term comparison of quality of life in laparoscopic versus open ventral hernia repair. Ann Surg. 2012;256:714–22.
5. Liang MK, Clapp M, Li LT, Berger RL, Hicks SC. Patient satisfaction, chronic pain, and functional status following laparoscopic ventral hernia repair. World J Surg. 2013;37:530–7.

Robotic Transanal Resection

Giovanni Dapri

Introduction

Transanal minimally invasive surgery (TAMIS) gained interest in the last decade [1], after the introduction in the laparoscopic era of the natural orifice transluminal endoscopic surgery (NOTES) [2].

TAMIS represents an evolution of laparoscopic surgery applied to the transanal approach and commonly known as transanal endoscopic microsurgery (TEM) [3]. TAMIS has been described using conventional or specially designed laparoscopic instruments and conventional telescope through dedicated transanal ports/platforms [4–5]. The robotic platform can be applied as well to realize the transanal procedures. The main advantage of the robot application is offered by the 360° robotic extremities' rotation in a small and limited space, like appears to be the rectal lumen. Furthermore, the other already reported advantages of robot-assisted laparoscopy, like the surgeon's comfort, the surgeon's ergonomy, the camera stability, the 3D view, and the double console for teaching and training [6], are added.

Different TAMIS applications are nowadays feasible and safe, like the middle and giant rectal polypectomy, the down-to-up total mesorectal excision (TME), and the treatment of colorectal anastomotic complications (leak/fistula, bleeding, stricture). The transanal approach during polypectomy allows the polyps removal, difficult to be removed through the endoscopic submucosal dissection, and the final flap/rectal wall closure. During the transanal down-to-up TME, more benefits are achieved like the exact localization of the intraluminal tumor, the precise distance between the tumor and the anal margin, the transmural rectal section started just few cm below the tumor, the improved lateral nerves' exposure, and the specimen's extraction through the natural orifice (which avoids additional abdominal incisions and consequent risk of ventral hernia). Transanal robot-assisted laparoscopy can also be adopted to treat and repair difficult situations like the colorectal anastomotic leak/fistula, bleeding, and stricture.

In this chapter the robot-assisted transanal technique for these procedures is described in details.

Technique

Patient and Robotic Platform Positioning

The patient, under general anesthesia, is placed supine with the legs apart in gynecologic positioning. The anal canal and rectal ampulla are cleaned by multiple disinfectant lavages. The transanal platform is inserted through the anal margin into the rectal lumen, and the robotic platform is connected to this latter. The console is placed close to the operative table as well. The trocars (Fig.19.1) are inserted through the transanal platform, keeping in mind one rule of conventional laparoscopy, which is the optical system in the middle of the created triangulation by the two working instruments [7]. Hence, the scope is placed in the central trocar at 6 o'clock position, the left-hand instrument (grasper) at the 9 o'clock position trocar, and the right hand instrument (cautery, harmonic, needle driver, shears, clip applier) at the 3 o'clock position trocar. An added instrument is inserted through a fourth trocar at the 12 o'clock position. A continuous CO_2 insufflation is required and applied through the transanal platform.

Polypectomy

The procedure starts with the rectal lumen exploration allowing the identification of the exact location of the polyps from the anal margin. Once the distance is measured, the mucosal layer around the lesion is marked by superficial scores with the cautery, inserted at 3 o'clock position, keeping some mm

G. Dapri
Saint-Pierre University Hospital, European School of Laparoscopic Surgery, Department of Gastrointestinal Surgery, Brussels, Belgium
e-mail: giovanni@dapri.net

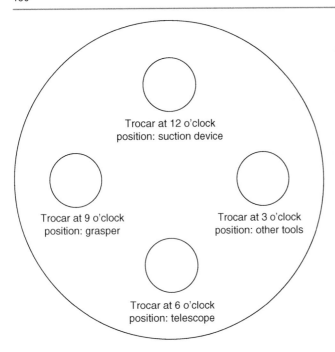

Fig. 19.1 Transanal trocars and robotic instruments positioning. (Published with kind permission of © Giovanni Dapri MD, PhD, FACS, 2018. All Rights Reserved)

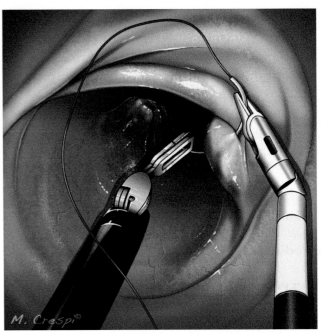

Fig. 19.2 Transanal TME: beginning of intraluminal lumen closure. (Published with kind permission of © Giovanni Dapri MD, PhD, FACS, 2018. All Rights Reserved)

free margins. The grasper, inserted at 9 o'clock position, is used to retract the mucosal tissue during the cautery or harmonic incision. The resection is started at 6 o'clock position, going laterally on the patient's right side and left side. Finally, the two lateral dissections are joined together at 12 o'clock position. The resection is performed with the removal of the mucosal and submucosal tissue, skeletonizing the below muscular layer or removing the lesion in full-thickness way. If perioperative bleeding occurs, the suction device, introduced through the fourth trocar at 12 o'clock position, is used. This latter tool is useful during the entire procedure to remove the smoke created with the cautery dissection. Once the resection is completed, the specimen is removed transanally. The mucosal-submucosal flap or the entire rectal wall is subsequently closed using two converging running sutures, keeping the grasper at the 9 o'clock position and the needle driver at the 3 o'clock position. Polydioxanone (PDS) 2/0 or V-lock 3/0 sutures are implemented. The shears are inserted through the fourth trocar at the end of the suturing. The suture line is checked, and the robotic instruments are removed.

Down-to-Up TME

The procedure starts with the rectal lumen exploration and with the tumor identification. The distance between the inferior edge of the malignant lesion and the pectineal line is measured. A purse-string suture around the rectal lumen is started at 3 o'clock position, and it goes to 6, 9, and 12 o'clock positions

(Fig. 19.2). This suture, placed 1 cm down the inferior edge of the malignant lesion, is performed using the grasper on the left side of the transanal port/platform and the needle driver on the right side of the transanal port/platform. Polypropylene 2/0 suture is used. Once tied, the suture is cut by the scissors, introduced through the fourth trocar. The rectal stump is completely insufflated. The cautery or the harmonic is introduced at the 3 o'clock position trocar. The mucosal layer is marked with a tattoo around the suture knot, staying 1 cm laterally. Then, the transmural rectal incision is started at 6 o'clock position, and it follows the previous tattoo around the suture knot. The mesorectal excision is started at the posterior plane, going deeply and searching the presacral fascia (Fig. 19.3). Once the correct and avascular plane is found, the dissection is completed for a length of 5–10 cm. Then, it goes laterally on the patient's right side and left side. Frequently the inferior and the middle rectal arteries are identified during the dissection. These latter vessels are freed, clipped by clip applier introduced at 3 o'clock position, and cut by shears introduced at 12 o'clock position. The sacral lateral nerves are maintained laterally, and the dissection is continued going upper in the direction of the promontory. The anterior dissection, sectioning the rectoprostatic fascia (Denonvilliers' fascia) or the rectovaginal septum, is performed, only after completing the posterior and the lateral dissections (Fig. 19.4). Douglas' pouch is opened, after freeing the fatty tissue below the rectoprostatic fascia or the rectovaginal septum, and the transanal dissection joins the peritoneal cavity. The posterior mesorectal plane is finished with the mobilization of the mesorectum from the promontory. The lat-

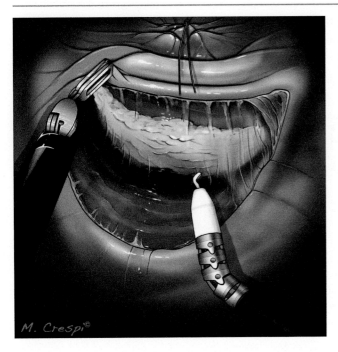

Fig. 19.3 Transanal TME: posterior dissection. (Published with kind permission of © Giovanni Dapri MD, PhD, FACS, 2018. All Rights Reserved)

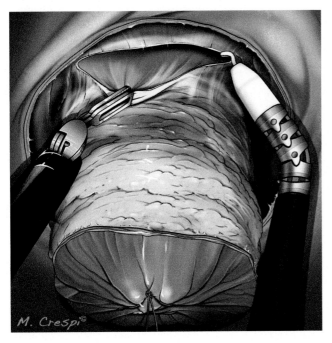

Fig. 19.4 Transanal TME: anterior dissection and Douglas' pouch opening. (Published with kind permission of © Giovanni Dapri MD, PhD, FACS, 2018. All Rights Reserved)

eral dissections are finalized as well. At this point the rectal resection can be performed completely through the anus, with the inferior mesenteric artery and vein sections from below, associated to the sigmoid/left colon mobilization. Usually colorectal surgeons join the transanal approach to the abdomi-

nal approach in one or two steps, realizing the abdominal approach through robot-assisted laparoscopy or conventional multi-port laparoscopy or single-incision laparoscopy [8]. During the abdominal approach, the vascular dissection, the sigmoid/left colon mobilization, and the splenic flexure downloading are performed. Once these different steps are finished, the specimen is ready to be extracted through the anus, after have encircled the rectum in a plastic protection, inserted through the anal platform. The robotic instruments are temporally removed from the patient. Externally to the patient, the sigmoid/left colon is cut at the appropriate distance from the tumor, and the specimen is sent to the pathologist for analysis. A circular stapler anvil, appropriate in diameter, is inserted into the sigmoid/left colon lumen. A purse-string suture is applied, and the anvil is pushed into the pelvis, through the anal canal. The transanal platform is reinserted through the anus, and the robotic instruments are repositioned. The rectal stump is closed using the grasper at 9 o'clock position and the needle driver at 3 o'clock position. A polypropylene 2/0 suture is adopted to close the rectal stump, and it is started at 6 o'clock position. Once the suture is tied and cut, the robotic instruments are removed, and the circular stapler is introduced through the anal canal, joining the anvil. A colorectal circular mechanical anastomosis is performed. This latter is checked with the reintroduction of the transanal port/platform through the anus and the patient's connection to the robot. If no evidence of anastomotic complications is apparent, the platform and the robotic instruments are removed.

Colorectal Anastomotic Complication Repair

In front of an evidence of immediate colorectal anastomotic leak or bleeding, a direct repair by transanal approach can be realized. The instruments adopted are the grasper through the 9 o'clock position, the needle driver through the 3 o'clock position, and the shears through the 12 o'clock position. The defect is repaired using separated Vicryl 2/0 suture, keeping in mind to avoid potential postoperative strictures. As well, delayed colorectal fistula can be treated in the same method through robot-assisted transanal laparoscopy.

Author's Recommendations

Polypectomy

The cautery is useful to perform this procedure, and the suction device helps with the smoke's evacuation created during the dissection. The final flap/rectal wall closure can be easily performed, starting with the first suture at one lateral corner and joining the other suture, coming from the opposite lateral corner, at the middle suture line.

Down-to-Up TME

The TME plane has to be started posteriorly, going deeply in the direction of the coccyx. The anterior dissection, which includes the rectoprostatic fascia (Denonvilliers' fascia) or the rectovaginal septum sectioning, is performed only after the posterior and the lateral dissections have been realized. This strategy permits avoiding potential injuries of the urethra, prostate, and vagina. The anterior dissection and rectal mobilization have to be performed keeping in mind that the length in male patients is longer than in female patients; hence Douglas' pouch opening can be reached fastly and suddenly more in female patients than in male patients.

Colorectal Anastomotic Complication Repair

This philosophy to treat colorectal anastomotic complications through transanal approach is quite new, and it has increased, thanks to the TAMIS introduction in colorectal surgery [9]. It allows the immediate or the delayed treatment of anastomotic complications, which usually are difficult to treat. Since the robotic instruments allow the surgeon a simplified method performing intraluminal 360° rotation, suturing and knotting techniques are easier through robot-assisted transanal approach.

References

1. deBeche-Adams T, Nassif G. Transanal minimally invasive surgery. Clin Colon Rectal Surg. 2015;28(3):176–80.
2. Rattner D. Introduction to NOTES white paper. Surg Endosc. 2006;20(2):185.
3. Buess G, Theiss R, Gunther M, Hutterer F, Pichlmaier H. Transanal endoscopic microsurgery. Leber Magen Darm. 1985;15(6): 271–9.
4. Dapri G, Guta D, Cardinali L, Mazzetti C, Cadenas Fabres A, Grozdev K, Sondji SH, Surdeanu I, Cadière GB. A new reusable platform for transanal minimally invasive surgery: first experience. Surg Technol Int. 2016;28(4):85–95.
5. Kim MJ, Park JW, Ha HK, Jeon BG, Shin R, Ryoo SB, Choi SJ, Park BK, Park KJ, Jeong SY. Initial experience of transanal total mesorectal excision with rigid or flexible transanal platforms in cadavers. Surg Endosc. 2016;30(4):1640–7.
6. Herron DM, Marohn M, SAGES-MIRA Robotic Surgery Consensus Group. A consensus document on robotic surgery. Surg Endosc. 2008;22(2):313–25.
7. Hanna GB, Drew T, Clinch P, Hunter B, Cuschieri A. Computer-controlled endoscopic performance assessment system. Surg Endosc. 1988;12(7):997–1000.
8. Dapri G, Marks JH, editors. Surgical techniques in rectal cancer : transanal, laparoscopic and robotic approach. Tokyo: Springer; 2017.
9. Dapri G, Guta D, Grozdev K, Antolino L, Bachir N, Jottard K, Cadière GB. Colorectal anastomotic leakage corrected by transanal laparoscopy. Color Dis. 2016;18(6):O210–3.

Robotic Parastomal Hernia

Peter A. Walker and Shinil K. Shah

Introduction

Parastomal hernias represent a challenging complication following many common surgical procedures such as colon resections and radical cystectomies. Early literature included descriptive case series [1] and retrospective reviews [2] indicating a 10% incidence of parastomal hernia formation. The majority of these hernias were not believed to be clinically significant with only 10–20% undergoing repair. More recent literature reviews indicate a much more significant incidence of parastomal hernia formation (up to 50%) [3]. In addition, the incidence of associated complications including bowel obstruction, urinary obstruction, chronic pain, and intestinal ischemia were found to be higher than initially belived [4]. Furthermore, quality of life scoring showed parastomal hernia formation to be associated with decreased physical function, increased pain, and decreased perception of general health [5]. For these reasons, the potential role of risk factor optimization prior to index operation and the need for elective parastomal hernia repairs need to be considered.

Review of the risk factors for parastomal formation shows many similarities to incisional hernia data. Evaluation of 165 patients who underwent elective colectomy with end colostomy formation with 36-month follow-up showed parastomal hernia formation in 37.8% of cases. Furthermore, multivariate analysis showed body mass index (BMI) > 25, hypertension, female gender, and age > 60 to be independent risk factors for the development of parastomal hernia [6]. Similarly, Donahue et al. reviewed 433 consecutive patients undergoing open radical cystectomy with ileal conduit formation and found the incidence of parastomal hernia formation to be 48% at 2 years. In addition, multivariate analysis once again showed female gender and increasing BMI to be independent risk factors for hernia formation as well as poor nutrition as indicated by lower serum albumin levels [7].

A large cross-sectional survey of 2854 patients with varying stoma types (colostomy, ileostomy, and urostomy) was also completed via a detailed questionnaire to evaluate potential risk factors for the development of parastomal hernias. The results indicated that preoperative risk factors such as cirrhosis, increased abdominal girth, active smoking, and previous hernias were associated with increased risk [8].

Evaluation of the risk factors for parastomal hernia formation is imperative to allow for potential optimization prior to operation. Attempts at weight reduction, improved nutrition, and smoking cessation could potentially lead to better outcomes. While many stomas are required at the time of emergency surgical procedures, the ones that are created on a more elective or planned basis may allow for time to decrease risk and optimize outcomes.

Despite patient optimization and improving techniques, the incidence of parastomal hernia formation remains significant. As previously stated, the development of a parastomal hernia increases the risk of bowel and urinary obstruction as well as decreases abdominal wall functionality and overall health. For these reasons, operative repair is often indicated. A review of common parastomal hernia repair techniques via open, laparoscopic, and robotic approaches is provided below.

Open Parastomal Hernia Repair

Symptomatic parastomal hernias can greatly increase patient morbidity, and up to half of patients require operative repair. Systematic reviews have evaluated different open repair techniques and found that non-mesh primary fascial repair was associated with an approximately 50% incidence of recurrence. Mesh reinforcement was found to

P. A. Walker (✉)
Department of Surgery, McGovern Medical School, University of Texas Health Science Center at Houston, Houston, TX, USA

S. K. Shah
Department of Surgery, McGovern Medical School, University of Texas Health Science Center at Houston, Houston, TX, USA

Michael E. DeBakey Institute for Comparative Cardiovascular Science and Biomedical Devices, Texas A&M University, College Station, TX, USA

© Springer Nature Switzerland AG 2019
S. Tsuda, O. Y. Kudsi (eds.), *Robotic-Assisted Minimally Invasive Surgery*, https://doi.org/10.1007/978-3-319-96866-7_20

decrease recurrence rates to 7.9–14.8% [9]. An additional review completed by Hansson et al. mirrored these results showing primary suture repair to be associated with increased recurrence rates when compared to mesh repair (odds ratio 8.9, 95% CI 5.2–15.1, $p < 0.0001$). Overall, evaluation of the available literature indicates that mesh repair is associated with acceptable rates of infection (approximately 3%) while offering improved long-term repair durability [10].

Literature discussing open parastomal hernia repair with mesh is somewhat limited with early publications consisting of small case series or case reports [11, 12]. Later reviews evaluated the commonly utilized "keyhole" technique. The technique involves lysis of adhesions followed by primary fascial closure at the time of parastomal hernia repair. Next, the stoma is pulled through a slit cut in the center of the mesh which is either placed in an onlay or sublay position. Fifty-eight patients undergoing keyhole repair were reviewed by Steele et al. and found to have a 36% incidence of morbidity (recurrence, obstruction, prolapse, wound infection, fistula, and erosion) with recurrence rates of 26% at a mean follow-up of 50.6 months [13].

Another commonly deployed repair is the "Sugarbaker" technique. The Sugarbaker repair involves lysis of adhesions followed by intraperitoneal sublay mesh with broad coverage of the stoma. Stelzner et al. completed a retrospective review of 30 patients undergoing open parastomal hernia repair via the Sugarbaker technique with a mean follow-up of 3.5 years showing a 15% incidence of parastomal hernia recurrence [14].

An additional consideration during parastomal hernia repair is the potential for resiting of the stoma to either the ipsilateral or contralateral side of the abdominal wall. An early retrospective review compared parastomal hernia repair via primary fascial closure and stoma relocation in 94 patients. The incidence of recurrence was 76% in the primary fascial closure cohort compared to 33% in the stoma relocation cohort ($p < 0.01$) [15]. An additional small review completed of 50 patients by Riansuwan et al. compared stoma relocation and fascial repair during recurrent parastomal hernia repair. The findings were similar with decreased rates of recurrence in the stoma relocation group (38% versus 74%, $p = 0.02$) [16]. Overall, the literature available evaluating stoma relocation is limited; however, the results indicate potential improvement in outcomes when compared to primary fascial closure alone.

Review of the literature available for open parastomal hernia repair shows significant recurrence rates with an incidence surpassing 50% in some studies. Primary fascial closure with mesh placement has been associated with a decrease in recurrence and is indicated in most cases. With the development of improved laparoscopic imaging and techniques, the role of laparoscopic parastomal hernia repair and the associated potential decreased wound complications needs to be considered.

Laparoscopic Parastomal Hernia Repair

Improvements in laparoscopic techniques have led to their widespread utilization for both ventral and incisional hernias, including parastomal hernias. Early case reports described the feasibility of the technique with intraperitoneal mesh placement [17]. More recently, a systemic review was completed on the American College of Surgeons National Surgical Quality Improvement Project (ACS-NSQIP) data comparing all patients that underwent open or laparoscopic hernia repair from 2005 to 2011. A total of 2167 cases were reviewed; only 10.4% of cases were completed laparoscopically. After adjusting for confounding variables, laparoscopic repair was associated with shorter operative times (137.5 vs. 153.4 min; $p < 0.05$), shorter length of hospital stay by 3.32 days ($p < 0.001$), and lower risks of overall morbidity (OR = 0.42, $p < 0.01$) and surgical site infections (OR 0.35, $p < 0.01$) [18]. Unfortunately, a paucity of published longer term recurrence data comparing open and laparoscopic repair exists at the time of this chapter.

Later retrospective case reviews evaluated laparoscopic keyhole repairs in 29 patients (Fig. 20.1). Findings confirmed the feasibility of the technique; however, the incidence of parastomal hernia recurrence was noted to be 46.4% with mean follow-up of 28 months [19]. An additional review of 55 patients undergoing laparoscopic keyhole repair completed by Hansson et al. showed similar recurrence rates of 37% at 36 months after repair. Observations included the unacceptably high recurrence rate associated with the technique and need to consider alternate approaches [20].

A multicenter cohort study was completed evaluating 61 consecutive patients undergoing laparoscopic parastomal hernia repair with the modified Sugarbaker technique using

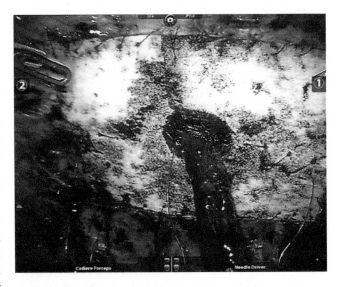

Fig. 20.1 Keyhole repair of parastomal hernia. Appearance of stoma site after minimally invasive (robotic-assisted laparoscopic) keyhole repair of parastomal hernia using bioabsorbable mesh

prosthetic mesh. The incidence of recurrence at 26 months was found to be 6.6% with an overall morbidity of 19% (ileus, wound infection, trocar site bleeding, and pneumonia) [21]. These findings suggest improve outcomes using the Sugarbaker as opposed to the keyhole technique. DeAsis et al. recently completed a meta-analysis of 15 manuscripts consisting of 469 patients comparing laparoscopic keyhole and Sugarbaker repairs. Recurrence rates were found to be decreased with the Sugarbaker technique (10.2%, 95% CI, 3.9–19.0) as compared to the keyhole repair (27.9%, 95% CI, 12.3–46.9). Postoperative complications included surgical site infection (3.8%, 95% CI, 2.3–5.7), infected mesh (1.7%, 95% CI, 0.7–3.1), and obstruction (1.7%, 95% CI, 0.7–3.0) [22].

The utilization of laparoscopic techniques for parastomal hernia could potentially offer decreased length of stay as well as surgical site infections with equivalent recurrence rates when compared to open repairs. Furthermore, the laparoscopic Sugarbaker technique seems to offer improved outcomes when compared to keyhole repair. As the overall incidence of laparoscopic repair remains low (10.4%), novel robotic platforms could offer avenues toward decreasing the technical learning curve and encouraging more widespread utilization of minimally invasive techniques.

Areas of Debate in Parastomal Hernia Repair

Prophylactic Mesh Placement

Secondary to the elevated incidence of parastomal hernia occurrence, some surgeons have employed the use of prophylactic mesh placement at the time of an index operation. Gogenur et al. completed an early prospective study evaluating the placement of a synthetic onlay mesh at the time of index colorectal procedures. This early trial enrolled only 24 patients and showed potential as the incidence of parastomal hernia at 12 months was only 8% [23]. Since that time, several randomized trials have been completed with mixed results. Recently, Pianka et al. completed a systematic literature search and meta-analysis of controlled trials comparing prophylactic mesh placement with standard controls. A total of 755 patients were included with results from the included randomized controlled trials showing a significant reduction in the incidence of parastomal hernia with prophylactic mesh placement (OR 0.24; 95% CI 0.1 to 0.58, $p = 0.034$). Furthermore, no significant differences were noted in postoperative complication rates indicating the safety of prophylactic mesh placement [24]. While additional trials are needed, preliminary data supports the utilization of prophylactic mesh placement at the time of index operation to decrease the incidence of parastomal hernia.

Utilization of Prosthetic Versus Biologic Mesh

Secondary to concern for potential mesh related complications such as infection, biologic or absorbable mesh is often used in parastomal hernia repair and/or for prophylactic placement in clean contaminated or contaminated cases. A recent systematic review of randomized trials consisting of 129 patients utilizing prophylactic composite or biologic mesh showed a reduction in parastomal hernia formation (RR 0.23, 95% CI 0.06 to 0.81; $p = 0.02$) and a decrease in the hernias requiring surgical repair (RR 0.13, 95% CI 0.02 to 1.02; $p = 0.05$) indicating the potential efficacy of these materials [25]. The increased cost associated with biologic materials has led to additional investigation comparing mesh types. A recent meta-analysis including 569 patients from 9 randomized trials showed similar results with prophylactic mesh leading to a decreased incidence of parastomal hernia as well as the need for hernia repair. Interestingly, a subgroup analysis comparing synthetic and biologic mesh types showed that the lower incidence of parastomal hernia formation was not appreciated in the biologic mesh group without any difference in morbidity from utilization of prosthetic material [26]. While review of the data indicates that prophylactic prosthetic mesh placement provides improved results with equal morbidity, additional trials are required to more clearly identify optimal mesh material.

Robotic Parastomal Hernia Repair

Robotic platforms offer increased degrees of freedom and the potential for a decreased learning curve during minimally invasive cases. While not mainstream, the utilization of such platforms has gained popularity over the previous years. Early literature consisted of small case series describing the technical feasibility of robotic-assisted laparoscopic ventral and incisional hernia repair [27]. More recently, larger retrospective reviews have been completed showing and confirming the safety of the procedure [28]; however, to date there is a paucity of long-term outcome data utilizing a robotic platform for ventral or incisional hernia repair. In addition, at the time of this review, there are zero publications specifically discussing the potential role of robotics for parastomal hernia repair. Therefore, this chapter will additionally review the preoperative planning, setup, and technical aspects of completing a robotic-assisted parastomal hernia repair.

Preoperative Planning

Parastomal hernias can often be associated with complex defects in the abdominal wall and, in many times, be present in the setting of concomitant midline incisional hernias.

Therefore, it is recommended to proceed with preoperative imaging to include a CT scan of the abdomen and pelvis in order to assess the abdominal wall musculature and size of the hernia defects.

As previously discussed, prior to any elective procedure attempts at risk factor optimization should be completed to decrease the risk of morbidity. Ensuring adequate nutrition, tobacco cessation, diabetic management, and weight management are cornerstones to this process. Elective parastomal hernia repair should not be considered in patients who are actively using nicotine products. It is our practice to require 4 weeks cessation and check for urine nicotine metabolites prior to proceeding with operation.

Obesity is also an important risk factor for recurrence with data showing increased incidence of recurrence when BMI surpasses 30 kg/m^2 [29]. Recent consensus statements and research has also highlighted the potential benefit of weight loss surgery prior to elective hernia repair with an initial BMI > 40 kg/m^2 [30, 31].

Finally, prior to the operation, we recommend attempts at multimodal pain management utilizing regional anesthesia and narcotic sparing pain regimens to include pretreatment with medications such as gabapentin, pregabalin, and celexicob. Improved perioperative pain control can lead to improved mobilization and recovery times. In addition, secondary to the potential for prolonged case duration, intraoperative decompression of the bladder with a Foley catheter is recommended in most cases.

Setup

The location of port placement is very important to avoid any external interference during the case. As most stoma sites are through the rectus muscle at approximately the level of the umbilicus, placing the trocars in the side contralateral to the stoma is key. Typically, we place the ports as previously described for ventral hernia repair (Fig. 20.2). A 12-mm camera port is placed with two 8-mm working ports on either side. It is important to allow 8–10 cm between ports to avoid external interference.

The patient is placed in supine position after induction, and the arm contralateral to the stoma site is tucked, leaving the arm on the side of the stoma out to ease the docking process. After draping, the abdomen can be entered per surgeon preference (optical entry, Veress needle, direct cutdown). The ports are placed in the previously stated configuration. While we do not routinely use an assist port (opting to complete suture exchange via the camera port), the operating surgeon can opt to place a 5–12-mm assist port for suctioning, retraction, and placement of suture and mesh during the case. At this point the patient is rotated slightly toward the side of the stoma.

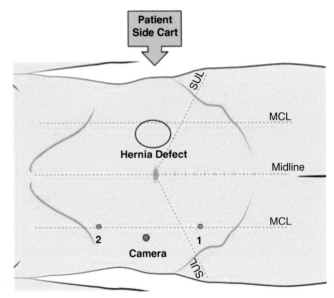

Fig. 20.2 Port placement The location of port placement is very important to avoid any external interference during the case. As most stoma sites are through the rectus muscle at approximately the level of the umbilicus, placing the trocars in the side contralateral to the stoma is key. Typically, we place the ports as previously described for ventral hernia repair (Fig. 20.2). A 12-mm camera port is placed with two 8-mm working ports on either side. It is important to allow 8–10 cm between ports to avoid external interference. for robotic parastomal hernia repair. A perpendicular dock is typically used for the patient side cart (SI). With the Xi system, there is more flexibility for positioning of the patient side cart. Typically two working ports (5 or 8 mm, depending on robotic system and instruments utilized) and an 8- or 12-mm camera port are placed on the side opposite to the hernia defect. For smaller patients, breaking the bed can allow for more room between ports. Additionally, a bump can be placed on the side of the ports to allow for more lateral placement if necessary. In general, an assist port is not necessary, as needles and mesh can be placed through the camera or instrument ports

The robot is then docked via a direct side dock bringing the platform over the side of the patient containing the stoma. The arms are then docked, and a 30° camera is used in the "up" position. In most cases a combination of needle drivers, monopolar shears, and a grasping device (bowel graspers, Cadiere Forceps, or ProGrasp™ forceps) is used. To avoid elevated costs, we typically find three instruments which are sufficient for each case (monopolar shears, grasping device, and a single needle driver).

Procedure

Once docked, we begin the dissection using a grasping instrument in the left-sided arm and the monopolar shears in the right-sided arm. The insufflation is kept at 15 mmHg, and extensive lysis of adhesions occurs to free any tissue from the anterior abdominal wall remote from the hernia. Gentle external traction is then used in an attempt to reduce the parastomal hernia contents. Next, a combination of sharp dissection with the shears and traction is used to completely free and reduce the hernia contents.

At this point the preperitoneal space is entered on the side of the fascial defect ipsilateral to the camera, and the preperitoneal plane is developed toward the hernia. This plane is extended into the hernia defect circumferentially to mobilize and attempt to completely reduce and excise the hernia sac. If the hernia sac is unable to be completely reduced, the sac is cut or released from the fascia circumferentially. After the adhesions are released, hernia contents are reduced and hernia sac excised or released; the intraabdominal pressure is reduced to 10–12 mmHg.

A ruler is then placed into the abdomen, and the width of the hernia defect is measured in order to select an appropriate-sized mesh. At this point we recommend attempted primary fascial closure secondary to a developing body of literature showing decreased adverse outcomes [32] when utilizing the technique. While any suture material can be used, we recommend a running closure utilizing an absorbable 0 barbed suture (Fig. 20.3). Of note, it is important to ensure an adequate opening for the existing stoma to avoid potential issue with obstruction or interference of blood flow.

As previously discussed, the existing data indicates the safety of synthetic mesh utilization for parastomal hernia repair [26]. Therefore, we recommend completing the hernia repair via the Sugarbaker technique with a medium weight macroporous mesh. Mesh size is calculated using the previously measured fascial defect, accounting for 5 cm of underlay in all directions. The mesh is inserted via the camera port after the center has been marked. The fascial closure suture is then used as a chandelier stitch to pull the mesh against the anterior abdominal wall. At this point the mesh is fixed to the posterior fascia of the anterior abdominal wall with a series of running

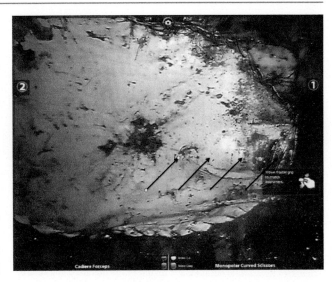

Fig. 20.4 Sugarbaker parastomal hernia repair. Intraoperative appearance after completion of parastomal hernia repair using the Sugarbaker technique. For this case, Dualmesh (W.L. Gore & Associates, Flagstaff, AZ) was utilized. Arrows indicate position of stoma

absorbable 0 barbed sutures. We recommend setting two separate sutures in place initially to anchor the mesh (one on the side contralateral to the camera and one adjacent to the tract of the stoma). After the mesh is anchored, fixation to the anterior abdominal wall is completed. Of note, avoid deep penetration when sewing to the posterior fascia. This can involve the overlying muscle and lead to bleeding with increased postoperative pain (Fig. 20.4). Once the mesh is fixed in place, conversion back to laparoscopic equipment occurs. The needles and ruler are removed, and the fascia of the 12-mm camera port site was closed per surgeon preference. We then place an abdominal binder at the end of the case for patient comfort.

Postoperative Care

After robotic parastomal hernia repair, patients are closely monitored in the postanesthesia care unit to ensure adequate pain control. Operations for smaller defects often allow patients to be discharged the same day with special instruction to ensure proper ambulation once home. For larger repairs or the need for improved pain control, the patients are placed in overnight observation. It is important to avoid large quantities of narcotics via the utilization of intravenous acetaminophen, gabapentin, and pregabalin in association with preoperative regional anesthesia.

Conclusions

Parastomal hernias are a common complication of operations requiring fecal or urinary diversion with an incidence approaching 50%. Patients with parastomal hernias can experience issues with obstruction, pain, and decreased functional mobility often necessitating opera-

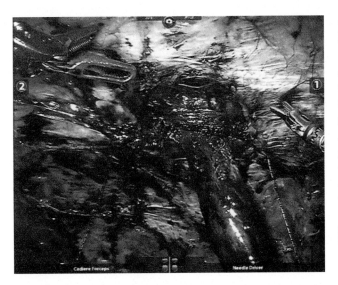

Fig. 20.3 Primary fascial closure. Intraoperative appearance of stoma site after primary fascial closure with barbed suture during robotic-assisted laparoscopic repair of a parastomal hernia

tive repair. The review of the available literature suggests that the laparoscopic modified Sugarbaker repair offers improved recurrence rates with decreased wound complications associated with open approaches. However, only approximately 10% of hernias are repaired via minimally invasive techniques. Robotic platforms offer increased degrees of freedom and could potentially decrease the learning curve for laparoscopic repair.

References

1. Leslie D. The parastomal hernia. Surg Clin North Am. 1984;64(2):507–15.
2. Pearl RK. Parastomal hernias. World J Surg. 1989;13(5):569–72.
3. Hotouras A, Murphy J, Thaha M, Chan CL. The persistent challenge of parastomal herniation: a review of the literature and future developments. Color Dis. 2013;15(5):e202–14.
4. Liu NW, Hackney JT, Gellhaus PT, Monn MF, et al. Incidence and risk factors of parastomal hernia in patients undergoing radical cystectomy and ileal conduit diversion. J Urol. 2014;191(5):1313–8.
5. Van Dijk SM, Timmermans L, Deerenberg EB, Lamme B, et al. Parastomal hernia: impact on quality of life? World J Surg. 2015;39(10):2595–601.
6. Sohn YJ, Moon SM, Shin US, Jee SH. Incidence and risk factors of parastomal hernia. J Korean Soc Coloproctol. 2012;28(5):241–6.
7. Donahue TF, Bochner BH, Sfakianos JP, Kent M. Risk factors for the development of parastomal hernia after radical cystectomy. J Urol. 2014;191(6):1708–13.
8. Temple B, Farley T, Popik K, Ewanyshyn C, et al. Prevalance of parastomal hernia and factors associated with its development. J Wound Ostomy Continence Nurs. 2016;43(5):489–93.
9. Al Shakarachi J, Williams JG. Systemic review of open techniques for parastomal hernia repair. Tech Coloproctol. 2014;18(5):427–32.
10. Hansson BM, Slater NJ, van der Velden AS, Groenewoud HM, et al. Surgical techniques for parastomal hernia repair: a systemic review of literature. Ann Surg. 2012;255(4):685–95.
11. Franks ME, Hrebinko RL Jr. Technique of parastomal hernia repair using synthetic mesh. Urology. 2001;57(3):551–3.
12. Kasperk R, Klinge U, Schumpelick V. The repair of large parastomal hernias using a midline approach and a prosthetic mesh in the sublay position. Am J Surg. 2000;179(3):186–8.
13. Steele SR, Lee P, Martin MJ, Mullenix PS, et al. Is parastomal hernia repair with polypropylene mesh safe? Am J Surg. 2003;185(5):436–40.
14. Stelzner S, Hellmich G, Ludwig K. Repair of paracolostomy hernias with a prosthetic mesh in the intraperitoneal onlay position: modified Sugarbaker technique. Dis Colon Rectum. 2004;47(2):185–91.
15. Rubin MS, Schoetz DJ Jr, Matthews JB. Parastomal hernia. Is stoma relocation superior to fascial repair? Arch Surg. 1994;129(4):413–8.
16. Riansuwan W, Hull TL, Millan MM, Hammel JP. Surgery of recurrent parastomal hernia: direct repair of relocation? Color Dis. 2010;12(7):681–6.
17. Pekmezci S, Memisoqlu K, Karahasanoglu T, Alemdaroglu K. Laparoscopic giant parastomal hernia repair with prosthetic mesh. Tech Coloproctol. 2002;6(3):187–90.
18. Halabi WJ, Jafari MD, Carmichael JC, Nguyen VQ, et al. Laparoscopic versus open repair of parastomal hernias: an ACS-NSQIP anaylsis of short term data. Surg Endosc. 2013;27(11):4067–72.
19. Mizrahi H, Bhattacharya P, Parker MC. Laparoscopic slit mesh repair of parastomal hernia using a designated mesh: long-term results. Surg Endosc. 2012;26(1):267–70.
20. Hasnsson BM, Bleichrodt RP, de Hingh IH. Laparoscopic parastomal hernia repair using a keyhole technique results in a high recurrence rate. Surg Endosc. 2009;23(7):1456–9.
21. Hansson BM, Morales-Conde S, Mussack T, Valdes J, et al. The laparoscopic modified Sugarbaker technique is safe and has a low recurrence rate: a multicenter cohort trial. Surg Endosc. 2013;27(2):494–500.
22. DeAsis FJ, Lapin B, Gitelis ME, Ujiki MB. Current state of laparoscopic parastomal hernia repair: a meta-analysis. World J Gastroenterol. 2015;21(28):8670–7.
23. Gogenur I, Mortensen J, Harvald T, Rosenberg J, et al. Prevention of parastomal hernia by placement of a polypropylene mesh at primary operation. Dis Colon Rectum. 2006;49(8):1131–5.
24. Pianka F, Probst P, Keller AV, Saure D, et al. Prophylactic mesh placement for the PREvention of paraSTOmal hernias: the PRESTO systemic review and meta-analysis. PLoS One. 2017;12(2):e0171548.
25. Wijeyekoon SP, Gurusamy K, El-Gendy K, Chan CL. Prevention of parastomal hernia with biologic/composite mesh: a systemic review and meta-analysis of randomized controlled trials. J Am Coll Surg. 2010;211(5):637–45.
26. Patel SV, Zhang L, Chadi SA, Wexner SD. Prophylactic mesh to prevent parastomal hernia: a meta-analysis of randomized controlled studies. Tech Coloproctol. 2017;21(1):5–13.
27. Allison N, Tieu K, Snyder B, Pigazzi A, et al. Technical feasibility of robot-assisted ventral hernia repair. World J Surg. 2012;36(2):447–52.
28. Gonzalez A, Escobar E, Romero R, Walker G, et al. Robotic-assisted ventral hernia repair: a multicenter evaluation of clinical outcomes. Surg Endosc. 2017;31(3):1342–9.
29. Nardi M Jr, Millo P, Brachet Contul R, et al. Laparoscopic ventral hernia repair with composite mesh: analysis of risk factors for recurrence in 185 patients with 5 years follow-up. Int J Surg. 2017;40:38–44.
30. Liang MK, Holihan JL, Itani K, et al. Ventral hernia management: expert consensus guided by systematic review. Ann Surg. 2017;265(1):80–9.
31. Pernar LI, Pernar CH, Dieffenbach BV, Brooks DC, Smink DS, Tavakkoli A. What is the BMI threshold for open ventral hernia repair? Surg Endosc. 2017;31(3):1311–7.
32. Tandon A, Pathak S, Lyons NJ, Nunes QM, et al. Meta-analysis of closure of the fascial defect during laparoscopic incisional and ventral hernia repair. Br J Surg. 2016;103(12):1598–607.

Robotic Flank Hernia Repair

Sean B. Orenstein

Introduction and Clinical Anatomy

Flank hernias represent a challenging entity for general surgeons. Repair of such hernias are plagued by higher recurrence rates, higher potential for chronic pain, as well as difficult anatomy compared to midline ventral hernia repairs. While the majority of flank hernias have traditionally been repaired by open means, laparoscopic and robotic approaches have been developed to offer patients the benefits of minimally invasive surgery [1]. Compared to traditional open flank hernia repairs, minimally invasive approaches offer several advantages including reduced infections, reduced length of hospital stay, quicker return to normal function, as well as potential for improved cosmesis [2–4]. However, not everyone is a candidate for a minimally invasive flank repair. Attributes like size and complexity of the hernia, history of infection, prior hernia repairs or abdominal surgeries, active skin pathology, body habitus, and comorbidities are all factors that should be weighed to determine if a minimally invasive repair is appropriate.

An essential component of repairing flank hernias takes place during the preoperative visit. It is important to set expectations with the patient when discussing postoperative outcomes. Notably, patients with sizeable flank bulging may continue to have asymmetric bulging despite defect closure and mesh reinforcement. Bulging will likely persist, to some degree, due to denervation as well as possible muscle atrophy from previous surgery(ies) or traumatic injury in the flank region [1, 5]. Loss of adequate nerve impulses and muscle tone leads to laxity of the musculature, resulting in chronic bulging that may not recover despite adequate hernia repair. Another important component of discussion involves postoperative pain. While chronic pain is a risk of any hernia repair, the lateral abdominal wall contains numerous nerves that typically traverse the region of flank hernia repair. Patients with severe preoperative pain may be disappointed by lack of resolution of such pain with their repair. Using the robotic platform, most suturing takes place intracorporeally, with limited to no transabdominal mesh fixation sutures. Therefore, some sources of chronic pain should be reduced with the use of robotic-assisted suturing.

Robotic-assisted flank hernia repair parallels that of its laparoscopic counterpart, both of which share principles used in open repairs. This includes the tenets of wide mesh overlap with some form of mesh fixation to the abdominal wall. As with most flank repairs, the mesh is typically placed intra-abdominally or within the pre-peritoneal plane. If placed intra-abdominally, a mesh with an anti-adhesion barrier is required to reduce visceral adhesions to the mesh.

Traditionally, minimally invasive ventral hernia repairs have been performed without hernia defect closure. While the data supporting defect closure over bridged repairs are more clear for open hernia repair, there is conflicting data on the benefits of defect closure for laparoscopic repairs [6, 7]. Nonetheless, surgeons should strive to close all hernia defects to maximize outcomes and reduce postoperative complications. Defect closure allows obliteration of the dead space above the mesh which lead to a reduction in postoperative seromas. Additionally, the Law of Laplace dictates that there will be increased tension on the bridged portion of mesh from a hernia repair without defect closure. This may ultimately lead to mesh "eventration," or bulging of the mesh within the hernia sac. Thus, closing the defect would equalize pressure across the mesh, based on Pascal's principle. The use of robotic-assisted repairs has allowed more concise tissue approximation using intracorporeal suturing. This is in contrast to laparoscopic-based defect closure, which is typically accomplished using transabdominal suturing and a suture passer. While this technique is highly useful for defect closure and mesh fixation when performed laparoscopically, it lacks a degree of accuracy and tissue approximation seen in robotic-assisted repairs, though modern barbed sutures make intracorporeal laparoscopic defect suturing more appealing.

S. B. Orenstein
Oregon Health & Science University, Department of Surgery, Division of Gastrointestinal and General Surgery, Portland, OR, USA
e-mail: orenstei@ohsu.edu

© Springer Nature Switzerland AG 2019
S. Tsuda, O. Y. Kudsi (eds.), *Robotic-Assisted Minimally Invasive Surgery*, https://doi.org/10.1007/978-3-319-96866-7_21

Preoperative Considerations

When considering who is a candidate for a robotic-assisted flank hernia repair, certain patient characteristics must be considered. Contraindications include:

- Inability to tolerate general anesthesia
- Inability to tolerate lateral decubitus positioning
- Hypercoagulability
- Active infection
- Loss of abdominal domain
- Poor skin quality overlying hernia (ulceration, skin graft)
- Patient expectations (scar revision or concomitant abdominal procedure)

Surgeon skill, including comfort level and competence using the robotic platform, needs to be weighed in before proceeding with robotic-assisted flank hernia repair. Because of the inherent challenges that flank hernia repair entails, inexperienced users of the robot should consider gaining additional proficiency before embarking on challenging flank hernia repair cases.

Preoperative evaluation and consultation are crucial aspects for patients undergoing robotic-assisted flank hernia repair (RAFHR). Such consultation should set expectations regarding the repair itself, mesh implantation and its ramifications, postoperative pain and recovery, as well as various abdominal wall changes following repair. Despite a minimally invasive approach, RAFHR can result in significant postoperative pain which may not differ much from traditional open repairs. However, robotic suturing of defects intracorporeally and limiting transabdominal sutures should, theoretically, reduce postoperative discomfort. One of the principal benefits of minimally invasive approaches is the well-documented reduction in wound- and mesh-related infectious complications. The likelihood of postoperative seroma formation should be discussed. The need for conversion to an open repair and the possibility of an enterotomy should be considered as well. The anticipated options if an enterotomy occurs should be explained to the patient, including staged repair of the hernia defect until the abdomen is free from contamination. Patients should be made aware that, although the hernia defect will be repaired and reinforced, persistent abdominal wall bulging may still be present following repair. Such abdominal wall changes, including persistent laxity and bulging, likely result from denervation at the time of previous operation(s) or traumatic injury.

High-resolution preoperative imaging, typically in the form of a CT scan of the abdomen and pelvis, is helpful in preoperative planning. Evaluation of hernia defect size, location, remaining abdominal wall musculature, adjacent viscera, incarcerated contents, etc. are valuable pieces of information that help plan out repair and determine feasibil-

ity of a robotic-assisted repair. For example, a flank defect extending inferiorly into the pelvic brim may alert the surgeon that bone anchors or other bony fixation devices are required. Additionally, evaluation of other ventral hernias (e.g., umbilical hernia) and signs of previous repairs allow for modification in trocar placement and items necessary for repair (e.g., additional mesh, laparoscopic retrieval bag, etc.).

Patients who have undergone previous failed repairs can be challenging. The reasons for recurrence are not always known, and every effort should be made to obtain all operative reports that pertain to prior hernia repairs in an attempt to determine the mesh used and tissue plane disrupted by prior repairs. Before embarking on a recurrent defect, the surgeon should feel extremely confident with adhesiolysis and have a low threshold to convert to open. Patients who have had previous mesh infections that required removal of the prosthesis pose an extremely difficult challenge and should be considered for open repair.

Standard preoperative orders consisting of antibiotic and deep venous thrombosis prophylaxis are given. A first-generation cephalosporin (e.g., cefazolin) is typically given, ensuring adequate weight-based dosing. Sequential compression devices should be utilized, and subcutaneous heparin can be employed preoperatively for high-risk patients.

Operative Steps

Patient Positioning

Following intubation and securing of endotracheal and IV tubes, the patient is positioned in a lateral decubitus position, or semilateral position, based on the size and location of the flank hernia. A beanbag and/or gel rolls are helpful to keep the patient in the desired lateral position. Great care should be taken to protect all pressure points with adequate gel and foam pads as well as axillary roll to ensure no pressure ulcer or nervous injury occurs. The upward arm can be secured to an adjustable arm sling or wrapped around several pillows to reduce brachial plexus injuries. The patient should be well-secured to the bed with a combination of straps and tapes to the bed itself. Warming drapes are applied, per hospital protocols. Once the patient is positioned, padded, and secured to the bed, the bed should be tested in various positions to ensure the patient is fully secure and does not move with repositioning during the case (Fig. 21.1).

While a Foley catheter is standard for bladder decompression and volume monitoring during the case, a three-way Foley should be considered to insufflate the bladder for identification in the repair of low defects that extend out to the suprapubic region or if the patient has received previous pelvic surgery (e.g., prostatectomy). Gastric decompression

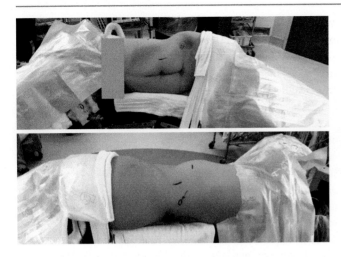

Fig. 21.1 Patient positioning. Patient with traumatic left flank hernia has been positioned in right lateral decubitus position with the aid of a suction beanbag and other gel pads

via orogastric tube is useful to decompress the stomach as well as help reduce aspiration events during lateral and Trendelenburg positioning.

The patient should be prepped and draped very widely to allow trocar placement and access to the defect itself in the event of open conversion. An iodine-impregnated adhesive drape applied to the skin of the prepped and draped patient is a useful way to keep drapes in place and seal the corners of the sterile field to limit contamination; however, data do not support a marked reduction in surgical site infection with use of such adhesive drapes.

Abdominal Access

Selecting the location for abdominal access can be challenging, as many of these patients have had multiple previous abdominal operations. The extent of previous operation(s) is not always known by the patient; therefore, attention should be made to abdominal scars on physical exam. Abdominal entry should be achieved via whichever technique the surgeon is most comfortable and familiar with, be it Hassan cutdown, optical trocar, or Veress needle entry.

Once safe abdominal cavity is achieved, three trocars will be placed in the contralateral abdominal wall. The trocars are commonly located near the anterior axillary line but should be staggered to triangulate the ports opposite from the hernia. The central, most lateral, trocar will be the camera port, while the superior and inferior ports are for working arms (e.g., dissecting, suturing, retracting, etc.). Trocar planning includes ensuring at least one non-camera port which contains a CO_2 insufflation port as excessive fogging may result if CO_2 is attached to the camera port. However, a separate 10-/12-mm assist port may simplify the CO_2 insufflation

port choice. If using the daVinci Si system, extended/bariatric-sized trocars are useful to extend the length of the console arms near bony prominences such as the pelvis and ribs and limit console-patient collisions.

Adhesiolysis

The Achilles' heel of minimally invasive ventral and flank hernia repair is lysis of adhesions. This step can be the most time-consuming and usually determines the length and complexity of the case. For patients without previous midline procedures, only minor adhesiolysis may be necessary. However, many patients have had prior central and midline surgical explorations, with resultant central adhesions that necessitate careful dissection before proceeding with the actual hernia repair. An upward-facing 30° camera is necessary to adequately visualize the anterior abdominal wall.

Attempts should be made to limit the use of energy sources during adhesiolysis, as thermal injuries seal at the time of dissection and may not be apparent for 3–5 days postoperatively. Sharp, cold, scissor dissection should be the principal method of adhesiolysis to reduce the risk of thermal injury. Atraumatic graspers are helpful in providing adequate countertraction during dissection, typically with a fenestrated bipolar device or cadiere grasper. Typically, during lysis of adhesions, the outer rim of adhesions may be sharply cut, giving way to "cotton candy" loose areolar tissue that is easily dissected using blunt dissection with gentle, short sweeps.

Bleeding during adhesiolysis can be problematic. Slight oozing that typically occurs should be largely ignored. It rarely continues, and chasing it, especially with cautery, may lead to a bowel injury. If the area of oozing can be isolated from viscera, judicious cautery may be used. An oozing area of adipose tissue can be lifted away from underlying bowel and cauterized. Fenestrated bipolar graspers are useful to direct focused cautery to omental bleeding, provided the bowel is far away to eliminate thermal spread.

Sizing the Hernia Defect

Measuring the defect is an important step in the procedure, as a durable repair relies on adequate mesh overlap with proper placement, which are both directly a result of accurately measuring the defect.

The edges of the hernia defect are best delineated with the aid spinal needles placed at each edges of the defect. Under direct visualization, insert the needle into the abdominal wall perpendicularly, so the needle can emerge at the edge of the defect. However, for very lateral defects, one should avoid spinal needle placement at the most lateral edge to avoid any lateral abdominal wall nervous or retroperitoneal injury; this edge can be estimated during measuring. A disposable plastic ruler can be cut lengthwise and inserted via the assist port to accurately measure intra-abdominal measurements of the defect based on the spinal needles. Other methods of defect measuring exist, including spinal needle placement and external markings. While this simplifies internal measuring with a ruler, the external measuring techniques overestimate the defect, which is more pronounced in larger defects and obese patients with thick anterior abdominal walls. Therefore, one should adjust their mesh sizing accordingly if using external measurements.

Tissue Plane Dissection and Hernia Defect Closure

Prior to defect closure and deciding which mesh to use, it is important to determine which plane of dissection will be utilized. For most robotic repairs, two tissue plane locations exist for mesh placement: pre-peritoneal (i.e., transabdominal pre-peritoneal, or TAPP, repair) or intraperitoneal underlay (i.e., intraperitoneal onlay mesh, or IPOM, repair). While abdominal wall reconstruction with component separation techniques may apply to very large or complex defects, such a repair is beyond the purview of this chapter. The tissue plane greatly affects which mesh one can use, as a mesh with an anti-adhesion barrier is necessary if placed as an intraperitoneal underlay to reduce visceral adhesions. Whereas, raw, uncoated meshes can be placed within the pre-peritoneal plane.

If feasible, TAPP flank repair is preferred as this allows mesh to be excluded from the abdominal viscera. The flap consists of peritoneum, and possibly the overlying transversalis fascia, though it may be hard to discern the differences between these two layers. It is important to avoid violating the posterior rectus sheath medially, as disruption may create focal weakness and ensuing herniation. The hernia defect should be in good view to assess the size and complexity of the defect(s) (Fig. 21.2). The most challenging aspect of TAPP dissection is creation of a complete peritoneal flap

without disruption, as any rent in the flap can lead to mesh exposure or interparietal hernia, whereby the bowel can herniate between layers of the abdominal wall. Recommended equipment includes a high-strength grasper (e.g., ProGrasp or a needle driver) and monopolar scissors. While other grasping forceps can be used (e.g., fenestrated bipolar, cadiere), the limited grip strength of these may lead to grazing and tearing of the flap. The planned dissection line runs vertically near the midline, but this line of dissection can be started off-midline for small or very lateral defects. To start pre-peritoneal dissection, it is recommended to start fairly medially in order to allow extra peritoneum to utilize for mesh coverage. As the peritoneum is quite thin, this extra amount of peritoneal tissue may help overcome any initial tears as dissection commences. Using cold or hot scissors, the pre-peritoneal plane is entered; this is carried superiorly and inferiorly far enough to eventually provide space for mesh that would overlap the defect at least 4–5 cm in all directions (Fig. 21.3). Using a combination of blunt, sharp, and light cautery dissection, the pre-peritoneal plane is dissected out laterally until reaching the hernia defect. The plane is continued within the hernia defect, bringing the hernia sac down as part of the flap. Excess hernia sac helps provide adequate coverage of the mesh, especially if thinned and denuded areas are created during dissection. The plane is then continued out laterally past the hernia defect at least 5–6 cm to allow for 4–5-cm mesh overlap. Under-sizing of the flap can lead to mesh edge curling; therefore, it is better to err on the side of creating a larger flap to cover the entire mesh without catching mesh edges during flap closure. Because the colon is typically in the vicinity of the lateral dissection, it is important to take care when completing the lateral flap. This can be accomplished with gentle blunt dissection of the continuous peritoneal flap without any electrocautery. Any fenestrations created in the peritoneum necessitate closure; small rents can be closed with simple figure-of-eight sutures using 2–0 resorbable suture, while larger rents may require a running suture using 2–0 resorbable suture (Fig. 21.4)

Intraperitoneal underlay mesh dissection is much simpler, as the only principal dissection involves dissecting the colon from the retroperitoneum. Using sharp dissection using scissors along with an atraumatic grasper (e.g., bowel grasper, cadiere grasper), the white line of Toldt is taken down and extended superiorly and inferiorly to fully medialize the colon. This maneuver allows for adequate mesh overlap laterally and posteriorly. After adequate medialization of the colon to ensure adequate mesh overlap, one can proceed with mesh placement and fixation.

As previously discussed, hernia repair should include appropriate defect closure prior to mesh reinforcement. The use of robotic-assisted surgery facilitates concise suturing of the fascial edges compared to its laparoscopic counterpart.

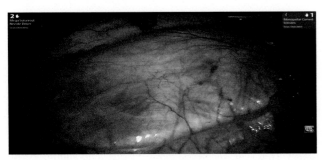

Fig. 21.2 Intracorporeal view of a large left flank hernia

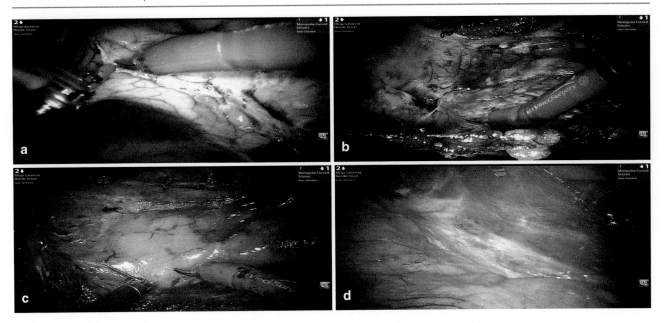

Fig. 21.3 Pre-peritoneal flap creation for TAPP flank hernia repair. (**a–d**) represent various stages of flap creation as dissection was carried out laterally

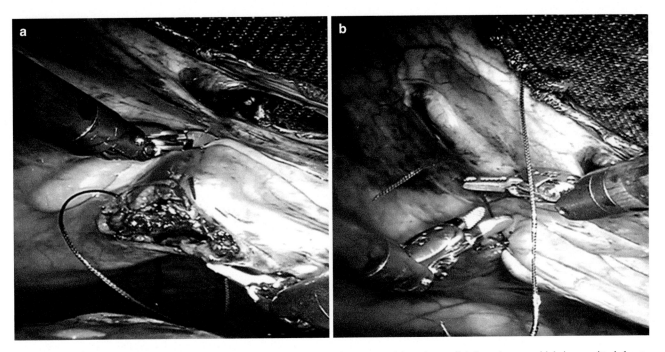

Fig. 21.4 Peritoneal flap fenestration closure. (**a**) Figure-of-eight stitch using 2–0 resorbable suture. (**b**) Closed fenestration. Note the unclosed fenestrations on the medial aspect of the flap; these will be incorporated into the medial flap closure, which is permitted due to excess peritoneum and hernia sac mobilized during flap dissection

After ensuring hemostasis, the hernia defect is closed. Several suture options exist for defect closure, including continuous versus interrupted sutures, permanent versus resorbable sutures, as well as traditional non-barbed sutures versus newer locking barbed sutures (e.g., V-Loc sutures, Medtronic, Minneapolis, MN, and Stratafix sutures, Ethicon, Somerville, NJ). Despite these many options, the use of lock-ing barbed sutures adds great ease of closing hernia defects, as one can sequentially tighten the suture without spontane-ous loosening of the suture during closure. For defect closure I prefer to use a larger-caliber, permanent monofilament barbed suture, either a #0 or #1 permanent polypropylene barbed suture. The defect is closed in the orientation that allows for the least tension upon closure. This may be in a

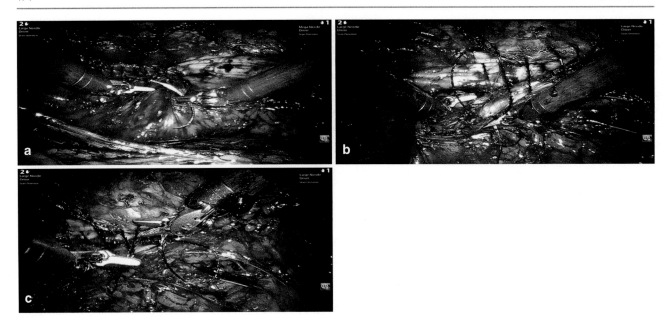

Fig. 21.5 Defect closure with locking barbed suture. (**a**) Superior (screen left) defect undergoing closure, while inferior defect (screen right) remains open. (**b**) Inferior (screen right) defect undergoing closure. (**c**) Sequential tightening of the locking barbed suture

vertical, transverse, or oblique orientation and should be tailored to the hernia defect based on intraoperative findings. For small defects, a single running barbed suture can be used to approximate the fascial edges, while larger defects should be closed from the ends with two separate sutures, sequentially tightening the defect from ends toward the center (Fig. 21.5). It is important to grasp and suture fascial tissue to assist with a durable repair, as suturing flimsy tissue such as the hernia sac will likely result in dehiscence. Small bites (~ 5 mm) and short travel (~ 5 mm) during closure are also recommended, though a larger bite may be necessary for friable or denuded tissue. One should ensure the sutures have been tightened throughout every throw before proceeding with mesh placement. When complete, the defect should be well approximated without gaps. However, one should note any fascial gaps or disruptions, as appropriate mesh selection is required to overcome these bridged areas. Additional local anesthetic can be infused into the fascia to assist with immediate postoperative analgesia.

Mesh Selection and Insertion

The type of mesh chosen for repair depends on whether pre-peritoneal or intraperitoneal placement has been chosen. As already stated, a TAPP repair allows the use of raw uncoated mesh prosthetics. The most commonly utilized meshes are manufactured from polypropylene or polyester, with multiple varieties of these based on weight/density, porosity, weave/knit structure, as well as other various characteristics. Because of the extreme tensile forces applied to the lateral abdominal wall/flank, larger defects should be considered for a medium or heavyweight mesh, as too light of a mesh can accompany postoperative laxity of the abdominal wall. That said, macroporous lightweight meshes have shown improved ingrowth, less mesh contraction, and more resilience in the setting of infection. Intraperitoneal underlay mesh placement requires the use of an anti-adhesion barrier, with the raw uncoated side facing the peritoneum to facilitate ingrowth, while the anti-adhesion surface faces the viscera. There are multiple meshes on the market with various anti-adhesions barriers. One should be familiar with different manufactures, materials, and sizes to best pick the appropriate mesh for your patient's repair. There is much good debate as to which mesh is the best or ideal for various hernia repairs; this debate is beyond the purview of this chapter.

The size of the mesh depends on the defect size as well as tissue plane dissected. In general, a generous 4–5 cm or more overlap in all directions is recommended to ensure adequate coverage of the (closed) defect. Prior to mesh insertion, the pre-peritoneal space should be measured to ensure the space will accommodate the appropriately sized mesh for the repair (Fig. 21.6). Part of mesh oversizing pertains to some degree of mesh shrinkage following mesh integration and fibrosis. Heavyweight meshes tend to induce more fibrosis; therefore, more shrinkage may result with the use of such meshes. Adequate secure fixation can help reduce such shrinkage and overcome the limitations of heavier weight meshes. It is commonly asked if mesh sizing depends on the open or

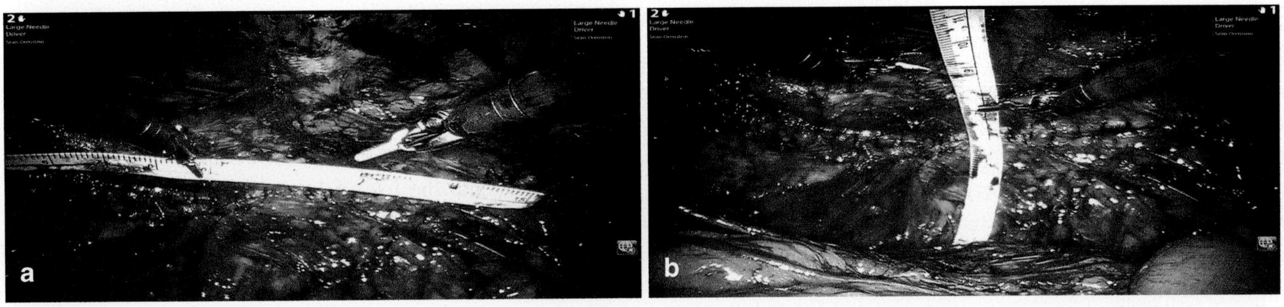

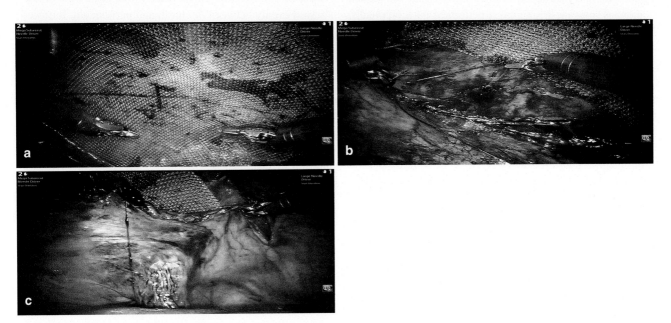

Fig. 21.6 Sizing of the pre-peritoneal flap space prior to mesh insertion shown in (**a**) longitudinal and (**b**) transverse dimensions

Fig. 21.7 (**a**) Mesh placement within the pre-peritoneal space. Note the black lines drawn prior to insertion for mesh orientation. A heavy-weight polypropylene mesh was utilized to provide additional stability for this large flank hernia. (**b**) Simple U-stitch for mesh fixation. (**c**) Testing flap coverage over mesh; note the redundant peritoneum from hernia sac dissection

closed hernia defect. While there is no straightforward answer, it is recommended to utilize a mesh with a minimum of 10–15 cm width or more in the event of fascial dehiscence. If a TAPP flank hernia repair is chosen, rounding the mesh corners by trimming some material off the four corners of the mesh helps prevent folding of the mesh following placement, as most pre-peritoneal pockets are not perfectly dissected at 90° angles within the corners.

Mesh insertion typically requires placement through a 12-mm trocar, as placing mesh through a smaller trocar can lead to mesh disruption or tearing. A separate 12-mm assist port makes mesh and suture insertion more simplified than removal of the camera that typically occupies the larger port. Very large meshes may even require a 15-mm trocar, though this would only be for some of the larger ventral hernia meshes on the market. Raw uncoated meshes can be carefully rolled up and inserted through the trocar, while coated meshes typically require a quick soak in sterile saline to

active the anti-adhesion barrier. Meshes with anti-adhesion barriers should be rolled with the barrier on the inside of the roll to prevent the barrier from scraping off during passage through the trocar.

Prior to insertion it is helpful to mark the mesh with a grid using a marker (Fig. 21.7a). Such lines down the vertical and horizontal axes can aid mesh positioning due to differing oblique or off-center angles of flank hernias. Alternatively, mesh manufacturers have developed laparoscopic mesh-positioning devices that may obviate the need for precise external measurements as well as eliminate the need to pre-place sutures. It is still important, however, to determine the center of the defect as well as to gain an accurate internal measurement of the defect in order to implant an appropriately sized mesh. Such devices are introduced within the abdomen and stabilize the mesh against the anterior abdominal wall with balloons and/or semirigid frames and then are removed following mesh fixation.

Mesh Fixation

Multiple options exist for securing the mesh to the abdominal wall, and one or more of these options are used to ensure a durable repair. The decision of where to fixate also plays an important role in flank hernia repairs, as there is a limit to the amount of deep fixation allowed posterolaterally due to the nerve distribution of this portion of the abdominal wall. Fixation options include intracorporeal sutures, transabdominal sutures, tacks, glues/adhesives, bone anchors, as well as self-gripping meshes. Robotic suturing obviates the need for transabdominal fixation, as most mesh suturing is performed intracorporeally. Therefore, pre-placed sutures are typically not required.

For TAPP flank hernia repairs, the raw uncoated mesh is oriented to cover the entire closed defect (Fig. 21.7a). A number (six or more) of simple U-stitches using 2–0 resorbable sutures are used to provide initial mesh fixation and prevent the mesh from sliding within the pre-peritoneal plane (Fig. 21.7b). Some surgeons advocate the use of fibrin sealant to limit mesh sliding and promote ingrowth during the initial healing phase following repair. Following mesh fixation, the peritoneal flap is closed over the mesh, ensuring the entire mesh is covered by peritoneum. It is helpful to test the flap coverage of the mesh by gently pulling the flap over the mesh (Fig. 21.7c). Insufficient peritoneal coverage over the mesh necessitates further dissection of the peritoneal flap or mesh trimming if an excess amount of mesh was utilized. Closure of the flap can be accomplished robotically using a running suture at the flap edge, typically using a resorbable 2–0 locking barbed suture. Alternatively, the flap can be closed using laparoscopic tacks, taking care to avoid tack placement of the posterolateral wall to limit the risk of nerve injury and chronic pain sequelae (Fig. 21.8). One must ensure the flap is closed in its entirety to prevent interparietal herniation and mesh exposure to the viscera.

Intraperitoneal mesh placements (i.e., IPOM) can be affixed using sutures as well as laparoscopic tacks. As discussed, modern meshes with positioning systems can aid in mesh placement positioning, by assisting with mesh apposition against the abdominal wall during fixation. After positioning the coated mesh over the closed defect, the mesh is robotically secured into place with circumferential sutures around the mesh edge, ensuring adequate bites of mesh, peritoneum, and fascia. However, caution should be used to ensure that bites are not too deep, as this can lead to suturing deeper nerves of the posterolateral abdominal wall. Some surgeons advocate the use of laparoscopic tacks instead of intracorporeal suturing in an effort to reduce operative time. Alternatively, one can suture or tack the most medial 1/2–2/3 of mesh depending on hernia location and complete the most posterolateral fixation with the use of a fibrin sealant or other adhesive. This takes some coordination to ensure the glue is sprayed evenly between the mesh and peritoneum, followed quickly by pressure against the mesh to ensure proper adhesion of the mesh to the abdominal wall.

One aspect of repair that is unique to hernias immediately adjacent to bony structures such as flank and suprapubic hernias is the need for bony fixation. Many flank hernias lie very close to the pelvis, with little to no high-quality fascia and soft tissue available for securing the mesh. The use of bone anchors is a way to help provide such durable fixation at the most inferior portion of the repair [8, 9]. While several options exist for bone anchors, Mitek bone anchors (5-mm Mitek Fastin RC Titanium Anchors, DePuy Mitek Inc, Raynham, MA) are relatively straightforward to insert and use for bony fixation (Fig. 21.9). To implant the

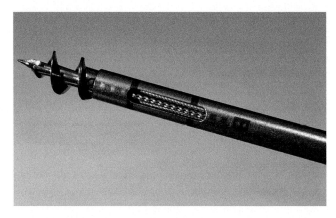

Fig. 21.9 Mitek bone anchor (5-mm Mitek Fastin RC Titanium Anchor, DePuy Mitek Inc, Raynham, MA)

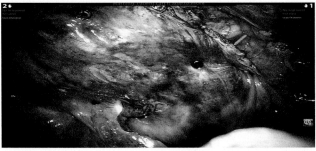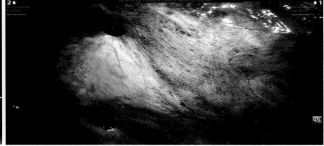

Fig. 21.8 Peritoneal flap coverage of mesh, with resorbable tacks used for flap fixation and quilting of the flap to reduce seroma formation

bone anchors, the site of bone anchor insertion is chosen – this is typically at the iliac crest near the anterior superior iliac spine (ASIS). A small skin incision is made over the ASIS, and subcutaneous tissues are dissected down to expose the bony prominence of the ASIS or other desired location for fixation. Before insertion of the bone anchor, confirm that all soft tissue has been removed to ensure complete bony exposure so that the anchor sits well within the cancellous bone and not catching any soft tissue between the anchor screw and adjacent bone. While some self-drilling bone anchors are produced, many require an initial pre-drilling with a specified drill bit size and to a desired depth according to the product's instructions for use (IFU). Care should be taken to ensure that pre-drilling and insertion of the bone anchor is into the thicker part of the iliac crest, in line with the bone so that anchor seats well within the body of the cancellous bone. The anchor is screwed into place to the proper depth according to the product's IFU, followed by removal of the outer plastic and metal sheathing of the inserter. Mitek anchors commonly contain two pairs of braided suture; one of the two pairs of sutures is kept, while the other pair is discarded. Using a laparoscopic suture passer, the two tails of the suture are brought separately through the subcutaneous tissues and delivered through the mesh into the peritoneal cavity under direct visualization, spacing them approximately 1 cm apart to create a U-stitch. The tails are then tied intracorporeally, completing bony fixation at the desired site. Frequently, two to three anchors are used; however, the number of required sutures is variable and should be tailored according to the size and location of the hernia. Multiple anchors should be spaced apart by 2 cm or more to limit deeper bone disruption or fracture. A sufficient number of bone anchors should be used to ensure adequate bony fixation inferiorly.

When fixation is complete, the bed should be rotated to ensure that the colon moves back to its normal anatomic site in the paracolic gutters, which typically overly the most posterolateral portion. This may also help compress the mesh and/or peritoneal flap shut against the abdominal wall. Prior to completion of the case, one last inspection of the abdominal cavity is performed to rule out active bleeding and evaluate for visceral injury. The fascia at trocars larger than 8 mm should be closed with sutures, along with closure of any overly-stretched 8 mm trocar sites. The skin at the trocar sites is closed with subcuticular stitches, followed by dermal adhesive or steri-strips. An abdominal binder may be placed for patient comfort. One method of compressing the area of interest (i.e., flank region) is to place a couple Kerlix gauze rolls overlying the flank, followed by the abdominal binder. This helps focus the binder compression over the flank instead of spread out over the entire abdomen. However, the role of binders in seroma reduction is unclear.

Postoperative Care

Perioperative Concerns

Appropriate pain management is crucial in the immediate postoperative period. Many patients undergoing robotic-assisted flank hernia repair are admitted. Multimodal analgesic regimens are highly beneficial and can include IV and/or PO narcotics, scheduled acetaminophen, and NSAIDS such as intravenous ketorolac for patients without renal disease. Additionally, because muscle spasms are common, muscle relaxants can be a beneficial adjunct. Scheduled diazepam with its antispasmodic properties is one option; however, judicious use is warranted with elderly patients and those with sleep apnea due to its sedative effects.

Activity restrictions are more stringent for flank repairs compared to typical ventral hernia repairs. Because of the challenging nature of flank hernia repairs and higher potential for fascial disruption, I routinely prohibit any heavy weight lifting (<25 lbs) or abdominal-pelvic-flank activities for 2–3 months postoperatively. Such limitations allow the defect closure and mesh integration to gain near-complete fibrosis and limit any potential disruption with heavy Valsalva, lifting, or twisting activities. That said, the patient is allowed to perform typical activities of daily living (ADLs), including ambulation, stairs, etc. It can be very helpful for the patient to receive guidance from physical and/or occupational therapy during their hospitalization for education on transferring in and out of a bed or car, lifting bags or other objects, navigating stairs, getting dressed, or other ADLs.

The postoperative diet depends on the degree of adhesiolysis. Without significant adhesiolysis the diet can be advanced rapidly. Following procedures where there is a lengthy lysis of adhesions or when bowel is densely involved, the diet is advanced slower, typically ensuring that the patient can tolerate clear liquids without nausea before progressing to a regular diet.

Hospitalization in the immediate postoperative period also allows the surgeon to monitor for any signs of missed enterotomy. There should always be an index of suspicion, particularly in difficult cases. Any unexplained tachycardia, leukocytosis, or persistent fever should be evaluated to rule out the presence of a bowel injury. Plain abdominal films or CT can be used; however, if there is any concern, the patient should be returned to the operating room for diagnostic laparoscopy or laparotomy.

Long-Term Concerns

Persistent pain can be seen beyond 6 weeks following flank hernia repair. Focal pain sites can be injected with a mixture of lidocaine and bupivacaine for diagnostic and therapeutic relief. However, this treatment is rarely required, especially with limited use of trans-fascial sutures in robotic-assisted repairs.

Almost all patients undergoing minimally invasive ventral or flank hernia repairs develop some degree of seroma at the hernia repair site, though several case series show reduced seromas with defect closure of ventral hernias [7]. However, most seromas rarely, if ever, require intervention such as drainage or aspiration. The risk of contaminating the mesh with drainage should be weighed against the benefits of relieving the fluid. Indications for aspiration include failure to resolve after a long period (e.g., 6 months), significant patient discomfort, or pressure on the skin causing necrosis or excoriation.

Mesh infection is one of the dreaded complications of any hernia repair. This complication is fortunately low in minimally invasive repairs; however, the consequences are grave. The management of mesh contamination is extensive and many times requires mesh removal. In patients that present with erythema or fluctuance of the flank and abdominal wall, CT imaging of the abdomen should be obtained. Fluid collection above or deep to the prosthetic that contains air is a mesh infection and is treated as such. The fluid may be aspirated and sent for gram stain and culture. The mesh should be removed if it has a component of ePTFE or multifilament polyester, as these mesh prosthetics have limited ability for salvage [10]. Attempts to salvage the mesh should involve open drainage of the fluid collection with negative pressure vacuum therapy. This maneuver may be successful with lightweight macroporous polypropylene materials but is less so with polyester-based materials.

Follow-up in patients after minimally invasive flank hernia repair has been poorly reported in the literature. The postoperative schedule could include appointments at 2–4 weeks, 3–6 months, 1 year, and possibly yearly thereafter depending on the severity of hernia and repair. Ideally, hernia patients should be examined at least up to 2 years for complications of seroma, persistent pain, and hernia recurrence.

References

1. Hope WW, Hooks WB 3rd. Atypical hernias: suprapubic, subxiphoid, and flank. Surg Clin North Am. 2013;93(5):1135–62. https://doi.org/10.1016/j.suc.2013.06.002.
2. Cobb WS, Kercher KW, Heniford BT. Laparoscopic repair of incisional hernias. Surg Clin North Am. 2005;85(1):91–103, ix. https://doi.org/10.1016/j.suc.2004.09.006.
3. Novitsky YW, Paton BI, Heniford BT. Laparoscopic ventral hernia repair. In: Operative techniques in general surgery: techniques of laparoscopic hernia repair. New York: Elsevier, Inc; 2006. p. 4–9.
4. Zhang Y, Zhou H, Chai Y, Cao C, Jin K, Hu Z. Laparoscopic versus open incisional and ventral hernia repair: a systematic review and meta-analysis. World J Surg. 2014;38(9):2233–40. https://doi.org/10.1007/s00268-014-2578-z.
5. Moreno-Egea A, Carrillo-Alcaraz A. Management of non-midline incisional hernia by the laparoscopic approach: results of a long-term follow-up prospective study. Surg Endosc. 2012;26(4):1069–78. https://doi.org/10.1007/s00464-011-2001-x.
6. Orenstein SB, Dumeer JL, Monteagudo J, Poi MJ, Novitsky YW. Outcomes of laparoscopic ventral hernia repair with routine defect closure using "shoelacing" technique. Surg Endosc. 2011;25(5):1452–7. https://doi.org/10.1007/s00464-010-1413-3.
7. Nguyen DH, Nguyen MT, Askenasy EP, Kao LS, Liang MK. Primary fascial closure with laparoscopic ventral hernia repair: systematic review. World J Surg. 2014;38(12):3097–104. https://doi.org/10.1007/s00268-014-2722-9.
8. Ali AA, Malata CM. The use of Mitek bone anchors for synthetic mesh fixation to repair recalcitrant abdominal hernias. Ann Plast Surg. 2012;69(1):59–63. https://doi.org/10.1097/SAP.0b013e31822128c6.
9. Yee JA, Harold KL, Cobb WS, Carbonell AM. Bone anchor mesh fixation for complex laparoscopic ventral hernia repair. Surg Innov. 2008;15(4):292–6. https://doi.org/10.1177/1553350608325231.
10. Rosen MJ. Polyester-based mesh for ventral hernia repair: is it safe? Am J Surg. 2009;197(3):353–9. https://doi.org/10.1016/j.amjsurg.2008.11.003.

Robotic Transversus Abdominis Release

Heidi J. Miller and Yuri W. Novitsky

Introduction

The ultimate goal of ventral hernia repair is to provide an excellent and durable repair with as low of recurrence rates as possible. We work to reconstruct the abdominal wall and restore function of the abdominal musculature. This is achieved through re-creation and reinforcement of the visceral sac, as well as restoration of the linea alba. We believe this is best accomplished with a tissue-based reconstruction, without bridging of fascia, and using mesh as reinforcement.

The transversus abdominis release (TAR) was described by Novitsky in 2012 [1] and is an extension of the Rives-Stoppa posterior rectus release, providing a true posterior component separation. Benefits of the TAR include a wide lateral dissection, preservation of perforating nerves and vessels to the anterior abdominal wall, and medial advancement of both posterior and anterior fascial layers for re-creation of the linea alba. It potentially reduces the risk of wound complications as no skin flaps are required and also reduces the risk of developing lateral hernias compared to other posterior component separation techniques, as there is no need to separate the linea semilunaris. The TAR provides excellent space for mesh placement in order to reinforce the visceral sac and is applicable to many patients and many hernias.

Traditionally the TAR has been an open procedure, requiring a large midline laparotomy incision, significant potential wound morbidity, and multiple-day hospital stays. Although laparoendoscopic approaches to TAR have been recently described, those approaches remain technically quite difficult to replicate [2]. The adoption and increased utilization of surgical robotics have allowed minimally invasive TAR to become much more widespread as the dissection and suturing are much less technically challenging with the EndoWrist technology of the robot, as well as improved visualization. Pioneering work by Abdalla, Carbonell, and Ballecer have led to the development and introduction of the robotic approach to TAR.

Literature Review

Novitsky et al. [3] evaluated outcomes of over 400 TAR procedures completed between 2006 and 2015. They reported a surgical site event rate of 19% and surgical site infection rate of 9%, with three patients requiring mesh debridement but no mesh explantations required. The median LOS of this series was about 6 days and a recurrence rate of 3.7% at 33 months average follow-up. This data has essentially cemented the TAR approach as one of the more effective open reconstructive techniques today.

The feasibility of robotic hernia repair has been well documented, starting in 2003 with individual cases being completed with intracorporeal suturing in both animal models and actual patients [4–7]. As robotics was taking off in the gynecologic and urologic fields, it has been lacking in evidence for benefit in the field of general surgery. However, it was slowly adopted for ventral hernia repair with the hope that using intracorporeal suturing instead of tacks and transfascial sutures may reduce postoperative pain, and that the visualization and EndoWrist dissection ability would accommodate preperitoneal dissections and allow for extraperitoneal mesh placement [8–10]. The data collected so far has shown that robotic ventral hernia repair is feasible and safe and has similar complication rates and outcomes to open and laparoscopic approaches to ventral hernia repairs.

In 2012, Abdalla et al. proved the feasibility of a retromuscular Rives-Stoppa-type minimally invasive repair with the use of robotic assistance [11]. This allowed an MIS approach to hernia repair using the principles of re-creation of the linea alba, retromuscular mesh placement, and minimal subcutaneous dissection in a procedure that had

H. J. Miller, MD, MPH (✉)
Department of Surgery, University of New Mexico, Albuquerque, NM, USA

Y. W. Novitsky, MD
Department of Surgery, Columbia University, New York, NY, USA

© Springer Nature Switzerland AG 2019
S. Tsuda, O. Y. Kudsi (eds.), *Robotic-Assisted Minimally Invasive Surgery*, https://doi.org/10.1007/978-3-319-96866-7_22

otherwise always been completed open. This has since been expanded by surgeons to include the posterior component separation by employing a robotic-assisted TAR [12]. Thus, an application for robotics in general surgery and hernia repair was uncovered by allowing a MIS approach to a procedure that had previously only been performed open. The laparoscopic TAR has since been attempted and shown to be feasible and safe, but its adoption has been limited due to the technical difficulty of the procedure without the benefit of the EndoWrist capability of the robotic instruments.

Warren et al. [13] compared 103 standard laparoscopic ventral hernia repairs (LVHRs) to 53 robotic retromuscular ventral hernia repairs (RRVHRs). The LVHR group had mostly (90%) intraperitoneal mesh placements with barrier-coated meshes, with or without defect closure, and using permanent transfascial sutures and permanent tacks for fixation. In the RRVHR group, all defects were closed, and the mesh was placed extraperitoneally in 96.2% of all cases; 70% of meshes were placed in the retromuscular space and 27% were place in the preperitoneal space. A myofascial release in the form of the TAR was required in 43% of cases, the remainder of retromuscular meshes being placed with a Reeves-Stoppa technique. The groups were similar, although the laparoscopic patients were older. All cases were CDC wound class 1 or 2. The RRVHR group had longer mean operating times, almost doubling the times for LVHR. From an outcome perspective, surgical site occurrences (SSO) were more common after RRVHR with a seroma rate of 47% vs 16% after LVHR. Two seromas required drainage after RRVHR and one after LVHR. The surgical site infection (SSI) rates were similar across the groups with two events after RRVHR and one following LVHR. Bowel injury was more common during the LVHR; however, one of the SSI complications following RRVHR was due to a missed bowel injury that led to intraabdominal sepsis. Reoperation rates were the same between both groups. Four LVHR were converted to open, compared to none of the RRVHR. Readmissions and other medical complications were similar across both groups. Narcotic use was not different between groups; however, the RRVHR group had a significantly shorter hospital length of stay of 1 day vs 2 for the LVHR group. The cost comparison was not statistically significant with LVHR hospital costs averaging nearly $14,000 and RRVHR nearly $20,000 [13].

More recently, Carbonell et al. [14] looked to compare open retromuscular ventral hernia repair (OVHR) to RRVHR in 1205 patients. In their study, 39 surgeons contributed the OVHR cases, and 14 surgeons contributed the RRVHR cases. Robotic cases that converted to open were analyzed in an intent-to-treat approach and were included in the RRVHR cases. A "propensity score" matching identified 111 RRVHR cases and 222 OVHR suitable for comparison. Differences between groups showed the OVHR group received more regional block anesthesia, which had shorter operative times and more drain usage. The RRVHR cases were more likely to use a running stitch or permanent suture to close the defect, and there were four conversions to open. RRVHR had a shorter LOS by 1 day than OVHR. There were no differences in clinically relevant surgical site events. SSI, reoperation, readmission, and other complications also occurred similarly between the two groups. There was no difference in the number of intraoperatively recognized complications, although one robotic case had one aforementioned unrecognized bowel injury leading to reoperation [14].

Preoperative Planning

Preoperative patient optimization is an important factor for success in abdominal wall reconstruction. We have good evidence that smoking cessation will reduce risk in hernia repair, and thus we require our patients to have abstained from smoking for at least 1 month prior to repair; nicotine testing is routinely undertaken. Preoperative weight loss is also an important risk reducer, and similarly to our open TAR patients, we mandate weight reduction to at least BMI < 45 to reduce the risk of systemic and wound infections. Patients who are candidates for screening colonoscopy should have this complete prior to repair. Finally, we recommend nutritional optimization with 5 days of arginine and omega-3 supplements, such as Impact ™ protein shakes or similar products prior to repair as well. Given the reduction in risk for wound infections that minimally invasive approaches provide, we find these recommendations to more pliable when we are using the robotic approach and might expand our ability to provide repairs for patients with greater BMIs and other risk factors while reducing their risk of postoperative complications.

Patient selection is another important factor for success in abdominal wall reconstruction, and choosing the right patient and hernia for the minimally invasive approach to TAR is still under evaluation. Currently we utilize robotic TAR for incisional hernias with widths between 8 and 15 cm, although this could be extended depending on the compliance of the abdominal wall and ratio of the volume of the hernia compared to the volume of the abdomen. We will also utilize the robotic TAR for patients with recurrent hernias where an underlay or onlay mesh had been previously placed.

Setup

The success of a robotic approach to a complex ventral hernia repair with separation of components relies on thoughtful preoperative setup, and this will depend slightly on which robotic platform is being used.

The da Vinci® Xi platform allows for slightly more flexibility in the room setup, as well as potentially extends the ability to perform the robotic transversus abdominis release procedure on a wider selection of patients given the shorter distance required between ports, thus potentially allowing for smaller patients or shorter torsos. Also, less space in the physical operating room is required as the boom can be rotated the full 180° needed for redocking and thus does not require that the patient or the robot be repositioned for a contralateral dock.

The da Vinci® Si platform will require more space, as the robot will physically need to be moved to the contralateral side of the patient for the 2nd dock and also requires more space (10 cm) between ports to avoid arm collisions. Room setup here will likely require that the patient be turned at least 45–90° away from anesthesia, to allow access for the robot to be brought in perpendicular to the patient and over the hip on the working side.

The patient is positioned supine on the operating table. A Foley catheter and orogastric tube are placed after the induction of general anesthesia. The patient's waist is positioned over on the bed where it can be flexed in order to open up the space between the costal margin and the iliac crest to create more working space. Both arms should be tucked to allow working space to avoid external collisions and to allow for the bedside assistant (Fig. 22.1).

We prefer to use long trocars, and for the Xi platform we use six long 8-mm cannulas. At least one will require an insufflation port unless the access port is to remain. When using the Si system we use four long 8-mm cannulas and two long 12-mm laparoscopic ports. Instrumentation remains the same across both platforms, using the robotic scissor with monopolar cautery in the right hand and the fenestrated bipolar grasper in the left. The Mega SutureCut™ Needle Driver will be placed in the right hand for suturing when that step of the procedure is reached.

Procedure

As with any minimally invasive procedure, safe access to the abdomen is the first key step to the procedure. We prefer an optical view trocar entry at the costal margin, just lateral to the midclavicular line. If possible, the right side is preferable, but this will vary depending on the location of the patient's hernia and previous operative history. Once access is obtained, the lower trocar is placed 2 cm medially and cephalad from the anterior superior iliac spine (ASIS). The camera port is placed in between at approximately anterior axillary line (Fig. 22.2). The next step is to reduce the hernia contents and complete an adhesiolysis to clear the abdominal wall. Adhesiolysis should be completed, carefully taking advantage of the pneumoperitoneum and sharp dissection to prevent unintended bowel injury. If there is mesh in place from prior hernia repairs, mesh excision is typically undertaken.

Once the adhesions are taken down, the hernia defect is visible, and the posterior myofascial dissection can be started. We first identify the medial edge of the rectus abdominis

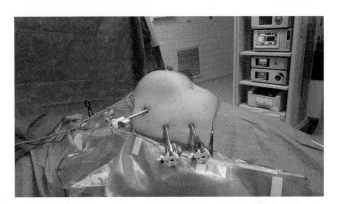

Fig. 22.2 Our typical trocar strategy. The lower port could be slightly shifted cephalad for upper abdominal hernias

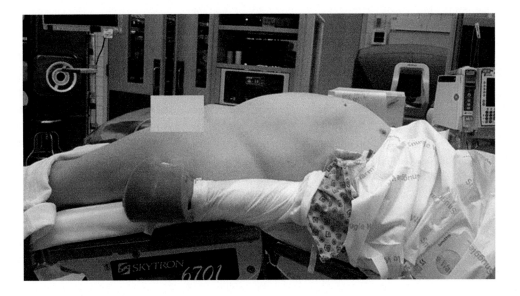

Fig. 22.1 Patient positioning. The legs are flexed to minimize external collisions with thighs. The arms are tucked

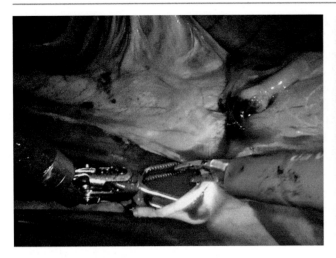

Fig. 22.3 Initial incision of the medial aspect of the posterior rectus sheath. It is important to confirm/visualize the fibers of the rectus muscle

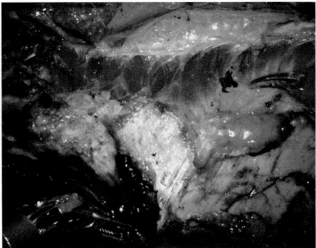

Fig. 22.4 Incision of the lateral aspect of the posterior rectus sheath (posterior lamella of the internal oblique aponeurosis) just medial to the neurovascular bundles

muscle on the contralateral side to port placement. The underlying medial aspect of the posterior rectus sheath is incised for the entire length of the rectus abdominis (Fig. 22.3), and the posterior sheath is then dissected off of the rectus muscle laterally until the lateral perforating neurovascular bundles are identified. The cranio-caudal extent of the dissection is adjusted for smaller defects. During this dissection, the left hand is providing tension and traction, and the right hand (scissors) is using cautery and blunt dissection to create this space. It is not necessary to dissect all the way to the semilunar line, as we aim to preserve the neurovascular bundles in order to avoid denervation and devascularization of the rectus muscle.

Once the posterior rectus sheath release and retrorectus dissection are complete, the lateral aspect of the posterior sheath is incised approximately 1 cm medial to the perforating neurovascular bundles. This exposes the transversus abdominis muscle (TA) (Fig. 22.4). We typically initiate this step at the cephalad aspect of the field, as TA extends more medial in that area and is easier to identify. The TA is transected using electrocautery while lifting it away from the underlying tissue with the grasper (Fig. 22.5). This provides access to the pre-transversalis plane, which will then be dissected bluntly laterally into the retroperitoneum and toward the lateral edge of the psoas muscle. Superiorly, the interdigitation of the diaphragm with the TA can be visualized as the preperitoneal plane cephalad to the costal margin is developed. As the dissection moves caudally along the aponeurotic TA, the arcuate line is reached, and it is transected. Here, the dissection plane must transition through the transversalis fascia to a preperitoneal plane in order to complete the dissection in the space of Retzius. This dissection can also be completed in a "bottoms-up" technique by identifying the arcuate line (Fig. 22.6), dissecting laterally and

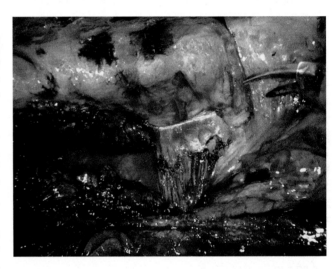

Fig. 22.5 Incision of the transversus abdominis muscle. Care must be taken not to divide the underlying transversalis fascia and peritoneum

underneath it to raise it away from the underlying tissues and starting the transversus abdominis transection in the aponeurotic TA and continuing the dissection cranially into the more muscular TA. The lateral dissection is complete when the posterior layer is lying flat against the abdominal viscera. Any disruptions to the posterior sheath can be repaired with a 2–0 absorbable suture at this time.

Mirrored ports are then placed on the contralateral side. The robot is then undocked at this time. The boom of the Xi can be rotated and redocked on the contralateral side, or for an Si, the patient is rotated 45–90° to allow the robot to be brought in over the contralateral hip and is then redocked.

Once the 2nd dock is complete, the hernia defect is again identified, any further adhesiolysis can be completed, and the dissection as described above is undertaken, again starting

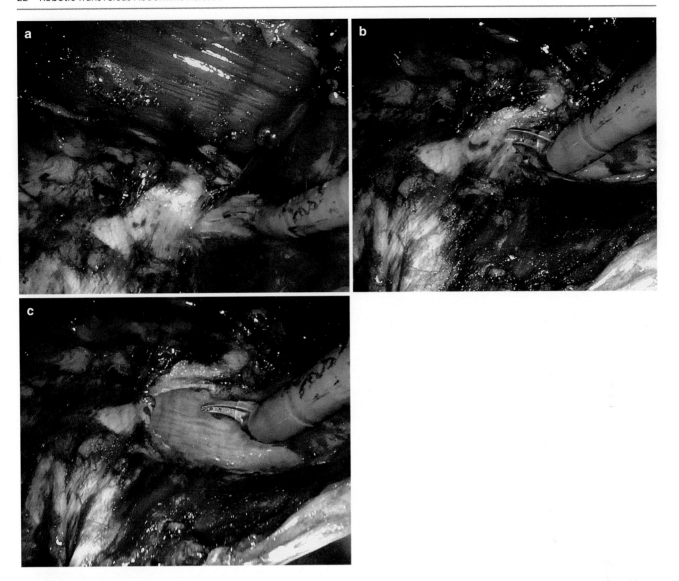

Fig. 22.6 rTAR "bottoms up": (**a**) identification of the arcuate line at its junction with linea semilunaris; (**b**) incision of the arcuate line; (**c**) retromuscular dissection facilitating cephalad progression and incision of the posterior rectus sheath and transversus abdominis muscle

by identifying the medial edge of the rectus abdominis muscle. The lateral dissection is completed after the transecting the transversus abdominis muscle and taken out laterally to the psoas muscle. The two planes are connected inferiorly by identifying bilateral Cooper's ligaments after complete dissection of the myopectineal orifices in the space of Retzius and dropping the preperitoneal fat pad off of the pubic symphysis. Superiorly by following the retromuscular plane that leads to the diaphragm and is deep to the ribs (Fig. 22.7), the subxiphoid fat pad can be identified and transected to connect the bilateral dissection planes. This plane can then be exploited for further dissection all the way to the central tendon of the diaphragm, which is important and useful for hernias that extend superiorly to achieve adequate mesh overlap. The dissection is complete when the entire posterior layer lies flat on the abdominal contents.

Closure of the posterior layer is then undertaken, using 2–0 absorbable self-locking sutures (Fig. 22.8), which are started from either apex and can be tied together in the middle. Any rents or defects can be closed with 2–0 Vicryl sutures or clips. There will be at least three small defects from the original ports placed transabdominally on the original docking side. These should be closed to reduce the risk of intraparietal hernias.

The next step is closure of the anterior fascia and restoration of the linea alba. To facilitate this closure under minimal tension, the pneumoperitoneum can be dropped to 8–10 mmHg. The anterior closure is completed with a 0 or #1 self-locking suture running from both directions (Fig. 22.9). This suture is also used to imbricate the hernia sac into the closure in order to reduce the risk of seroma formation. Generally, the suture is brought through one side

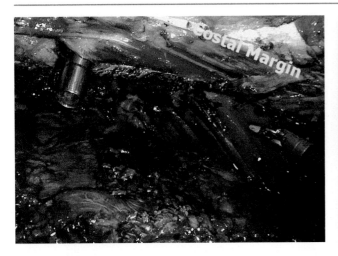

Fig. 22.7 Superior extension of the retromuscular dissection in the preperitoneal plane on the diaphragm

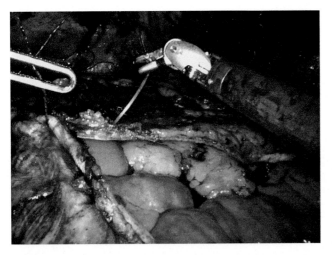

Fig. 22.8 Restoration of the visceral sac via closure of the posterior layers. We utilize a running 2–0 absorbable barbed suture

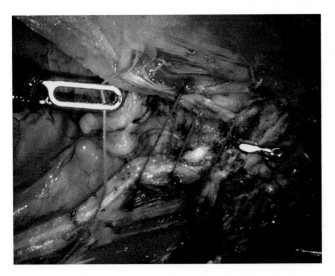

Fig. 22.9 Restoration of the linea alba via approximation of the medialized anterior rectus sheaths using #1 nonabsorbable barbed suture

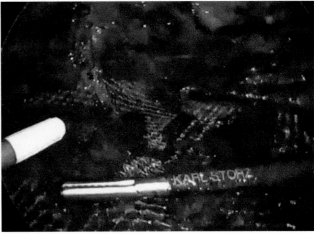

Fig. 22.10 Laparoscopic placement of a sublay mesh. Fibrin glue fixation is optional

of the anterior fascia, then a bite of hernia sac is taken, and finally the suture is brought through the contralateral side of the fascia. Care must be taken not to include full thickness bites of the anterior abdominal wall skin.

After the sutures are placed, they are tightened up under reduced pneumoperitoneum (5–6 mmHg). It is important to inspect the entire linea alba for any gaps or improper sutures. If any are found, we suggested placing additional figure-of-eights intracorporeally or transabdominally.

Following closure of both anterior and posterior layers, a ruler is introduced to measure the dissected space as well as the hernia defect. A spinal needle placed at the edges of the defect can facilitate accurate measurements. The robot is then undocked as mesh is placed laparoscopically (Fig. 22.10). A mesh is cut to size to fill the entire retromuscular space, rolled into a single scroll. We use a macroporous, midweight polypropylene mesh of approximately 30x30 cm in size. We typically add no additional suture fixation. Occasionally a fibrin glue is used. Drains are used selectively.

Postoperative Care

We have adopted an Enhanced Recovery After Surgery (ERAS) [15] protocol for our open TARs, and this is accelerated for the minimally invasive approach. Most patients will be kept overnight in the hospital, started on clear liquids, and advanced to a regular diet as tolerated. The patient is given minimal narcotics, and a multimodal pain medication approach is used and includes an intraoperative transversus abdominis plane (TAP) block with liposomal bupivacaine, Tylenol, NSAIDs, and gabapentin.

Patients are discharged with minimal activity restrictions, advancing to light activity immediately as tolerated. We expect them to be out of bed on the evening of POD 0. Driving and strenuous activities are typically limited until seen in the clinic at the 2-week post op visit. We prefer to follow our abdominal wall reconstruction patients long term to monitor for recurrence and complications. The patients are seen back at 6 weeks, 6 months, 1 year postoperatively, and then annually.

Discussion

Although there is currently a lot of enthusiasm for the robotic TAR, there remain a lot of unanswered questions regarding its indication, overuse, complications, and outcomes. There is a limited amount of short-term data that has recently become available, which is promising that the robotic TAR offers economic value over open TAR, but long-term outcomes are still awaited. Areas of research will be to define the most appropriate patients and hernias to be approached with the robotic TAR in order to limit the number of unnecessary component separations done, reduce cost, and limit potential complications. Long-term outcome data will also be necessary to evaluate for recurrence rates and procedure-specific complications, such as the intraparietal hernias that have been documented [11, 13]. The best pathway for surgeons to become competent and to provide a safe and successful procedure to their patients is also unknown, although we recommend clear understanding of the anatomy and procedure from an open approach prior to attempting the robotic approach. This will help with intraoperative trouble shooting as well as in the case of conversion to open TAR.

References

1. Novitsky YW, Elliott HL, Orenstein SB, Rosen MJ. Transversus abdominis muscle release: a novel approach to posterior component separation during complex abdominal wall reconstruction. Am J Surg 2012;204(5):709–716. Available from: https://doi.org/10.1016/j.amjsurg.2012.02.008.
2. Belyansky I, Zahiri HR, Park A. Laparoscopic transversus abdominis release, a Novel minimally invasive approach to complex abdominal wall reconstruction. Surg Innov. 2016;23(2):134–41. Available from: http://www.ncbi.nlm.nih.gov/pubmed/26603694
3. Novitsky YW, Fayezizadeh M, Majumder A, Neupane R, Elliott HL, Orenstein SB. Outcomes of posterior component separation with transversus abdominis muscle release and synthetic mesh sublay reinforcement. Ann Surg. 2016;264(2):226–32. Available from: http://content.wkhealth.com/linkback/openurl?sid=WKPTLP:landingpage&an=00000658-900000000-97031
4. Schluender S, Conrad J, Divino CM, Gurland B. Robot-assisted laparoscopic repair of ventral hernia with intracorporeal suturing. Surg Endosc. 2003;17(9):1391–5.
5. Ballantyne GH, Hourmont K, Wasielewski A. Telerobotic laparoscopic repair of incisional ventral hernias using intraperitoneal prosthetic mesh. JSLS. 2003;7(1):7–14. Available from: http://www.ncbi.nlm.nih.gov/pubmed/12722992
6. Beldi G. Technical feasibility of a robotic-assisted ventral hernia repair. World J Surg. 2012;36(2):453–4.
7. Allison N, Tieu K, Snyder B, Pigazzi A, Wilson E. Technical feasibility of robot-assisted ventral hernia repair. World J Surg. 2012;36(2):447–52.
8. Tayar C, Karoui M, Cherqui D, Fagniez PL. Robot-assisted laparoscopic mesh repair of incisional hernias with exclusive intracorporeal suturing: a pilot study. Surg Endosc. 2007;21(10):1786–9.
9. Gonzalez A, Escobar E, Romero R, Walker G, Mejias J, Gallas M, et al. Robotic-assisted ventral hernia repair: a multicenter evaluation of clinical outcomes. Surg Endosc. 2017;31:1342–9.
10. Sugiyama G, Chivukula S, Chung PJ, Alfonso A. Robot-assisted transabdominal preperitoneal ventral hernia repair. JSLS J Soc Laparoendosc Surg. 2015;19(4):e2015.00092. Available from: http://www.ncbi.nlm.nih.gov/pmc/articles/PMC4756357/
11. Abdalla RZ, Garcia RB, da Costa RID, de Luca CRP, Abdalla BMZ. Modified robot assisted Rives/Stoppa videosurgery for midline ventral hernia repair. Arq Bras Cir Dig. 2012;25(2):129–32.
12. Ballecer C. Robotic ventral hernia repair. In: Novitsky YW, editor. Hernia surgery: current principles. Cham: Springer International Publishing; 2016. p. 273–86.
13. Warren JA, Cobb WS, Ewing JA, Carbonell AM. Standard laparoscopic versus robotic retromuscular ventral hernia repair. Surg Endosc Other Interv Tech. 2017;31(1):324–32.
14. Carbonell AM, Warren JA, Prabhu AS, Ballecer CD, Janczyk RJ, Herrera J, et al. Reducing length of stay using a robotic-assisted approach for retromuscular ventral hernia repair: a comparative analysis from the Americas Hernia Society Quality Collaborative. Ann Surg. 2017. Available from: http://insights.ovid.com/crossref?an=00000658-900000000-96161
15. Majumder A, Fayezizadeh M, Neupane R, Elliott HL, Novitsky YW. Benefits of multimodal enhanced recovery pathway in patients undergoing open ventral hernia repair. J Am Coll Surg. 2016. Available from: http://linkinghub.elsevier.com/retrieve/pii/S1072751516001903

Robotic Suprapubic Hernias

Shinil K. Shah, Erik B. Wilson, and Peter A. Walker

Introduction

Suprapubic ventral/incisional hernias (SPH, also sometimes referred to as parapubic hernias [1]), due to their location and associated anatomic factors, frequently offer challenges to durable repair. SPH are most frequently incisional and may be associated with suprapubic laparoscopic trocar placement, sites of suprapubic catheter placement, and Pfannenstiel-, Maylard-, or Cherney-type incisions [2]. One of the early descriptions in the literature of this subset of hernias was offered by el Mairy in 1974 [3]. The incidence of SPH tends to be significantly less than other types of incisional hernias, with estimates ranging from about 0.5–2%. The relationship to the pubic arch, bladder, and retroperitoneal vasculature as well as the lack of a posterior rectus sheath represents the key anatomic issues that have to be considered when contemplating an operative strategy.

Laparoscopic Suprapubic Hernia Repair

Multiple operative approaches including open, laparoscopic, and robotic have been reported, and the relative rarity of this type of hernia makes it difficult to determine which approach is superior [4, 5]. Overlay and underlay (retromuscular/retrorectus, pre-peritoneal (either transabdominal or totally extraperitoneal), or intraperitoneal) techniques have been described in the repair of these hernias. Given that these types of hernias are typically 4–5 cm or less from the pubic arch [6], pre-peritoneal or retromuscular placement of mesh tends to facilitate mesh fixation to the pubic arch and Cooper's ligament [7–9]. Overlay techniques tend to be associated with higher recurrence rates [8]. Lack of fixation of the mesh to Cooper's ligament has also been associated with higher recurrence rates and should be considered one of the key technical points of repair [6]. Familiarity with minimally invasive inguinal hernia repair should be considered mandatory prior to surgeons attempting repair of SPH [6].

One of the earliest series reported of laparoscopic intraperitoneal repair of SPH was published by Hirasa et al. A series of seven patients with recurrent SPHs were described utilizing intraperitoneal mesh placement with underlay of the mesh of 2–3 cm and fixation utilizing laparoscopic tacks. With a mean follow-up of 5.8 months, one recurrence was noted [10]. A report of laparoscopic pre-peritoneal repair of SPH was actually published several years prior, reporting a single case of a transabdominal pre-peritoneal repair of a SPH after prostatectomy, and included description of the now well-accepted principle of fixation of the mesh to Cooper's ligament [11].

Since then, a number of small series describing laparoscopic repair incorporating some pre-peritoneal dissection to allow for fixation to the pubis and Cooper's ligament have been published. Ferrari et al. reported a series of 18 patients undergoing laparoscopic SPH repair with 2 recurrences noted at the inferior border with 37 months of follow-up. Mesh was fixed with laparoscopic tacks only [12]. Most of the other published series describing pre-peritoneal dissection report fixation with transfascial sutures as well as laparoscopic tacks. Carbonell et al. reported a series of 36 patients (22/36 patients with recurrent hernias) undergoing laparoscopic SPH repair, including pre-peritoneal dissection to allow for fixation of the mesh to Cooper's ligament and the pubis. There were two noted recurrences over a mean follow-up of 21.1 months (5.5%), with both occurring in the first nine cases, and were attributed to lack of appropriate inferior fixa-

S. K. Shah (✉)
Department of Surgery, McGovern Medical School, University of Texas Health Science Center at Houston, Houston, TX, USA

Michael E. DeBakey Institute for Comparative Cardiovascular Science and Biomedical Devices, Texas A&M University, College Station, TX, USA
e-mail: shinil.k.shah@uth.tmc.edu

E. B. Wilson
Department of Surgery, McGovern Medical School, University of Texas Health Science Center at Houston, Houston, TX, USA

P. A. Walker
Health First Medical Group, Rockledge, FL, USA

© Springer Nature Switzerland AG 2019
S. Tsuda, O. Y. Kudsi (eds.), *Robotic-Assisted Minimally Invasive Surgery*, https://doi.org/10.1007/978-3-319-96866-7_23

tion [1]. Other series have described similar technique as well as results, including series by Palanivelu et al. (17 patients (1 recurrent hernia), 5.8% recurrence over 9 months of mean follow-up) [6] and Varnell et al. (47 patients (27 patients with recurrent hernias), 6.3% recurrence rate over 2.6 months of mean follow-up) [2]. Varnell et al. described a pre-peritoneal approach, starting with dissection inferior to the umbilicus, reduction of the hernia sac with the pre-peritoneal defect, and with at least partial re-peritonealization of the mesh in some cases [2]. The largest series of laparoscopic SPH described a review of 72 patients, including 5 patients with a previous incisional hernia repair, reporting no recurrences over a mean follow-up of 4.8 years. A partial pre-peritoneal approach was utilized, with the pre-peritoneal flap starting at the level of the anterior superior iliac spine and continuing inferiorly. After fixation of the mesh with tacks as well as transfascial sutures, the mesh was partially re-peritonealized [9]. Fixation of the mesh with bone anchors has also been reported for the repair of SPHs. Yee et al. reported a series of 17 patients with SPHs, in which a similar technique as reported by Carbonell et al. was utilized [1], but in addition to laparoscopic tacks and transfascial sutures, bone anchors were placed into the pubis to additionally secure the mesh. This study included patients with both lumbar hernias (13 patients) as well as SPH; recurrence was noted in 2 patients in both groups over a mean follow-up of 13.2 months [13].

There has been increasing interest in the extended view totally extraperitoneal (eTEP) approach to abdominal wall reconstruction, and some authors have reported its use in the repair of SPH; however there are no large series published for this subset of ventral/incisional hernias [4].

Robotic Ventral/Incisional Hernia Repair

There continues to be increasing interest in robotics for the repair of ventral/incisional hernias. There is limited data specifically reporting on robotics and SPH repair; however, a review of the current literature in ventral/incisional hernia repair is certainly important. The initial report of robotic-assisted ventral hernia repair described two patients in which robotic technology was utilized to facilitate laparoscopic repair. Transfascial sutures and tacks were utilized for fixation; robotics was utilized for adhesiolysis, intraperitoneal handling of the mesh, and suture presentation to a suture passing device [14]. Schluender et al. first published the use of robotics to facilitate circumferential suturing of mesh in a porcine model of laparoscopic ventral hernia repair [15].

The initial clinical report of intracorporeal suture fixation of mesh was published by Tayar et al. and described a series of 11 patients [16]. Allison et al. reported a series of 13 patients in which similar mesh fixation was utilized; however, they included primary fascial closure as part of the described technique [17]. Other case series have demonstrated techniques of robotic transabdominal pre-peritoneal ventral hernia repair with primary defect closure (3 patients) [18] and robotic intraperitoneal mesh placement with primary defect closure (106 patients) [19] demonstrating acceptable short-term results. Recently, a series of 368 patients describing a multi-institutional experience of robotic ventral and incisional hernia repair has been reported. In this series, 69.3% of patients had primary defect closure, and 58.2% of patients had fixation of mesh with sutures alone [20]. Details specifically regarding robotic repair of SPH were not discussed.

There is limited data comparing laparoscopic to robotic ventral hernia repair. Gonzalez et al. compared robotic-assisted ventral hernia repair with primary fascial closure to laparoscopic ventral hernia repair without primary fascial closure (67 patients in each group). Surgical time was longer, and median follow-up time was shorter in the robotics group, without any statistically significant differences in overall complications or recurrence [21]. Chen et al. compared 39 patients undergoing robotic-assisted repair to 33 patients undergoing laparoscopic repair of small ventral and incisional hernias. Accounting for a larger defect size in the robotic group (3.07 cm as compared to 2.02 cm, $p < 0.001$) and limited follow-up (mean 47 days), robotics was associated with increased operative time without any differences in outcomes [22]. Recently, Warren et al. described a comparison of laparoscopic ventral hernia repair (103 patients) to robotic retromuscular repair (53 patients). The robotic group was associated with higher incidence of fascial closure (96.2% versus 50.5%, $p < 0.001$), larger size of mesh placed, mesh placement in the extraperitoneal position, increased use of transversus abdominis release, increased operative times, and increased surgical site occurrences (seromas) (47.2% vs 16.5%, $p < 0.001$). There was decreased intraoperative bowel injury (one patient versus nine patients, $p = 0.011$) and decreased median length of stay (1 versus 2 days, $p = 0.004$) in the robotic group. Recurrence rates were not compared [23]. Most recently, Carbonell et al. published an analysis of 333 patients from the Americas Hernia Society Quality Collaborative (2013–2016), comparing 111 robotic retromuscular ventral hernia repairs to 222 open retromuscular repairs, using propensity score matching to compare median length of stay. Median length of stay was noted in to be lower and surgical site occurrences higher (mostly seromas) in the robotics group as compared to the open approach.

Preoperative Planning

When dealing with hernias in atypical locations, preoperative imaging, typically computed tomography (CT), should be considered [8]. As with other types of complex abdominal wall reconstruction/incisional hernia repairs, attention in the preoperative period should be paid to factors that are associated with recurrence, including nutritional optimization, tobacco use, and morbid obesity.

Elective repair of SPHs should not be considered in patients who are actively smoking, and most guidelines recommend at least 4 weeks of smoking cessation prior to surgery. In high-risk patients, consider testing for nicotine metabolites preoperatively.

Morbid obesity is a known risk factor for recurrence, and similar to other types of ventral/incisional hernias, elective surgery should be avoided in patients with morbid obesity. Increased risks for recurrence have been seen in patients with a BMI over 30 kg/m^2 [24]. In patients with a BMI over 40–50 kg/m^2, aggressive means for preoperative weight loss, including consideration for weight loss surgery, should be considered prior to hernia repair [25, 26]. Elective surgery should also be avoided in patients with uncontrolled diabetes (glycosylated hemoglobin >8%) [25]. In patients with glycosylated hemoglobin greater than 6.5%, preoperative optimization of diabetes management should be considered [25].

Given the need to mobilize the bladder off the abdominal wall when repairing SPH, Foley catheter placement should be considered to decompress the bladder [8]. Aggressive use of regional anesthesia and multimodal, narcotic sparing, pain regimens, including pretreatment with medications such as gabapentin, pregabalin, and/or celecoxib, should be utilized. In patients with a history or major risk factors for urinary retention, considerations including preoperative tamsulosin and a restrictive intraoperative fluid strategy should be employed.

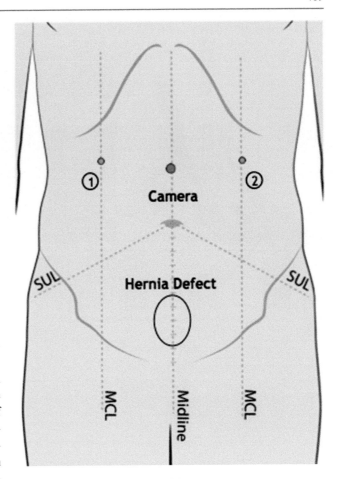

Fig. 23.1 Port placement for robotic suprapubic hernia repair. Generally the camera port is placed in the supraumbilical or epigastric location depending on the location of the superior aspect of the hernia fascial defect. Instrument arms (either 5 mm or 8 mm depending on the choice of instruments and or the robotic platform being utilized) are placed laterally, typically 8–10 centimeters from the camera port

Setup

The setup for robotic SPH repair is similar to that of robotic inguinal and femoral hernia repair, with the exception that ports should be placed somewhat higher to allow for preperitoneal or retromuscular flap creation several centimeters superior to the edge of the fascial defect. Initial peritoneal entry should occur with either optical entry techniques, Veress needle, or cutdown techniques as per the experience and comfort level of the operating surgeon. Typically, a camera port is placed in the epigastric location, and two working ports are placed on either side, allowing for 8–10 centimeters of distance between the trocars (Fig. 23.1). We typically do not utilize an accessory trocar and usually place mesh and sutures through the camera port; however a 5–12-mm accessory trocar for suctioning, suture, and mesh placement may be advisable early on in the learning curve or as part of an individual surgeon's preference.

Unless utilizing a platform with integrated table motion, the patient should be placed in Trendelenburg prior to docking to facilitate access and pelvic dissection. Routine or selective Foley catheter placement should be considered, especially in recurrent or anticipated difficult cases. Docking of the robotic patient side cart can either be done in the midline with the patient in lithotomy position or as a parallel side dock from either the right or left hip (Fig. 23.2). If feasible, tucking both arms aids in docking of the robotic patient side cart, instrument exchanges, placement of mesh and/or sutures, as well as facilitating activities of bedside assistants and surgical technologists.

Typical instruments utilized include monopolar shears or hook cautery, needle drivers, and grasping instruments (bowel graspers (tip-up fenestrated graspers, bowel graspers, Cadiere forceps), ProGrasp™ forces, bipolar forceps (fenestrated or Maryland)) of the surgeons choice should be available. As cost is an increasingly important concern, all attempts should be made to minimize the number and type of instruments utilized. Typically, three instruments, including a needle driver, monopolar shears, and some type of grasping instrument, are sufficient for the majority of cases.

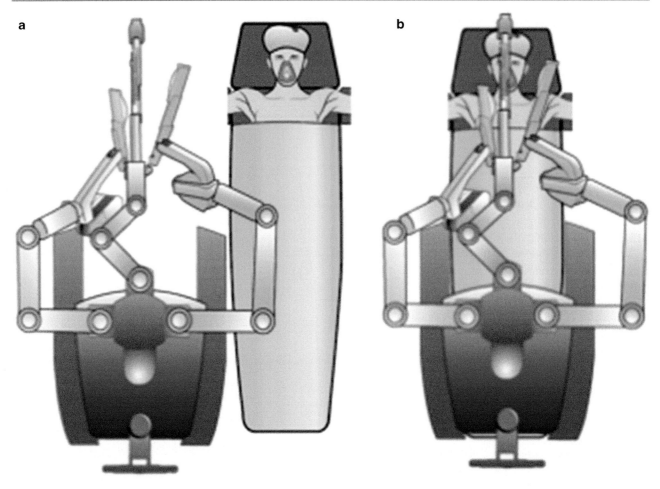

Fig. 23.2 Docking of the patient side cart is easiest either as a parallel side dock from the right or left side (**a**) or in the midline if the patient is in lithotomy position (**b**). With the da Vinci Xi platform (Intuitive Surgical), docking can be done from any position

Procedure

When considering the number of approaches for robotic suprapubic hernia repair, unless considering a total extraperitoneal approach, there are number of common key steps. After safe peritoneal entry and port placement, lysis of adhesions is carefully undertaken. The borders of the hernia fascial defect are determined and measured. Relationships to key anatomical structures, including distance from the pubic arch, should carefully be noted. If there is difficulty identifying the position of the bladder, fluid can be instilled via a Foley catheter to aid intraoperative visualization. Distending the bladder may also help with operative dissection [1].

Pure intraperitoneal mesh repair of SPHs is difficult and is not advised as it does not tend to allow for adequate inferior coverage of the facial defects. To achieve adequate mesh overlap, repair almost always requires takedown of the bladder to identify the pubic arch and Cooper's ligament. Failure to release the bladder can result in iatrogenic injury utilizing a pure intraperitoneal approach. For this reason, a pre-peritoneal dissection should be considered mandatory to expose the pubis and Cooper's ligament.

Complete as well as partial transabdominal pre-peritoneal repairs have been described. Additionally, totally extraperitoneal as well as eTEP approaches have been discussed, but to date, series describing the use in SPH repair have not been published [4]. For complete pre-peritoneal or eTEP type repairs, dissection of the pre-peritoneal plane generally starts in the midline inferior to the umbilicus and continues inferiorly. Generally, the hernia sac will be reduced during the pre-peritoneal dissection. With partial pre-peritoneal repairs, typically, the pre-peritoneal plane is entered at the level of the anterior superior iliac spine, and dissection is carried to the opposite side. This dissection is similar to that which is performed during transabdominal pre-peritoneal repairs of inguinal or femoral hernias. Dissection is carried inferiorly to release the bladder, identify both Cooper's ligaments as well as the pubic arch, and continue to the space of Retzius. Care should be taken to identify and prevent injury to the inferior epigastric as well as location of the iliac vessels [2]. This dissection allows for adequate inferior coverage of the mesh and the ability to secure the mesh to Cooper's ligaments (Figs. 23.3 and 23.4). Pre-peritoneal dissection also allows for placement of a larger mesh, as the borders of this space tend not to be restricted by the lateral rectus [8]. In the case of partial pre-peritoneal repairs, the mesh can then be partially re-peritonealized, and the intraperitoneal portion of the mesh can be fixed to the abdominal wall using the technique of the surgeon's choice, including transfascial sutures, absorbable or permanent tacks, or circumferential suturing to the posterior abdominal wall with absorbable or nonabsorbable sutures [9].

One of the potential advantages of robotic ventral/incisional hernia repair is the ability to fixate mesh without transfascial sutures and, in many cases, laparoscopic tacks. Depending on the surgeon's preference, absorbable or permanent sutures can be utilized to fixate the mesh to Cooper's ligament and the pubis as well as to the anterior abdominal wall using interrupted or running techniques. Barbed sutures can facilitate running fixation of the mesh.

The role of fascial closure during the repair of SPH is currently a topic of debate. There is some suggestion that primary fascial closure during ventral/incisional hernia repair may be associated with decreased seroma and wound complication rates [27], as well as potentially lower recurrence rates [28]. Fascial closure can be difficult in SPH and traditional anterior component separation techniques may not assist in repair or in promoting primary anterior fascial closure [8]. In difficult or larger hernias, retromuscular dissection with or without transversus abdominis release may allow for release of the anterior fascia, allow for primary fascial closure, and allow for placement of adequate-sized mesh prosthesis [8]. Primary fascial closure is typically accomplished in robotic ventral/incisional hernia repair with the use of interrupted or running barbed or non-barbed sutures.

Choice of mesh is generally left to the individual surgeon. With a completely pre-peritoneal dissection and complete re-peritonealization of the mesh, uncoated meshes can be utilized; however, if there is exposed mesh, coated meshes

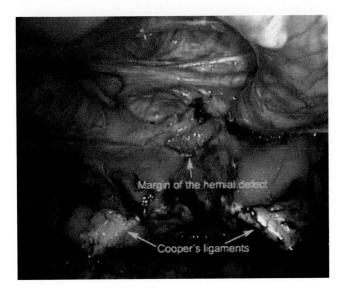

Fig. 23.3 Demonstrated is the inferior view that should be visualized prior to mesh placement and fixation. Cooper's ligament and the pubis should be dissected completely, with care taken to avoid injury to the inferior epigastric and iliac vessels, to allow for adequate inferior overlap of the mesh. Note in this case, a partial pre-peritoneal dissection was utilized. Figure reproduced with permission. (From Sharma et al. [9], with permission of Springer)

a

b

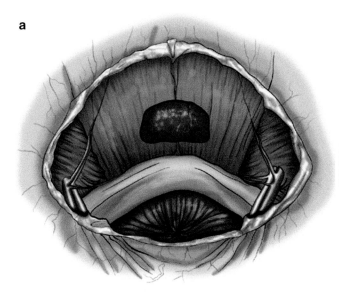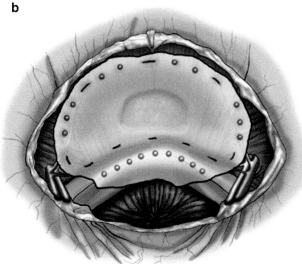

Fig. 23.4 After full dissection and exposure (**a**), mesh is placed with care taken to ensure it is adequately fixated to Cooper's ligament and the pubis (**b**). This can be accomplished with sutures, laparoscopic tacks, or a combination of both. Although not depicted in this figure, consideration should be given for primary closure of the hernia defect. Figures reproduced with permission. (From Varnell et al. [2], with permission of Elsevier)

should be considered. Generally, medium-weight meshes should be utilized for repair, and ultra-light, light-weight or super heavy-weight meshes are associated with worse outcomes [25].

Conclusions

The repair of SPH represents a challenge, secondary to primarily anatomic reasons. There is increasing data supporting the use of minimally invasive means of repair. Careful attention to preoperative optimization as well as intraoperative technique, particularly adequate inferior fixation of the mesh, is likely to result in best outcomes. Although continued further study is required, robotic surgery may be a valuable tool to facilitate pre-peritoneal dissection as well as mesh fixation.

References

1. Carbonell AM, Kercher KW, Matthews BD, Sing RF, Cobb WS, Heniford BT. The laparoscopic repair of suprapubic ventral hernias. Surg Endosc. 2005;19(2):174–7.
2. Varnell B, Bachman S, Quick J, Vitamvas M, Ramshaw B, Oleynikov D. Morbidity associated with laparoscopic repair of suprapubic hernias. Am J Surg. 2008;196(6):983–7; discussion 987–988.
3. el Mairy AB. A new procedure for the repair of suprapubic incisional hernia. J Med Liban. 1974;27(6):713–8.
4. Ramana B. Suprapubic incisional hernias: is open surgery a standard? World J Surg. 2017;41(6):1475.
5. Renard Y, Simonneau AC, de Mestier L, et al. Standard of open surgical repair of suprapubic incisional hernias. World J Surg. 2017;41(6):1466–74.
6. Palanivelu C, Rangarajan M, Parthasarathi R, Madankumar MV, Senthilkumar K. Laparoscopic repair of suprapubic incisional hernias: suturing and intraperitoneal composite mesh onlay. A retrospective study. Hernia: J Hernias Abdom Wall Surg. 2008;12(3):251–6.
7. Lal R, Sharma D, Hazrah P, Kumar P, Borgharia S, Agarwal A. Laparoscopic management of nonmidline ventral hernia. J Laparoendosc Adv Surg Tech A. 2014;24(7):445–50.
8. Hope WW, Hooks WB 3rd. Atypical hernias: suprapubic, subxiphoid, and flank. Surg Clin North Am. 2013;93(5):1135–62.
9. Sharma A, Dey A, Khullar R, Soni V, Baijal M, Chowbey PK. Laparoscopic repair of suprapubic hernias: transabdominal partial extraperitoneal (TAPE) technique. Surg Endosc. 2011;25(7):2147–52.
10. Hirasa T, Pickleman J, Shayani V. Laparoscopic repair of parapubic hernia. Arch Surg. 2001;136(11):1314–7.
11. Matuszewski M, Stanek A, Maruszak H, Krajka K. Laparoscopic treatment of parapubic postprostatectomy hernia. Eur Urol. 1999;36(5):418–20.

12. Ferrari GC, Miranda A, Sansonna F, et al. Laparoscopic repair of incisional hernias located on the abdominal borders: a retrospective critical review. Surg Laparosc Endosc Percutan Tech. 2009;19(4):348–52.
13. Yee JA, Harold KL, Cobb WS, Carbonell AM. Bone anchor mesh fixation for complex laparoscopic ventral hernia repair. Surg Innov. 2008;15(4):292–6.
14. Ballantyne GH, Hourmont K, Wasielewski A. Telerobotic laparoscopic repair of incisional ventral hernias using intraperitoneal prosthetic mesh. JSLS: J Soc Laparoendosc Surg/Soc Laparoendosc Surg. 2003;7(1):7–14.
15. Schluender S, Conrad J, Divino CM, Gurland B. Robot-assisted laparoscopic repair of ventral hernia with intracorporeal suturing. Surg Endosc. 2003;17(9):1391–5.
16. Tayar C, Karoui M, Cherqui D, Fagniez PL. Robot-assisted laparoscopic mesh repair of incisional hernias with exclusive intracorporeal suturing: a pilot study. Surg Endosc. 2007;21(10):1786–9.
17. Allison N, Tieu K, Snyder B, Pigazzi A, Wilson E. Technical feasibility of robot-assisted ventral hernia repair. World J Surg. 2012;36(2):447–52.
18. Sugiyama G, Chivukula S, Chung PJ, Alfonso A. Robot-assisted transabdominal preperitoneal ventral hernia repair. JSLS: J Soc Laparoendosc Surg/Soc Laparoendosc Surg. 2015;19(4): e2015.00092.
19. Kudsi OY, Paluvoi N, Bhurtel P, McCabe Z, El-Jabri R. Robotic repair of ventral hernias: preliminary findings of a case series of 106 consecutive cases. Am J Robot Surg. 2015;2(1):22–6.
20. Gonzalez A, Escobar E, Romero R, et al. Robotic-assisted ventral hernia repair: a multicenter evaluation of clinical outcomes. Surg Endosc. 2017;31(3):1342–9.
21. Gonzalez AM, Romero RJ, Seetharamaiah R, Gallas M, Lamoureux J, Rabaza JR. Laparoscopic ventral hernia repair with primary closure versus no primary closure of the defect: potential benefits of the robotic technology. Int J Med Robot + Comput Assisted Surg: MRCAS. 2015;11(2):120–5.
22. Chen YJ, Huynh D, Nguyen S, Chin E, Divino C, Zhang L. Outcomes of robot-assisted versus laparoscopic repair of small-sized ventral hernias. Surg Endosc. 2017;31(3):1275–9.
23. Warren JA, Cobb WS, Ewing JA, Carbonell AM. Standard laparoscopic versus robotic retromuscular ventral hernia repair. Surg Endosc. 2017;31(1):324–32.
24. Nardi M Jr, Millo P, Brachet Contul R, et al. Laparoscopic ventral hernia repair with composite mesh: analysis of risk factors for recurrence in 185 patients with 5 years follow-up. Int J Surg. 2017;40:38–44.
25. Liang MK, Holihan JL, Itani K, et al. Ventral hernia management: expert consensus guided by systematic review. Ann Surg. 2017;265(1):80–9.
26. Pernar LI, Pernar CH, Dieffenbach BV, Brooks DC, Smink DS, Tavakkoli A. What is the BMI threshold for open ventral hernia repair? Surg Endosc. 2017;31(3):1311–7.
27. Tandon A, Pathak S, Lyons NJ, Nunes QM, Daniels IR, Smart NJ. Meta-analysis of closure of the fascial defect during laparoscopic incisional and ventral hernia repair. Br J Surg. 2016;103(12):1598–607.
28. Nguyen DH, Nguyen MT, Askenasy EP, Kao LS, Liang MK. Primary fascial closure with laparoscopic ventral hernia repair: systematic review. World J Surg. 2014;38(12):3097–104.

Robotic Proctocolectomy

24

Volkan Ozben and Bilgi Baca

Abbreviations

IPAA   Ileal pouch-anal anastomosis
SMA   Superior mesenteric artery
SMV   Superior mesenteric vein

Introduction

Total proctocolectomy with ileal pouch-anal anastomosis (IPAA) is the procedure of choice for the surgical treatment for ulcerative colitis and familial adenomatous polyposis [1–3], Although a three-stage procedure (total colectomy, completion proctectomy with IPAA and diverting ileostomy, and ileostomy closure) is performed in the emergency setting in patients with ulcerative colitis, this operation is usually carried out in two stages in which total proctocolectomy is combined with an IPAA and diverting ileostomy as the first stage, followed by ileostomy closure as the second stage. Since its initial description in 1978 [4], the surgical techniques have evolved over the years with respect to pouch construction and operative approach. In terms of operative approach, since the first laparoscopic proctocolectomy was reported in 1992 [5], multiple studies have now shown that laparoscopy provides favorable postoperative outcomes, such as faster recovery, shorter hospital stay, and good functional outcomes when compared to open proctocolectomy [3, 6, 7].

The introduction of robotic surgery with its technical advantages over laparoscopy, including three-dimensional vision, better dexterity with stable wristed instrumentations, and improved ergonomics. Has revolutionized minimal invasive approach [8]. As a result, robotic surgery has become the preferred choice for many colorectal procedures in the hope to further optimize surgical outcomes [9]. Although robotic proctocolectomy is a relatively new concept, there is a growing body of evidence suggesting the safety and effectiveness of the use of the robot in this procedure. In this chapter, we present a literature review and describe the technical aspects of robotic proctocolectomy procedure and perioperative patient care.

Literature Review

Since 2011, when Pedraza et al. [10] first described the application of the robotic system for proctectomy during the proctocolectomy procedure, seven studies including two comparative studies [11, 12], two case series [13, 14], and two cases [15, 16] have been reported regarding the use of the robot in the abdominal and/or pelvic stage of this operation (Table 24.1).

In the initial three reports [10, 11, 13], the general trend was to use the robot primarily for the pelvic stage (proctectomy) of the procedure. In their series including five ulcerative colitis patients undergoing proctocolectomy procedure, Pedraza et al. [10] reported the feasibility and safety of hybrid robotic-assisted laparoscopy procedure combining conventional laparoscopy for colectomy and robotic approach for proctectomy. The mean operative time was 330 min with a robot docking time of 16.8 min and surgeon console time of 122 min. The mean estimated blood loss was 200 ml. There were no intraoperative complications, and none of the procedures required conversion to open or another minimally invasive modality. Postoperatively, the mean time to return of bowel function was 2.4 days, length of hospital stay was 5.6 days, and no patients developed major postoperative complications. Shortly after this study, McLemore et al. [13] reported the technical advantages of the robotic approach for pelvic dissection during the stage II procedure (completion proctectomy with ileoanal pouch reconstruction) in three patients with toxic ulcerative colitis who had prior laparoscopic total colectomy. In a different

V. Ozben · B. Baca (✉)
Department of General Surgery, Acibadem Mehmet Ali Aydinlar University, School of Medicine, Istanbul, Turkey

© Springer Nature Switzerland AG 2019
S. Tsuda, O. Y. Kudsi (eds.), *Robotic-Assisted Minimally Invasive Surgery*, https://doi.org/10.1007/978-3-319-96866-7_24

Table 24.1 The number of robotic proctectomy, colectomy, and proctocolectomy procedures reported in the literature

Author	Publication year	Total number of robotic procedures	Robotic colectomy (*n*)	Robotic proctectomy (*n*)	Laparoscopic colectomy and robotic proctectomy (*n*)	Robotic proctocolectomy (*n*)
Pedraza et al. [10]	2011	5 (UC: 5)	–	–	5	–
McLemore et al. [13]	2011	3 (UC: 3)	–	3	–	–
Miller et al. [11]	2012	17 (UC: 13, IC: 2, CD: 2)	–	17	–	–
Juo and Obias [15]	2015	1 (FAP: 1)	1	–	–	–
Roviello et al. [14]	2015	4 (UC: 4)	–	–	–	4
Baca et al. [16]	2015	1 (UC: 1)	–	–	–	1
Mark-Christensen et al. [12]	2016	81 (UC: 81)	–	79	–	2

UC ulcerative colitis, *IC* indeterminate colitis, *CD* Crohn's disease, *FAP* familial adenomatous polyposis

study, Miller et al. [11] matched 17 robotic proctectomies (10 with IPAA and 7 with completion proctectomy) to laparoscopic proctectomies for inflammatory bowel diseases. Overall, there were no conversions to open surgery, and the postoperative complication rates were similar in this study. With respect to the completion proctectomy subgroup, all the perioperative outcomes were similar between the two approaches except operative times were longer (351 vs 238 min), return of bowel function was slower (3.0 vs 1.7 days), and length of stay was longer (6.4 vs 4.1 days) in the robotic procedures. With respect to the IPAA subgroup, the authors noted no difference in perioperative outcomes between the two approaches, including operative times (370 vs 316 min), return of bowel function (3.6 vs 2.6 days), and length of hospital stay (8.5 vs 6.1 days). Quality of life and sexual function after IPAA were also equivalent between the groups. The authors conclude that robotic surgery is comparable to laparoscopy with respect to perioperative outcomes, complications, and short-term functional outcomes.

In the following years, the trend in the use of robotic approach shifted from the pelvic side of the operation to abdominal colectomy. In 2015, Juo and Obias [15] reported the feasibility of robotic single incision total colectomy in a patient with familial adenomatous polyposis and demonstrated the possibility of access to the entire abdominal cavity through a single umbilical incision. Eventually, in the same year, the first totally robotic proctocolectomy was reported by Roviello et al. [14] in a series of four patients with ulcerative colitis. To date, this has been the largest series of totally robotic proctocolectomy procedure ever reported. In this study, the authors described the robotic single-docking technique. The mean operative time and blood loss were 235 min and 100 ml, respectively. There were no conversions. The overall postoperative morbidity was 75% including one patient who required reoperation due to small bowel obstruction secondary to internal herniation. The authors conclude that the single-docking technique to perform total proctocolectomy is safe and feasible and also time-saving as opposed to a multiple docking approach.

Lastly, Mark-Christensen et al. [12] compared a series of 81 robot-assisted laparoscopic IPAA with 170 open IPAA procedures. Of the 81 robotic procedures, completion proctectomy and restorative proctocolectomy were performed in 79 and 2 patients, respectively. The operative time was longer for the robotic procedures, and there were no differences in the distribution of complications. Pouch failure occurred in one patient following robotic and two patients following open surgery. On multivariate analyses, robotic surgery was associated with longer operative times and more readmissions.

As seen, data on totally robotic proctocolectomy procedure is still very limited with a total number of seven patients reported in the literature [12, 14, 16]. Nevertheless, all these reports provide essential data on the safety and efficacy of robotic approach to guide further investigations. With any complex procedure gaining gradual acceptance, the technique should be expected to evolve. Considering this, the technical details of the totally robotic proctocolectomy procedure in our practice will be described in the following section.

Preoperative Planning

In patients with well-controlled colitis or familial adenomatous polyposis, we prefer a two-stage procedure with a combined total proctocolectomy, IPAA, and diverting loop ileostomy followed by subsequent ileostomy closure. The patient's general condition and nutritional status should be optimized prior to surgery. The patient is counselled by the colorectal nurse who marks the site of ileostomy. Mechanical bowel preparation is administered 1 day before surgery. Low molecular weight heparin is administered 12 h. before the operation for venous thrombosis prophylaxis, and intravenous antibiotic prophylaxis is given 1 h. before surgical incision. After induction of general anesthesia, a nasogastric tube and a urinary catheter are placed.

Setup

Under general anesthesia, the patient is fixed on the operating table in the modified lithotomy position with both arms tucked alongside the body. The Allen Yellofin stirrups™ and shoulder supports should be used for secure patient positioning. The patient cart is draped in a sterile fashion. The robotic console is positioned in a way that the surgeon can effectively see the operating table and communicate with the bedside assistant throughout the procedure. The vision cart is positioned outside the sterile field and should be visible to the bedside assistant.

Procedure

The operation is performed via a medial-to-lateral approach using the da Vinci Xi robotic system (Intuitive Surgical Inc., Sunnyvale, CA, USA) [16]. A total number of seven trocars are used: four 8-mm, one 12-mm robotic, and two 5-mm assistant trocars. A Veress needle is introduced through an 8-mm skin incision in the supraumbilical region, and pneumoperitoneum with an intra-abdominal pressure of 12 mmHg is established. An 8-mm robotic trocar is placed through this incision, and a 30° camera is introduced into the abdomen via this trocar. The remaining four robotic trocars are placed under direct vision, as follows: one 8-mm trocar in the right iliac fossa, one 12-mm trocar with a reducer cap in the right lower quadrant at the premarked ileostomy site, and two 8-mm trocars in the left upper quadrant. All the five robotic trocars are positioned at least 6 cm apart from each other and arranged in a line, as shown in Fig. 24.1. Then, two assistant trocars are placed: one is at the premarked suprapubic incision site and the other one in the right upper quadrant. These assistant trocars are used by the bedside assistant for suction and retraction.

The operation is completed in two stages: the first stage involves dissection of the right colon up to the level of the mid-transverse colon, and for this, four robotic trocars (the right lower quadrant, supraumbilical and two left upper quadrant trocars) and the suprapubic assistant trocar are used. The second stage is for the dissection of the remaining colon and rectum. In this stage, four robotic trocars (the right iliac, right lower quadrant, supraumbilical and one left upper quadrant trocars) and the right upper quadrant assistant trocar are used (Fig. 24.1). The 12-mm robotic trocar at the premarked ileostomy site serves for stapler insertion to perform bowel transection in both stages of the operation.

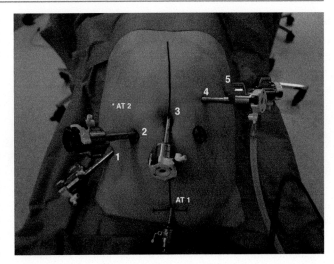

Fig. 24.1 Trocar placement in robotic proctocolectomy. Four 8-mm robotic, one 12-mm robotic and two 5-mm assistant trocars are used. Robotic trocar # 1 (8 mm) is in the right iliac fossa, trocar # 2 (12 mm) in the right lower quadrant, trocar # 3 (8 mm) in the supraumbilical area, and trocars 4 and 5 (each 8 mm) in the left upper quadrant. AT 1, assistant trocar in the suprapubic area. AT 2, assistant trocar in the right upper quadrant. The robotic trocars # 2, 3, 4, and 5 and AT 1 are used for dissection of the right colon up to the level of mid-transverse colon. For the dissection of the remaining colon and rectum, the robotic trocars # 1, 2, 3, and 4 and AT 2 are used

In the first stage, the patient is placed in a 15° Trendelenburg position with the operating table tilted 30° to the left side. The small bowel loops are retracted medially and the omentum above the transverse colon with a laparoscopic grasper, exposing the ventral side of the ascending and transverse mesocolon. The robotic cart is docked from the right side of the patient, the camera is positioned at arm 3, and the robotic system is targeted to the right colon. Then, the other robotic arms are mounted to the trocars and instruments are inserted, as follows: double fenestrated tip-up grasper at arm 1, double fenestrated bipolar forceps at arm 2, and monopolar curved scissors at arm 4. The assistant surgeon positions on the left side of the patient.

Dissection is initiated by retracting the ascending mesocolon laterally with the tip-up grasper near the ileocecal junction. The peritoneum overlying the ileocolic vascular pedicle is lifted up with bipolar forceps and incised with monopolar scissors. The ileocolic vein and artery are isolated individually, clipped with Hem-o-lok clips (Weck Closure Systems, Research Triangle Park, NC) near its origin from the superior mesenteric vein (SMV) and artery (SMA), and divided between the clips using scissors. A robotic vessel sealer can also be used to divide the vascular structures. Mesenteric dissection is performed staying between the embryological planes just anterior to the Toldt's and Gerota's fasciae and the duodenum. During this dissection process, the right colic vessels, if present, are clipped and divided near their origins in the same fashion. Mesenteric dissection is continued up to the root of the middle colic vessels, which are then divided between clips. While the assistant applies gentle traction on the transverse colon caudally, the bursa omentalis is entered and the gastrocolic ligament divided from right to left along the greater curvature of the stomach up to the hepatic flexure, preserving the gastric vascular arcade. Hem-o-lok clips or a vessel sealer can be used for vascular control during this dissection. With inferiomedial traction, the hepatic flexure is taken down, and lateral attachments of the ascending colon are mobilized craniocaudally using scissors.

For the dissection of mesocolon, the most common technique employed by surgeons is that the mesocolon is resected near the bowel wall without performing vascular high ligation. However, in our early experience with laparoscopic proctocolectomy procedures, we noticed that dissection in this plane required ligation of numerous mesenteric vascular branches and was sometimes difficult in the presence of pericolonic inflammation especially in patients with chronic ulcerative colitis. On the other hand, vascular high ligation and dissection along the embryological planes may provide better vascular control and a clearer surgical field which, in turn, help improve visualization and ease preservation of the retroperitoneal structures. In addition to this, any incidental colorectal cancer could be treated using this technique without a need for further lymphadenectomy especially in patients with familial adenomatous polyposis [17].

Following full mobilization of the right colon, transection of the ileum is performed. The terminal ileum 2 cm away from the ileocecal valve is dissected free of its mesentery and divided using a robotic EndoWrist® stapler with a blue cartridge (Intuitive Surgical Inc., Sunnyvale, CA, USA). For this, the reducer cap is temporarily removed from the 12-mm trocar in order to introduce the robotic stapler. Demounting of the robotic arms completes the first stage of the operation.

In the second stage, without moving the robotic cart, the boom of the robotic system is rotated from the right side of the patient to left for the dissection of the left colon and rectum. The angle of Trendelenburg position is increased from 15° to 30°, and the operating table is tilted 30° to the right. The small bowel loops are retracted out of the pelvis to the right side of the abdomen with a laparoscopic grasper. The camera is inserted in the supraumbilical trocar at arm 2, and the robotic system is targeted to the left inguinal region. The other robotic arms are mounted to the trocars and instruments are inserted, as follows: double fenestrated bipolar forceps at arm 1, monopolar curved scissors at arm 3, and double fenestrated tip-up grasper at arm 4. The assistant surgeon moves to the right side of the patient.

Again, the mesentery of the left colon is approached in a medial-to-lateral fashion. With anterior traction on the sigmoid colon with the tip-up grasper, the peritoneum is incised at the sacral promontorium level, and the aorta-mesenteric window is entered using the monopolar scissors and bipolar forceps. Following identification of the inferior mesenteric artery, the artery is clipped and transected 1 cm away from its origin in order to preserve the inferior mesenteric nerve plexus. The inferior mesenteric vein is divided in the same manner. The mesocolon is separated from the anterior surface of the pancreas, the omental bursa is entered, and dissection is continued to the level of the splenic flexure. Then, dissection is directed into the embryological planes over Gerota's and Toldt's fasciae, preserving the left ureter, gonadal vessels, and autonomic nerves. After completing medial dissection, the distal transverse colon is retracted caudally, the bursa omentalis is reentered and the remaining gastrocolic ligament divided from right to left, separating the omentum completely from the stomach and spleen. We prefer removing the omentum in this operation in order to decrease the risk of postoperative adhesion formation. In addition to this, the omentum may harbor foci of microabscesses in the presence of active inflammation; thus removal of the omentum may prevent the risk of intra-abdominal septic complications postoperatively. The left colon is retracted medially, the lateral attachments of the colon are divided, and the splenic flexure is taken down completely.

Following completion of the abdominal portion of operation, attention is directed to the pelvis. The same trocar configuration is used for both left colectomy and pelvic dissection. The rectum is dissected according to the total mesorectal excision principles. Although not essential in a benign disease, total mesorectal excision provides an almost bloodless plane of dissection and allows us to create a better pouch configuration. First, the peritoneal reflection just below the sacral promontory is incised, and the rectum is mobilized posteriorly by sharp dissection in the "holy plane" between the fascia propria recti and the presacral fascia. This dissection is achieved by pulling gently the sigmoid colon anteriorly and cranially by the assistant. Dissecting the posterior mesorectum first enables the surgeon to hold the mesorectum easily, thus facilitates its lateral dissection. Then, the right lateral side of the mesorectum is mobilized, and this is followed by the mobilization of the left side of the mesorectum. Care should be taken to preserve the right and left hypogastric nerves during posterior dissection and inferior hypogastric plexus during lateral dissection (Fig. 24.2). After adequate mobilization is achieved bilaterally, attention is directed to the anterior mesorectum. In the absence of malignancy, we perform mesorectal dissection behind the Denonvillier's fascia in order to avoid postoperative sexual dysfunction. The mesorectal dissection is continued down to the pelvic floor. At this stage, the surgeon changes the angle of the robotic camera from "down" to "up" position in order to see the intersphincteric area. After full mobilization of the mesorectum is completed, the assistant surgeon performs a digital rectal examination to determine the level of rectal transection. The tip of a finger placed in the anus with the

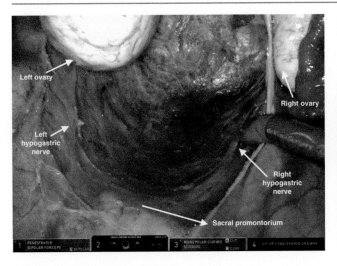

Fig. 24.2 Completion of the mesorectal dissection

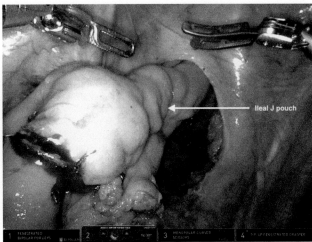

Fig. 24.4 View of the ileal J-pouch

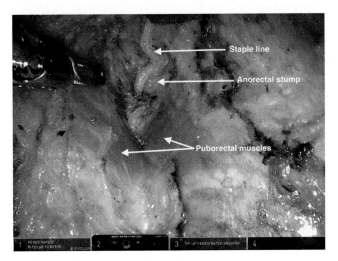

Fig. 24.3 View of the anorectal stump and staple line following distal rectal transection

proximal interphalangeal joint at the level of the anal verge provides a useful estimate of the appropriate level of transection. The rectum is divided using a robotic stapler(s) with green cartridge introduced through the 12-mm trocar (Fig. 24.3).

Following rectal transection, the robotic system is undocked, and a suprapubic incision is performed at the suprapubic assistant trocar site to a length of 6–8 cm. This incision is used to extract the proctocolectomy specimen and to carry out ileal J-pouch creation (Fig. 24.4). A J-pouch of 18–20 cm is constructed in a usual fashion using linear staplers. An anvil of a 29-mm or 31-mm circular stapler is secured in the distal end of the pouch, and the bowel is returned into the abdomen. The suprapubic incision is closed and pneumoperitoneum is re-established. The patient is placed to a reverse Trendelenburg position with a slight left tilt. If there are concerns about a tension-free IPAA, then suf-

ficient mesenteric length is generally achieved with peritoneal relaxing incisions. If reach issue is still of concern, extra length can be obtained by releasing the mesenteric attachments up to the third portion of the duodenum. The robotic system is re-docked and the pouch-anal anastomosis is carried out using a circular stapler placed transanally. Care is taken not to twist the intestine and not to entrap the vagina in the staple line in female patients.

An air-leak test is performed to ensure anastomotic and suture-line integrity. The pelvis is copiously irrigated. After hemostasis is assured, a silicone drain is placed into the pelvis through the right flank trocar site. Finally, the ileum approximately 30 cm away from the pouch is brought through the abdominal incision at the 12-mm trocar site in the right lower quadrant. All trocars are removed, skin incisions are closed, and the diverting loop ileostomy is matured in a standard fashion.

Postoperative Care

Postoperative intravenous narcotics and nonsteroidal anti-inflammatory medication are given as needed for postoperative pain control. Venous thrombosis prophylaxis is continued for 7 days postoperatively. Removal of nasogastric tube and start of oral intake are determined on the basis of return of bowel movement. Patients are discharged from the hospital when sufficient oral intake, full ambulation, and adequate pain control with oral analgesics are achieved. Within 2 months after surgery, the integrity of anastomosis is confirmed with a contrast enema study and then the patient is scheduled for ileostomy closure.

Conflicts of Interest The authors, Volkan Ozben and Bilgi Baca, declare that they have no conflicts of interest.

References

1. Fazio VW, Ziv Y, Church JM, Oakley JR, Lavery IC, Milsom JW, Schroeder TK. Ileal pouch-anal anastomoses complications and function in 1005 patients. Ann Surg. 1995;222:120–7.
2. Farouk R, Pemberton JH, Wolff BG, Dozois RR, Browning S, Larson D. Functional outcomes after ileal pouch-anal anastomosis for chronic ulcerative colitis. Ann Surg. 2000;231:919–26.
3. Konishi T, Ishida H, Ueno H, Kobayashi H, Hinoi T, Inoue Y, Ishida F, Kanemitsu Y, Yamaguchi T, Tomita N, Matsubara N, Watanabe T, Sugihara K. Feasibility of laparoscopic total proctocolectomy with ileal pouch-anal anastomosis and total colectomy with ileorectal anastomosis for familial adenomatous polyposis: results of a nationwide multicenter study. Int J Clin Oncol. 2016;21:953–61.
4. Parks AG, Nicholls RJ. Proctocolectomy without ileostomy for ulcerative colitis. Br Med J. 1978;2:85–8.
5. Peters WR. Laparoscopic total proctocolectomy with creation of ileostomy for ulcerative colitis: report of two cases. J Laparoendosc Surg. 1992;2:175–8.
6. Seshadri PA, Poulin EC, Schlachta CM, Cadeddu MO, Mamazza J. Does a laparoscopic approach to total abdominal colectomy and proctocolectomy offer advantages? Surg Endosc. 2001;15:837–42.
7. Schiessling S, Leowardi C, Kienle P, Antolovic D, Knebel P, Bruckner T, Kadmon M, Seiler CM, Büchler MW, Diener MK, Ulrich A. Laparoscopic versus conventional ileoanal pouch procedure in patients undergoing elective restorative proctocolectomy (LapConPouch Trial)-a randomized controlled trial. Langenbeck's Arch Surg. 2013;398:807–16.
8. Ballantyne GH, Moll F. The da Vinci telerobotic surgical system: the virtual operative field and telepresence surgery. Surg Clin North Am. 2004;83:1293e1304.
9. Damle A, Damle RN, Flahive JM, Schlussel AT, Davids JS, Sturrock PR, Maykel JA, Alavi K. Diffusion of technology: trends in robotic-assisted colorectal surgery. Am J Surg. 2017;214:820–4. pii: S0002-9610(16)30934-5.
10. Pedraza R, Patel CB, Ramos-Valadez DI, Haas EM. Robotic-assisted laparoscopic surgery for restorative proctocolectomy with ileal J pouch-anal anastomosis. Minim Invasive Ther Allied Technol. 2001;20:234–9.
11. Miller AT, Berian JR, Rubin M, Hurst RD, Fichera A, Umanskiy K. Robotic-assisted proctectomy for inflammatory bowel disease: a case-matched comparison of laparoscopic and robotic technique. J Gastrointest Surg. 2012;16:587–94.
12. Mark-Christensen A, Pachler FR, Nørager CB, Jepsen P, Laurberg S, Tøttrup A. Short-term outcome of robot-assisted and open IPAA: an observational single-center study. Dis Colon Rectum. 2016;59:201–7.
13. McLemore EC, Cullen J, Horgan S, Talamini MA, Ramamoorthy S. Robotic-assisted laparoscopic stage II restorative proctectomy for toxic ulcerative colitis. Int J Med Robot. 2012;8:178–83.
14. Roviello F, Piagnerelli R, Ferrara F, Scheiterle M, De Franco L, Marrelli D. Robotic single docking total colectomy for ulcerative colitis: first experience with a novel technique. Int J Surg. 2015;21:63–7.
15. Juo YY, Obias V. Robot-assisted single-incision total colectomy: a case report. Int J Med Robot. 2015;11:104–8.
16. Baca B, Aghayeva A, Ozben V, Bayraktar O, Atasoy D, Erguner I, Karahasanoglu T, Hamzaoglu I. Robotic total proctocolectomy for ulcerative colitis – a video vignette. Color Dis. 2015;17:736.
17. Atasoy D, Aghayeva A, Bayraktar O, Ozben V, Baca B, Hamzaoglu I, Karahasanoglu T. Vascular high ligation and embryological dissection in laparoscopic restorative proctocolectomy for ulcerative colitis. J Laparoendosc Adv Surg Tech A. 2017;27:33–5.

Robotic Hysterectomy

25

Erica Stockwell, Jasmine Pedroso, and K. Warren Volker

History

Minimally invasive surgery is the one of most ground-breaking surgical innovations in the past 30 years. Laparoscopic surgery was initially introduced in 1901 when Von Ott inspected the abdominal cavity of a pregnant woman. It did not gain widespread popularity, however, until 1987 when French gynecologist, Mouret, performed the first laparoscopic cholecystectomy [3]. It was around this time that the first generation of robots was created to perform image-guided precision tasks. The technology evolved and in 2005 the FDA approved Intuitive Surgical's da Vinci® surgical system for use in gynecologic surgery.

Robotic surgery in gynecology is one of the fastest growing fields of robotic surgery. This includes the use of the da Vinci surgical system in benign gynecology and gynecologic oncology. Robotic surgery can be used to treat fibroids, abnormal periods, endometriosis, ovarian tumors, pelvic organ prolapse, and female cancers and perform hysterectomies, myomectomies, and lymph node biopsies. A 2013 JAMA study reported that robotic hysterectomy increased almost 1000% between 2007 and 2010 (from 0.5% to 9.5% of all hysterectomies), while rates of laparoscopic hysterectomy increased much more slowly (from 24.3% to 30.5%) [4].

Robotic-assisted surgery has demonstrated clear advantages over conventional laparoscopy for gynecologic oncology, specifically for lymph node dissection, but its superiority in benign surgery is contested as complication rates tend to be similar between robotic-assisted and conventional laparoscopy. Benefits of robotic-assisted surgery for benign gynecologic conditions include increased dexterity, improved ergonomics, three-dimensional optics, reduced blood loss, decreased postoperative pain, shorter hospital stay, and quicker learning curve than with conventional laparoscopy [5–7]. Drawbacks include increased operative time, increased operative cost, and potentially increased rate of vaginal cuff dehiscence [7, 8]. While robotic-assisted surgery has been shown to be safe and feasible in gynecologic surgery, additional randomized controlled trials are required to determine specific indications for use. Robotic-assisted hysterectomy is potentially most beneficial for obese patients, in those with large uteri, those with complex surgical pathology (such as advanced endometriosis and extensive pelvic adhesions), and in those with pelvic organ prolapse. In addition, surgical advancements such as single-site hysterectomy may change the relative advantages and disadvantages of laparoscopic versus robotic hysterectomy.

Patient Positioning

A successful robotic-assisted hysterectomy begins with proper and secure patient positioning. Once the robot is docked, the patient is, for the most part, unable to be repositioned. The first step is therefore to secure an anti-slip pad or beanbag positioner to the table to prevent the patient from sliding backward while in steep Trendelenburg position. Draw sheets underneath the patient should be minimized, and a gel donut or foam pillow should also be placed under the patient's occiput to avoid ischemic necrosis and alopecia while in Trendelenburg.

The patient is placed in a low dorsal lithotomy position using stirrups (see Fig. 25.1). Heels should be flush with the back of the stirrup, and all pressure points should be well padded. Extreme flexion, extension, and abduction should be avoided to minimize neuromuscular injuries. The buttocks should be positioned just off the edge of the table with the sacrum fully supported. If the patient is not placed down far enough on the table, then uterine manipulation will be lim-

E. Stockwell · K. W. Volker (✉)
Las Vegas Minimally Invasive Surgery, WellHealth Quality Care, a DaVita Medical Group, Las Vegas, NV, USA
e-mail: wvolker@hcpnv.com

J. Pedroso
Obstetrics and Gynecology, MountainView Hospital, Centennial Hills Hospital, Las Vegas, NV, USA

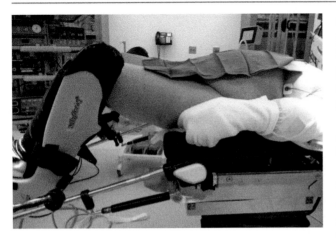

Fig. 25.1 Positioning in low dorsal lithotomy

ited during the case. On the other hand, if the patient is too far down, this will put increased pressure on the patient's lower back resulting in possible injury.

Both arms should be padded and tucked at the patient's sides in a thumbs-up position in order to provide space for the surgeon to operate from the level of the patient's shoulder to angle directly toward the pelvis and to prevent nerve injury to the patient. It is a good practice to tuck the arms even for short procedures as any procedure carries the possibility of taking longer than anticipated. For obese patients, plastic sleds, arm rests, or bed extenders may be placed lateral to the patient to provide enough room to tuck the arms.

A strap may be placed across the patient's chest to further prevent patient slippage. Alternatively, shoulder pads may be placed, but extreme caution should be taken to place them directly over the acromions and padded so as not to impinge upon the neck or create a brachial plexus injury through stretch or compression.

The eyes should be closed and covered to prevent corneal abrasions. A protective barrier such as a metal cage attached to the bed frame, or a foam pillow, should be placed over the patient's head to prevent dislodging of the endotracheal tube, injury from instruments resting on the face, or robotic arm collision.

Lastly, the patient is slowly tipped into Trendelenburg position. This should be done prior to prepping and draping to ensure the patient does not slide too far backward, that arms stay tucked in place, and that legs are not over extended and to ensure that the patient is able to tolerate anesthesia in a Trendelenburg position. The degree of Trendelenburg should be enough to allow for mobilization of the bowel out of the pelvis to adequately visualize pelvic anatomy. It often does not require the maximum Trendelenburg position of 30–40°. A pilot study in which surgeons were blinded to degree of Trendelenburg used demonstrated a mean of only 16° required to adequately visualize the pelvis [9]. Overall, the total time the patient spends in Trendelenburg position

should be minimized to avoid injury secondary to slippage or physiologic changes associated with Trendelenburg positioning. Steep Trendelenburg position for more than 3 h may predispose a patient to potential brachial plexus injury, corneal abrasions, laryngeal edema, cerebral edema, and posterior ischemic optic neuropathy [10].

Uterine Manipulation

Good uterine manipulation is also key in performing a successful hysterectomy, and there are a variety of uterine manipulators available for use. Uterine manipulators help to provide adequate exposure, afford proper triangulation, and avoid injury to the ureters and bladder. There are uterine positioning systems available as well to hold the manipulator in place and maintain uterine position. There are no randomized control trials comparing the variety of uterine manipulators head-to-head to prove brand superiority. Choice is largely dependent on surgeon preference and availability. The author prefers to use a manipulator with a disposable lighted cervical cup, pneumo-occluder, and reusable metal intrauterine rod.

Trocar Placement

Proper port placement is the next imperative step to a successful robotic-assisted hysterectomy. First, the surgeon must decide how may robotic arms to use and whether to also place an assistant port. A two-arm system is more cost-effective, but a three-arm system can provide static counter traction in difficult cases. With the placement of an assist port, the surgeon's assistant can irrigate, suction, provide counter traction, take mesh or suture in and out of the field, and provide tactile feedback. Straightforward hysterectomies can often be performed via two arms without need for an assistant port (Fig. 25.2a) as suture can be introduced through the vagina.

Typically, the camera port is placed first in the midline at the level of the umbilicus. This site may be adjusted 2–3 cm superiorly for large uterine size or just to the left of the midline for thin patients to avoid clashing with the first and third robotic arms. Alternatively, for patients with prior midline vertical incisions or umbilical hernias, the left upper quadrant (Palmer's point) may serve as a better initial entry point to avoid injury to the bowel. The camera port is 8 or 12 mm in diameter on the Si da Vinci robotic platform or 8 mm on the Xi da Vinci robotic platform. All robotic trocars are 8 mm in diameter.

The remaining trocar placement is determined after pneumoperitoneum is achieved, and an assessment of the patient's anatomy has been performed. Ideally, robotic ports are

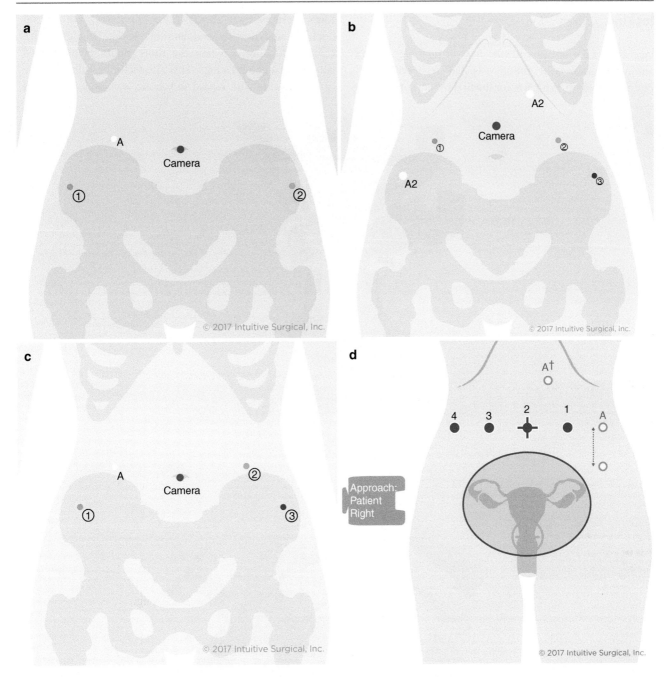

Fig. 25.2 (**a**) Si configuration of two arms. 1, robotic arm 1; 2, robotic arm 2; A, accessory port placement. ((Alternatively can place on the patient's left side if docking on the patient's right) ©2018 Intuitive Surgical, Inc.). (**b**) Si configuration of three arms, semilunar. 1, robotic arm 1; 2, robotic arm 2; 3, robotic arm 3; A1/2, alternative accessory port placements. ((Alternatively, robotic arm 2 can place on the patient's right side for a right-handed surgeon) ©2018 Intuitive Surgical, Inc.). (**c**) Si configuration of three arms, "W". 1, robotic arm 1; 2, robotic arm 2; 3, robotic arm 3; A, accessory port. ((Alternatively, robotic arm 2 and accessory port placement may be switched) ©2018 Intuitive Surgical, Inc.). (**d**) Xi configuration (trocars in horizontal line). (©2018 Intuitive Surgical, Inc.)

placed at least 8–10 cm lateral to the camera port with the third arm lateral to arm one. This can either be placed in an arc around the umbilicus (Fig. 25.2b), in a "W" conformation (Fig. 25.2c) for the Si da Vinci robotic platform, or straight across or slight arc for the Xi da Vinci robotic platform (Fig. 25.2d).

For right-handed surgeons, arm three should be placed on the right to provide traction-counter traction while operating with the right hand and vice versa for left-handed surgeons. The assistant port, if used, is then placed opposite the third robotic arm in the upper quadrant or the lateral-most location.

Docking

Once all trocars are placed, the next critical step in performing a successful robotic-assisted hysterectomy is docking the robot. Typically for the Si da Vinci robotic plat-

form, there are three options for docking the robot: central docking, side docking, and parallel docking (Fig. 25.3a, b). Central docking is when the robot boom is positioned between the patient's legs. This allows for best direct angle of instruments with regard to robotic arm attachments but

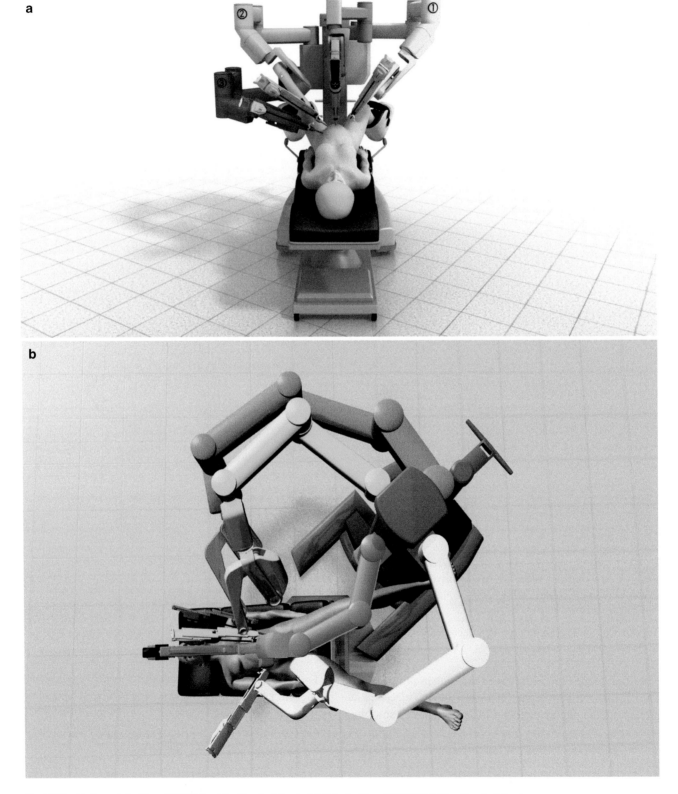

Fig. 25.3 (**a**) Central docking. (©2018 Intuitive Surgical, Inc.). (**b**) Side docking. (©2018 Intuitive Surgical, Inc.)

prohibits ease of access to the vagina for uterine manipulation or tissue extraction. Side docking involves the robot being positioned at angle in line with the camera port and contralateral shoulder, on the patient's right for right-handed surgeons, vice versa for left-handed surgeon. This allows for adequate angulation of the robotic instruments and access to the vagina, but is often difficult and more time-consuming to direct the team for positioning. Lastly, parallel docking involves positioning the robot parallel to the bed (on the right for right-handed surgeons and vice versa for left-handed surgeons). For the Xi da Vinci robotic platform, docking position is less important as the instruments rotate around an adjustable central boom and contain a targeting positioning system for optimization of robotic arm angles. The instrument arms should be positioned to achieve the greatest angle between instruments in order to prevent collision and maximize pitch and aft movements (Fig. 25.4).

Instrumentation

Proper instrumentation is also important to perform robotic surgery successfully. A bipolar grasper or PK dissector is placed in arm 2 in the contralateral non-dominant hand to grasp, coagulate, and seal vessels. A monopolar scissors, harmonic scalpel, or vessel sealer is typically placed in arm 1 in the dominant hand to facilitate dissection. Prograsp forceps or a small retractor is typically placed in arm 3 to provide static counter traction to facilitate dissection. The Prograsp should not be used on the bowel whereas the small retractor may be used to hold bowel back.

Procedural Details

The steps involved in a robotic-assisted hysterectomy are the same steps as in a conventional laparoscopic hysterectomy. First, the round ligament is incised and the anterior leaf of

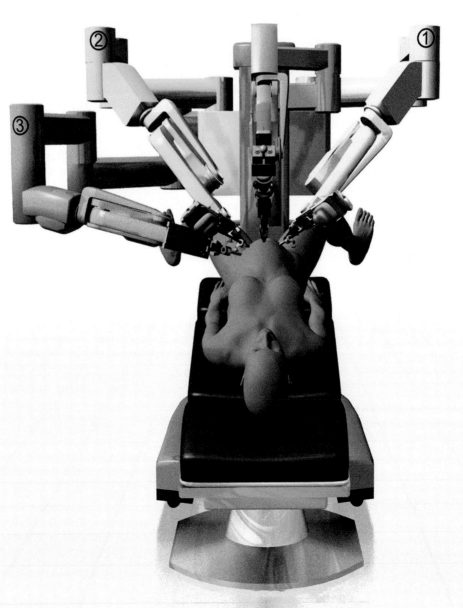

Fig. 25.4 Robotic arm angles. (©2018 Intuitive Surgical, Inc.)

the broad ligament is transected down to the level of the cervical isthmus, then dissected medially to create a bladder flap. Next, the posterior leaf of the broad ligament is incised and the ureter and internal iliac artery and vein are identified. The infundibulopelvic (IP) ligament is isolated by creating a window in the middle leaf of the broad ligament. This maneuver drops the ureter posterior and lateral from the area of dissection. If performing an oophorectomy, the IP ligament is then desiccated and transected. If no oophorectomy is performed, then the utero-ovarian ligament is desiccated and transected. It is current recommendation to perform a salpingectomy at the time of hysterectomy regardless of oophorectomy to reduce the risk of ovarian cancer in the future. This is easily performed by coagulating and transecting the mesosalpinx laterally to medially to the level of the uterine cornua. The fallopian tube can be left attached to the uterus or removed separately to prevent obscuration of the uterine artery. Next, the uterine artery is skeletonized using blunt and sharp dissection. This procedure is repeated similarly on the contralateral side. The bladder flap is brought down further over the level of the cervicovaginal junction, and bilateral uterine arteries are desiccated and transected. The uterine arteries are then lateralized to the cervix, and colpotomy is carried out in a layered fashion. Bipolar energy use should be minimized during colpotomy to minimize char and decrease risk of vaginal cuff dehiscence.

A bag for tissue containment and extraction is then placed through the vagina, and the uterine specimen is placed within the bag for retrieval through the vagina. In cases where tissue extraction is difficult, the robot may be undocked to allow for increased space for retraction, better visualization, and changes in patient position. After the specimen is removed, the vaginal cuff is then repaired with interrupted or running suture. We recommend the use of an absorbable 0-barbed suture to close the cuff in a running fashion in two layers, with fixation of the cuff to the bilateral uterosacral ligaments for pelvic support. After this step, the pelvis is irrigated and a *low-pressure check* is performed by temporarily desufflating the abdomen and then reinflating to ensure hemostasis under physiologic pressures. The robot is then undocked. Cystoscopy is performed to evaluate for patency of the bilateral ureters and bladder injury. We recommend making cystoscopy a routine part of any laparoscopic or robotic-assisted hysterectomy. Lastly, the surgeon may choose to apply an adhesion barrier or fibrin sealant, but routine use of these products is controversial.

Special Surgical Considerations

Not all hysterectomies are straightforward, and the surgical approach described in the prior section may need to be modified based on anatomy encountered at the time of surgery. As approximately 1/3 of babies are delivered via cesarean section, it is common to encounter scarring from a prior cesarean section at the time of hysterectomy. This scarring is usually located anteriorly and can involve the bladder and the anterior abdominal wall. Other than prior surgery, endometriosis, prior appendicitis, diverticulitis, and pelvic infection can also lead to significant scarring. Usually the best approach to hysterectomy in the face of significant scarring is to start from normal anatomy rather than initially tackling the scar directly. This technique allows one to identify normal anatomy and avoid organ injury as tissue planes are often disrupted and malpositioned in the setting of significant scar tissue. In the setting of anterior adhesions, as commonly found after a cesarean section, it may be easiest to start laterally or posteriorly. As the bladder is often involved in the adhesion, it is often helpful to backfill the bladder with fluid to demarcate its position. When performing adhesiolysis near the bowel or bladder, it is best to minimize the use of cautery as to avoid thermal injury. Saline may be used to perform hydrodissection with a laparoscopic suction irrigator device. When anticipating significant scarring posterolaterally, it may be prudent to place lighted ureteral stents prior to starting the procedure.

One benefit of robotic-assisted laparoscopy over conventional laparoscopy is the availability of wristed instruments. This proves useful when operating on large specimens such as a uterus with large fibroids. There are several techniques that may help when operating on a large uterus. As aforementioned, trocar placement should be based on the patient's anatomy, which includes the surgical pathology. If a uterus extends to the umbilicus, the trocars should be placed more superiorly to best triangulate and target the anatomy. The specimen may also be pulled down into the pelvis during the operation rather than being pushed out of the pelvis to allow greater distance between the camera, operating arms, and specimen. The greater the distance from the camera and instruments, the greater the availability for triangulation. Manipulation is key. Sometimes it is difficult to manipulate a large specimen from uterine manipulation alone. It may help to provide some manipulation from the assistant port with the use of a single- or double-tooth tenaculum. We suggest the use of a dilute vasopressin injection prior to the use of a tenaculum to reduce bleeding at the site of puncture. Lastly, a 30° camera may be of use rather than a 0° camera when attempting to visualize structures obscured by large fibroids, such as the uterine artery or bladder flap. With the Xi da Vinci robot, the camera can be placed through any of the robotic trocars and can be moved to see around structures.

In minimally invasive surgery, when the uterine specimen is too large to be removed intact through the vagina, it must be cut into smaller pieces to either fit through the vagina or through small incisions. This process is called morcellation. Morcellation has recently come under scrutiny regarding the risk of disseminating occult malignancy, specifically leiomyosarcoma, which is difficult to diagnose preoperatively, to other parts of the abdomen and pelvis. The FDA issued a warning against the use of power morcellation in laparoscopic surgery in 2014 [11]. Since then, many surgeons have reverted to open incision, or "abdominal hysterectomy," for large uterine specimens. This however does not need to be the case. During laparoscopy, large specimens can be placed within a containment system, as described above, and manually extracted within that system to avoid spillage of tissue. This is done by either cutting the specimen up into small pieces with a scalpel or coring the specimen out into one long continuous piece, within a containment system such as a bag.

During prolonged tissue extraction (>5 min), we recommend undocking the robot, taking the patient out of steep Trendelenburg position, and desufflating the abdomen to minimize intracranial and intrathoracic pressure. The uterine specimen may be removed through the vagina or through a minilaparotomy incision either suprapubically or through the umbilicus. Typically, a C-shaped incision or bivalve technique is used, and the uterine specimen is allowed to rotate to provide fresh edges to grasp as extraction is carried out. The contained extraction system bag is adjusted and pulled tauter as more specimen is removed. The scalpel blade should be changed often as calcified fibroids can dull an edge quickly. Care should be taken to avoid lacerating the bag or any structures that may be adjacent to the bag, such as bowel or vagina. Lastly, a circumferential retraction device, such as Applied Medical's Alexis retractor, may be used outside of the bag to retract and protect the tissue at the opening. This may be performed either vaginally or through a minilaparotomy incision.

The use of routine bowel prep prior to hysterectomy is controversial. We find it is most helpful to decompress and move the bowel when performing a sacrocolpopexy or lysing adhesions involving the bowel.

Single Site

More recently single-site robotic-assisted hysterectomy has become popular. In general, each step of the single-port procedure has been found to be equivalent in time to a multiport approach to robotic-assisted hysterectomy, except for vaginal cuff closure [12]. The advantages of single-site robotic hysterectomy include improved aesthetics for the patient, allowance for surgeon independence while minimizing the need for a bedside assistant, and automatic reassignment of the robotic arm controls as compared to single-site conventional laparoscopy. Disadvantages include non-wristed instruments, decreased degrees of freedom and triangulation, longer suturing time, restricted assistant port use, and limited

scope of pathology (surgeons tend to feel more comfortable with less complex and smaller pathology).

While there are a variety of single-site ports available that are compatible with the robotic arms, Intuitive® has a single port that is meant to be used with their single-site instruments. To place the trocar, you first make a 2–3 cm incision either vertically through the base of the umbilicus or in a "C" or "Ω" around the umbilicus. We recommend tagging the apices of the fascia with 0-vicryl or PDS suture to use for closure at the end. A circumferential retractor, such as Applied Medical's Alexis O retractor, may be used to reduce distance from the skin to fascia in those patients with a larger amount of subcutaneous tissue and may ease placement. We then moisten and fold the port to allow ease of entry into the small incision (Fig. 25.5). Once secured, the abdomen is insufflated. Since the arms cross in single-port surgery, the instrument for operating from the right side needs to come down the left trocar and vice versa for the left (Fig. 25.6).

Next, we list several tips and tricks to help overcome some of the barriers described of single-port robotic-assisted hysterectomy. First, we recommend using an angled 30° scope to avoid collision with the other instrument arms. Second, triangulation is improved somewhat by aiming the camera slightly to the side of the targeted anatomy and not directly at the target. Third, good uterine manipulation is key to provide optimal angles for the surgeon. Fourth, each arm should be working opposite of each other, providing traction-

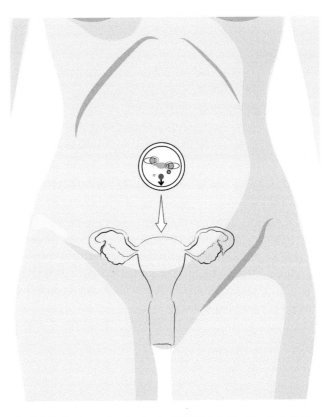

Fig. 25.5 Configuration single site. (©2018 Intuitive Surgical, Inc.)

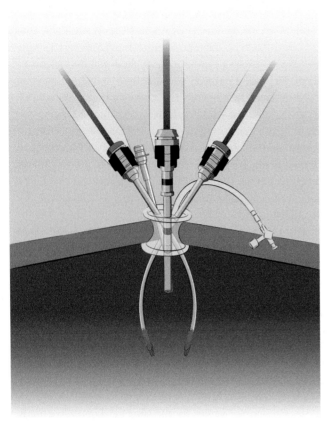

Fig. 25.6 Single-site port. (©2018 Intuitive Surgical, Inc.)

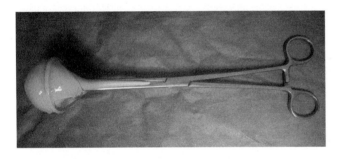

Fig. 25.7 Cut nasal bulb syringe on a ring forceps, containing suture for the vaginal cuff

counter traction. Fifth, a straighter cutting needle should be used with barbed suture for the vaginal cuff. Lastly, this needle may be placed in a cut nasal bulb syringe on a ring forceps through the vagina after the uterine specimen is removed (Fig. 25.7). Once the needle is retrieved, this contraption doubles as a pneumo-occluder.

Summary

In summary, there are several steps to a successful robotic-assisted hysterectomy. The first step is proper patient and equipment positioning. The next step is correct trocar placement. The third step is appropriate docking of the robot. Lastly, the surgeon must be prepared to adapt and alter their technique for larger and/or complicated anatomy. Single-port approach to robotic-assisted hysterectomy is also a feasible option for robotic-assisted hysterectomy for properly selected patients.

References

1. Centers for Disease Control and Prevention Website. Key statistics from the national survey of family growth. Atlanta: Centers for Disease Control and Prevention; 2015. Retrieved on June 23, 2017 from: http://www.cdc.gov/nchs/nsfg/key_statistics/h.htm#hysterectomy.
2. Whiteman M, Hillis S, Jamieson D, et al. Inpatient hysterectomy surveillance in the United States 2000–2004. Am J Obstet Gynecol. 2008;198(1):34.
3. Wright JD, Ananth CV, Lewin SN, Burke WM, Lu YS, Neugut AI, et al. Robotically assisted vs laparoscopic hysterectomy among women with benign gynecologic disease. JAMA. 2013;309(7):689–98.
4. Vecchio R, MacFayden BV, Palazzo F. History of laparoscopic surgery. Panminerva Med. 2000;42(1):87–90.
5. Stylopoulos N, Rattner D. Robotics and ergonomics. Surg Clin North Am. 2003;83:1321.
6. Smorgick N. Robotic-assisted hysterectomy: patient selection and perspectives. Int J Women's Health. 2017;9:157–61.
7. Uccella S, Ghezzi F, Mariani A, Cromi A, Bogani G, Serati M, et al. Vaginal cuff closure after minimally invasive hysterectomy: our experience and systematic review of the literature. Am J Obstet Gynecol. 2011;205(2):119.e1–12.
8. Swenson CW, Kamdar NS, Harris JA, Uppal S, Campbell DA Jr, Morgan DM. Comparison of robotic and other minimally invasive routes of hysterectomy for benign indications. Am J Obstet Gynecol. 2016;215:650.e1–8.
9. Ghomi A, Kramer C, Askari R, Chavan NR, Einarsson JI. Trendelenburg position in gynecologic robotic surgery. J Minim Invasive Gynecol. 2012;19(4):485–9.
10. Gainsburg DM. Anesthetic concerns for robotic-assisted laparoscopic radical prostatectomy. Minerva Anestesiol. 2012;78:596–604.
11. Laparoscopic uterine power morcellation in hysterectomy and myomectomy: FDA safety communication. [April 17, 2014]; Food and Drug Administration; 2014 (at http://www.fda.gov/MedicalDevices/Safety/AlertsandNotices/ucm393576.htm).
12. Truong M, Advincula A. Understanding the spectrum of multiport and single-site robotics for hysterectomy. OBG Manage. 2014;26(8):53.

Robotic Myomectomy

Antonio R. Gargiulo

Myomectomy: Moving Forward

Myomectomy is one of the most common gynecologic operations in women of reproductive age: what once was a highly morbid, controversial, and even heroic alternative to hysterectomy has now become a very safe surgery [1]. This operation arguably represents the quintessence of reproductive surgery, as it allows fertility preservation in the face of neoplastic pathology striking at the very core of a woman's reproductive tract. In all of its forms, be them invasive or minimally invasive (hysteroscopy aside), myomectomy is a microsurgical operation: myometrial, endometrial and tubal preservation, hemostasis, precise tissue apposition, reconstruction in layers, and absence of exposed suture are all essential to its success. There is one fundamental point that must be acknowledged by surgeons on both sides of the robotic controversy: there is only one myomectomy, regardless of access modality. We are held to identical operative standards whether or not we open the abdominal wall to perform this operation. Our patients do not expect to undergo a "simplified" uterine surgery when they agree to minimally invasive surgery. Regrettably, not all minimally invasive myomectomies are completed according to microsurgical principles, because accurate laparoscopic intracorporeal suturing of an actively bleeding uterus is out of the reach of most gynecologic surgeons [2].

It is now well established that minimally invasive myomectomy is clinically superior to open myomectomy [3–8]: this is an irrefutable modern medical reality, for which parallels can be drawn with many common abdominal surgeries, such as hysterectomy, appendectomy, and cholecystectomy.

A. R. Gargiulo
Department of Obstetrics, Gynecology and Reproductive Biology, Harvard Medical School, Center for Infertility and Reproductive Surgery, Brigham and Women's Hospital, Boston, MA, USA

Center for Robotic Surgery, Brigham and Women's Hospital, Boston, MA, USA

Exeter Hospital, Exeter, NH, USA
e-mail: agargiulo@bwh.harvard.edu

In spite of this, our main qualm is not with those surgeons who continue to offer open myomectomy as their primary operative modality. Open surgery remains an honest professional choice, based on personal surgical aptitude and in respect of the current standards of care. Also, when an open myomectomy is prospected nowadays, savvy patients should seek a second opinion (and eventually chose minimally invasive myomectomy), while less savvy ones may face the reproductive consequences of an outdated operation, in a somewhat Darwinian model. Instead, we unequivocally criticize those surgeons who perform a simplified version of myomectomy in order to perform it laparoscopically. These colleagues stand to gain an unfair market advantage over their peers, because even well informed patients are not able to appreciate the technical inferiority of their technique. For example, single-layer closure of uterine incisions is not at all described for classic open myomectomy, yet it represents the prevailing type of repair in laparoscopic myomectomy, as highlighted by a recent study (in contrast to a two- and three-layer closure prevalence in robotic myomectomy) [9]. One can easily argue that the "need-for-speed" implicit in the repair of a bleeding myometrium may induce surgeons with limited laparoscopic suturing skills to opt for a mass closure of the myometrium. This is the negation of microsurgery: it results in uterine wall hematoma formation and healing by secondary intention, and is associated with an increased chance of postoperative adhesions because of wound protrusion [10]. In our opinion, one of the most significant contributions of robotics to minimally invasive myomectomy is the ability to provide a consistently high quality of suturing. One of the striking findings of the first large multicenter study on reproductive outcomes following robotic myomectomy was the unusually low rate of adhesions (11%) found at the time of subsequent cesarean section [11].

Of course, there are several exceptional laparoscopists who will perform a microsurgical laparoscopic myomectomy just as well, or maybe better, than what many can perform with robotic assistance. We have seen these true champions emerge in all fields of minimally invasive surgery and have been mesmerized by their surgical feats on videos and at conferences. Their techniques are objectively hard to emulate and – after three decades of unsuccessful attempts to adequately standardize advanced laparoscopy – have now also become largely unnecessary. That is because robotic surgical platforms offer a more consistent and widespread access to reliable minimally invasive surgery, unencumbered by the anti-ergonomic challenges of conventional laparoscopy. Health systems no longer seek a few uber-surgeons but rather the standardization of safe minimally invasive surgery through enabling digital technology and intensive virtual reality simulation programs. In order to survive as surgery centers, hospitals need to be able to offer a consistently high rate of outpatient surgery, with a consistently low rate of complications and readmissions. Robotic surgery can answer this need. Before the results of ongoing studies will lend final support to our hypothesis that the widespread use of robotic platforms will change many of the current surgical paradigms, we would like to share our specific experience as it relates to myomectomy. Based on recent publications, we can say that an acceptable risk of conversion to open surgery in advanced benign gynecologic laparoscopy is somewhere around 5% (this is based on hysterectomy, which is arguably less complex than myomectomy). In contrast, our team has experienced a single conversion to open surgery in our first one thousand robotic myomectomies [12, 13]. Moreover, an internal cost analysis comparing readmission rates for hundreds of robotic and laparoscopic myomectomies at our institution in 2014 calculated values of 0% and 9%, respectively (personal communication: Brigham and Women's Hospital Robotic Safety and Steering Committee). Lack of unplanned surgical admissions and readmissions is the type of consistency that successful health systems are striving toward: a standard that humans are unlikely to accomplish without help from a robot.

Standardization of surgery though robotics is a very real paradigm shift in health care: it may seem futuristic, but it is already happening. Ultimately, when facing surgery, a patient should be able to choose her hospital based on transparent statistics, much like we do for other high-stakes decisions in our daily lives. For example, when boarding a commercial aircraft, we hardly care to inquire about the credentials of our captain and first officer. Rather, we trust the airline itself, with its strict credentialing system, and we take this level of safety for granted. This is clearly not yet the case for surgery and particularly for elective surgery. Many patients will travel long distances in search of the surgeon who will perform the best surgery. The diffusion of robotic surgery will make these long-distance treatment endeavors less and less common. The biggest value of robotic surgery, even now, before automation or artificial intelligence is applied to this field, is that of making a reliably good standard of minimally invasive surgery available to most patients at their own

regional hospital. We have already witnessed what can be achieved in medicine when standardization, computer assistance, and digital simulation converge: the dramatic decline in anesthesia-related morbidity and mortality of the past two decades should serve as an inspiration for all of us on the "other side" of the operating table.

Following pioneering work by Arnold Advincula and his team, published in 2004, the safety and efficacy of robotic myomectomy have been well established: its perioperative outcomes are similar to those of laparoscopic myomectomy, and its long-term reproductive outcomes are excellent [14–18]. Similar to what has been observed for conventional laparoscopic myomectomy, case-matched comparisons between patients undergoing open and robotic myomectomy have shown lower blood loss, fewer complications, and shorter hospital stay for this new minimally invasive procedure [19, 20].

Standardization of Robotic Myomectomy Across Multiple Robotic Platforms

The merits, safety record, and bright future of robotic myomectomy are well established. This second, more clinical, section of our chapter is based on the understanding that robotic platforms will continue to evolve at an accelerated pace but that – barring a revolution in tissue biotechnology – the myomectomy operation itself will remain unchanged. Therefore, optimal application of a few constant surgical principles to current and future robotic technology will be the basis of a successful practice. In a short Baconian inductive exercise, we shall endeavor to dissect the myomectomy operation into basic steps and assess how robotic platforms may impact each of these steps. This way, our didactic effort may continue to be relevant as surgical robots evolve.

Giving the indication for surgery is the first surgical act. The decision of whether to proceed with a myomectomy is often a complex one, beyond the scope of this volume. We have long argued that, aside from scenarios where fibroids impair the quality of life, only a trained fertility expert should establish the indication for myomectomy [21–24]. Access to a surgical robot never changes the indications for myomectomy. However, there is no question that, in a field where indications can be controversial and the surgery is often "elective," having reliable and consistent access to a minimally invasive option can ease patients' decision toward intervention. This may result in long-term advantages to patients, because it contributes to avoid delayed intervention on a pathology that generally continues to grow and can result in more invasive and less conservative operations.

The quality of imaging technique determines the ability to provide a confident indication for myomectomy. For this step also, the availability of robotic surgery does not make things easier. Au contraire, minimally invasive myomectomy removes the ability to palpate the uterus to locate fibroids. This lack of haptic feedback is partial for conventional laparoscopy and complete for robotic surgery. This will change in future robotic platforms [25]. However, haptic feedback obtained through the tip of a laparoscopic instrument is not comparable to that obtained by palpation of the uterus between the fingers of one hand. Because of this, all forms of minimally invasive laparoscopy will always require high-quality preoperative imaging. Magnetic resonance imaging's (MRI) ability to locate smaller fibroids is superior to ultrasound, and so is its accuracy in ruling out adenomyosis [26, 27]. A good quality three-dimensional ultrasound (ideally performed by the surgeon) can gather adequate preoperative anatomical information for small tumor loads. However, approaching a large myomectomy without the advantage of MRI mapping is likely to result in a high residual fibroid burden in minimally invasive myomectomy, compared to the abdominal approach. The above notwithstanding, there is no published evidence to date of an increased risk of reoperation after minimally invasive myomectomy compared to abdominal myomectomy [28]. Moreover, there is evidence to suggest that even the palpation allowed by open myomectomy cannot compete with imaging techniques in terms of the ability to detect residual myomas [29, 30]. This suggests that the role of haptic feedback in myomectomy is overrated. Definitive technological improvement for myomectomy in future generations of surgical platforms may reside in real-time image fusion, rather than in haptic feedback. We consider MRI to be an essential preoperative imaging requirement for robotic myomectomy, in all but the smallest cases. MRI is an operator-independent technique: skillful reading of a standard pelvic MRI is a professional imperative for advanced minimally invasive gynecologists. It has been our experience that surgeons can always predict which myomectomies can be completed robotically through a combination of pelvic examination and careful study of high-quality imaging. Big surgical surprises should basically no longer happen.

If the anatomical challenges ahead are deemed commensurate to the skills of the surgical team, planning may begin for a successful minimally invasive myomectomy. Here, the advantages provided by the robotic approach become more evident. Myomectomy involves three main steps: hysterotomy, enucleation, and reconstruction in layers. Blood loss begins with hysterotomy and ends with the completion of uterine reconstruction. Two factors have to be optimized to limit blood loss: speed of execution and pharmacological preparation of the uterus. This is a fundamental microsurgical concept in myomectomy: hemostasis is not achieved by cauterization of the myometrium (an irreplaceable reproductive tissue) but by enucleating and suturing with speed and precision.

Speed of execution is aided by robotic assistance at many levels. The ability to suture from absolutely any angle around the uterus means that hysterotomy for enucleation can be placed in the location and with the slant that will assure best access through least myometrial depth. For example, a large posterior FIGO 5 myoma for which MRI shows that the thinnest free margin is deep in the posterior lower segment is best enucleated through an oblique low posterior incision. This type of incision is notoriously the hardest to repair with conventional laparoscopy: this could result in a poor choice of incision location, in order to facilitate repair.

Hysterotomy is commonly carried out with monopolar cautery instruments on the current robotic platforms. Monopolar curved scissors, permanent cautery hook, and spatula are all employed for this goal. While these tools are practical and familiar to all surgeons, they are not ideal in terms of their tissue sparing characteristics. To date, all reported uterine ruptures following laparoscopic and robotic myomectomy have occurred following monopolar or bipolar electrocautery use [11, 31]. At a very minimum, these tools should never be used in coagulation mode but exclusively in cutting mode. Ideal instruments for hysterotomy, with more contained lateral thermal spread, include the ultrasonic scalpel and the CO_2 laser. Both of these energy forms are not adequately optimized for use with current surgical platforms and require significant technical adjustments that limit their acceptance and popularity [32–34]. Future optimization of ultrasonic energy and CO_2 laser energy for their inclusion in the standard robotic armamentarium will represent a significant technological improvement for robot-assisted reproductive surgery.

The key to successful enucleation is the prompt recognition of entry into the elusive space between the edge of the actual myoma and the fibrous pseudocapsule that separates it from the normal surrounding myometrium. The pseudocapsule must remain in situ for proper myometrial healing: hence, the anatomically correct myomectomy is always intracapsular. Robotic myomectomy allows high-definition three-dimensional magnification of the fibroid pseudocapsule. The correct enucleation technique bears similarities to the nerve-sparing robotic radical prostatectomy technique, as it allows gentle uterine leiomyoma detachment from the pseudocapsule neurovascular bundle, with reduction in blood loss and myometrial trauma [35] (Fig. 26.1). When the correct cleavage plane has been entered and an adequate width of the hysterotomy is established, the myoma is grasped with a robotic tenaculum and placed under traction. The vector of this traction is determined by the location of the myoma, not of the tenaculum (another advantage of robotic technology, where the tenaculum has a 90° wristing ability). The surrounding myometrium is then carefully detached from the myoma, mostly with blunt dissection: this is accomplished with a motion that pushes the uterus away

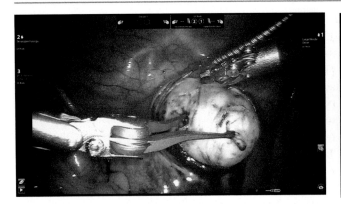

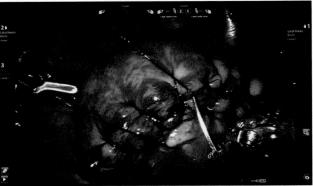

Fig. 26.1 Correct myoma enucleation technique. Similar to the nerve-sparing robotic radical prostatectomy technique, it allows gentle detachment from the pseudocapsule neurovascular bundle, with reduction in blood loss and myometrial trauma. Robotic tenaculum is used to steady the tumor, and a blunt instrument (the tip of a flexible CO2 laser guide, in this particular case) is used to push the myometrium away from the immobilized myoma. Notice the lack of thermal damage on the myometrium: hemostasis is assured by mechanical and chemical means in robotic myomectomy

Fig. 26.2 The outermost layer of closure in myomectomy uses barbed suture in either subserosal or imbricating "baseball" stitch fashion, so that no barbs are left exposed. This figure shows a classic example of the "baseball" stitch. This is our default superficial myometrial closure because we do not burn the myometrium; hence, we need better mechanical compression of the edges for hemostasis

from the immobilized myoma, and not vice versa. Bipolar coagulation can be applied sparingly to particularly vascular areas, making sure that they are well away from the endometrium and tubes. Chromopertubation with methylene blue or indigo carmine (depending on availability) is performed in most of our myomectomies to identify any breach into the uterine cavity in a timely fashion. Maintaining the area hemostatic by destroying the myometrium and the pseudocapsule with cautery should be absolutely avoided, because it has the potential to permanently compromise reproductive function. Hemostasis in robotic myomectomy is based on suturing.

The mechanics of suturing with a fully wristed instrument are very different from those employed in conventional laparoscopy and have to be acquired and perfected on a virtual reality simulator, with its objective scoring software. Nondominant hand suturing and backhand suturing should also be mastered on a simulator, as they are often essential in complex myomectomy scenarios. Barbed sutures on CT-1- and CT-2-type needles are employed for myomectomy: substantial needle drivers (such as the Mega Needle Driver for the da Vinci Surgical System) are usually best suited to drive these particular needles. We recommend using two robotic needle drivers for myomectomy, rather than using nondedicated instruments such as graspers, in order to limit costs. That is because time wasted equals wasted blood in myomectomy. Efficient suturing mandates that the uterus is adequately positioned and that it remains steady, so that the force applied to the needle will not be dispersed in moving the uterus. Effective uterine manipulation by an expert bedside assistant is ideal. However, in the case of a large uterus, manipulators offer limited support. We use the robotic tenac-

ulum for enucleation and for uterine positioning and immobilization during suturing. Running sutures are adequate to close the deep layers, whereas the most superficial layer has to be either subserosal or imbricating "baseball" stitch, so that no barbs are left exposed. If an endometrial breach is noted, the myometrium just above the breach is carefully reapproximated, to limit the chance for intrauterine synechiae (Fig. 26.2).

Adequate visualization under rapidly changing anatomical circumstances (morphological changes occurring with tumor enucleation) and rapid and safe suture exchanges in and out of the patient are two key aspects of minimally invasive myomectomy. In terms of adequate visualization, independent camera control and three-dimensional vision, a basic feature of all robotic platforms, are an obvious advantage. However, the basic measure to optimize visualization in minimally invasive myomectomy consists in placing the camera port cephalad to the uterine fundus (please note that even if new generations of robots allow the camera to be used in all robotic arms, a "camera port" is still clearly identifiable at the beginning of the case). This is quite different from hysterectomy, where the camera port can be placed caudal to the uterine fundus regardless of uterine size because the surgical targets remain close to the pelvic brim and to the cervix. The target in myomectomy usually changes with myoma size. Consequently, we make sure that the camera port is about 10 cm above the level of a palpable fundus. In the case of very large uterine pathology, the trocar may transfix the falciform ligament of the liver [36]. We carefully survey this entry point after trocar removal at the end of the case, and no complications from laceration of this ligament have been encountered by us nor have they been reported in the literature. Maybe more important is to maintain a very clear communication with the anesthesiologist regarding the need for full decompression of the stomach since induction.

Once the camera port has been set at the appropriate height on the abdomen, large myomas can be adequately visualized throughout their enucleation and tackled successfully. Indeed, the fastest way to effectively "shrink" a large fibroid, and make it more manageable by laparoscopy, is to move the camera port up a few centimeters. Robotic instrument ports for myomectomy can be two or three: our default number is three, but we do use two ports for our more straightforward cases. These ports are also placed in the upper abdomen: at the same height of the umbilicus (or higher) and at 8 cm distance minimum from each other.

Rapid and safe suture exchanges in and out of the patient are accomplished by placing the assistant port in a lower quadrant location just medial to the anterior-superior iliac spine (ASIS), on the side where the assistant will stand (which is generally the side opposite to the location of the robotic cart, where only one of the robotic instrument ports is present). Let me enumerate the many reasons for this unusually caudal assistant port location (most gynecologic operations place an assistant port in the upper abdomen). First, myomectomy is suture-intensive, and many needles must travel in and out of the abdomen in full view: losing a needle because the assistant port is situated out of the reach of the laparoscope is not an excusable mistake. Second, the right lower quadrant port can be effectively used as a point of extraction for the specimen (see below) and remains mostly hidden from view, adding some cosmetic value to this operation. Third, a bedside assistant working through a low quadrant port can remain in a safer location (away from the swinging of the robotic arms) and can reach the uterine manipulator at the same time. This provides an ergonomic advantage and decreases the occupational hazards of this operation. Fourth, any conventional laparoscopic actions needed before or after the docking of the robot are performed easier if at least two access ports are found in a sagittal plane, as they always are in this configuration. Hence, there is no question in our mind that the only rational location for the assistant port in robotic myomectomy is in one of the lower quadrants (Fig. 26.3).

Pharmacological preparation of the uterus includes long-term and short-term interventions: all of them are extremely important. A myomectomy in a patient who has been poorly prepared pharmacologically is an unnecessarily risky operation that should only be done in an emergency situation. Long-term pharmacologic interventions include iron therapy (by oral or by intravenous infusion) to correct preoperative anemia, timely suspension of medications known to negatively affect coagulation (such as nonsteroidal anti-inflammatory agents, other platelet inhibitors, and anticoagulants), and hormonal treatments to shrink fibroids and their aberrant vascularity (GnRH-agonists and possibly selective progesterone-receptor modulators) [37]. Most importantly, patients must be reminded that the safety of

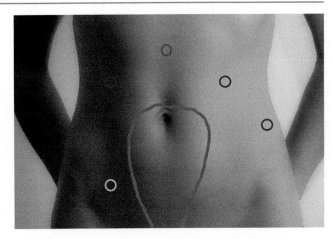

Fig. 26.3 This is the schematic representation of our preferred laparoscopic port placement for a large robotic myomectomy. Please note the location of the robotic ports in the upper abdomen and the bedside assistant port in the lower quadrant

many herbal products and other dietary supplements on blood parameters has not been established. Therefore, the use of these preparations should be discontinued long before undergoing any surgical procedure [38]. Short-term pharmacologic interventions utilize compounds that act on the uterus in different ways and may be used as single agent or in combination. The hormone vasopressin causes rapid onset and persistent vasoconstriction. We infiltrate 5 IU of vasopressin in the myometrium (no untoward events have ever been reported with doses under 5 IU) a few minutes before hysterotomy and repeat the injection every 30–60 min as needed (plasma half-life of 10–20 min). The degree of dilution has no effect on the efficacy of vasopressin [39]. The synthetic prostaglandin misoprostol induces uterine contractions as well as causing vascular constriction. Preoperative administration of misoprostol (vaginal or rectal) has been shown to decrease intraoperative bleeding in abdominal myomectomy. We administer a 400 mcg rectal dose of misoprostol following induction of anesthesia. A double dose (400 mcg 3 h before and 1 h before surgery) has been shown to be more effective but can cause diarrhea and cramping [40, 41]. The antifibrinolytic tranexamic acid has an emerging and very promising role in decreasing intraoperative blood loss in uterine surgery [42]. Its proven safety, even at high dose (>25–50 mg/kg) in orthopedic surgery patients with prior history of deep venous thrombosis, should dispel every safety concerns regarding its use in myomectomy [43]. Combined use of misoprostol and vasopressin is the current protocol for all our robotic myomectomies. Intravenous tranexamic acid, as a single dose of 1000 mg at the beginning of surgery, is used in those cases where preoperative hematocrit is suboptimal, the tumor load is particularly large, or a tendency to abnormal coagulation is suspected or observed.

Once closure of hysterotomy is completed and hemostasis is confirmed with low-pressure test, the robotic myomectomy is complete. However, the specimen still needs to come out of the patient. This step of the operation is not robot-assisted. It currently employs conventional laparoscopic or classic surgical skills, depending on whether your hospitals legal team has ruled in favor or against the use of electromechanical laparoscopic morcellators. Every surgeon should be familiar with the US Food and Drug Administration (FDA) position statements of 2014 and 2017 regarding the use of electromechanical morcellators for uterine tissue extraction and with the infamous "black box warning" that this agency has placed on the morcellator. Briefly, following several reports of morcellated uterine malignancy, which can upstage the disease and shorten the disease-free interval of patients, the FDA has explicitly discouraged the use of this technology in postmenopausal women and has recommended prudent use in premenopausal women [44, 45]. De facto, the "black box warning" has resulted in the disappearance of morcellators from most hospitals' surgical armamentarium, rather than in a more discriminate use. The FDA position has heavily influenced the medical-legal climate in the USA and in many other nations and has led to the development of many techniques for extraction of the uterine tissue in a containment system [46, 47].

Avoiding the use of the morcellator in the case of myomectomy has no biological rationale, because tumor fragments and innumerable free cells escape the uterus during the enucleation (rather than extraction) of the presumed myoma. Contrary to hysterectomy, myomectomy does not give any possibility to removal of the tumor en bloc. We can somewhat console ourselves with the knowledge that contained uterine tissue extraction in myomectomy will minimize the seeding of myoma fragments. This should limit the risk of two rare complications of morcellation: parasitic myomas and disseminated leiomyomatosis [48].

Tissue extraction is a step of the procedure that is not currently assisted by robotic technology (although it is, in our view, a field ripe with technical development opportunities). Not being able to effectively extract myomas at the end of a robotic myomectomy makes this procedure impossible to perform in a minimally invasive fashion, no matter how advanced the robotic technology at our disposal may be. Indeed, the FDA "black box warning" is responsible for an acute rebound of open gynecologic surgery and for the morbidity and mortality that this has entailed [49]. But it needn't be that way. Being the first health system in the world to deal with the lack of available electromechanical morcellation, our hospital has developed sophisticated extraction techniques that keep robotic myomectomy a minimally invasive procedure [46, 50]. Our techniques employ large endoscopic specimen extraction bags that are inserted and extracted through a 2.5 cm open laparoscopy umbilical incision or through a 2.5 cm incision in either lower quadrant. Tissue extraction is accomplished using a #10 blade in a semicircular motion while applying direct traction of tissue with standard towel clips. The cosmetic effect of these incisions is exceptionally good (Fig. 26.4), and our robotic myomectomy practice has thrived in the post-morcellation age thanks to our tissue extraction abilities at a time when many other minimally invasive surgeons are offering minilaparotomy for tissue extraction instead.

The choice of whether to employ adhesion prevention barriers after robotic myomectomy is a personal one: we feel that a review of the vast literature on this subject is not immediately relevant to this chapter. We universally apply oxidized regenerated cellulose to all of the uterine incisions and all deperitonealized areas following myomectomy.

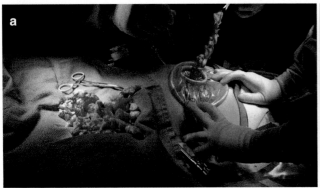 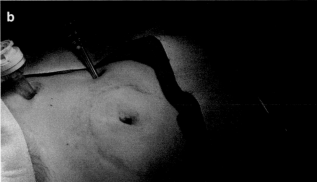

Fig. 26.4 Umbilical skin incision for contained uterine tissue extraction: during active extraction (**a**) and at completion of extraction (**b**). We insert and extract endoscopic specimen bags through a 2.5 cm open laparoscopy umbilical incision or a 2.5 cm incision in either lower quadrant, medial to the anterior-superior iliac spine. In our experience, minilaparotomy for tissue extraction is never needed in robotic myomectomy, and its use should be abandoned

Special Scenarios in Robotic Myomectomy

Many reproductive surgeons have a love-hate relationship with myomectomy: it is a challenging operation because of the protean nature of the pathology at hand, but it has an undeniable technical appeal precisely due to the challenges it presents. Approaching myomectomy with the level of preparation outlined above, and with a good command of the robotic platform, can be easily compared to heading out on an off-road expedition armed with a GPS and an all-terrain vehicle. There should be no technical obstacle that cannot be circumvented or overcome. This section will discuss special scenarios, where specific maneuvers apply.

Robotic myomectomy for very large myomas (over 10 cm in diameter) poses unique challenges because the pathology will slowly emerge from the uterus to create an elongated "hourglass" structure, larger than the original surgical target. We should admit at the outset that robotic platforms are not currently optimized for large myomectomies. The available robotic tenaculum is a delicate instrument, not allowing substantial traction on tumors that often weigh 500 g or more. More importantly, the current cantilever-based robotic platforms are two-quadrant operators, but a robotic myomectomy where the uterine size reaches or surpasses the umbilicus is a four-quadrant operation. This said, there are steps one can take to keep this technology enabling even under these circumstances. High placement of the camera port has been discussed above. The bedside assistant can help on the other end by providing optimal exposure. This is achieved by lateralizing the uterus with the uterine manipulator and the assistant tenaculum, so that it lies at a right or left angle in the abdomen, which can keep the operative target more caudal. Clearly, this myomectomy uses all four robotic arms, with no exceptions.

We sometimes execute our largest cases with a hybrid technique: conventional laparoscopic myoma enucleation with ultrasonic scalpel, followed by docking of the robot for microsurgical uterine reconstruction. Conventional laparoscopy provides a more substantial tenaculum and unlimited four-quadrant action, while the robot provides better suturing ability for a pristine reconstruction in layers [32].

Robotic myomectomy for small myomas (<7 cm) is a common occurrence in reproductive surgery. In these cases, we strive to provide a robotic myomectomy with minimal cosmetic impact, building on the technical advantages provided by the robotic platform [33, 50, 51]. Hopefully, all reproductive surgeons are acutely aware of their patients' cosmetic concerns [52–54] and strive to provide patient-centered, yet effective, surgical care. In this context, we have developed robotic single-site myomectomy, which remains a technique with limited applicability in terms of myoma size

and number and involves the use of special equipment. The main steps of our technique can be summarized as follows. A primary port is placed in the umbilicus, and an anatomy survey is carried out to confirm that the surgery can be accomplished via single site. The primary port is extended to a size of 2.5 cm (similar to the classic open laparoscopy technique). A multi-lumen silicone port is set in the umbilical incision. A camera cannula is placed through the dedicated lumen of the silicone port; the robotic patient-side cart is docked. Two curved instrument cannulas are inserted under continuous laparoscopic guidance and connected to robotic arms. An assistant cannula is placed through the dedicated assistant cannula lumen of the silicone port. Semirigid 5 mm robotic instruments are loaded through the curved cannulas. We use a flexible CO2 laser for hysterotomy, but monopolar energy can also be used through a cautery hook. Wristed needle drivers are used for reconstruction in layers of the hysterotomy with barbed sutures (Fig. 26.5). Tissue extraction is accomplished with conventional single-incision laparoscopy technique. A self-retaining wound retractor is set in the umbilical incision, if not already set at the beginning of the case. A silicone gel top allows for pneumoperitoneum to be maintained. An endoscopic specimen bag is placed in the abdominal cavity through the gel. Myomas are loaded into endoscopic bag. The bag is retrieved through the Alexis retractor, and a contained sharp tissue extraction technique (described above) is employed. The merit of our technique in the age of contained uterine tissue extraction is that of sparing the patient three extra laparoscopic entry points while assuring exceptionally favorable cosmetic outcome and an uncompromised myomectomy technique (Fig. 26.6). Not all

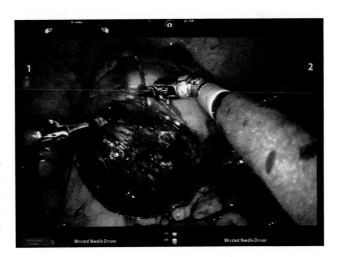

Fig. 26.5 Single-site robotic myomectomy employing dedicated da Vinci Surgical System semirigid 5 mm wristed needle drivers. This is an advanced robotic procedure, only recommended for expert robotic surgery teams and well selected patients

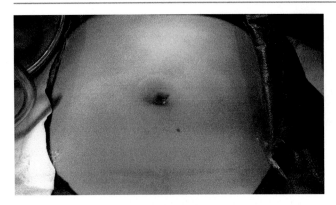

Fig. 26.6 Single-site robotic myomectomy. Patient photographs immediately and 3 weeks after surgery. In well selected cases with myomas under 7 cm in diameter, this technique spares two or three additional abdominal incisions and leaves no appreciable scar

patients can fully accommodate a 2.5 cm incision within the umbilicus: this is a technique that should be proposed only to those who can. For those who cannot, an excellent cosmetically conscious multi-port alternative exists. A camera port is placed at the umbilicus, and two robotic instrument cannulas are placed just medial and slightly cephalad to the left and right ASIS. A 5 mm bedside assistant port can be placed in the suprapubic area (but can be omitted in most cases). Needles travel through the assistant or instrument ports and tissue extraction in an endoscopic bag can be accomplished through one of the lateral ports, after the incision is expanded to 2.5 cm.

Cervical and retroperitoneal myomas comprise about 10% of cases in our practice [13]. Cervical myomas are always identified at MRI, but retroperitoneal myomata can escape detection. Our only conversion to open myomectomy in over 1000 robotic myomectomies to date was a vascular large anterior cervical retroperitoneal myoma filling the paravesical space. We consider this the most challenging robotic myomectomy scenario. There is no substitute for great knowledge of retroperitoneal anatomy in this type of surgery. The robot allows us to concentrate on this more complex anatomy and on surgical strategy, instead of being distracted with how to move our hands to achieve the effect we desire. Retroperitoneal myomas are most often exophytic; hence, they do not require a large hysterotomy and repair. Rather, the challenge is to safely remove them from their location without avulsing a ureter, vein, or artery. All available hemostatic agents should be used at once in such cases (see above): for very large cervical myomas, we have occasionally requested transient uterine artery embolization by our interventional radiology team before robotic myomectomy [55, 56] with excellent results. Another strength of the robotic approach for

this specific operation resides in its improved ability to provide a high-quality, steady image in the crevices where a safe plane can be developed between the tumor and its surroundings. We recommend having the bedside assistant ready on the suction irrigator the entire time and pushing the uterus out of the pelvic as much as possible, with a well-placed manipulator. The general strategy involves pulling the myoma away from the pelvic sidewall and eventually rotating the uterus as much as possible to expose the pedicle of the myoma. Surgeons who are particularly comfortable with retroperitoneal dissection will follow the ureter to the base of the retroperitoneal or cervical myoma and incise the medial leaflet of the broad ligament, so the ureter can fall medial and posterior, away from the action. Locating the ureter will also make it easier to locate the proximal portion of the uterine artery, which can be safely clipped if necessary. The robotic platform renders these complex minimally invasive techniques more accessible.

Conclusions: Robotic Myomectomy in Five Take-Home Points

1. Minimally invasive myomectomy is one of most challenging gynecologic operations, with an extremely low adoption at over 25 years of its introduction as a conventional laparoscopic operation. Because of the evidence pointing to the superiority of laparoscopic over open myomectomy, robotic myomectomy is the much needed breakthrough in this unsustainable scenario.
2. Robotic myomectomy has a 15-year track record of safety and can be applied to most clinical scenarios, thereby limiting the need for open myomectomy to a minimum. Robotic myomectomy is the alternative to open myomectomy, but it is also the ethical alternative to all simplified non-microsurgical versions of laparoscopic myomectomy.
3. Port number and location vary with myoma number and size: Skilled robotic surgeons must pick the best approach based on high-quality preoperative imaging.
4. Robotic technology is not a substitute for anatomical expertise and pharmacologic management of intraoperative blood loss. Tissue extraction techniques are also not robotic and need to be mastered by all surgeons offering robotic myomectomy.
5. Specific future developments in robotic technology that may favorably affect robotic myomectomy would be image fusion, better integration of CO_2 laser and ultrasonic scalpel into the robotic platform, autonomous suturing, and contained robotic morcellation.

References

1. Bortoletto P, Hariton E, Gargiulo AR. The evolution of myomectomy: from laparotomy to minimally invasive surgery. BJOG. 2018;125(5):586.
2. Liu G, Zolis L, Kung R, Melchior M, Singh S, Cook EF. The laparoscopic myomectomy: a survey of Canadian gynaecologists. J Obstet Gynaecol Can. 2010;32(2):139–48.
3. Seracchioli R, Rossi S, Govoni F, et al. Fertility and obstetric outcome after laparoscopic myomectomy of large myomata: a randomized comparison with abdominal myomectomy. Hum Reprod. 2000;15:2663–8.
4. Seracchioli R, Manuzzi L, Vianello F, et al. Obstetric and delivery outcome of pregnancies achieved after laparoscopic myomectomy. Fertil Steril. 2006;86:159–65.
5. Mais V, Ajossa S, Guerriero S, Mascia M, Solla E, Melis GB. Laparoscopic versus abdominal myomectomy: a prospective, randomized trial to evaluate benefits in early outcome. Am J Obstet Gynecol. 1996;174:654–8.
6. Holzer A, Jirecek ST, Illievich UM, Huber J, Wenzl RJ. Laparoscopic versus open myomectomy: a double-blind study to evaluate postoperative pain. Anesth Analg. 2006;102:1480–4.
7. Practice Committee of the American Society of Reproductive Medicine. Pathogenesis, consequences, and control of peritoneal adhesions in gynecologic surgery. Fertil Steril. 2007;88:21.
8. Jin C, Hu Y, Chen XC, Zheng FY, Lin F, Zhou K, Chen FD, Gu HZ. Laparoscopic versus open myomectomy – a meta-analysis of randomized controlled trials. Eur J Obstet Gynecol Reprod Biol. 2009;145:14–21.
9. Puchino N, Litta P, Freschi L, Russo M, Santoro AN, Gadducci A, Cela V. Comparison of the initial surgical experience with robotic and laparoscopic myomectomy. Int J Med Rob. 2014;10(2):208–12.
10. Kumakiri J, Kikuchi I, Kitade M, Matsuoka S, Kono A, Ozaki R, Takeda S. Association between uterine repair at laparoscopic myomectomy and postoperative adhesions. Acta Obstet Gynecol Scand. 2012;91(3):331–7.
11. Pitter MC, Gargiulo AR, Bonaventura LM, Lehman JS, Srouji SS. Pregnancy outcomes following robot-assisted myomectomy. Hum Reprod. 2013;28:99–108.
12. Patzkowsky KE, As-Sanie S, Smorgick N, Song AH, Advincula AP. Perioperative outcomes of robotic vs. laparoscopic hysterectomy for benign disease. JSLS. 2013;17(1):100–6.
13. Choussein S, Srouji SS, Missmer SA, Farland LV, Gargiulo AR. Perioperative outcomes and complications of robot-assisted laparoscopic myomectomy (RALM). J Minim Invasive Gynecol. 2015;22(6S):S70.
14. Advincula AP, Song A, Burke W, Reynolds RK. Preliminary experience with robot-assisted laparoscopic myomectomy. J Am Assoc Gynecol Laparosc. 2004;11(4):511–8.
15. Gargiulo AR, Srouji SS, Missmer SA, Correia KF, Vellinga TT, Einarsson JI. Robot-assisted laparoscopic myomectomy compared with standard laparoscopic myomectomy. Obstet Gynecol. 2012;120(2 Pt 1):284–91. Erratum in: Obstet Gynecol. 2013;122(3):698.
16. Bedient CE, Magrina JF, Noble BN, Kho RM. Comparison of robotic and laparoscopic myomectomy. Am J Obstet Gynecol. 2009;201(6):566 e1–5.
17. Nezhat C, Lavie O, Hsu S, Watson J, Barnett O, Lemire M. Robotic-assisted laparoscopic myomectomy compared with standard laparoscopic myomectomy-a retrospective matched control study. Fertil Steril. 2009;91(2):556–9.
18. Pitter M, Srouji S, Gargiulo A, Kardos L, Seshadri-Kreaden U, Hubert HB, Weitzman GA. Fertility and symptom relief following robot-assisted laparoscopic myomectomy. Obstet Gynecol Int. 2015. https://doi.org/10.1155/2015/967568. Epub 2015 Apr 19.
19. Advincula AP, Xu X, Goudeau S, Ransom SB. Robot-assisted laparoscopic myomectomy versus abdominal myomectomy: a comparison of short-term surgical outcomes and immediate costs. J Minim Invasive Gynecol. 2007;14(6):698–705.
20. Barakat EE, Bedaiwy MA, Zimberg S, Nutter B, Nosseir M, Falcone T. Robotic-assisted, laparoscopic, and abdominal myomectomy: a comparison of surgical outcomes. Obstet Gynecol. 2011;117(2 Pt 1):256–29.
21. Gargiulo AR. Fertility preservation and the role of robotics. Clin Obstet Gynecol. 2011;54(3):431–48.
22. Lipskind ST, Gargiulo AR. Computer-assisted laparoscopy in fertility preservation and reproductive surgery. J Minim Invasive Gynecol. 2013;20(4):435–45.
23. Gargiulo AR. Computer-assisted reproductive surgery: why it matters to reproductive endocrinology and infertility subspecialists. Fertil Steril. 2014;102(4):911–21.
24. Lewis EI, Gargiulo AR. Uterine fibroids in the setting of infertility: when to treat, how to treat. Curr Obstet Gynecol Rep. 2017;6(1):1–10.
25. Fanfano F, Reistano S, Rossitto C, Gueli Alletti S, Costantini B, Monterossi G, Cappuccio S, Perrone E, Scambia G. Total laparoscopic (S-LPS) versus TELELAP ALF-X robotic-assisted hysterectomy: a case-control study. J Minim Invasive Gynecol. 2016;23(6):933–8.
26. Shwayder J, Sakhel K. Imaging for uterine myomas and adenomyosis. J Minim Invasive Gynecol. 2014;21(3):362–76.
27. Moghadam R, Lathi RB, Shahmohamady B, Saberi NS, Nezhat CH, Nezhat F, Nezhat C. Predictive value of magnetic resonance imaging in differentiating between leiomyoma and adenomyosis. JSLS. 2006;10(2):216–9.
28. Bhave Chittawar P, Franik S, Pouwer AW, Farquhar C. Minimally invasive surgical techniques versus open myomectomy for uterine fibroids. Cochrane Database Syst Rev. 2014;10:CD004638.
29. Angioli R, Battista C, Terranova C, Zullo MA, Sereni MI, Cafà EV, Panici PB. Intraoperative contact ultrasonography during open myomectomy for uterine fibroids. Fertil Steril. 2010;94(4):1487–90.
30. Battita C, Capriglione S, Guzzo F, Luvero D, Sadun B, Cafa EV, Sereni MI, Terranova C, Plotti F, Angioli R. The challenge of preoperative identification of uterine myomas: is ultrasound trustworthy? A prospective cohort study. Arch Gynecol Obstet. 2016;293(6):1235–41.
31. Parker WH, Einarsson J, Istre O, Dubuisson JB. Risk factors for uterine rupture after laparoscopic myomectomy. J Minim Invasive Gynecol. 2010;17(5):551–4.
32. Quaas AM, Einarsson JI, Srouji SS, Gargiulo AR. Robotic myomectomy: a review of indications and techniques. Rev Obstet Gynecol. 2010;3(4):185–91.
33. Choussein S, Srouji SS, Farland LV, Gargiulo AR. Flexible carbon dioxide laser fiber versus ultrasonic scalpel in robot-assisted laparoscopic myomectomy. J Minim Invasive Gynecol. 2015;22(7):1183–90.
34. Bailey AP, Lancerotto L, Gridley C, Orgill DP, Nguyen H, Pescarini E, Lago G, Gargiulo AR. Greater surgical precision of a flexible carbon dioxide laser fiber compared to monopolar electrosurgery in porcine myometrium. J Minim Invasive Gynecol. 2014;21(6):1103–9.
35. Tinelli A, Malvasi A, Hurst BS, Tsin DA, Davila F, Dominguez G, Dell'edera D, Cavallotti C, Negro R, Gustapane S, Teigland CM,

Lettler L. Surgical management of neurovascular bundle in uterine fibroid pseudocapsule. JSLS. 2012;16(1):119–29.

36. Bedaiwy MA, Zhang A, Henry D, Falcone T, Soto E. Surgical anatomy of supraumbilical port placement: implications for robotic and advanced laparoscopic surgery. Fertil Steril. 2015;103(4):e33.

37. De Milliano I, Twisk M, Ket JC, Huirne JA, Hehenkamp WJ. Pretreatment with GnRHa or ulipristal acetate prior to laparoscopic and laparotomic myomectomy: a systematic review and meta-analysis. PLoS One. 2017;12(10):e0186158. https://doi.org/10.1371/journal.pone.0186158. eCollection 2017.

38. Cordier W, Steenkamp V. Herbal remedies affecting coagulation: a review. Pharm Biol. 2012;50(4):443–52.

39. Celik H, Sapmaz E. Use of a single preoperative dose of misoprostol is efficacious for patients who undergo abdominal myomectomy. Fertil Steril. 2003;79:1207–10.

40. Ragab A, Khaiary M, Badawy A. The use of single versus double dose of intra-vaginal prostaglandin E2 "misoprostol" prior to abdominal myomectomy: a randomized controlled clinical trial. J Reprod Infertil. 2014;15:152–6.

41. Cohen SL, Senapati S, Gargiulo AR, Srouji SS, Tu FF, Solnik J, Hur HC, Vitonis A, Jonsdottir GM, Wang KC, Einarsson JI. Dilute versus concentrated vasopressin administration during laparoscopic myomectomy: a randomized controlled trial. BJOG. 2017;124(2):262–8.

42. Topsoee MF, Settnes A, Ottesen B, Bergholt T. A systematic review and meta-analysis of the effect of prophylactic tranexamic acid treatment in major benign uterine surgery. Int J Gynaecol Obstet. 2017;136(2):120–7.

43. Jansen JA, Lameijer JRC, Snoeker BAM. Combined intravenous, topical and oral tranexamic acid administration in total knee replacement: evaluation of safety in patients with previous thromboembolism and effect on hemoglobin level and transfusion rate. Knee. 2017;24(5):1206–12.

44. U.S. Food and Drugs Administration. UPDATED laparoscopic uterine power morcellation in hysterectomy and myomectomy: FDA safety communication. November 24, 2014. http://www.fda.gov/MedicalDevices/Safety/AlertsandNotices/ucm424443.htm.

45. U.S. Food and Drugs Administration. FDA in brief: FDA releases new findings on the risks of spreading hidden uterine cancer through the use of laparoscopic power morcellators. December 14, 2017. https://www.fda.gov/NewsEvents/Newsroom/FDAInBrief/ucm589137.htm.

46. Srouji SS, Kaser DK, Gargiulo AR. Techniques for contained morcellation in gynecologic surgery. Fertil Steril. 2015;103(40):e34.

47. Clark NV, Cohen SL. Tissue extraction techniques during laparoscopic uterine surgery. J Minim Invasive Gynecol. 2018;25(2):251–6.

48. Cohen A, Tulandi T. Long-term sequelae of unconfined morcellation during laparoscopic gynecological surgery. Maturitas. 2017;97:1–5.

49. Harris JA, Swenson CW, Uppal S, Kamdar N, Mahnert N, As-Sanie S, Morgan DM. Practice patterns and postoperative complications before and after US Food and Drug Administration safety communication on power morcellation. Am J Obster Gynecol. 2016;214(1):98.e1–98.e13.

50. Gargiulo AR, Lewis EI, Kaser DJ, Srouji SS. Robotic single site myomectomy: a step by step tutorial. Fertil Steril. 2015;104(5):e13.

51. Lewis EI, Srouji SS, Gargiulo AR. Robotic single site myomectomy: initial report and technique. Fertil Steril. 2015;103:1370–7.

52. Bush AJ, Morris SN, Millham FH, et al. Women's preferences for minimally invasive incisions. J Minim Invasive Gynecol. 2011;18:640–3.

53. Yeung PP Jr, Bolden CR, Westreich D, et al. Patient preferences of cosmesis for abdominal incisions in gynecologic surgery. J Minim Invasive Gynecol. 2013;20:79–84.

54. Goebel K, Goldberg JM. Women's preference of cosmetic results after gynecologic surgery. J Minim Invasive Gynecol. 2014;21:64–7.

55. Hawa N, Robinson J, Chahine BE. Combined preoperative angiography transient uterine artery embolization makes laparoscopic surgery for massive myomatous uteri a reasonable option: case reports. J Minim Invasive Gynecol. 2012;19(3):386–90.

56. Liu L, Li Y, Xu H, Chen Y, Zhang G, Liang Z. Laparoscopic transient uterine artery occlusion and myomectomy for symptomatic uterine myoma. Fertil Steril. 2011;95(1):254–8.

Robotic Tubo-Ovarian Surgery

27

Erica Stockwell

Introduction

Robotic-assisted gynecologic surgery has been implemented in all fields of gynecology, including reproductive endocrinology and infertility, urogynecology, and gynecologic oncology. The most common procedures performed are hysterectomy, myomectomy, sacrocolpopexy, and excision of endometriosis. According to the American College of Obstetrics and Gynecology Committee Opinion, robot-assisted cases should be appropriately selected based on the available data and expert opinion [1]. American Association of Gynecologic Laparoscopists states in their Position Statement that robotic-assisted and conventional laparoscopic techniques for benign gynecologic surgery are comparable regarding perioperative outcomes, intraoperative complications, length of hospital stay, and rate of conversion to open surgery. However, published reports demonstrate that robotic-assisted laparoscopic surgery has similar or longer operating times and higher associated costs [2]. The use of the robot does not add much benefit over conventional laparoscopic surgery for most straightforward benign gynecologic cases, but does provide benefit in complex cases. Endowristed movement of robotic instruments allows for better and more precise suturing compared to conventional laparoscopy. The robotic platform also offers superior visualization and allows the surgeon to rely less on a bedside assistant.

Indications for use of the robotic platform in adnexal surgery include endometriosis, moderate-to-severe adhesive disease, malignancy, and tubal reanastomosis. It does not provide a cost benefit to utilize the robot for straightforward bilateral salpingectomies, salpingo-oophorectomies, or ovarian cystectomies, unless an adequate surgical assist is not available.

Preprocedural Details

Patient positioning, trocar placement, and robotic docking follow the same guidelines as stated in the robotic-assisted hysterectomy chapter. Please reference this chapter for further details. Regarding instrumentation, we recommend use of a bipolar and a monopolar instrument, such as a fenestrated bipolar grasper or a PK dissector in arm 2 and a monopolar scissors in arm 1. We also recommend routine use of a uterine manipulator.

Endometriosis and Adhesive Disease

Endometriosis is a chronic and progressive gynecologic disorder that affects women of reproductive age. Chronic pain and infertility are the most debilitating problems associated with endometriosis. When medical therapies fail, patients may benefit from surgical treatment. The robot offers distinct advantages over conventional laparoscopy for use in the approach of endometriosis and moderate-to-severe adhesive disease (Figs. 27.1, 27.2, 27.3, and 27.4). Enhanced three-dimensional visualization, 10× magnification, and EndoWrist instruments with seven degrees of freedom facilitate precise and careful dissection. In addition, Firefly Technology using indocyanine (ICG) green dye has been shown to improve detection of lesions that are difficult to visualize with the naked eye [3]. ICG turns endometriotic implants, associated with increased neovascularization, dark green and aids in complete resection of the targeted tissue [4]. The goal of surgical treatment of endometriosis is to take down adhesions, release tethered tissues, remove endometriomas, and, when possible, completely resect any endometriotic nodules. Often, retroperitoneal dissection is necessary to remove deeply infiltrating endometriotic nodules. When full resection is not possible, such as in the case of numerous scattered implants studding peritoneal surfaces, endometriotic implants should be fulgurated. For this, we evoke the use of the argon beam coagulator.

E. Stockwell
Las Vegas Minimally Invasive Surgery, WellHealth Quality Care, a DaVita Medical Group, Las Vegas, NV, USA
e-mail: estockwell@wellhealthqc.com

© Springer Nature Switzerland AG 2019
S. Tsuda, O. Y. Kudsi (eds.), *Robotic-Assisted Minimally Invasive Surgery*, https://doi.org/10.1007/978-3-319-96866-7_27

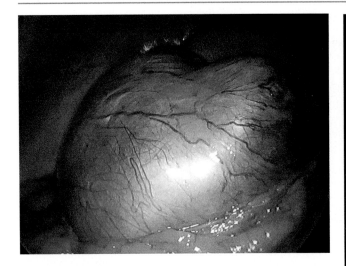

Fig. 27.1 Endometrioma

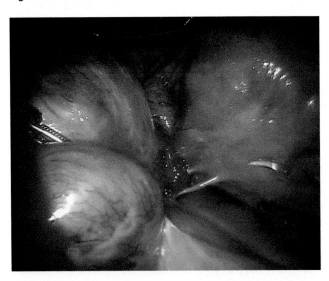

Fig. 27.2 Severe adhesions involving endometrioma, uterus, fallopian tube, and bowel

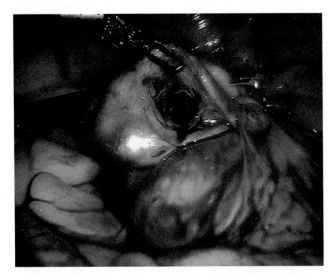

Fig. 27.3 Ruptured endometrioma and "chocolate" cystic fluid

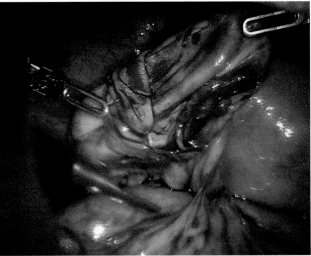

Fig. 27.4 Removing endometrioma cyst wall (right instrument) from ovarian stroma (left instrument)

Tubal Reanastomosis

Tubal ligation is a medical procedure that closes or cuts the fallopian tubes, blocking the female egg from reaching the uterus and consequently preventing pregnancy. Between 1% and 26% of women who undergo tubal ligation later experience regret [5]. Young women are much more likely to feel regret than older women. Although tubal sterilization procedures are considered to be permanent, requests for reversal of the procedure are common. Most tubal ligation procedures can be reversed. If the fallopian tube is fulgurated extensively, missing the fimbriated portion, or completely removed, tubal reanastomosis may not be possible, and the patient may be better served through in vitro fertilization. However, if the method of tubal ligation used previously followed tubal ligation and resection, or utilized a ring or clip, tubal reanastomosis may be attempted and often performed successfully (Fig. 27.5).

Sterilization reversal is the most successful surgical reconstructive procedure for improving fertility. Often, the cost of a tubal reanastomosis surgery is similar to cost of in vitro fertilization, and patients must be counseled thoroughly regarding chances of success when deciding between performing one or another. Factors that influence the success rate of tubal reanastomosis include age of the patient, time from sterilization, sterilization technique, and remaining tubal length. Ideally, resulting tubal length should be 4 cm or more with less success demonstrated in those with shorter tubes [6].

The purpose of tubal reanastomosis is to reconnect the proximal cornual tubal segment to the distal fimbriated tubal segment. First, the blocked ends of each tubal segment are incised, exposing patent tubal lumen (Figs. 27.6 and 27.7). The newly opened tubal ends are drawn to each other by placing

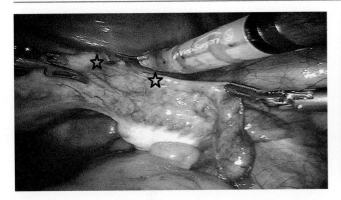

Fig. 27.5 Portion of fallopian tube removed from prior tubal ligation (between the two stars)

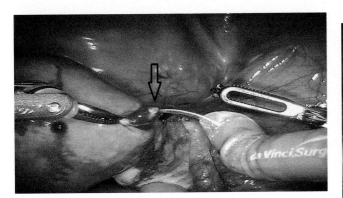

Fig. 27.6 Scar excised, exposing proximal tubal lumen (arrow)

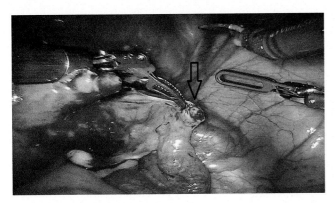

Fig. 27.7 Scar excised, exposing distal tubal lumen (arrow)

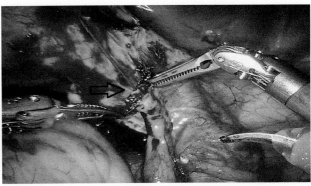

Fig. 27.8 Urologic wire (arrow) is used to gently thread through the tubal segments and into the uterine cavity to line the tubes up for reconnection

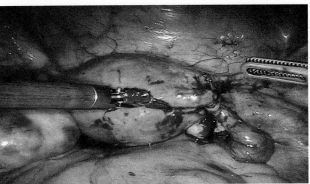

Fig. 27.9 Completed tubal reanastomosis of right fallopian tube with patency demonstrated via chromopertubation

Summary

In summary, though robotic-assisted surgery has been shown to be beneficial in complex cases, such as with endometriosis, scar tissue, malignancy, or microsurgery, the additional operating costs do not lend to utilization for most laparoscopic benign adnexal surgery. This chapter discusses two cases in which utilization of the robotic platform may be beneficial. In excision of endometriosis, the fine dissection, magnified three-dimensional view, and utilization of Firefly Technology aid in procedural success. In tubal reanastomosis, the delicate movements and magnified three-dimensional view enable microsurgery success.

sutures in the connective tissue of the mesosalpinx. This retention suture prevents the tubal segments from pulling apart while the tube heals. Microsurgical 6-0 sutures are used to precisely align the tubal lumens, the muscularis externa, and the serosa layer of the tube. This is done in a circumferential fashion in 4-5 sutures. A narrow flexible stent may be used to gently thread through the tubal segments and into the uterine cavity to line the tubes up for reconnection (Fig. 27.8), but care must be taken to not damage the delicate cilia that line the tube. At the conclusion of the procedure, chromopertubation should be performed to ensure patency of each tube (Fig. 27.9).

References

1. Robotic surgery in gynecology. Committee Opinion No. 628. American College of Obstetricians and Gynecologists. Obstet Gynecol. 2015;125:760–7.
2. AAGL position statement: robotic-assisted laparoscopic surgery in benign gynecology. J Minim Invasive Gynecol. 2013;20(1):2–9.
3. Sinha R, Sanjay M, Bana R, Jeelani F, Kumari S. Robotic assisted surgery for endometriosis – "is the way forward?". Open J Obstet Gynecol. 2016;6:93–102. https://doi.org/10.4236/ojog.2016.62011.

4. Nezhat FR. Sirota perioperative outcomes of robotic assisted laparoscopic surgery versus conventional laparoscopy surgery for advanced-stage endometriosis. JSLS. 2014;18(4). pii: e2014.00094. doi: https://doi.org/10.4293/JSLS.2014.00094.

5. George K, Kamath MS, Tharyan P. Minimally invasive versus open surgery for reversal of tubal sterilization. Cochrane Database Syst Rev. 2013;(2). Art. No.: CD009174. https://doi.org/10.1002/14651858.CD009174.pub2.

6. Boeckxstaens A, Devroey P, Collins J, Tournaye H. Getting pregnant after tubal sterilization: surgical reversal or IVF? Hum Reprod. 2007;22:2660.

Part IV

Urology

Robotic Intracorporeal Ileal Conduit

Jayram Krishnan and Daniel Groves

History of Urinary Diversion

Urinary diversion was pioneered by Sir John Simon in 1851, when he performed an ureteroproctostomy in an exstrophy patient. With continued advancements in the ureterointestinal anastomosis occurring throughout the late nineteenth century, Zaayer is credited with performing the first ileal conduit in 1911 [1]. Bricker and Wallace later repopularized this method of urinary diversion with continued modifications of the ureterointestinal anastomosis. Bricker's technique for the ureteroileal anastomosis involved separate anastomoses for each ureter to the serosa of the ileum during the 1950s [2]. Wallace popularized the technique of suturing each ureter's medial wall to one another and then an end-end anastomosis to the proximal end of the ileal conduit [3]. As minimally invasive surgery has progressed from urinary diversion being performed as a hybrid procedure to a complete intracorporeal procedure with the innovation of the robot, approximately 18% of surgeons were using the intracorporeal approach in 2014 [4].

Preoperative Evaluation

Patients undergoing robotic ileal conduit must be candidates for laparoscopic surgery. Patients with chronic obstructive pulmonary disease, restrictive lung disease, morbid obesity, or decreased cardiac output are at increased risk for complications with pneumoperitoneum [5] and may not be candidates for minimally invasive intracorporeal urinary diversion. Patients with inflammatory bowel disease, radiation to the ileum, and short gut syndrome may not be candidates for ileal conduit [6]. Continent urinary diversion is contraindicated in patients with chronic renal failure, patients with hepatic dysfunction, patients without the mental capacity of physical dexterity to perform self-catheterization, or patients requiring a urethrectomy [7].

Mechanical bowel preparation has been shown to be unnecessary in ileal urinary diversion. Raynor et al. retrospectively reviewed two separate cohorts undergoing radical cystectomy and ileal urinary diversion [8]. The first cohort was instructed to complete a clear liquid diet 24 h prior to surgery, 8 ounces of magnesium citrate, and an enema 2 h prior to the procedure, while the other cohort was instructed to eat a regular diet and undergo an enema 2 h prior to the procedure. Their results revealed no difference with return to bowel function, time to discharge, or overall complications, and no patients in either cohort experienced bowel anastomotic leak, fistula, abscess, peritonitis, or surgical site infection [8]. Shi Deng performed a systematic review and meta-analysis of the literature in 2013 including two randomized controlled trials and five cohort studies and found no increase in complications comparing patients undergoing a mechanical bowel preparation versus those who did not [9]. Recently, many institutions are implementing an Enhanced Recovery After Surgery (ERAS) program prior to and after the surgical procedure. This program generally includes a preoperative nutrition evaluation, carbohydrate loading prior to surgery, and continuing a regular diet up until the time of surgery. This program is expected to enhance recovery after surgery and shorten the hospital length of stay.

Choice of Urinary Diversion

Patients must be given their options regarding the type of urinary diversion that will be performed. Urologists choose urinary diversions based on the patient's health and medical status as well patient preference. There is a psychologic adjustment that a patient must undergo prior to urinary diversion surgery. An ileal conduit will result in an ostomy to be placed on the abdomen. This is in contrast to the common

J. Krishnan (✉) · D. Groves
Department of Urology, Cleveland Clinic, Akron, OH, USA
e-mail: KRISHNJ2@ccf.org

© Springer Nature Switzerland AG 2019
S. Tsuda, O. Y. Kudsi (eds.), *Robotic-Assisted Minimally Invasive Surgery*, https://doi.org/10.1007/978-3-319-96866-7_28

alternative, known as the orthotopic neobladder. Based on quality-of-life measures, there is no long-term difference between these two types of urinary diversions [10]. It is a healthy practice to have patients meet with an enterostomal therapist, who will provide ostomy education as well as perform optimal stomal site marking.

Operative Technique

Gill demonstrated the first completely intracorporeal laparoscopic ileal ureter in the literature in 2000 [11]. Menon and his colleagues described the first robotic radical cystectomy with ileal conduit urinary diversion in the literature [12]. In many cases, the urinary diversion is created in combination with removal of the bladder, so techniques reported in the literature will often describe both procedures. Hemal has provided an updated technique in more recent literature that reviews many aspects of this surgical procedure [13].

After induction of general anesthesia, the patient is positioned in either dorsal lithotomy or supine based on which robotic platform is used. We generally prefer the Intuitive Xi system, where the patient is placed in the supine position. All pressure points and areas of compression are adequately padded to prevent nerve injuries and compartment syndromes.

Patient's arms are tucked to the sides and upper body is secured to the table to prevent movement while in steep Trendelenburg. Shoulder pads or adhesive tape can be used to secure the patient to the table. The Xi robotic system can be coupled with the Table Motion bed that communicated with the robotic console, so that the optimum position is selected by the surgeon and anesthesiologist.

Sterile field is created between the xiphoid process and the entire groin. In females, vagina is completed prepped as well as the penis in males. Port placement is described in Fig. 28.1. Ports are placed in a similar fashion to robotic pelvic surgery.

Camera port is placed at the midline, 4 cm above the umbilicus. The robotic stapler trocar is placed in the left abdomen, 5–6 cm away from the camera port, and similarly on the right, the robotic trocar is placed 5–6 cm away. This port can be adjusted in order to accommodate for the eventual stoma site if feasible. 12 mm assistant port is placed in the right abdomen. We prefer to use the AirSeal, valveless trocar system as our assistant port. The final robotic trocar is placed in the left upper abdomen, 5–6 cm away from the robotic stapler trocar.

Creation of the intracorporeal ileal conduit is performed similarly to an open surgical fashion [14]. Fifteen centimeters of ileum is isolated, approximately 15–20 cm away from the ileocecal valve. This prevents electrolyte issues that can present when involving the terminal ileum (Fig. 28.2).

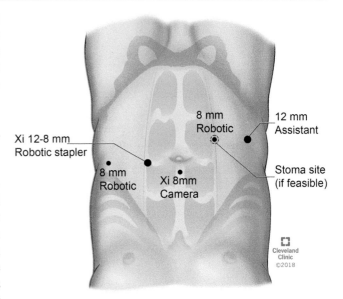

Fig. 28.1 Camera port is placed at the midline, 4 cm above the umbilicus. The robotic stapler trocar is placed in the left abdomen, 5–6 cm away from the camera port, and similarly on the right, the robotic trocar is placed 5–6 cm away. This port can be adjusted in order to accommodate for the eventual stoma site if feasible. 12 mm assistant port is placed in the right abdomen. We prefer to use the AirSeal, valveless trocar system as our assistant port. The final robotic trocar is placed in the left upper abdomen, 5–6 cm away from the robotic stapler trocar. (Reprinted with permission, Cleveland Clinic Center for Medical Art & Photography ©2018. All Rights Reserved)

We place a number of 2-0 vicryl stay sutures on the bowel to provide adequate manipulation while performing intracorporeal stapling. Guru and his colleagues describe the Marionette where a long suture is placed at the distal aspect of the isolated bowel segment and using that to manipulate the bowel segment [15]. Once the 15 cm ileal conduit is isolated, bowel continuity is restored by performing and end-to-side anastomosis. Mesentery can be divided using a Vessel Sealer or robotic stapler. We generally use the Firefly, ICG identification system to identify adequate blood flow to the bowel segments. The mesenteric defect is closed using a 2-0 vicryl suture. Oversewing the bowel anastomosis with a Lembert suture is optional and based on surgeon preference. The ileal conduit is then opened, irrigated, and prepared for ureteroileal anastomosis. Ureteroileal anastomosis can be performed using either the Bricker [2] or the Wallace [3] techniques. Pruthi and his colleagues reported no differences in stricture rate and complications between the two techniques [16]. We perform a Bricker style anastomosis using 2 interlocked 3-0 V-Loc sutures in a running fashion. The goal is a watertight, tension-free anastomosis.

Intracorporeal ureteral stent placement is performed with the coordination of your bedside assistant. We secure our stents to the skin side of the conduit with a 3-0 chromic suture to prevent migration of the stents. Prior to undocking the robot, a laparoscopic grasper is placed in the distal aspect

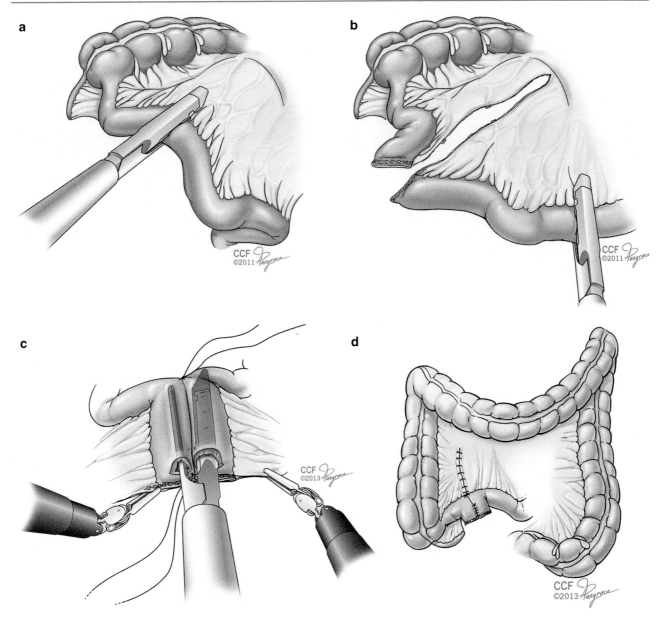

Fig. 28.2 Loop isolation and bowel anastomosis. (**a**): distal segment. (**b**): proximal segment. (**c**): Latero-lateral anastomosis using an Endo GIA. (**d**): Final aspect. (Reprinted with permission, Cleveland Clinic Center for Medical Art & Photography ©2018. All Rights Reserved)

of the conduit and brought extracorporeally through the medial right-sided robotic port if feasible for ostomy creation (Fig. 28.3).

Finally, the stoma is matured in the standard fashion according to surgeon preference. Final diagram is shown below (Fig. 28.4).

Postoperative Outcomes

Ahmed et al. reviewed outcomes of cystectomy performed with intracorporeal versus extracorporeal urinary diversion between 2003 and 2011 in 2014 [4]. A retrospective review

of 935 patients who underwent cystectomy with urinary diversion was performed using the International Robotic Cystectomy Consortium's (IRCC) multi-institutional, prospectively maintained database. One hundred sixty-seven patients underwent intracorporeal urinary diversion, and 768 patients underwent extracorporeal urinary diversion. Of the patients who underwent intracorporeal diversion, 106 patients underwent ileal conduit formation, and 61 patients underwent neobladder creation. Ahmed et al. found that operative time, estimated blood loss, and length of stay were similar between the groups [4]. The 30-day and 90-day readmission rate was significantly higher in the extracorporeal urinary diversion group [4]. The 90-day mortality rate was

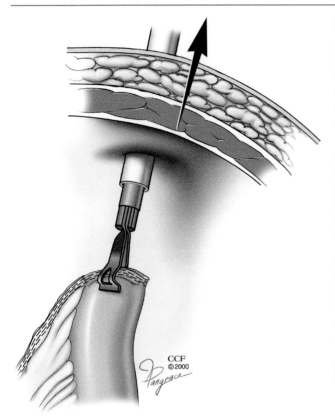

Fig. 28.3 A laparoscopic grasper is used to bring the distal aspect of the conduit extracorporeally through the medial right-sided robotic port. (Reprinted with permission, Cleveland Clinic Center for Medical Art & Photography ©2018. All Rights Reserved)

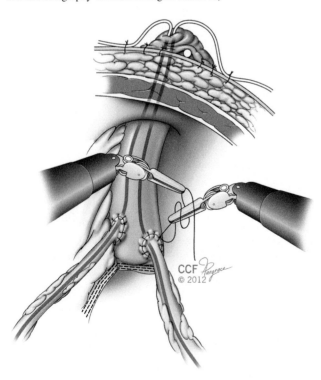

Fig. 28.4 Maturation of the ileal conduit stoma with ureteral stents sutured in placed and the conclusion of the ureteral intestinal anastomosis. (Reprinted with permission, Cleveland Clinic Center for Medical Art & Photography ©2018. All Rights Reserved)

higher in the extracorporeal urinary diversion group [4]. Ahmed et al. found no difference in Clavien-Dindo grades III–V complications between the groups and a lower wound infection and gastrointestinal complication rate in the intracorporeal urinary diversion group [4]. Overall, Ahmed et al. concluded that intracorporeal urinary diversion is safe and offers improved outcomes.

Hussein et al. performed an updated review of the IRCC's database of intracorporeal vs extracorporeal urinary diversion after cystectomy [17]. Their review included 2125 patients with 1094 who underwent intracorporeal urinary diversion. The results included a significantly shorter operative time (357 vs 400 min) and less blood loss with fewer blood transfusions [17]. Hussein et al. found a higher high-grade complication rate in the intracorporeal urinary diversion group of 13% vs 10% [17]. In their review Hussein et al. found that intracorporeal urinary diversion increased from 9% in 2005 to 97% in 2015 [17]. The complication rate of intracorporeal urinary diversion decreased significantly with time [17].

Conclusion
Robotic intracorporeal ileal conduit is a feasible, reproducible technique that can be performed routinely by interested and experienced surgeons. Adherence to open surgical principles while translating to the robotic platform will provide successful outcomes with decreased complications.

References

1. Saber A. Urinary diversion: historical aspect and patient's satisfaction. Urol Nephrol Open Access J. 2014;1(3):00020. https://doi.org/10.15406/unoaj.2014.01.00020.
2. Bricker EM. Bladder substitution after pelvic evisceration. Surg Clin North Am. 1950;30:1511.
3. Wallace DM. Ureteric diversion using a conduit: a simplified technique. Br J Urol. 1966;38:522.
4. Ahmed K, Khan SA, Hayn MH, et al. Analysis of intracorporeal compared with extracorporeal urinary diversion after robot-assisted radical cystectomy: results from the International Robotic Cystectomy Consortium. Eur Urol. 2014;65:340–7.
5. Ost MC, Tan BJ, Lee BR. Urological laparoscopy: basic physiological considerations and immunological consequences. J Urol. 2005;174:1183–8.
6. Wein A, Kavoussi LR, Partin AW, Peters CA. Chapter 97: Use of intestinal segments in urinary diversion. In: Campbell walsh urology. 11th ed. Elsevier, Philadelphia, PA; 2016. p. 2281–316.
7. Colombo R, Naspro R. Ileal conduit as the standard urinary diversion after radical cystectomy for bladder cancer. Eur Urol Suppl. 2010;9:736–44.
8. Raynor MC, Lavien G, Nielsen M, et al. Elimination of preoperative mechanical bowel preparation in patients undergoing cystectomy and urinary diversion. Urol Oncol. 2013;31:32.
9. Deng S, et al. The role of mechanical bowel preparation before ileal urinary diversion: a systematic review and meta-analysis. Urol Int. 2014;92:339–48.
10. Goldberg H, Baniel J, Mano R, Rotlevy G, Kedar D, Yossepowitch O. Orthotopic neobladder vs. ileal conduit urinary diversion: a

long-term quality-of-life comparison. Urol Oncol. 2016;34(3):121. e1–7. https://doi.org/10.1016/j.urolonc.2015.10.006. Epub 2015 Dec 3.

11. Gill IS, Fergnany A, Klein EA, et al. Laparoscopic radical cysto-prostatectomy with ileal conduit performed completely intracorporally (the initial 2 cases). Urology. 2000;56:26–30.

12. Menon M, Hemal AK, Tewari A, Shrivastava A, Shoma AM, El-Tabey NA, et al. Nerve-sparing robot-assisted radical cystoprostatectomy and urinary diversion. BJU Int. 2003;92:232e6.

13. Sandberg JM, Hemal AK. Robot-assisted laparoscopic radical cystectomy with complete intracorporeal urinary diversion. Asian J Urol. 2016;3(3):156–66.

14. Balaji KC, Yohannes P, McBride CL, Oleynikov D, Hemstreet GP 3rd. Feasibility of robot-assisted totally intra- corporeal laparoscopic ileal conduit urinary diversion: initial results of a single institutional pilot study. Urology. 2004;63:51e5.

15. Guru K, Seixas-Mikelus SA, Hussain A, Blumenfeld AJ, Nyquist J, Chandrasekhar R, et al. Robot-assisted intra-corporeal ileal conduit: marionette technique and initial experience at Roswell Park Cancer Institute. Urology. 2010;76:866e71.

16. Kouba E, Sands M, Lentz A, Wallen E, Pruthi RS. A comparison of the Bricker versus Wallace ureteroileal anastomosis in patients undergoing urinary diversion for bladder cancer. J Urol. 2007;178(3 Pt 1):945–8; discussion 948–9. Epub 2007 Jul 16.

17. Hussein AA, May PR, Jing Z, et al. Outcomes of intracorporeal urinary diversion after robot-assisted radical cystectomy: results from the International Robotic Cystectomy Consortium. J Urol. 2017;199:1302–11.

Robotic Partial Nephrectomy

Kemal Ener and Abdullah Erdem Canda

Introduction

Currently, most renal cell carcinomas are detected incidentally as small renal masses because of the widespread use of radiological imaging [1]. Radical nephrectomy is still the gold standard treatment of renal tumors. When feasible, partial nephrectomy (PN) is recommended as a gold standard treatment for patients with small renal tumors, since it might have less renal function impairment and equivalent oncological survival compared to radical nephrectomy [2]. There is still no size threshold beyond which PN should not be performed. Currently, if it is technically feasible, PN may be performed for tumors up to 7 cm in major dimensions [3].

Laparoscopic partial nephrectomy (LPN) and robotic partial nephrectomy (RAPN) are the main mini-invasive alternatives to open partial nephrectomy (OPN), aimed at reducing the added morbidity of an open incision and potential rib resection. Since the introduction of RAPN in 2004 [4], it has been proposed as an alternative to other surgical approaches as a minimally invasive treatment option. Robotic surgery provides the advantages of eliminating hand tremor, leads to three-dimensional and magnified view, and fulfills the requirements of laparoscopic surgery. The utilization of the robot in this field has facilitated the PN procedure, especially during the renal dissection, reconstruction, and intracorporeal suturing. Recently, RAPN has become the preferred surgical method with oncological safety for small renal masses [5].

In conventional PN procedures, clamping the renal artery cuts off the blood flow to the entire kidney with a possible ischemic damage to the kidney. It is expected that postopera-

tive renal function may worsen especially in patients with underlying chronic renal diseases. The inability of cooling the kidney during robotic and laparoscopic approaches is also a debated issue. Zero-ischemia PN technique avoids complete renal ischemia and may provide better postoperative renal function. The number of studies on the topic of zero-ischemia PN is increasing in the literature favoring the technique in terms of preserving the postoperative kidney function [6–11]. Especially in patients with underlying renal diseases, for whom functional kidney reserve is more essential, implementation of this method should be encouraged. Nonetheless, even if the patient has no renal disease, zero ischemia may be the first method of choice in patients with peripherally located exophytic masses, considering that every patient with renal tumors who is undergoing renal surgery can be a potential candidate for renal failure. We have previously published the results of zero-ischemia RAPN series of our institution and stated that it was a safe and feasible minimally invasive method with acceptable functional outcomes in peripherally located small and even in selected larger renal masses [12].

Hemostatic agents are widely used in PN procedures to achieve a better hemostasis. The use of hemostatic agents (e.g., fibrin sealant, oxidized regenerate cellulose) leads to immediate and durable hemostasis [13, 14]; therefore, they were adopted for use in PNs [14–17]. In a recent study by Morelli et al., 31 patients underwent RAPN for 33 renal tumors [18]. Twenty-seven of 33 lesions (82%) did not require vascular clamping and therefore were treated in the absence of ischemia. The authors suggested systematic use of hemostatic agents in RAPN procedures which may be a safe and effective method to avoid ischemia in the treatment of selected renal masses.

To identify anatomic characteristics of renal tumors in CT and MRI and ensure a more objective and standard preoperative evaluation, RENAL nephrometry and the PADUA scoring systems have been developed. These scoring systems may help to predict the oncological success and perioperative and postoperative complications of PN. Regarding RENAL nephrometry, the complexity of the tumor is

All of the surgical figures included in this chapter are obtained from Prof. Canda's own robotic surgical cases.

K. Ener
Umraniye Training and Research Hospital,
Department of Urology, Istanbul, Turkey

A. E. Canda (✉)
Koc University, School of Medicine,
Department of Urology, Istanbul, Turkey

© Springer Nature Switzerland AG 2019
S. Tsuda, O. Y. Kudsi (eds.), *Robotic-Assisted Minimally Invasive Surgery*, https://doi.org/10.1007/978-3-319-96866-7_29

classified as low (4–6) or medium–high (7–12). In the PADUA classification, renal tumors are given scores from 6 to 14 according to their anatomical localization. Tumors with a score of 8–9 have 14-fold of higher complication risk than tumors with a score of 6–7, and tumors with a score of over 10 have 30-fold of higher complication risk than those with a score of 6–7.

Literature Review

Open Versus Robotic Approach

In the literature, there are several retrospective and prospective studies comparing RAPN and OPN [19–21]. Retrospectively, unifocal clinical T1 renal masses in non-solitary kidneys were reviewed in a past study [19]. In this study, tetrafecta was evaluated between the groups which was defined as negative surgical margins, freedom from perioperative complications, ≥80% renal functional preservation, and no chronic kidney disease upstaging. For T1a masses, tetrafecta achievement was similar between approaches, but for T1b masses, the robotic approach achieved significantly higher tetrafecta rates (43.0% vs 21.3%) that were primarily due to lower perioperative morbidity, specifically related to wound complications. Positive surgical margin rates and renal functional preservation were comparable between open and robotic approaches.

In another retrospective study, Sprenkle PC et al. compared the outcomes for 53 minimally invasive PN (16 robotic and 37 laparoscopic PN) and 226 OPN procedures for tumors >4–7 cm in size [20]. The authors concluded that OPN and minimally invasive PN procedures performed in patients with tumors >4–7 cm offer acceptable and comparable results in terms of operative, functional, and convalescence measures, regardless of approach. A retrospective review was performed to compare 69 RAPNs with 234 OPNs in terms of clinicopathologic variables, operative parameters, and renal functional outcomes [21]. The mean operative time and the mean warm ischemia time were longer in the RAPN group. But there were no significant differences in the postoperative estimated glomerular filtration rate (eGFR) and change in the eGFR. There were six patients with positive surgical margins in the OPN group, while there are no patients with positive surgical margins in the RAPN group. The intraoperative and overall postoperative complication rates were similar between the groups. The authors concluded that RAPN was a viable option small renal tumor as a nephron-sparing surgery approach.

In a multicenter study, perioperative results and complications of open and robotic PN procedures were compared [3].

In this study, the open PN group consisted of 198 patients, and robotic PN group consisted of 105 patients. No difference was observed in terms of tumor nephrometry, renal function, ischemia time, positive surgical margin, and intra- and postoperative complications. Nonetheless, less bleeding and surgical complications and shorter hospital stay were found in the robotic PN group. However, the operative time was found longer for the patients in the robotic group.

In a systematic review and meta-analysis, 16 comparative studies including 3024 cases were evaluated and compared regarding perioperative outcomes of RAPN and OPN [22]. Although operative time and warm ischemia time were longer in the RAPN group, estimated blood loss, hospital stay, and perioperative complications were less than the open group. Besides, there were no differences in positive surgical margin, the change of glomerular filtration rate, transfusion rate, and conversion rate between the two groups. In conclusions the authors suggested RAPN as an effective alternative to OPN.

In a single-center study, Mearini et al. compared the results of zero-ischemia OPN, LPN, and RAPN in terms of complete removal of tumor, preservation of renal function, and having no grade ≥ 3 complications according to Clavien-Dindo classification [23]. In this study, 80 patients underwent OPN, 66 LPN, and 31 RAPN procedures. All of the techniques were found to be safe and effective; moreover, RAPN and LPN offered benefits of a reduced operative time, blood loss, on-demand ischemia, and rate of high-grade complications.

Both LPN and RAPN can be performed through transperitoneal or retroperitoneal approaches. However, retroperitoneal LPN is less utilized than transperitoneal LPN because of its technical difficulties [24]. Kieran et al. compared the intraoperative parameters and perioperative complications of retroperitoneal and transperitoneal approaches to LPN [25]. They concluded that the retroperitoneal approach reduced the operative time, hospital stay, and complications without compromising the oncologic outcomes. One meta-analysis showed that retroperitoneal LPN had a shorter operative time and a shorter length of stay, which led to the conclusion that retroperitoneal approach might be faster and equally safe compared with the transperitoneal approach [26]. In a meta-analysis, Xia et al. compared the outcomes of transperitoneal and retroperitoneal RAPN regarding complications, conversion, operative time, warm ischemia time, estimated blood loss, and positive surgical margins [27]. The meta-analysis suggested that retroperitoneal RAPN was equally safe and efficacious in terms of complications, conversion, warm ischemia time, estimated blood loss, and positive surgical margins compared with transperitoneal RAPN. In addition, retroperitoneal RAPN had a marginally significant advantage of shorter operative time.

Laparoscopic Versus Robotic Approach

Initially, PN was performed solely with an open approach. More recently, minimally invasive approaches (laparoscopic or robotic) have been increasingly used for PN. LPN has been shown to offer better cosmetic results, less postoperative pain, shorter length of hospital stay, and faster postoperative recovery than OPN. However, the spread of laparoscopic PN has been limited due to the difficulties of the technique and surgeons' long learning curve and is more applicable to the small and less complex renal tumors [28]. On the contrary, RAPN is a more reproducible technique and provides the superiority of bridging the technical difficulties of LPN. Hanzly et al. evaluated the learning curves of RAPN and LPN by examining the operative times, warm ischemia times, estimated blood loss, the postoperative eGFR, and intra- and postoperative complications [29]. Intraoperative and postoperative complications were similar in both groups. In the RAPN group, operative time and warm ischemia time were shorter, and postoperative stay was longer. The percentage decrease in postoperative eGFR was lower in the RAPN group compared with the LPN. The authors stated that variables of the learning curve for RAPN can be obtained earlier than the same variables for LPN.

In a multicenter comparative study (the RECORd Project), perioperative results and predictive factors of trifecta achievement (absence of perioperative complications, negative surgical margins, and ischemia time) of OPN (133 patients), LPN (57 patients), and RAPN (95 patients) were evaluated for clinical T1b renal tumors [30]. In this study, median estimated blood loss was significantly lower at RAPN patients compared to other groups. Consistently with the literature, median ischemia time was significantly shorter during OPN than the other approaches (RAPN had significantly shorter ischemia time compared to LPN). Intraoperative and postoperative complications were significantly less in RAPN group compared to OPN group. LPN (1.9%) and RAPN (2.5%) showed a lower rate of positive surgical margins than OPN (6.8%). Trifecta was achieved in 62.4%, 63.2%, and 69.5% OPN, LPN, and RAPN, respectively. The predictive factors for trifecta achievement were exophytic tumor growth pattern, estimated blood loss, and high-volume centers.

A meta-analysis including 4919 patients who underwent robotic and laparoscopic PN (2681 RAPN, 2238 LPN) procedures favoured robotic approach in terms of conversion to open surgery, complication rates, ischemia time, and positive surgical margins, despite having larger tumor size and higher mean RENAL nephrometry scores in the robotic group [31]. In this meta-analysis, both approaches had similar operative time, estimated blood loss, and postoperative change in eGFR. In a multicenter study, perioperative and long-term renal functional outcomes of RAPN versus LPN procedures were compared [32]. The matched-pair comparison of 195 RAPNs and 195 LPNs showed no significant differences with regard to overall change in eGFR or positive surgical margin rates. However, the amount of renal functional recovery was found higher in the RAPN group. Operative time and warm ischemic time were significantly shorter in the RAPN group.

In a retrospective study, patients who underwent LPN (n = 52) or RAPN (n = 48) performed by a single surgeon were compared [33]. In contrast to the existing literature, no significant differences were found between groups with regard to mean estimated blood loss, operation time, ischemia time, intraoperative and postoperative complication rates, hospital stay, percent reduction of hemoglobin, positive margins, or changes in renal function. The authors concluded that RAPN was a comparable and alternative option to LPN, with equivalent oncological and functional outcomes, as well as comparable morbidity to LPN. Our institution's initial experience with RAPN was previously published [34]. The study included 42 patients undergoing transperitoneal RAPN. During a median follow-up period of 15.5 months, there was no distant metastasis or local recurrence. According to our experience, RAPN is a safe minimally invasive surgical approach, with excellent surgical and oncological outcomes in T1 kidney tumors.

Preoperative Planning

In order to determine the location and size of the renal tumors, abdominal computed tomography (CT) or magnetic resonance imaging (MRI) is performed. The RENAL nephrometry and PADUA scores of the patients are calculated from the examination of the CT and MRI scans. In line with our current practice, patients with small renal masses are considered for zero-ischemia RAPN. If an accessory lower pole artery is present and the tumor is located peripherally as an exophytic mass lesion <3 cm in size, we selectively occlude the lower pole artery by applying a laparoscopic bulldog clamp. Then, in the presence of an accessory artery selectively supplying the renal mass, we apply a polymer ligation clip to block the blood supply to the mass and perform zero-ischemia RAPN.

In patients with a solitary kidney and in those with the tumor characteristics described above, zero-ischemia RAPN could be performed that might have a positive impact on residual postoperative kidney function. Another important tool that might be required during this type of surgery is intraoperative endoscopic ultrasound, which might be helpful for showing the depth of the tumor before starting excision.

Antiaggregant and anticoagulant treatments are discontinued at least 1 week prior to surgery in order to minimize the risk of bleeding. Subcutaneous low-molecular-weight heparin is initiated. Two units of erythrocyte suspension are prepared for a possible blood transfusion. Antibiotic prophylaxis is administered to all patients during anesthesia induction. Before the administration of the anesthesia, high-thigh antiembolism stockings are applied to both legs to prevent deep vein thrombosis and embolization. After intratracheal general anesthesia, a urethral Foley catheter is inserted, and the patient is then placed in the 60° flank position with the surgical bed flexed that allows a clear view of the surgical field. The surgical field is cleaned with povidone-iodine.

Setup

In regard to the surgeon's preference, an intraperitoneal incision is performed by inserting a Veress needle or with the open Hasson's method, approximately 1 cm superolateral to the umbilicus to begin surgical access. Pneumoperitoneum at 15 mmHg is maintained with CO_2 insufflation by placement of an 8-mm robotic camera trocar (Fig. 29.1). Then, an 8-mm port is placed approximately 4 cm craniomedial to the spina iliaca anterior superior (SIAS) for the first robotic arm, and an 8-mm robotic port is placed at the arcus costarum at the midclavicular line under direct vision for the second robotic arm. A 12-mm assistant port is placed 2 cm medial to the line connecting the robotic port and the camera port. Finally, at the surgeon's discretion, if an extra robotic arm is to be used, an 8-mm robotic port is placed approximately 2 cm below the SIAS under direct vision. The port placements are similarly performed for the right and left kidneys. Some of the robotic surgeons routinely prefer the application of an extra arm that might facilitate the procedure by providing the console surgeon a better kidney retraction, hilar dissection, and vascular control independent from the bedside assistant. For the next step, the robotic unit was docked at a 15° angle from the back of the patient, and the operation is begun by connecting the robotic arms and introducing the robotic instruments through the ports.

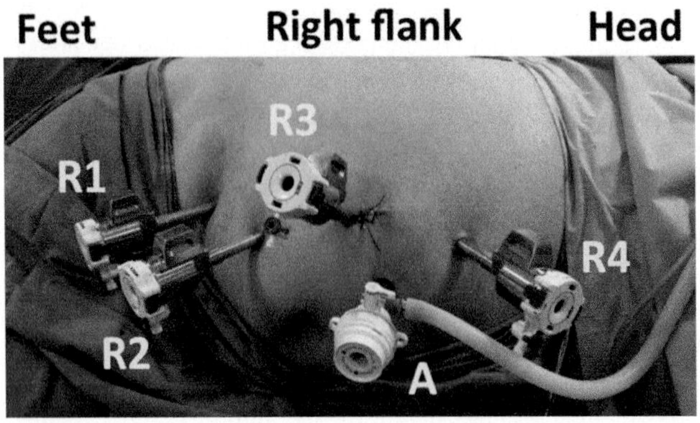

Procedure

During surgery, the standard PN procedure is followed as we previously described [35]. Initially, the white line of Toldt is identified, the colon is mobilized medially, and the retroperitoneal space is entered. The ureter is identified in the retroperitoneum and followed up to the renal hilum, where the renal vessels are identified. The renal vein and renal artery are dissected, encircled, and secured with vascular tapes (Fig. 29.2). Gerota's fascia is opened, and the perirenal fatty tissue is dissected off to expose the kidney and the renal mass. The line of excision for the renal lesion is marked on the renal capsule using monopolar curved scissors and cautery (Fig. 29.3). An absorbable suture is introduced into the abdominal cavity for performing renorrhaphy and parked in the abdomen appropriately (Fig. 29.4).

An endoscopic bulldog clamp is prepared for use if needed. If the dissection of the renal hilum, including the renal artery and vein, is not performed, it may be difficult for the assistant surgeon to apply a laparoscopic bulldog clamp in the event of unexpected and excessive bleeding while performing zero-ischemia RAPN. Therefore, we always suggest identification and securing the renal artery and vein with vascular tapes at the beginning of the surgery.

In the on-clamp approaches, the laparoscopic bulldog clamp is applied on the renal artery (Fig. 29.5). Excision of the renal mass lesion is initiated using monopolar curved

Fig. 29.1 Abdominal port sites. R1-4, 8-mm robotic ports; A, 11-mm assistant port

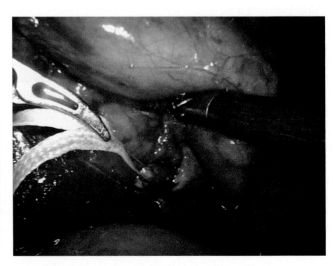

Fig. 29.2 Securing the renal artery with a vascular tape

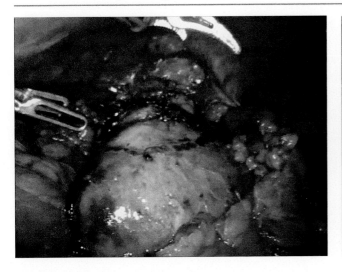

Fig. 29.3 Marking the renal capsule with cautery around the mass lesion with few millimeters safety margin

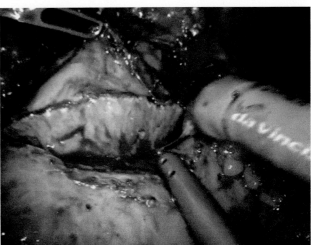

Fig. 29.6 Performing partial nephrectomy with monopolar curved scissors

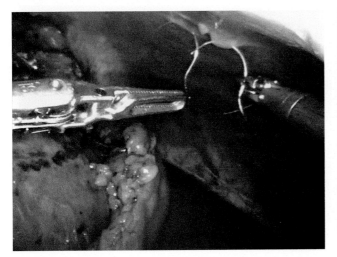

Fig. 29.4 Introduction of the sutures for renorrhaphy into the abdomen

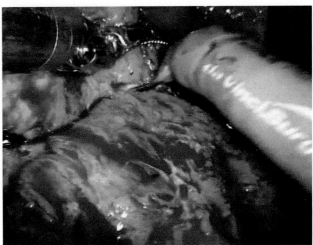

Fig. 29.7 Completion of partial nephrectomy

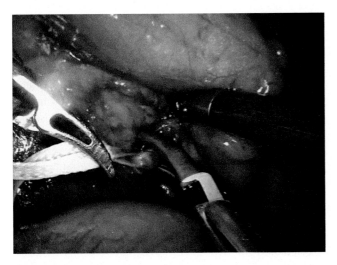

Fig. 29.5 Application of laparoscopic bulldog clamp on the renal artery

scissors with an adequate (few millimeters) parenchymal margin (Fig. 29.6). If no major bleeding is encountered, excision of the tumor can be completed (Fig. 29.7). If zero-ischemia RAPN is performed, the surgeon should keep in mind that this technique may have a risk of major bleeding. To address this, even in the zero-ischemia procedures, we introduce a laparoscopic bulldog clamp into the abdominal cavity and locate it close to the predissected renal artery and vein before starting excision of the tumor. If major bleeding occurs, a bulldog clamp can be easily applied on the renal artery and vein. In this situation, the level of experience of the assistant surgeon is extremely important. Therefore, we suggest having an available assistant surgeon who has experience with this type of surgery.

We use an absorbable poliglecaprone suture to perform internal renorrhaphy (Fig. 29.8). Each suture is kept tight

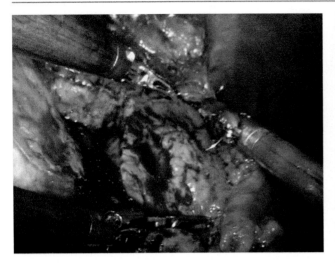

Fig. 29.8 Performing internal renorrhaphy with 3/0 monocryl suture

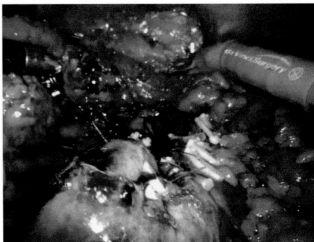

Fig. 29.11 Appearance of partial nephrectomy with internal and external renorrhaphy completed

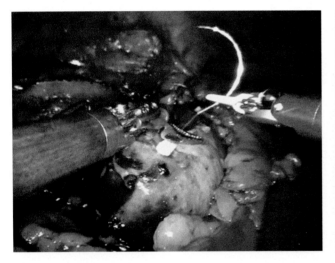

Fig. 29.9 Completion of internal renorrhaphy, applying polymer ligation clip

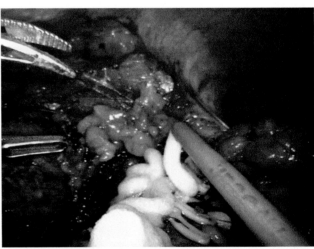

Fig. 29.12 Application of hemostatic agent over the partial nephrectomy surface

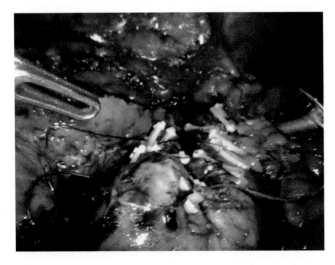

Fig. 29.10 Performing external renorrhaphy with 3/0 vicryl suture

by applying an absorbable endoclip on the renal capsule (Fig. 29.9). If the tumor bed is rather small, we proceed to external renorrhaphy using the same suture following completion of internal renorrhaphy (Figs. 29.10 and 29.11). The hemostatic agent may then be applied to the surgical area to achieve an adequate hemostasis (Fig. 29.12). Thereafter, the excised renal mass is placed into the endobag. After the vascular tapes are removed from the intra-abdominal cavity, the perirenal fat over the completed PN site is closed using a 3/0 polyglactin suture with an atraumatic needle (Fig. 29.13). The intra-abdominal pressure is decreased to 5 mmHg, and the surgical area is checked for bleeding. Following hemostasis, a drain is inserted into the abdominal cavity close to the surgical field. Abdominal ports are removed under direct vision and the port sites are closed.

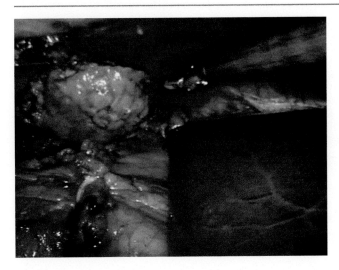

Fig. 29.13 Closure of perirenal fat tissue with a barbed suture over the partial nephrectomy area

Postoperative Care

Patients are given intravenous fluids, analgesics, and antibiotics postoperatively. Urethral catheters and drains are removed, and the patients are discharged from the hospital. Routine biochemistry and hemogram tests are carried out immediately after surgery and on the first day after surgery. A follow-up abdominal CT is carried out on all patients in the postoperative sixth month, after which patients are followed up with annual abdominal CT and chest radiography.

References

1. Kirkali Z, Canda AE. Open partial nephrectomy in the management of small renal Masses. Adv Urol. 2008;2008:309760. https://doi.org/10.1155/2008/309760. Published online 2008 Jul 15.
2. Ljungberg B, Bensalah K, Canfield S, et al. EAU guidelines on renal cell carcinoma: 2014 update. Eur Urol. 2015;67(5):913–24.
3. Minervini A, Vittori G, Antonelli A, Celia A, Crivellaro S, Dente D, et al. Open versus robotic-assisted partial nephrectomy: a multi-center comparison study of perioperative results and complications. World J Urol. 2014;32:287–93.
4. Fergany AF, Hafez KS, Novick AC. Long-term results of nephron sparing surgery for localized renal cell carcinoma: 10- year followup. J Urol. 2000;163:442–5.
5. Gettman MT, Blute ML, Chow GK, Neururer R, Bartsch G, Peschel R. Robotic-assisted laparoscopic partial nephrectomy: technique and initial clinical experience with DaVinci robotic system. Urology. 2004;64:914–8.
6. Abreu AL, Gill IS, Desai MM. Zero-ischaemia robotic partial nephrectomy (RPN) for hilar tumours. BJU Int. 2011;108:948–54.
7. Novak R, Mulligan D, Abaza R. Robotic partial nephrectomy without renal ischemia. Urology. 2012;79:1296–301.
8. Kaczmarek BF, Tanagho YS, Hillyer SP, Mullins JK, Diaz M, Trinh QD, et al. Off-clamp robot-assisted partial nephrectomy preserves renal function: a multi-institutional propensity score analysis. Eur Urol. 2013;64:988–93.
9. George AK, Herati AS, Srinivasan AK, Rais-Bahrami S, Waingankar N, Sadek MA, et al. Perioperative outcomes of off-clamp vs complete hilar control laparoscopic partial nephrectomy. BJU Int. 2013;111:E235–41.
10. Papalia R, Simone G, Ferriero M, Guaglianone S, Costantini M, Giannarelli D, et al. Laparoscopic and robotic partial nephrectomy without renal ischaemia for tumours larger than 4 cm: perioperative and functional outcomes. World J Urol. 2012;30:671–6.
11. Gill IS, Patil MB, Abreu AL, Ng C, Cai J, Berger A, et al. Zero ischemia anatomical partial nephrectomy: a novel approach. J Urol. 2012;187:807–14.
12. Ener K, Canda AE, Altınova S, Atmaca AF, Alkan E, Asil E, Özcan MF, Akbulut Z, Balbay MD. Impact of robotic partial nephrectomy with and without ischemia on renal functions: experience in 34 cases. Turk J Urol. 2016;42(4):272–7.
13. Dionigi G, Boni L, Rovera F, Dionigi R. Dissection and hemostasis with hydroxylated polyvinyl acetal tampons in open thyroid surgery. Ann Surg Innov Res. 2007;1:3.
14. Richter F, Schnorr D, Deger S, Trk I, Roigas J, Wille A, Loening SA. Improvement of hemostasis in open and laparoscopically performed partial nephrectomy using a gelatin matrix-thrombin tissue sealant (FloSeal). Urology. 2007;61(1):73–7.
15. Baumert H, Ballaro A, Shah N, Mansouri D, Zafar N, Molinie V, Neal D. Reducing warm ischaemia time during laparoscopic partial nephrectomy: a prospective comparison of two renal closure techniques. Eur Urol. 2007;52(4):1164–9.
16. Rouach Y, Delongchamps NB, Patey N, Fontaine E, Timsit MO, Thiounn N, Mejean A. Suture or hemostatic agent during laparoscopic partial nephrectomy? A randomized study using a hypertensive porcine model. Urology. 2009;73(1):172–7.
17. Gill IS, Ramani AP, Spaliviero M, Xu M, Finelli A, Kaouk JH, Desai MM. Improved hemostasis during laparoscopic partial nephrectomy using gelatin matrix thrombin sealant. Urology. 2005;65(3):463–6.
18. Morelli L, Morelli J, Palmeri M, D'Isidoro C, Kauffmann EF, Tartaglia D, Caprili G, Pisano R, Guadagni S, Di Franco G, Di Candio G, Mosca F. Robotic surgery and hemostatic agents in partial nephrectomy: a high rate of success without vascular clamping. J Robot Surg. 2015;9(3):215–22.
19. Simhan J, Smaldone MC, Tsai KJ, et al. Perioperative outcomes of robotic and open partial nephrectomy for moderately and highly complex renal lesions. J Urol. 2012;187(6):2000–4.
20. Sprenkle PC, Power N, Ghoneim T, et al. Comparison of open and minimally invasive partial nephrectomy for renal tumors 4–7 centimeters. Eur Urol. 2012;61(3):593–9.
21. Lee S, Oh J, Hong SK, et al. Open versus robot-assisted partial nephrectomy: effect on clinical outcome. J Endourol. 2011;25(7):1181–5.
22. Shen Z, Xie L, Xie W, Hu H, Chen T, Xing C, Liu X, Xu H, Zhang Y, Wu Z, Tian D, Wu C. The comparison of perioperative outcomes of robot-assisted and openpartial nephrectomy: a systematic review and meta-analysis. World J Surg Oncol. 2016;14(1):220.
23. Mearini L, Nunzi E, Vianello A, Di Biase M, Porena M. Margin and complication rates in clampless partial nephrectomy: a comparison of open, laparoscopic and robotic surgeries. J Robot Surg. 2016;10(2):135–44.
24. Ng CS, Gill IS, Ramani AP, Steinberg AP, Spaliviero M, Abreu SC, Kaouk JH, Desai MM. Transperitoneal versus retroperitoneal laparoscopic partial nephrectomy: patient selection and perioperative outcomes. J Urol. 2005;174(3):846–9.
25. Kieran K, Montgomery JS, Daignault S, Roberts WW, Wolf JS Jr. Comparison of intraoperative parameters and perioperative complications of retroperitoneal and transperitoneal approaches to laparoscopic partial nephrectomy: support for a retoperitoneal approach in selected patients. J Endourol. 2007;21(7):754–9.
26. Fan X, Xu K, Lin T, Liu H, Yin Z, Dong W, Huang H, Huang J. Comparison of transperitoneal and retroperitoneal laparoscopic

nephrectomy for renal cell carcinoma: a systematic review and meta-analysis. BJU Int. 2013;111(4):611–21.

27. Xia L, Zhang X, Wang X, Xu T, Qin L, Zhang X, Zhong S, Shen Z. Transperitoneal versus retroperitoneal robot-assisted partial nephrectomy: a systematic review and meta-analysis. Int J Surg. 2016;30:109–15.

28. Png KS, Bahler CD, Milgrom DP, Lucas SM, Sundaram CP. The role of R.E.N.A.L. nephrometry score in the era of robot-assisted partial nephrectomy. J Endourol. 2013;27:304–8.

29. Hanzly M, Frederick A, Creighton T, Atwood K, Mehedint D, Kauffman EC, Kim HL, Schwaab T. Learning curves for robot-assisted and laparoscopic partial nephrectomy. J Endourol. 2015;29(3):297–303.

30. Porpiglia F, Mari A, Bertolo R, Antonelli A, Bianchi G, Fidanza F, Fiori C, Furlan M, Morgia G, Novara G, Rocco B, Rovereto B, Serni S, Simeone C, Carini M, Minervini A. Partial nephrectomy in clinical T1b renal tumors: multicenter comparative study of open, laparoscopic and robot-assisted approach (the RECORd Project). Urology. 2016;89:45–51.

31. Leow JJ, Heah NH, Chang SL, Chong YL, Png KS. Outcomes of robotic versus laparoscopic partial nephrectomy: an updated meta-analysis of 4,919 patients. J Urol. 2016;196(5):1371–7.

32. Kim JH, Park YH, Kim YJ, Kang SH, Byun SS, Kwak C, Hong SH. Perioperative and long-term renal functional outcomes of robotic versus laparoscopic partial nephrectomy: a multicenter matched-pair comparison. World J Urol. 2015;33(10):1579–84.

33. Choi JD, Park JW, Lee HW, Lee DG, Jeong BC, Jeon SS, Lee HM, Choi HY, Seo SI. A comparison of surgical and functional outcomes of robot-assisted versus pure laparoscopic partial nephrectomy. JSLS. 2013;17(2):292–9.

34. Ener K, Canda AE, Altinova S, Atmaca AF, Alkan E, Asil E, Ozcan MF, Akbulut Z, Balbay MD. Robotic partial nephrectomy for clinical stage T1 tumors: experience in 42 cases. Kaohsiung J Med Sci. 2016;32(1):16–21.

35. Canda AE, Balbay MD. Robotic zero ischemia partial nephrectomy: step by step surgical technique with tips and tircks. Robot Surg Res Rev. 2014;1:1–9.

Radical Prostatectomy

Brett A. Johnson and Jeffrey A. Cadeddu

Introduction

Radical prostatectomy has been the gold standard for organ-confined prostate adenocarcinoma since its introduction over 100 years ago. While initially performed via a perineal approach, the retropubic approach quickly became the standard in the 1950s [1]. The first laparoscopic approach to radical prostatectomy was described in 1997 by Schuessler et al. [2]. At that time the minimally invasive prostatectomy was demonstrated to be feasible, but it was difficult and time-consuming and did not offer any benefits to the traditional open retropubic approach.

Since the introduction of the da Vinci surgical robot in 2000, there has been a revolutionary shift in the surgical approach to radical prostatectomy. Robotic-assisted laparoscopic prostatectomy (RALP) has become a de facto standard in the United States for management of localized prostate cancer. The advantages of stereoscopic vision, three-dimensional wrist movements, and an additional robotic arm have drastically decreased the difficulty of minimally invasive radical prostatectomy. It is important to note that the copious marketing by industry to facilities, providers, and patients also likely played a role in the rapid adoption of this modality. Compared to a laparoscopic radical prostatectomy, RALP primarily facilitates visualization, dissection, and suturing. Just as for radical retropubic prostatectomy, the goals of RALP are to maximize oncological control of prostate cancer and minimize risk of complication, morbidity, and functional loss.

Literature Review

As RALP has become more commonplace around the United States and Europe, numerous studies comparing it to the open approach have been completed. Retrospective comparisons between RALP and open surgery have demonstrated a significant decrease in operative blood loss and rate for transfusion [3]. Oncologically RALP delivers similar oncological control of prostate cancer. When comparing experienced surgeons at high-volume centers, the rate of positive margins is comparable between open and robotic prostatectomy [4]. Similarly, biochemical recurrence rates between open and robotic prostatectomy are comparable [5]. A Phase III prospective randomized control trial comparing open to robotic prostatectomy is underway in Australia. Six- and 12-week sexual function and continence outcomes are similar for both techniques. Neither open nor robotic technique demonstrated superior rate of positive margins [6].

Robotic surgery, in general, is more expensive than open surgery, and RALP is no exception [7]. This is due to the upfront and maintenance costs of the robotic surgical system as well as the large number of disposable and semi-disposable instruments required. RALP costs approximately $1155 per case more than open prostatectomy not including the upfront cost to purchase the device [8].

The biggest impact on patient quality of life following radical prostatectomy is the incidence of urinary incontinence and erectile dysfunction. Stress urinary incontinence following radical prostatectomy has been well described; however, some of the anatomical mechanisms are still being elucidated [9]. Several studies have demonstrated that recovery of continence by 12 months postoperatively is over 90% [10–12]. Furthermore, novel techniques to speed up the recovery of incontinence are continually being considered and evaluated [13]. Since the advent of better anatomical understanding of the neurovascular bundle, post-prostatectomy erectile dysfunction has decreased significantly [14]. A definitive conclusion regarding the difference in erectile function between open and robotic approach is

B.A. Johnson · J. A. Cadeddu (✉)
Department of Urology, University of Texas Southwestern, Dallas, TX, USA
e-mail: Jeffrey.Cadeddu@utsouthwestern.edu

© Springer Nature Switzerland AG 2019
S. Tsuda, O. Y. Kudsi (eds.), *Robotic-Assisted Minimally Invasive Surgery*, https://doi.org/10.1007/978-3-319-96866-7_30

difficult to reach. Various series have demonstrated that erectile function 12 months postoperatively ranges from 68% to 96% [3, 15, 16]. Although surgical technique is critical, preoperative erectile function and age are significant predictors of post-RALP erectile dysfunction, and patients must be counseled appropriately [17]. Many centers will utilize adjuvant phosphodiesterase-5 inhibitors (PDE5i) or vasoactive injections to decrease erectile dysfunction postoperatively. This is sometimes referred to as "penile rehabilitation." The basis of this treatment is the induction of nocturnal erections which may play a protective role in preserving erectile tissue [18, 19]. Some studies have demonstrated improvement in erectile function with daily administration of PDE5Is, while others have shown no difference [20, 21]. While our practice is to initiate daily tadalafil, overall, the literature is mixed.

Preoperative Planning

At its core, surgical indication for RALP is clinically localized prostate cancer in a patient whom the benefit of excision of the prostate outweighs the risks. Screening and diagnosis of prostate cancer are incredibly complex subjects and are beyond the scope of this chapter. Patients diagnosed with prostate cancer have a wide range of management options available to them including watchful waiting, active surveillance, radiotherapy with or without neoadjuvant androgen deprivation, or surgical excision. Carefully informed consent involving all options is necessary. The choice of management should be based on the clinical nature of the disease and the desires of the patient.

Clinical decision-making adjuncts may facilitate patient education and surgical planning. The Partin tables use clinical features of prostate cancer including Gleason score, serum PSA, and clinical stage to predict whether the tumor will be confined to the prostate [22]. Another important decision to make preoperatively is whether to perform a bilateral pelvic lymph node dissection (PLND). The role of PLND is not as clearly defined as it is for other malignancies. There is little doubt that PLND does convey a more accurate picture of cancer staging; however, the true impact on cancer-free survival is not fully elucidated. The Memorial Sloan Kettering Cancer Center developed a pre-radical prostatectomy nomogram that can help predict the chance of node positivity based on the patient's age, PSA, and biopsy details [23]. This can assist in discussion of the risks versus benefits of PLND. Many urologists will forego PLND if the chance of node positivity is less than 5%.

Preoperatively a full mechanical bowel preparation may be used but is usually unnecessary. Clear-liquid diet and one-half bottle of magnesium citrate the day prior to surgery are recommended to decompress the rectum. All anticoagulants should be held preoperatively. If the patient is systemically anticoagulated, they may be bridged with enoxaparin. Antiplatelet therapy should be held at least 5 days prior to surgery; however, for patients with high thromboembolic risk, RALP on low-dose aspirin has been described [24].

Setup

RALP is performed under general anesthesia with endotracheal intubation. An orogastric tube is necessary to decompress the stomach. The patient is positioned supine with the legs split. The arms are tucked to the side, and the patient is placed in steep Trendelenburg. The anesthesia team should be comfortable with the consequences of pneumoperitoneum including higher end-tidal CO_2 and oliguria. Adequate IV access must be obtained prior to positioning as the arms will not be accessible once they are tucked. The bedside assistant can be either on the left or the right of the operating table, but left is our preference. The robotic patient cart is aligned to be docked between the legs. In the discussion of port placement, we will refer to the assistant on the left and the fourth arm on the right; however, these may be reversed based on surgeon preference.

Most commonly, a transperitoneal approach is utilized for RALP; however, an extraperitoneal approach has been well described [25]. The extraperitoneal approach utilizes a balloon-dilating device to develop the space of Retzius. The operation then proceeds in essentially the same manner as transperitoneal. The benefit of an extraperitoneal approach is that the bowel is kept from the operative field, theoretically reducing the chance of injury. Also, in case of urine leak, urine is confined away from the abdominal viscera. Comparative studies have shown there is little to no difference in perioperative outcomes between these two approaches [26]. For the purposes of this chapter, we will describe the transperitoneal approach.

Pneumoperitoneum is typically obtained via the Veress technique. This is done either at the umbilicus or 2 cm above where the camera port will be placed. If there is concern for adhesions, an alternate Veress site or the Hasson technique may be used. The camera port is placed in the midline just above the umbilicus. An 8-mm robotic trocar is used for the camera port for the newest da Vinci Xi. For all previous versions of the robot, a 12-mm port is used for the camera port. Aside from the camera, three 8-mm robotic arm ports and two assistant ports (one 12 mm and one 5 mm) are used. The larger port allows for passing suture, clip appliers, and an entrapment sac. After placement of the camera port, the two medial robotic ports are placed 8–9 cm lateral to the umbilicus on either side. In the cranial-caudal axis, they should be either in line or just inferior to the umbilicus. On the left side, the third robotic port is placed 8–9 cm laterally to the medial robotic port and in line with it in the cranial-caudal axis.

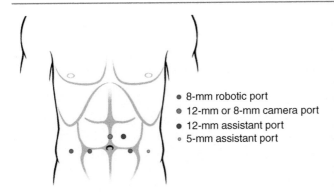

Fig. 30.1 Trocar placement for robotic-assisted laparoscopic prostatectomy with the bedside assistant on patient's left

- 8-mm robotic port
- 12-mm or 8-mm camera port
- 12-mm assistant port
- 5-mm assistant port

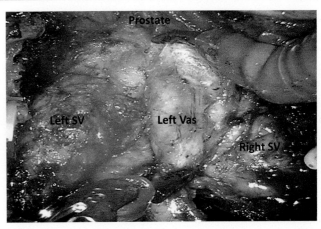

Fig. 30.2 The posterior approach begins with dissection of the vasa and seminal vesicles. These can be seen and dissected here

The 5-mm assist port is placed in the same location on the contralateral side. The 12-mm assist port should be on the same side as the 5-mm port and placed midway between the camera port and the ipsilateral robotic arm port in the medial-lateral axis and even with the umbilicus in the craniocaudal axis (Fig. 30.1). The distances should be measured after complete insufflation. In significantly obese patients, the ports should be placed slightly inferior to where the ports would be placed normally. A 0-degree lens is recommended for the entire case. Some surgeons will utilize the 30-degree down endoscope for apical dissection; however, it is usually not necessary.

Procedure

Open prostatectomy is performed in a retrograde approach (apex to bladder neck), and while this has been described via a robotic approach, the current standard for RALP is an antegrade dissection (bladder neck to apex). The antegrade approach allows for better identification of the neurovascular bundle.

There are two commonly described starting points of dissection, an anterior and a posterior (retrovesical) approach. Overall, the steps to the dissection are the same for each approach; however, the starting point differs. During the anterior approach, the initial step is to develop the space of Retzius and to release the bladder off of the anterior abdominal wall. Dissection of the seminal vesicles and vasa is performed after transection of the bladder neck. In the posterior approach, the initial steps are dissection of the seminal vesicles and vasa and then proceeding with release of the bladder from the anterior wall. The posterior approach is our preference and will be described here, but either approach is acceptable.

Any adhesions of the sigmoid colon to the anterolateral peritoneum should be released before beginning. The bowel then is gently retracted out of the pelvic cul-de-sac. Steep Trendelenburg will facilitate this. The peritoneum overlying the pouch of Douglas is incised transversely. By dissecting the fat underneath the peritoneum, the vasa can be identified bilaterally. The vasa are cauterized with bipolar current and transected with monopolar scissors. This should be done at least 3–4 cm from the prostate to allow the proximal end of the vas to become a handle for later dissection. The seminal vesicles can be identified lateral to the ampulla of the vas. A combination of cautery and blunt dissection should allow them to be exposed. Of note, the neurovascular bundle course just lateral to the tips of the seminal vesicles and monopolar current should be used sparingly in this area. The arteries of the seminal vesicles need to be identified and preferably cauterized with bipolar current. The seminal vesicles should be mobilized completely to their insertion into the prostate (Fig. 30.2).

Attention is then transitioned to release the bladder from the anterior abdominal wall. This begins with a transverse incision in the anterior peritoneum inferior to the umbilicus. An avascular areolar plane exists between the bladder and the anterior abdominal wall. Finding this plane will allow development of the space of Retzius. Utilizing the fourth arm for traction on the bladder cranially will facilitate the dissection. The longitudinally running cord-like medial umbilical ligaments will be encountered during this dissection. Cautery should be used to ligate and transect these to avoid bleeding. This space is developed down toward the pelvis until the prostate can be seen. Often there is periprostatic fat that needs to be dissected away to completely visualize the prostate. For high-risk patients, this fat can be sent for permanent pathology. An accessory pudendal artery will be present in approximately 25% of patients [25]. These can be seen typically just lateral to the puboprostatic ligament. If possible, these arteries should be preserved as they can contribute to erectile function.

Once the adequate visualization of the prostate, endopelvic fascia, puboprostatic ligaments, and pubic bone is obtained, dissection of the prostate itself may commence (Fig. 30.3). Bilaterally the endopelvic fascia is incised sharply. Pelvic floor musculature should be visualized laterally and the prostatic capsule medially. Careful sharp dissection without cautery is used to separate the muscle fibers off of the prostate on each side. Care should be taken toward the apex as the dorsal venous complex (DVC) can be unintendedly entered. The puboprostatic ligaments are then incised sharply. This exposes the DVC.

The DVC is a potential source for bleeding and should be approached with caution. Pneumoperitoneum will tamponade the DVC if it is entered unintentionally. This is one of the major reasons there is less bleeding in RALP compared to an open approach. The DVC is now suture ligated with a 2–0 or 0 polydioxanone suture (with or without barbs). The needle is passed underneath the DVC and above the urethra (Fig. 30.4). The non-sewing arm can be used to provide countertraction to better place and retrieve the needle. By ensuring the catheter moves freely when the needle is in the

DVC, accidentally piercing the urethra and catheter with the needle can be recognized and corrected. A figure-of-eight suture is adequate for ligation of the DVC. Some surgeons will opt to also place a figure-of-eight stitch to ligate the vessels on the anterior of the prostate. This is referred to as the "back-bleeder stitch" and can assist with hemostasis during dissection of the prostate. Attention can now be turned to the bladder neck.

The identification and transection of the bladder neck are one of the more nuanced aspects of this procedure. Without tactile feedback, the surgeon relies on visual clues for the development of the proper plane. The fourth arm is used to grasp the bladder and gentle cephalad traction is applied. Observing the balloon of the catheter as it is seated at the bladder neck can give a sense of where the bladder neck and prostate meet. Also, retracting the bladder neck medially can assist in visualization of the contour of the prostate as it meets the bladder neck [27]. The importance of this plane is paramount. If the incision is too distal, prostate tissue will be left behind. If too proximal, the bladder neck will have to be reconstructed and/or the ureteral orifices will extremely close to the vesicourethral junction and may interfere with the anastomotic suture.

Once the proper plane is identified, it is incised with monopolar scissors starting in the midline and moving laterally. The surgeon should be mindful of the bladder pedicle which can bleed if this incision is brought too laterally. Detrusor muscle appears visually much different than prostate tissue, so if prostate stroma is encountered, the incision should be moved more proximally. As dissection progresses deeper, the catheter is encountered. Once the catheter is seen, the balloon is deflated and retracted to the point that the fourth arm can grasp the tip of the catheter and pull toward the anterior abdominal wall. Gentle traction on the catheter from outside the body can tent the prostate up and away from the bladder (Fig. 30.5). If there is a very large median lobe,

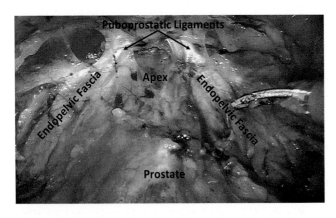

Fig. 30.3 Following dissection of the space of Retzius, the anatomical landmarks of the prostate can be seen

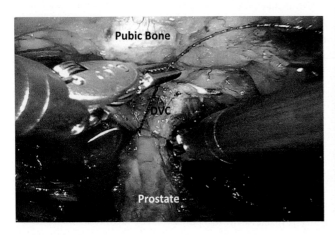

Fig. 30.4 After incising the endopelvic fascia bilaterally, the dorsal venous complex (DVC) is ligated with suture

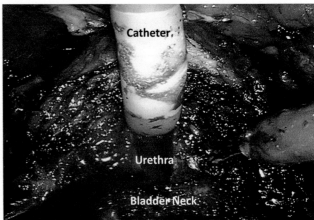

Fig. 30.5 The base of the prostate is incised and the urethra is exposed. The catheter is used for anterior traction during dissection

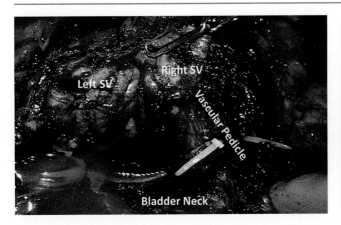

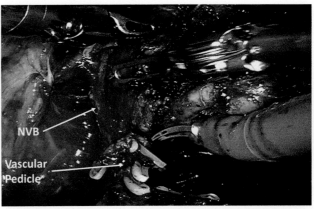

Fig. 30.6 The previously dissected seminal vesicles (SV) are brought through the incision in the base of the prostate. Using the fourth arm, the SVs are placed on anterior traction

Fig. 30.7 The left neurovascular bundle (NVB) is dissected away from the prostate capsule laterally, while the left vascular pedicle is taken with locking clips

this can be grasped with the fourth arm instead of the catheter. This traction/countertraction maneuver separates the prostate and bladder facilitating dissection of the posterior bladder neck. This dissection should be carried at a 45-degree downward angle to avoid a back wall injury to the bladder. It is important to stay in the midline for this step, as the vascular pedicles of the prostate lie laterally.

If the seminal vesical dissection is completed at the beginning as described above, the seminal vesicles will come into sight as the posterior bladder neck is dissected with monopolar scissors. The vasa and seminal vesicles can simply be brought through the opening in the posterior bladder neck (Fig. 30.6). If an anterior approach is performed, the vasa and seminal vesicles are dissected now in the same manner as described above. The fourth arm is utilized to grasp them and apply traction toward the anterior abdominal wall. This sets up dissection of the rectal plane and the pedicles.

Lifting the seminal vesicles and the vasa allows visualization of Denonvilliers' fascia. This fascia can be left on the anterior of the rectum or completely excised depending on severity of disease pathology and comfort of the surgeon. A transverse incision is made in this fascia, and blunt lateral dissection pulls the posterior prostate free from the anterior rectum. Posterior traction with the assistant's suction tip facilitates dissection of this plane. This plane should be brought close to the apex of the prostate as possible.

The next step is controlling of the vascular pedicles laterally. Many techniques have been described for control of the vascular pedicles. Techniques utilizing hemostatic sutures, locking clips, metallic clips, stapling devices, and bipolar electrosurgery have been described [27]. Regardless of the method, the key is appropriate isolation of the pedicle. Anterior and contralateral traction facilitates isolation of the pedicles. Blunt dissection is used to develop packets that are then ligated and divided. If a nerve-sparing approach is desired, the nerve bundles should be identified prior to liga-

tion of the pedicle. Control of the pedicle proceeds from base to apex on either side of the prostate.

Whether to utilize a nerve-sparing technique is dependent on the severity of the disease and the postoperative goals of the patient. If preservation of the neurovascular bundle (NVB) is desired, the levator fascia on the anteromedial aspect of the mid-prostate is incised. This develops an interfascial plane between the prostate capsule and the levator fascia. These layers are separated bluntly and carried from base to apex where the fascia separates from the capsule. The NBVs should be visualized and released before ligating the pedicle at that level (Fig. 30.7). Thermal energy is avoided during this dissection of the NVBs. The nerve fibers are highly susceptible to thermal injury as shown in both animal and human studies [28]. Most of the bleeding encountered during the NVB dissection is minimal and does not need thermal energy to control.

Once the NVB is released and the pedicles are divided, the DVC and the urethra are all that remain. This portion of the operation is critical as the apex is often a site of positive margins [29]. Also, excessive dissection at the apex can interfere with continence and erectile outcomes. Monopolar scissors are used to divide the DVC just proximal to the DVC stitch. Liberal use of cautery will minimize bleeding at the DVC. This should be taken down until the junction of the prostatic apex and urethra is visualized. Sharp dissection with minimal cautery is utilized to transect the urethra in an effort to prevent thermal injury to nerve fibers and sphincter muscle. As much urethral length as possible should be preserved, but incising too proximally on the prostate will lead to a positive apical margin. Once the urethra is incised, the catheter is pulled back so the posterior urethra can be identified (Fig. 30.8). Sharp dissection continues until the urethra is released. There is often a bridge of tissues (Denonvilliers' and posterior rhabdosphincter) below the urethra tethering the prostate to the anterior rectum. This area can be carefully

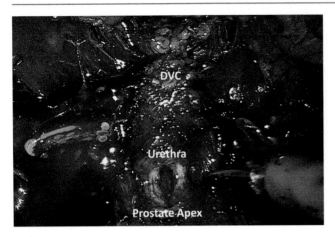

Fig. 30.8 After transecting the DVC, the apex of the prostate is incised revealing the urethra

dissected to release the specimen completely. Care is taken not to injure the rectum or NVBs.

The prostate and the prostatic fossa are then carefully inspected. If it appears there is residual prostate tissue in the fossa, this can be excised and sent for pathology. Residual bleeding at the pedicles is suture ligated to avoid cautery-induced thermal injury to the NVBs. If no nerve sparing is utilized, cautery can be used to achieve hemostasis. A 10-mm entrapment sac is inserted through the 12-mm assistant port, and the specimen is placed within it. The tether on the sac can be grasped through the 5-mm port and brought out through the trocar. This will facilitate retrieval of the entrapment sac from the camera port later.

If appropriate, the pelvic lymph node dissection is performed at this juncture. The peritoneum is typically already released from dissection of the bladder. The external iliac artery and vein are identified and vas deferens divided. The nodal packet is released from the medial aspect of the external iliac vein. It is bluntly dissected proximally to the iliac bifurcation and distally to the pubic bone. Gentle blunt dissection at the distal aspect of the nodal pack near the pelvic sidewall allows for visualization of the obturator nerve. Once the packet is dissected down to a pedicle, clips can be used to ligate and divide the pack. Clips should not be applied until the obturator nerve is visualized to avoid nerve injury or transection. The packet can be removed via the 10-mm assistant port or placed in a separate entrapment sac. While complications associated with lymph node dissection are rare, they are possible. Obturator nerve, external iliac artery, and external iliac vein are the most commonly injured structures (30). Small vascular injuries can be controlled with polypropylene suture; however, large injures require rapid conversion to open and intraoperative assistance from vascular surgery. Most obturator injuries lead to little functional impairment. If a complete transection occurs, the cut ends should be sutured together with the assistance of neurosurgeon [31].

Ureteral injury is very rare, but surgeons should be aware that the ureters pass over the common iliac vessels near the bifurcation.

The remaining steps involve reconstruction of lower urinary tract. The opening of the bladder is inspected. Depending on the dissection and the size of the prostate, the bladder neck opening may be considerably larger than the urethra. In this case, an absorbable suture can be used to narrow the opening to the bladder neck. The surgeon should take care not to occlude the ureteral orifices which enter the bladder posterolaterally.

One of the biggest challenges of traditional laparoscopic radical prostatectomy is the vesicourethral anastomosis. The advent of robotic surgery has greatly facilitated this portion of the operation by allowing greater visualization and wristed movements. The anastomosis is typically done with 3–0 or 4–0 double-armed absorbable suture. The anastomotic suture may be either barbed or non-barbed. The suture is initially placed at the posterior bladder neck, and each arm is run on one side from posterior to anterior. It is necessary to take deep bites of the urethra to prevent urine leak. Perineal pressure and intermittently advancing the catheter may facilitate visualization and access to the urethral stump. Once the suture has been run, the two arms meet at the anterior urethra. The throws are cinched progressively from posterior to anterior making a tight seal between the bladder neck and the urethra (Fig. 30.9). The two arms are tied to one another, and the final catheter is placed. It should irrigate freely with minimal extravasation of fluid. Figure-of-eight sutures may be placed at the site of leak if it is seen.

While preservation of the NVB during radical prostatectomy has been practiced for decades, modern advances in RALP technique often are related to return of continence. Various techniques have demonstrated improvement in overall continence. The "Rocco stitch" supplies posterior support for the vesicourethral anastomosis. A running absorbable

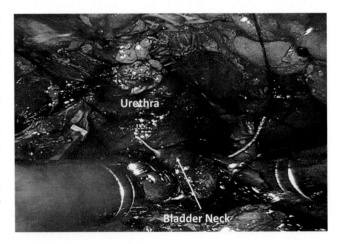

Fig. 30.9 Suture the vesicourethral anastomosis with a barbed absorbable suture

suture is used to approximate the remnant of Denonvilliers' fascia and posterior bladder neck to the posterior rhabdosphincter beneath the urethra [32]. There is evidence that a reduced angle of the membranous urethra related to the pubic symphysis facilitates urinary control [9]. Posterior urethral suspension (PUS) elevates the pelvic floor and reduces the membranous urethra-pelvic angle. Bilateral size 2–0 polyglactin sutures are preplaced into posterior urethral rhabdosphincter connective tissue at the 5 and 7 o'clock positions. Urethrovesical anastomosis is performed using a double-armed, running 3–0 barbed suture, careful to not incorporate suspension sutures into the anastomosis. After completion of the anastomosis, each suspension suture is secured to the ipsilateral pubic bone periosteum (Fig. 30.10). Canvasser et al. demonstrated that PUS patients had significantly improved objective measures of urinary control, including less use of protective incontinence products at 1 and 2 weeks after catheter removal. Patients also wore fewer pads and had less leakage on each pad from week 1 to week 4 after catheter removal. In this study, a 16 French suprapubic tube and an 18 French urethral catheter were placed postoperatively. The morning after surgery, the urethral catheter is removed. The suprapubic tube is capped at about 8–10 postoperative day, and the patient begins voiding. The suprapubic tube is subsequently removed at the first follow-up appointment on postoperative day 10–12 [13].

Once the urethrovesical anastomosis is complete, the operative field is carefully inspected. Some surgeons will decrease pneumoperitoneum to 8 mm Hg to inspect the pelvis prior to undocking. The pneumoperitoneum serves as a tamponade for venous bleeding. This can obscure large venous bleeders during intraoperative inspection and lead to postoperative bleeding. The bowel should also be inspected to make sure there was no injury during instrument exchange. A 15 French slit-lumen drain is optional and placed through any of the robotic ports and sutured in place.

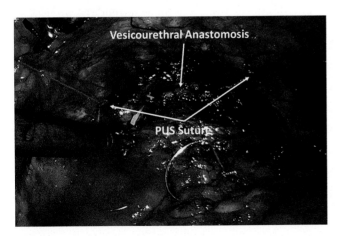

Fig. 30.10 With the vesicourethral anastomosis complete, the posterior urethral suspension (PUS) is performed

The patient cart may be undocked and then backed away. The 8-mm robotic ports typically do not need fascial closure, but the 12-mm assistant port should be closed with the Carter-Thomason fascial closure device. This can be accomplished robotically prior to the undocking or with the assistant holding the robotic camera as a laparoscope. The skin is closed and dressings are applied.

Intraoperative Complications

While RALP is, generally speaking, a safe operation, complications are possible. It is critical for the surgeon to immediately recognize and manage intraoperative complication. During any surgical procedure, proper positioning is critical to avoid neuropraxia and rhabdomyolysis. Prompt recognition of rhabdomyolysis postoperatively can prevent serious morbidity or death. Vascular or bowel injury is possible during peritoneal access or during dissection. The bedside assistant must be facile with exchanging robotic arms and passing in suture and be comfortable notifying the surgeon if resistance is felt. Any injury should be promptly recognized and managed to avoid more serious morbidity. Most small vascular or visceral injuries can be repaired robotically; however, open conversion may be required. Rectal injuries typically occur during posterior dissection. If they are recognized immediately, often a multilayer closure with absorbable suture is all that is required [27]. In patients with history of radiation, diverting colostomy should be considered. Any surgeon performing a RALP should be comfortable also performing an open radical prostatectomy in the case of a need to convert. While conversion is rare, it is an undeniable part of laparoscopic surgery (see Table 30.1).

Postoperative Care

Following postanesthesia care, patients are admitted to general care for one night (typically) in the hospital. A clear-liquid diet can be given the day of surgery, and the diet is advanced to generally the following day. If the drain output is less than 30 cc per 8 h, the drain can be removed on postoperative day 1. If the patient is tolerating general diet and their pain is well controlled with oral analgesia, he can be dis-

Table 30.1 RALP complications [30, 33–37]

Complication	Risk
Rectal injury	0.7–2.4
DVT/PE	0.5
Open conversion	<2%
Transfusion	<2%
Equipment malfunction	0.4%
Anastomotic complication	2%

charged at postoperative day 1. Flatus is not a requisite to discharge but is a good indication of return of bowel function. Patients are discharged with their catheter which is removed in 9–10 days. If the patient has both a urethral catheter and a suprapubic tube, the urethral catheter is removed day after surgery. The suprapubic tube is capped around postoperative day 8 and removed around postoperative day 10.

The surgeon must also observe carefully for postoperative complications. While the need for blood transfusion is commonplace for open prostatectomy, this risk is significantly decreased for RALP; nevertheless, checking a serum hematocrit level at postoperative day 0 and 1 is recommended. An anastomotic urine leak usually presents with elevated drain output and an elevated drain creatinine. Often these will resolve with prolonged catheter drainage; however, complete disruptions may require reoperation. If there is concern for urine leak, the drain should be left and a cytogram performed.

Conclusion

For many, RALP has become a preferred treatment modality for localized prostate adenocarcinoma. While not definitely proven to be superior to open prostatectomy, it has been shown to be safe and effective, and it offers technical facility to a nuanced operation. Robotic surgery is still evolving, and new advances are being made every day. There is little doubt that RALP continues to be a critical component for treatment of prostate cancer moving forward.

References

1. Denmeade SR, Isaacs JT. A history of prostate cancer treatment. Nat Rev Cancer. 2002;2(5):389–96.
2. Schuessler WW, Schulam PG, Clayman RV, Kavoussi LR. Laparoscopic radical prostatectomy: initial short-term experience. Urology. 1997;50(6):854–7.
3. Tewari A, Kaul S, Menon M. Robotic radical prostatectomy: a minimally invasive therapy for prostate cancer. Curr Urol Rep. 2005;6(1):45–8.
4. Brown JA, Garlitz C, Gomella LG, Hubosky SG, Diamond SM, McGinnis D, et al. Pathologic comparison of laparoscopic versus open radical retropubic prostatectomy specimens. Urology. 2003;62(3):481–6.
5. Schroeck FR, Sun L, Freedland SJ, Albala DM, Mouraviev V, Polascik TJ, et al. Comparison of prostate-specific antigen recurrence-free survival in a contemporary cohort of patients undergoing either radical retropubic or robot-assisted laparoscopic radical prostatectomy. BJU Int. 2008;102(1):28–32.
6. Yaxley JW, Coughlin GD, Chambers SK, Occhipinti S, Samaratunga H, Zajdlewicz L, et al. Robot-assisted laparoscopic prostatectomy versus open radical retropubic prostatectomy: early outcomes from a randomised controlled phase 3 study. Lancet [Internet]. 2016;388(10049):1057–66. Available from: https://doi.org/10.1016/S0140-6736(16)30592-X
7. Scales CD, Jones PJ, Eisenstein EL, Preminger GM, Albala DM. Local cost structures and the economics of robot assisted radical prostatectomy. J Urol. 2005;174(6):2323–9.
8. Lotan Y, Cadeddu JA, Gettman MT. The new economics of radical prostatectomy : cost comparison of open , Laparoscopic and Robot Assisted Techniques. J Urol. 2004;172(4 Pt 1):1431–5.
9. Soljanik I, Bauer RM, Becker AJ, Stief CG, Gozzi C, Solyanik O, et al. Is a wider angle of the membranous urethra associated with incontinence after radical prostatectomy? World J Urol. 2014;32(6):1375–83.
10. Menon M, Shrivastava A, Kaul S, Badani KK, Fumo M, Bhandari M, et al. Vattikuti institute prostatectomy: contemporary technique and analysis of results. Eur Urol. 2007;51(3):648–58.
11. Krambeck AE, DiMarco DS, Rangel LJ, Bergstralh EJ, Myers RP, Blute ML, et al. Radical prostatectomy for prostatic adenocarcinoma: a matched comparison of open retropubic and robot-assisted techniques. BJU Int. 2009;103(4):448–53.
12. Tewari A, Jhaveri J, Rao S, Yadav R, Bartsch G, Te A, et al. Total reconstruction of the vesico-urethral junction. BJU Int. 2008;101(7):871–7.
13. Canvasser NE, Lay AH, Koseoglu E, Morgan MSC, Cadeddu JA. Posterior Urethral Suspension During Robot-Assisted Radical Prostatectomy Improves Early Urinary Control: A Prospective Cohort Study. J Endourol. 2016;30(10):1089–94. end.2016.0220
14. Walsh PC, Schlegel PN. Radical pelvic surgery with preservation of sexual function. Ann Surg. 1988;208(4):391–400.
15. Menon M, Tewari A, Baize B, Guillonneau B, Vallancien G. Prospective comparison of radical retropubic prostatectomy and robot-assisted anatomic prostatectomy: the Vattikuti urology institute experience. Urology. 2002;60(5):864–8.
16. Kaul S, Savera A, Badani K, Fumo M, Bhandari A, Menon M. Functional outcomes and oncological efficacy of Vattikuti institute prostatectomy with veil of Aphrodite nerve-sparing: an analysis of 154 consecutive patients. BJU Int. 2006;97(3):467–72.
17. Briganti A, Gallina A, Suardi N, Capitanio U, Tutolo M, Bianchi M, et al. Predicting erectile function recovery after bilateral nerve sparing radical prostatectomy: a proposal of a novel preoperative risk stratification. J Sex Med. 2010;7(7):2521–31.
18. Montorsi F, Maga T, Strambi LF, Salonia A, Barbieri L, ScattonI V, et al. Sildenafil taken at bedtime significantly increases nocturnal erections: results of a placebo-controlled study. Urology. 2000;56(6):906–11.
19. Brock G, Tu LM, Linet OI. Return of spontaneous erection during long-term intracavernosal alprostadil (Caverject) treatment. Urology. 2001;57(3):536–41.
20. Montorsi F, Salonia A, Gallina A, Zanni G, Deho F, Briganti A, et al. There is no significant difference between on-demand PDE5-I vs PDE5-I as rehabilitative treatment in patients treated by bilateral nerve-sparing radical retropubic prostatectomy. J Urol. 2006;175(4):225.
21. Mulhall JP, Land S, Parker M, Waters WB, Flanigan RC, Burnett AL, et al. The use of an erectogenic pharmacotherapy regimen following radical prostatectomy improves recovery of spontaneous erectile function. J Sex Med. 2005;2(4):532–42.
22. Blute ML, Bergstralh EJ, Partina W, Walsh PC, Kattan MW, Scardino PT, et al. Validation of Partin tables for predicting pathological stage of clinically localized prostate cancer. J Urol. 2000;164(5):1591–5.
23. Stephenson AJ, Scardino PT, Eastham JA, Bianco FJ, Dotan ZA, Fearn PA, et al. Preoperative nomogram predicting the 10-year probability of prostate cancer recurrence after radical prostatectomy. J Natl Cancer Inst. 2006;98(10):715–7.
24. Binhas M, Salomon L, Roudot-Thoraval F, Armand C, Plaud B, Marty J. Radical prostatectomy with robot-assisted radical prostatectomy and laparoscopic radical prostatectomy under low-dose aspirin does not significantly increase blood loss. Urology. 2012;79(3):591–5.
25. Kirby R, Montorsi F, Gontero P, Smith Jr. J. Radical Prostatectomy: from open to robotic. Informa Healthcare; 2007.

26. Atug F, Castle EP, Woods M, Srivastav SK, Thomas R, Davis R. Transperitoneal versus extraperitoneal robotic-assisted radical prostatectomy: is one better than the other? Urology. 2006;68(5):1077–81.

27. Getzenberg RH, Partin AW. Campbell-Walsh Urology [Internet]. Campbell-Walsh Urology. 2012. 2748–2762.e6 p. Available from: https://doi.org/10.1016/B978-1-4160-6911-9.00098-0

28. Ong A, Su L, Varkarakis I, Inagaki T, Link R, Bhayani S, et al. Nerve sparing radical prostatectomy: effects of hemostatic energy sources on the recovery of cavernous nerve function in a canine model. J Urol. 2004;172(4):1318–22.

29. Touijer K, Kuroiwa K, Saranchuk JW, Hassen WA, Trabulsi EJ, Reuter VE, et al. Quality improvement in laparoscopic radical prostatectomy for pT2 prostate cancer: impact of video documentation review on positive surgical margin. J Urol. 2005;173(3):765–8.

30. Ficarra V, Novara G, Artibani W, Cestari A, Galfano A, Graefen M, et al. Retropubic, Laparoscopic, and Robot-Assisted Radical Prostatectomy: A Systematic Review and Cumulative Analysis of Comparative Studies. Eur Urol. 2009;55:1037–63.

31. Zhao W, Jiang W, He C, Tian Y, Wang J. Laparoscopic repair of obturator nerve transection during pelvic lymphadenectomy. Int J Gynecol Obstet. 2015;129(3 PG-273-274):273–4.

32. Rocco F, Carmignani L, Acquati P, Gadda F, Dell'Orto P, Rocco B, et al. Early continence recovery after open radical prostatectomy with restoration of the posterior aspect of the Rhabdosphincter. Eur Urol. 2007;52(2):376–83.

33. Lavery HJ, Thaly R, Albala D, Ahlering T, Shalhav A, Lee D, et al. Robotic equipment malfunction during robotic prostatectomy: a multi-institutional study. J Endourol. 2008;22(9):2165–8.

34. Secin FP, Jiborn T, Bjartell AS, Fournier G, Salomon L, Abbou CC, et al. Multi-institutional study of symptomatic deep venous thrombosis and pulmonary embolism in prostate cancer patients undergoing laparoscopic or robot-assisted laparoscopic radical prostatectomy. Eur Urol. 2008;53(1):134–45.

35. Webb DR, Sethi K, Gee K. An analysis of the causes of bladder neck contracture after open and robot-assisted laparoscopic radical prostatectomy. BJU Int. 2009;103(7):957–63.

36. Gonzalgo ML, Pavlovich CP, Trock BJ, Link RE, Sullivan W, Su L-M. Classification and trends of perioperative morbidities following laparoscopic radical prostatectomy. J Urol. 2005;174(1):135–9. discussion 139

37. Bhayani SB, Pavlovich CP, Strup SE, Dahl DM, Landman J, Fabrizio MD, et al. Laparoscopic radical prostatectomy: a multi-institutional study of conversion to open surgery. Urology. 2004;63(1):99–102.

Robotic Intracorporeal Urinary Diversion for Bladder Cancer

Abdullah Erdem Canda

Introduction

Robotic-assisted laparoscopic radical cystectomy (RARC) with extended pelvic lymph node (LN) dissection and intracorporeal urinary diversion is increasingly being performed in the management of invasive bladder cancer as a minimally invasive surgical approach, although open radical cystectomy (RC) is still the gold standard surgical approach in the management of muscle-invasive bladder cancer, in addition to high-grade, recurrent, noninvasive tumors [1].

In this chapter, an overview on this subject is given, and surgical technique is explained with preoperative and postoperative precautions.

Literature Review

Learning Curve

It was reported that, in order to reach an operative time of 6.5 h, at least 20 RARC procedures was required, and in order to obtain a LN yield of 20 or more, 30 cases were required [2]. International Robotic Cystectomy Consortium (IRCC) reported that learning curve for RARC demonstrated an acceptable level of proficiency following performing 30 procedures for proxy measures of RARC quality that included a series 496 RARC cases by 21 surgeons at 14 institutions [3]. Recently, Collins et al. concluded that totally intracorporeal RARC with intracorporeal neobladder is a complex procedure, but it can be performed safely, with a structured approach, at a high-volume established robotic surgery center without com-

promising perioperative and pathological outcomes during the learning curve for surgeons [4].

Oncologic Outcomes

Lymph node yield and surgical margins (SMs) in RC are considered as the most important parameters in surgical oncologic quality and efficacy. A positive SM rate of less than 10% [5, 6] and a LN yield of greater than 15 LNs [7–9] are recommended for oncological sufficiency in open RC. In the literature, the mean LN yield in RARC publications ranged between 15 and 21 and positive SM rate between 1.4% and 7% that suggest RARC has similar results compared to open surgery [10].

Recently, European Association of Urology (EAU) Robotic Urology Section (ERUS) Scientific Working Group carried out a multicenter study in order to evaluate if RARC with intracorporeal urinary diversion negatively impacts early recurrence patterns because of inadequate resection or pneumoperitoneum that included 717 patients. Early recurrence rates and locations appeared to be similar to those for open RC series [11]. Likewise, IRCC group that comprised a total of 1894 patients from 23 institutions in 11 countries concluded that the incidence of early oncologic failure following RARC has decreased with time. Disease-related rather than technical-related factors have a major role in early oncologic failure after RARC [12].

Nguyen et al. evaluated a series of 301 patients who underwent RARC for bladder cancer and concluded that predictors of distant recurrences, peritoneal carcinomatosis, and extrapelvic LN metastases after RARC did not significantly differ and were mainly related with pathological tumor characteristics and tumor biology rather than surgical aspects [13].

Because long-term follow-up time is not available for most of the published series, it is currently not possible to draw strict conclusions about the long-term oncologic efficacy of RARC. However, studies with short- and intermediate-term

All of the surgical figures included in this chapter are obtained from Prof. Canda's own robotic surgical cases.

A. E. Canda
Koc University, School of Medicine, Department of Urology, Istanbul, Turkey

follow-up demonstrated that RARC with intracorporeal urinary diversion has acceptable oncologic outcomes.

Complications

In our initial experience with RARC and intracorporeal urinary diversion, there were nine minor (grade 1 and 2) and four major (grades 3–5) complications in the perioperative (0–30 days) period and four minor and three major complications in the postoperative (31–90 days) period according to the modified Clavien system [14].

In a multi-institutional study with RARC performed in four institutions (n = 277), complications occurred in 68 patients (30%), with 7% having Clavien grade ≥ 3 complications. On multivariate analysis, decreased age and increased American Society of Anesthesiologists (ASA) score were detected as predictors of higher Clavien complication score [15]. In the IRCC multicenter study that involved 939 patients, 41% (n = 387) and 48% (n = 448) of patients had a complication within 30 and 90 days of robotic surgery, respectively. Of the complications, 52% were grade 0, 29% were grade 1–2, and 19% were grade 3–5. Most common complications occurred related with gastrointestinal system (27%). Remaining complications involved infectious (23%) and genitourinary (17%) systems. Multivariate analysis showed that increasing patient age, neoadjuvant chemotherapy, and blood transfusion were independent predictors of any and high-grade complications. During follow-up, 30- and 90-day mortality rates were identified as 1.3% and 4.2%, respectively [16].

Recently, Simone et al. evaluated outcomes of RARC and intracorporeal Padua ileal neobladders in 45 patients (17). The overall incidence of perioperative 30- and 180-day complications were 44.4%, 57.8%, and 77.8%, respectively, while severe complications occurred in 17.8%, 17.8%, and 35.5%, respectively [17]. IRCC evaluated outcomes of 1000 ≤ pT3 and 118 pT4 patients in a multicenter study who underwent RARC. The median blood loss was 350 mL. The complication rate was similar (54% vs 58%; P = 0.64) among ≤pT3 and pT4 patients, respectively. The overall 30- and 90-day mortality rate was 0.4% and 1.8% vs 4.2% and 8.5% for ≤pT3 vs pT4 patients (P < 0.001), respectively [18].

Due to the published literature, RARC with extracorporeal and intracorporeal seem to have acceptable complication rates. However, particularly series with intracorporeal urinary diversion have limited numbers of patients. Therefore, the outcomes should be interpreted cautiously.

Functional Outcomes

Functional outcomes include urinary continence and erectile functions in males following RARC. In our initial series of 27 patients with RARC and intracorporeal Studer pouch reconstruction, of the available 18 patients, 11 were fully continent, 4 had mild, and 2 had severe daytime incontinence [14].

Due to the results from the Karolinska Institutet that included 70 patients with RARC and totally intracorporeal modified Studer ileal neobladder formation, daytime continence and satisfactory sexual erectile function at 1 year were reported at 70% and 90%, respectively [19]. Torrey et al. also reported the functional outcomes of 34 patients who underwent RARC with Indiana pouch continent cutaneous urinary diversion (n = 31), and 30 patients (97%) had daytime and nighttime continence at a mean follow-up of 20.1 months [20]. Very recently, Asimakopoulos et al. reported the outcomes of 40 men with clinically localized bladder cancer whom underwent nerve and seminal vesicle sparing RARC with a modified Y-shaped orthotopic neobladder by the same surgeon [21]. The 1-year nocturnal continence rate was 72.5%. Erectile function returned to normal, defined as an IIEF-6 score greater than 17, in 77.5% of the patients within 3 months, while 72.5% of the patients returned to the preoperative IIEF-6 score within 1 year [21].

In summary, although the experience in the literature is limited with RARC with intracorporeal ileal neobladder formation, promising functional outcomes have been reported by few authors.

Open Versus Robotic Approach

The number of publications comparing open versus robotic approach is limited in the literature. In addition, the numbers of patients included in these studies are also limited.

Although some studies reported longer operation times in the robotic approach [22–25], others reported similar outcomes [26–28]. Many studies reported decreased intraoperative blood loss [22–25, 28, 29] and transfusion rates [25, 28] in the robotic group. Positive SM rates [22–24, 26, 28–31] and LN yields [22–24, 26, 28–31] were detected to be similar in most studies. In terms of complications, many studies suggested similar outcomes [22, 24–27, 30–32]. However, others reported decreased complication rates in the robotic group [28]. In a randomized clinical trial comparing open (n = 124) versus robotic (n = 128) radical cystectomy, Bochner et al. reported similar complication rates, hospital stay, pathologic outcomes, and quality-of-life outcomes between the groups. On the other hand, lower estimated blood loss and longer operating time were detected in the robotic arm [33].

Although some studies suggested an advantage in the robotic group in terms of quicker return of bowel function [22, 23] and decreased time to resumption of a regular diet [23, 30], others suggested similar outcomes [26].

Recently, Shen and Sun published the outcomes of randomized trials of perioperative outcomes comparing robot-assisted versus open radical cystectomy in a systematic review and meta-analysis [34]. In their study, significant differences were detected in terms of operative time favoring open group and estimated blood loss and time to diet favoring robotic group. No significant differences were detected in terms of complications, length of stay, positive SMs, and LN yield [34]. In a National Comparative Effectiveness Study by Hu et al. evaluating perioperative outcomes, health-care costs, and survival after robotic-assisted versus open radical cystectomy that included 439 patients in the robotic group and 7308 patients in the open group, greater LN yield and shorter hospital stay were identified in the robotic group, inpatient costs were similar, and overall survival and cancer-specific survival rates were similar [35].

In our own experience, we retrospectively compared open (*n* = 42) versus robotic (*n* = 32) radical cystectomy with intracorporeal Studer pouch and detected an advantages in the robotic group in terms of decreased blood loss, better preservation of neurovascular bundles, an increased lymph node yield, and a decreased rate of hospital readmissions for minor complication [36].

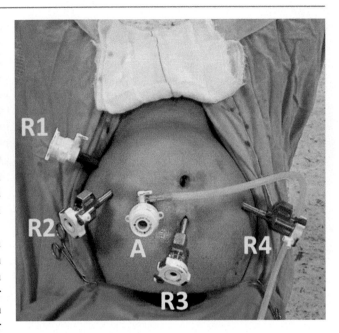

Fig. 31.1 Port sites, R1–4 are ports for robotic arms, and A is the port for assistant surgeon

Preoperative Planning

In our initial experience, although patients with a history of abdominopelvic radiotherapy and major abdominal surgery were excluded, currently we perform this complex procedure in this patient group in addition to patients older than 75 years old. Patients with comorbidities including pulmonary diseases, cardiovascular diseases, and endocrine diseases are consulted with these departments in the preoperative period. Therefore, optimization of the comorbid medical diseases including anemia in the preoperative period is provided.

Improved cystectomy care quality with enhanced recovery (ERAS) protocols has been suggested by many publications [37–39]. Preoperatively, patient counseling is carried out with detailed information given to the patients about postoperative outcomes that we think could reduce anxiety. Although in the past an osmotic laxative is given for mechanical bowel preparation, currently no mechanical or laxative bowel preparation is suggested. The day before the surgery, patients are given oral alvimopan and a clear liquid diet. In addition, a high carbohydrate diet 2–3 days prior to operation is suggested unless the patient is diabetic. Intravenous antibiotics (cefoxitin) are administered during induction of general anesthesia. Heparin is administered 1 h before the surgical procedure.

eral extended pelvic lymph node dissection, and transposition of the left ureter under the mobilized sigmoid colon to the right side. If a tension-free urethra-intestinal anastomosis could be performed, patient position might be changed to mild (5°) Trendelenburg position just before starting to perform intracorporeal Studer pouch reconstruction. Port sites are presented in Fig. 31.1. Overall, five ports are placed. Initially, an 8 mm robotic port is placed 5 cm above the umbilicus for robotic 0 degree camera for robotic arm 3. Then, an 8 mm robotic port is inserted about 11 cm from the umbilicus on the right side for robotic arm 4. Thereafter, another 8 mm robotic port is inserted about 9 cm from the umbilicus on the left side for robotic arm 2. Between this port and the camera port, a 12 mm assistant port is inserted about 1–2 cm above the line connecting them. Lastly, a 15 mm port is inserted about 2 cm above and medial to the left anterior superior iliac spine in order to introduce laparoscopic bowel staplers during division of the ileal segments. The rest of the time, an 8 mm robotic port is introduced through 15 mm port (port through port) for robotic arm 1. Maryland Bipolar Forceps, Tip-Up Fenestrated Grasper™, monopolar curved scissors (Hot Shears™), Large needle driver™, and a ProGrasp™ forceps are used. A 0° lens is used throughout the procedure.

Setup

Setup is explained for da Vinci Xi (Intuitive Surgical, Sunnyvale, California). Initially, patient is placed in deep (30°) Trendelenburg position until robotic cystectomy, bilat-

Procedure

Initially ileocecal valve and cecum are identified. A 10 cm or 15 cm sized vascular tape is introduced into the abdomen in order to measure the length of the ileal segments. A 15–20 cm

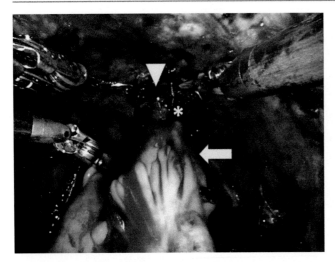

Fig. 31.2 Anastomosis between urethra and ileum. Arrowhead, urethra; arrow, ileum; *, anastomosis

terminal ileal segment starting from the cecum is spared. Starting from there, a 10 cm ileal segment is measured that is going to be anastomosed to the urethra. At that point on the ileum, an incision is made on the anti-mesenteric side with monopolar curved scissors. An anastomosis between the urethra and ileum is performed by using a double-armed bidirectional 3/0 PGA-PCL monofilament absorbable suture (17 mm, 1/2 circle, RB-1, taper point, 16x16 cm, STRATAFIX, Ethicon®) (Fig. 31.2). A 20 F Foley urethral catheter is inserted through the urethra, and its balloon is inflated with 3 cc sterile saline.

If the meso of the ileum is short, that will be anastomosed to the urethra, and for that reason if it is not possible to approximate the ileum to the urethra, several maneuvers could be done in order to overcome this problem including applying a perineal push and applying a vascular tape at the most dependent part of the segregated ileal segment for ureteroileal anastomosis that could be used for further traction; balloon of the Foley catheter could be further inflated and could be used for traction, and lastly transverse superficial peritoneal incisions on the meso could be made.

A 40 cm ileal segment on the left side of ureteroileal anastomosis is assigned for the pouch. Overall, a 50 cm ileal segment (10 cm on the right side and 40 cm on the left side on the ureteroileal anastomosis) is used for the Studer pouch. The first robotic arm is removed out though the 15-mm-sized port on the very left side, and laparoscopic ileal stapler is introduced in order to divide the ileal segments and perform side-to-side ileo-ileal anastomosis (overall, four 60 mm and two 45 mm EndoGia™ articulating medium/thick reload, Covidien® laparoscopic staplers are used). Laparoscopic ileal staplers are applied at the points sparing 40 cm ileum on the left side and 10 cm ileum on the right side starting from the anastomosis between urethra and ileum. Staplers are

placed perpendicular across the ileum and adjacent mesointestinum of approximately 2 cm (Fig. 31.3). Two 60 mm staplers are used here. Then, incisions by using monopolar curved scissors are made on the anti-mesenteric sides of the ileal segments to perform for side-to-side anastomosis (Fig. 31.4). Initially, a 60 mm stapler is introduced through the bowel openings and is fired, and thereafter a 45 mm stapler is also introduced and is fired in order to create enough space between ileo-ileal anastomosis (Fig. 31.5). Then, a 60 mm and an additional 45 mm stapler are applied in order to complete the side-to-side ileo-ileal anastomosis (Fig. 31.6). The remnant stapled bowel tissue is taken out through the 15 mm assistant port (Fig. 31.7).

Following completion of the side-to-side ileo-ileal anastomosis, the next step is to reconstruct the Studer pouch. The

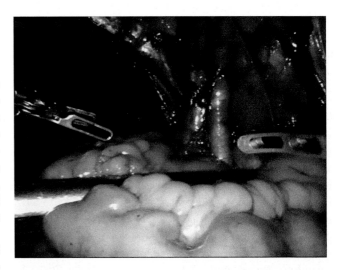

Fig. 31.3 Laparoscopic stapler is placed perpendicular across the ileum

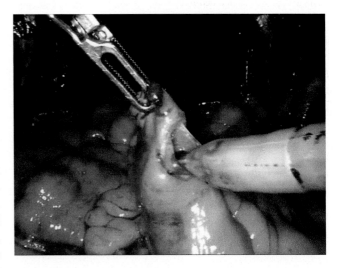

Fig. 31.4 Incision made by using monopolar curved scissors on the anti-mesenteric side of the ileal segment in order to perform a side-to-side anastomosis

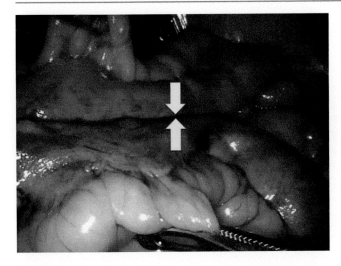

Fig. 31.5 A 60 mm laparoscopic bowel stapler is introduced through the ileal openings for ileo-ileal anastomosis. Arrow: stapler line

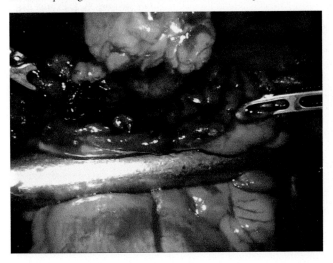

Fig. 31.6 A 60 mm laparoscopic bowel stapler is applied in order to complete the side-to-side ileo-ileal anastomosis

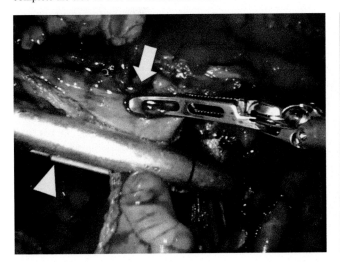

Fig. 31.7 A 45 mm laparoscopic bowel stapler (arrowhead) is applied, and the remnant stapled bowel tissue (arrow) will be taken out through the 15 mm assistant port on the left side of the abdomen

last (proximal) 10 cm ileal segment of the ileum to be used for the Studer pouch on the left side is spared as chimney/afferent loop, and the anti-mesenteric border of the remaining ileal segment is incised all the way long for detubularization (Fig. 31.8). It is important not to make the incision line close to the previously performed ureteroileal anastomosis in order to prevent disruption. Initially, closure of the posterior wall is completed by asymmetric closure. At the beginning, 4–5 interrupted 3/0 vicryl sutures are put for reinforcement. Thereafter, 2–3 V-LOC™ 180 absorbable wound closure device (3/0, 1/2 circle, 17 mm, taper point, CV-23, 30 cm, Covidien®) is used for posterior closure (Fig. 31.9).

In order to accomplish an asymmetric anterior wall closure, a 3/0 Vicryl suture is used in order to close the anterior wall of the pouch leaving the proximal redundant wall on the

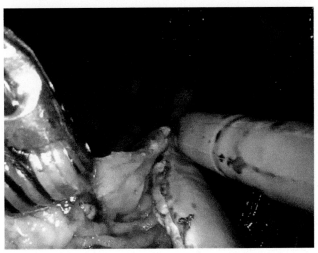

Fig. 31.8 Anti-mesenteric border of the ileal segment is incised all the way long for detubularization

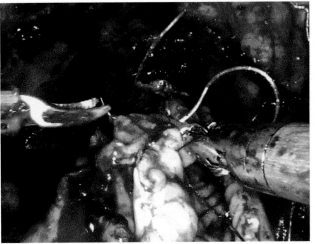

Fig. 31.9 A V-LOC™ 180 absorbable wound closure device (3/0, 1/2 circle, 17 mm, taper point, CV-23, 30 cm, Covidien®) is used for posterior closure

left open (Fig. 31.10). This opening will be closed at the end following introduction of the ureteral stents into the pouch. V-LOC™ 180 absorbable wound closure device (3/0, 1/2 circle, 17 mm, taper point, CV-23, 30 cm, Covidien®) is again used for anterior wall closure (Fig. 31.11).

The next step is performing a Wallace-type uretero-ureteral anastomosis. Ureters are spatulated longitudinally with monopolar curved scissors without applying any energy (Fig. 31.12). A 4/0 monocryl suture (15 mm, 1/2 circle, taper point, 15 cm, Tekmon®) is used to form the posterior plate (Fig. 31.13).

Thereafter, stapler line is excised at the proximal end of the afferent loop. Afterwards two ureteral stents (8F, 70 cm) are inserted in the midline through the abdominal wall by

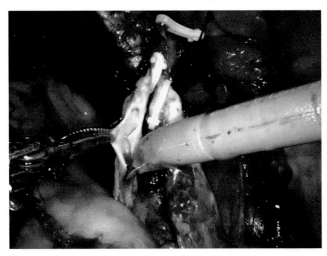

Fig. 31.12 Ureters are spatulated longitudinally in order to make a Wallace-type uretero-ureteral anastomosis

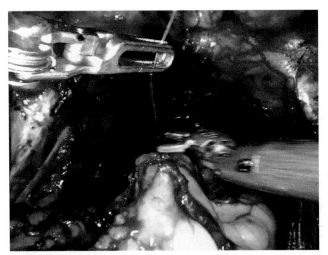

Fig. 31.10 An asymmetric anterior wall closure is accomplished by using a 3/0 vicryl suture or a V-LOC™ 180 absorbable wound closure device (3/0, 1/2 circle, 17 mm, taper point, CV-23, 30 cm, Covidien®) leaving the proximal redundant wall of the pouch left open

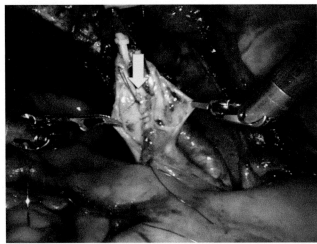

Fig. 31.13 A 4/0 monocryl suture is used to form the posterior plate (arrow)

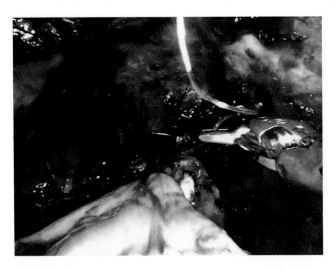

Fig. 31.11 V-LOC™ 180 absorbable wound closure device (3/0, 1/2 circle, 17 mm, taper point, CV-23, 30 cm, Covidien®) is again used for anterior wall closure

Seldinger method and into the abdominal cavity by the bed-side assistant surgeon. Initially, the soft end of the glide wire is introduced, and over the glide wire, the ureteral stent is advanced. They are taken through the anterior wall of the pouch (as proximal redundant wall on the left open afferent loop) and introduced into both renal pelvis (Fig. 31.14). An anastomosis is made between Wallace-type uretero-ureteral anastomosis and proximal end of the afferent loop by using a 17 mm, 1/2 circle, RB-1, taper point, 16x16 cm, STRATAFIX, Ethicon® suture starting from the 6 o'clock position with both needles. Alternatively, a double-armed 4/0 monocryl suture could also be used (Fig. 31.15).

Thereafter, the redundant ileal wall of the pouch is closed on itself with another running V-LOC™ 180 absorbable wound closure device (3/0, 1/2 circle, 17 mm, taper point, CV-23, 30 cm, Covidien®). While doing that, ureteral stents

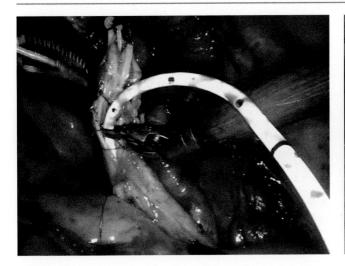

Fig. 31.14 Insertion of singe-J stents into the ureters and renal pelvis

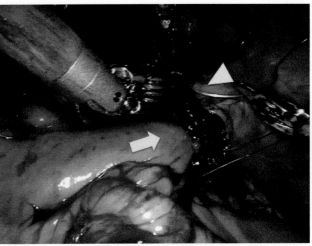

Fig. 31.16 Afferent loop fixed to the posterior peritoneum and is retroperitonealized. Arrow, afferent loop; arrowhead, peritoneum

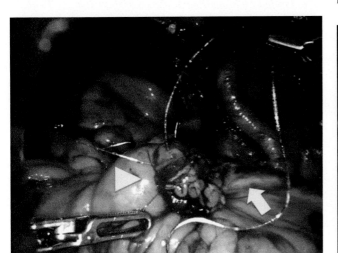

Fig. 31.15 Anastomosis between Wallace-type uretero-ureteral anastomosis (arrow) and proximal end of the afferent loop (arrowhead)

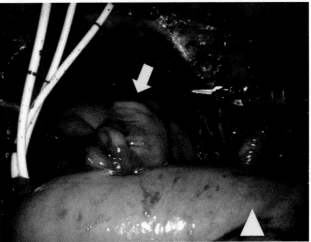

Fig. 31.17 Appearance of completed Studer pouch (arrow) filled with sterile saline in order to see a watertight pouch. Arrowhead: afferent loop. In this particular case, due to a right ureteric duplication, three singe-J stents were inserted

are kept between the sutures. Lastly, afferent loop is fixed to the posterior peritoneum and is retroperitonealized (Fig. 31.16) by using a 3/0 vicryl suture. Completed Studer pouch is filled with saline in order to see a watertight pouch (Fig. 31.17).

Postoperative Care

Nasogastric tube is removed on postoperative day 1 if no significant drainage is present. On postoperative day 1, early mobilization and early oral nutrition (with clear fluids and nutrition drinks) are suggested. Sugar-free chewing gum could also be suggested. For bowel function, medications including alvimopan and metoclopramide are suggested, and home medications are also started. For pain control, acetaminophen or NSAIDs could be used. Patient is taught how to irrigate the neobladder by herself/himself. Deep breathing exercises are suggested, and flutter valve is given to the patient in order to improve pulmonary function. Low-molecular-weight heparin is administered for vascular thromboembolic prophylaxis. Diet is advanced in the following days as tolerated. Following passing flatus, a regular diet is suggested. Drain is removed when there is no sufficient drainage (less than 100 cc). In case of a sufficient drainage, drain creatinine could be checked. At least 1000 mL fluid intake and normal diet are achieved before discharge. Stents are removed on postoperative day 14 [37, 38].

On postoperative day 21, cystography was performed by filling the bladder with 200 mL diluted contrast material. If no leakage was observed, the urethral catheter was removed; otherwise, the urethral catheter was kept for 1 more week for another cystography [40].

Postoperatively, patients were evaluated at 6 weeks, 3 months, and every 6 months thereafter with clinical examination and tests including serum creatinine, blood urea nitrogen, serum electrolytes, blood gas analyses, urine cytology, urine culture, and ultrasonography of the abdomen. Chest radiography, cystography, and urography were performed after 3, 6, and 12 months. Abdominopelvic CT was performed at 6 months and once a year thereafter [40].

References

1. Huang GJ, Stein JP. Open radical cystectomy with lymphadenectomy remains the treatment of choice for invasive bladder cancer. Curr Opin Urol. 2007;17(5):369–75.

2. Liss MA, Kader AK. Robotic-assisted laparoscopic radical cystectomy: history, techniques and outcomes. World J Urol. 2013;31(3):489–97.3.

3. Hayn MH, Hussain A, Mansour AM, et al. The learning curve of robot-assisted radical cystectomy: results from the international robotic cystectomy consortium. Eur Urol. 2010 Aug;58(2):197–202.

4. Collins JW, Tyritzis S, Nyberg T, Schumacher MC, Laurin O, Adding C, Jonsson M, Khazaeli D, Steineck G, Wiklund P, Hosseini A. Robot-assisted radical cystectomy (RARC) with intracorporeal neobladder - what is the effect of the learning curve on outcomes? BJU Int. 2014;113(1):100–7.

5. Herr H, Lee C, Chang S, Lerner S. Bladder Cancer Collaborative Group. Standardization of radical cystectomy and pelvic lymph node dissection for bladder cancer: a collaborative group report. J Urol. 2004;171(5):1823–8.

6. Skinner EC, Stein JP, Skinner DG. Surgical benchmarks for the treatment of invasive bladder cancer. Urol Oncol. 2007;25(1):66–71.

7. Stein JP, Cai J, Groshen S, Skinner DG. Risk factors for patients with pelvic lymph node metastases following radical cystectomy with en bloc pelvic lymphadenectomy: concept of lymph node density. J Urol. 2003;170(1):35–41.

8. Leissner J, Hohenfellner R, Thüroff JW, Wolf HK. Lymphadenectomy in patients with transitional cell carcinoma of the urinary bladder; significance for staging and prognosis. BJU Int. 2000;85(7):817–23.

9. Herr HW, Faulkner JR, Grossman HB, et al. Surgical factors influence bladder cancer outcomes: a cooperative group report. J Clin Oncol. 2004;22(14):2781–9.

10. Canda AE, Atmaca AF, Arslan ME, Keske M, Cakici OU, Cakmak S, Kamaci D, Urer E. Robotic radical cystectomy in bladder cancer: is it the future? Open Access Surgery. 2014;7:47–57.

11. Collins JW, Hosseini A, Adding C, Nyberg T, Koupparis A, Rowe E, Perry M, Issa R, Schumacher MC, Wijburg C, Canda AE, Balbay MD, Decaestecker K, Schwentner C, Stenzl A, Edeling S, Pokupić S, D'Hondt F, Mottrie A, Wiklund PN. Early recurrence patterns following totally Intracorporeal robot-assisted radical cystectomy: results from the EAU robotic urology section (ERUS) scientific working group. Eur Urol. 2017;71(5):723–6.

12. Hussein AA, Saar M, May PR, Wijburg CJ, Richstone L, Wagner A, Wilson T, Yuh B, Redorta JP, Dasgupta P, Khan MS, Menon M, Peabody JO, Hosseini A, Gaboardi F, Mottrie A, Rha KH, Hemal A, Stockle M, Kelly J, Maatman TJ, Canda AE, Wiklund P, Guru KA. Collaborators. Early oncologic failure after robot-assisted radical cystectomy: results from the international robotic cystectomy consortium. J Urol. 2017 Jun;197(6):1427–36.

13. Nguyen DP, Al Hussein A Awamlh B, O'Malley P, Khan F, Lewicki PJ, Golombos DM, Scherr DS. Factors impacting the occurrence of local, distant and atypical recurrences after robot-assisted

14. radical cystectomy: a detailed analysis of 310 patients. J Urol. 2016;196(5):1390–6.

14. Canda AE, Atmaca AF, Altinova S, Akbulut Z, Balbay MD. Robot-assisted nerve-sparing radical cystectomy with bilateral extended pelvic lymph node dissection (PLND) and intracorporeal urinary diversion for bladder cancer: initial experience in 27 cases. BJU Int. 2012 Aug;110(3):434–44.

15. Smith AB, Raynor M, Amling CL, et al. Multi-institutional analysis of robotic radical cystectomy for bladder cancer: perioperative outcomes and complications in 227 patients. J Laparoendosc Adv Surg Tech A. 2012;22(1):17–21.

16. Johar RS, Hayn MH, Stegemann AP, et al. Complications after robot- assisted radical cystectomy: results from the international robotic cystectomy consortium. Eur Urol. 2013;64(1):52–7.

17. Simone G, Papalia R, Misuraca L, Tuderti G, Minisola F, Ferriero M, Vallati G, Guaglianone S, Gallucci M. Robotic Intracorporeal Padua Ileal Bladder: Surgical Technique, Perioperative, Oncologic and Functional Outcomes. Eur Urol. 2016;pii: S0302–2838(16):30721–7. https://doi.org/10.1016/j.eururo.2016.10.018. [Epub ahead of print]

18. Al-Daghmin A, Kauffman EC, Shi Y, Badani K, Balbay MD, Canda E, Dasgupta P, Ghavamian R, Grubb R 3rd, Hemal A, Kaouk J, Kibel AS, Maatman T, Menon M, Mottrie A, Nepple K, Pattaras JG, Peabody JO, Poulakis V, Pruthi R, Palou Redorta J, Rha KH, Richstone L, Schanne F, Scherr DS, Siemer S, Stöckle M, Wallen EM, Weizer A, Wiklund P, Wilson T, Wilding G, Woods M, Guru KA. Efficacy of robot-assisted radical cystectomy (RARC) in advanced bladder cancer: results from the International Radical Cystectomy Consortium (IRCC). BJU Int. 2014;114(1):98–103. https://doi.org/10.1111/bju.12569. Epub 2014 May 22

19. Tyritzis SI, Hosseini A, Collins J, et al. Oncologic, functional, and com- plications outcomes of robot-assisted radical cystectomy with totally intracorporeal neobladder diversion. Eur Urol. 2013;64(5):734–41.

20. Torrey RR, Chan KG, Yip W, et al. Functional outcomes and complications in patients with bladder cancer undergoing robotic-assisted radical cystectomy with extracorporeal Indiana pouch continent cutaneous urinary diversion. Urology. 2012;79(5):1073–8.

21. Asimakopoulos AD, Campagna A, Gakis G, Corona Montes VE, Piechaud T, Hoepffner JL, Mugnier C, Gaston R. Nerve sparing, robot-assisted radical cystectomy with Intracorporeal bladder substitution in the male. J Urol. 2016 Nov;196(5):1549–57.

22. Nix J, Smith A, Kurpad R, Nielsen ME, Wallen EM, Pruthi RS. Prospective randomized controlled trial of robotic versus open radical cystectomy for bladder cancer: perioperative and pathologic results. Eur Urol. 2010;57(2):196–201.

23. Knox ML, El-Galley R, Busby JE. Robotic versus open radical cystectomy: identi cation of patients who bene t from the robotic approach. J Endourol. 2013;27(1):40–4.

24. Styn NR, Montgomery JS, Wood DP, et al. Matched comparison of robotic-assisted and open radical cystectomy. Urology. 2012;79(6):1303–8.

25. Sung HH, Ahn JS, Seo SI, et al. A comparison of early complications between open and robot-assisted radical cystectomy. J Endourol. 2012;26(6):670–5.

26. Parekh DJ, Messer J, Fitzgerald J, Ercole B, Svatek R. Perioperative outcomes and oncologic ef cacy from a pilot prospective randomized clinical trial of open versus robotic assisted radical cystectomy. J Urol. 2013;189(2):474–9.

27. Gondo T, Yoshioka K, Nakagami Y, et al. Robotic versus open radical cystectomy: prospective comparison of perioperative and pathologic outcomes in Japan. Jpn J Clin Oncol. 2012;42(7):625–31.

28. Ng CK, Kauffman EC, Lee MM, et al. A comparison of postoperative complications in open versus robotic cystectomy. Eur Urol. 2010;57(2):274–81.

29. Nepple KG, Strope SA, Grubb RL 3rd, Kibel AS. Early oncologic outcomes of robotic vs open radical cystectomy for urothelial cancer. Urol Oncol. 2013;31(6):894–8.

30. Wang GJ, Barocas DA, Raman JD, Scherr DS. Robotic vs open radical cystectomy: prospective comparison of perioperative outcomes and pathological measures of early oncological efficacy. BJU Int. 2008;101(1):89–93.

31. Kader AK, Richards KA, Krane LS, Pettus JA, Smith JJ, Hemal AK. Robot-assisted laparoscopic vs open radical cystectomy: comparison of complications and perioperative oncological outcomes in 200 patients. BJU Int. 2013;112(4):E290–4.

32. Sterrett S, Mammen T, Nazemi T, et al. Major urological oncological surgeries can be performed using minimally invasive robotic or laparoscopic methods with similar early perioperative outcomes compared to conventional open methods. World J Urol. 2007;25(2):193–8.

33. Bochner BH, Dalbagni G, Sjoberg DD, Silberstein J, Keren Paz GE, Donat SM, Coleman JA, Mathew S, Vickers A, Schnorr GC, Feuerstein MA, Rapkin B, Parra RO, Herr HW, Laudone VP. Comparing open radical cystectomy and robot-assisted laparoscopic radical cystectomy: a randomized clinical trial. Eur Urol. 2015 Jun;67(6):1042–50.

34. Shen Z, Sun Z. Systematic review and meta-analysis of randomised trials of perioperative outcomes comparing robot-assisted versus open radical cystectomy. BMC Urol. 2016 Sep 23;16(1):59.

35. Hu JC, Chughtai B, O'Malley P, Halpern JA, Mao J, Scherr DS, Hershman DL, Wright JD, Sedrakyan A. Perioperative outcomes, health care costs, and survival after robotic-assisted versus open radical cystectomy: a National Comparative Effectiveness Study. Eur Urol. 2016 Jul;70(1):195–202.

36. Atmaca AF, Canda AE, Gok B, Akbulut Z, Altinova S, Balbay MD. Open versus robotic radical cystectomy with intracorporeal Studer diversion. JSLS. 2015 Jan-Mar;19(1):e2014.00193.

37. Cerantola Y, Valerio M, Persson B, Jichlinski P, Ljungqvist O, Hubner M, Kassouf W, Muller S, Baldini G, Carli F, Naesheimh T, Ytrebo L, Revhaug A, Lassen K, Knutsen T, Aarsether E, Wiklund P, Patel HR. Guidelines for perioperative care after radical cystectomy for bladder cancer: Enhanced Recovery After Surgery (ERAS®) society recommendations. Clin Nutr. 2013;32(6):879–87.

38. Baack Kukreja JE, Kiernan M, Schempp B, Siebert A, Hontar A, Nelson B, Dolan J, Noyes K, Dozier A, Ghazi A, Rashid HH, Wu G, Messing EM. Quality Improvement in Cystectomy Care with Enhanced Recovery (QUICCER) study. BJU Int. 2017 Jan;119(1):38–49.

39. Collins JW, Patel H, Adding C, Annerstedt M, Dasgupta P, Khan SM, Artibani W, Gaston R, Piechaud T, Catto JW, Koupparis A, Rowe E, Perry M, Issa R, McGrath J, Kelly J, Schumacher M, Wijburg C, Canda AE, Balbay MD, Decaestecker K, Schwentner C, Stenzl A, Edeling S, Pokupić S, Stockle M, Siemer S, Sanchez-Salas R, Cathelineau X, Weston R, Johnson M, D'Hondt F, Mottrie A, Hosseini A, Wiklund PN. Enhanced Recovery After Robot-assisted Radical Cystectomy: EAU Robotic Urology Section Scientific Working Group Consensus View. Eur Urol. 2016;70(4):649–60.

40. Akbulut Z, Canda AE, Ozcan MF, Atmaca AF, Ozdemir AT, Balbay MD. Robot-assisted laparoscopic nerve-sparing radical cystoprostatectomy with bilateral extended lymph node dissection and intracorporeal Studer pouch construction: outcomes of first 12 cases. J Endourol. 2011;25(9):1469–79.

Part V

Cardiothoracic

Robotic CABG

32

Scott C. DeRoo and Micahel Argenziano

Introduction

Coronary artery disease (CAD) remains one of the leading causes of death, being responsible for over eight million deaths worldwide and greater than 600,000 deaths in the USA annually [1, 2]. Over the past several decades, the prevention and treatment of coronary artery disease have undergone significant change and improvement; however, the persistently high morbidity and mortality of this condition remain a challenging clinical problem. Current treatment of CAD focuses largely on primary medical prevention through the use of statin medications; however, severe or symptomatic CAD is subject to more invasive and definitive management. At present, there are two main options for the treatment of CAD: percutaneous coronary intervention (PCI) and/or surgical revascularization.

Surgical revascularization was first pioneered in the early 1960s when a saphenous vein was grafted from the aorta to a coronary vessel [3]. Since that time the procedure has undergone multiple refinements; however, the overall principle of restoring blood flow to an occluded coronary artery via a bypass graft has remained the same. In the modern era, the use of saphenous vein grafts has decreased in favor of arterial conduits and PCI, which have demonstrated improved patency when compared to saphenous veins. In particular, the unique physiologic properties of the internal mammary artery (IMA) have made it well-suited for use as a bypass conduit, and long-term patency rates in excess of 95% at 10 years supersede that of saphenous vein grafts and drug-eluting stents [4]. Use of the left IMA (LIMA) to bypass the left anterior descending artery has been demonstrated to confer a significant survival advantage when compared to both PCI and the use of vein grafts and continues to offer the greatest benefit to patients with regard to long-term survival.

Although LIMA-LAD has remained the "gold standard" for coronary revascularization, the use of additional arterial conduits or vein grafts to revascularize other coronary vessels has recently come under scrutiny. Current generation drug-eluting stents demonstrate equal or superior patency when compared to vein grafts used to bypass non-LAD targets and spare patients from a traumatic, open cardiac surgical procedure. The use of additional arterial conduits may result in patency rates similar to or greater than drug-eluting stents; however, the adoption of total arterial revascularization is not a widespread practice as it requires additional surgical expertise and comes with increased short-term risks such as a higher rate of sternal wound infection.

Given the significant survival advantage conferred by LIMA-LAD bypass, as well as improvements in DES and PCI, several clinicians have proposed a hybrid approach, in which LAD lesions are treated by LIMA-LAD bypass and all other coronary lesions with PCI in order to maximize the benefit and minimize risk associated with each procedure [5–7]. In order to minimize surgical risk as well as invasiveness of therapy, several groups began working toward a minimally invasive procedure through which an isolated LIMA-LAD bypass could be performed. Although initial attempts at minimally invasive LIMA harvest and coronary anastomosis were performed thoracoscopically, it was not until the advent of the surgical robot that enthusiasm for this minimally invasive technique began to grow [8–10].

Development and History of Robotic CABG

Minimally invasive CABG was initially developed in order to prevent patients from developing complications related to a full sternotomy and cardiopulmonary bypass. Initial

S. C. DeRoo
Cardiothoracic Surgery, Columbia University/New-York Presbyterian Hospital, New York, NY, USA

M. Argenziano (✉)
Department of Surgery, New-York Presbyterian Hospital, New York, NY, USA
e-mail: ma66@cumc.columbia.edu

© Springer Nature Switzerland AG 2019
S. Tsuda, O. Y. Kudsi (eds.), *Robotic-Assisted Minimally Invasive Surgery*, https://doi.org/10.1007/978-3-319-96866-7_32

attempts at minimally invasive CABG utilized either an inferior hemisternotomy with conventional IMA harvest or port-access thoracoscopic mammary artery harvest with LIMA-LAD anastomosis performed through a left anterior mini-thoracotomy [11]. Coronary anastomosis was then performed with or without the use of cardiopulmonary bypass depending on the nature of the specific case as well as surgeon preference. Given the complexity and steep learning curve of thoracoscopic mammary artery harvest, as well as the relatively superior results of CABG vs early-generation stents, enthusiasm for the procedure remained limited.

In the year 2000 the DaVinci© Surgical Robot was approved for use (Intuitive Surgical Systems, California) and simplified both the learning curve and process of minimally invasive mammary artery harvest. Despite initial enthusiasm, robotic multivessel CABG failed to gain significant traction in the cardiac surgical community. Though multifactorial, a still-significant learning curve as well as concerns regarding completeness of revascularization likely contributed to a lack of enthusiasm in the cardiac surgical community as a whole. Despite these concerns several groups maintained an interest in minimally invasive robotic CABG and over time have demonstrated conclusively that with experience, outcomes equivalent or superior to traditional CABG can be achieved [5–7, 12–14]. In part due to publicity achieved by these select groups, the total number of robotically performed CABG has been increasing, with the volume of robotic CABG as a percentage of total CABG increasing slightly from 0.59% in 2006 to 0.97% in 2012 [15]. With the continued emergence of increasingly efficacious drug-eluting stents and percutaneous techniques, there appears to be renewed interest in robotic and minimally invasive CABG, not as an isolated procedure but as a component of a "hybrid" approach which combines the benefits of PCI and CABG while minimizing risk and invasiveness.

Types of Robotic CABG

Robotic CABG can be classified into three main groups with regard to the invasiveness of the procedure as well as the need for cardiopulmonary bypass. These groups include minimally invasive direct access coronary bypass (MIDCAB), on-pump totally endoscopic coronary artery bypass (TECAB), and off-pump TECAB. Although similar, each approach carries a unique set of risks and benefits, and the choice of which type of robotic CABG to perform should be carefully tailored to each patient with regard not only to patient-specific factors but also to institutional and individual surgeon expertise.

Robotic MIDCAB

Robotic MIDCAB is performed similarly to thoracoscopic MIDCAB but relies on the use of the surgical robot for harvesting of the IMA. For harvest of the LIMA or RIMA, a robotic camera port is typically placed in the fourth intercostal space on the midclavicular line in the left chest. Carbon dioxide insufflation is used to create a controlled pneumothorax with pressures between 6 and 12 mmHg prior to introduction of the camera. Two additional instrument ports are created: one in the third or fourth ICS on the anterior axillary line and the other in the sixth or seventh ICS on the anterior axillary line [16]. (Fig. 32.1). This allows for full visualization and access of the LAD, as well as the LIMA and RIMA. Once ports are appropriately placed, the mediastinum is separated from the chest wall, and the LIMA or RIMA is harvested in a technique similar to open surgery. When the IMA harvest is complete, the center port is converted to a 4–5 cm anterior non-rib-spreading mini-thoracotomy. A soft tissue retractor is positioned, pericardiotomy is performed, and the target coronary artery is identified (Fig. 32.2). A suction stabilizer is passed through the inferior port incision and held by an attachment to the rib retractor, and standard off-pump CABG techniques are used to perform an open coronary anastomosis (Fig. 32.3). In some cases, multiple vessels may be bypassed if they are accessible via the anterior mini-thoracotomy. In general, this is limited to diagonal branches or a ramus branch (Fig. 32.4). In the event

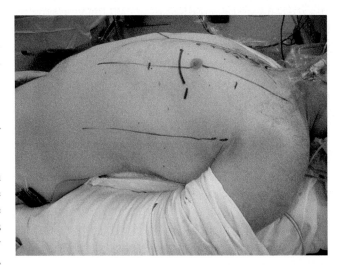

Fig. 32.1 Preoperative marking of MIDCAB patient. The sternum as well as all appropriate interspaces are identified and marked. The anterior axillary line is marked, as is the midclavicular line. Port sites as well as the location of the small anterior thoracotomy are identified and clearly demarcated. Careful preoperative planning is essential to the success of a MIDCAB procedure

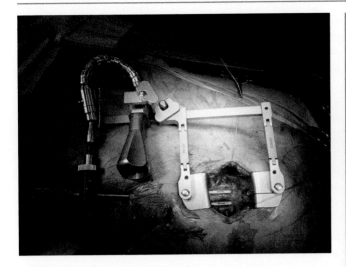

Fig. 32.2 Positioning for robotically assisted MIDCAB. A small approximately 4–5 cm anterior
thoracotomy is performed directly over the LAD. A soft tissue retractor is in place, and a suction stabilization device is employed to reduce movement of the LAD during anastomosis.

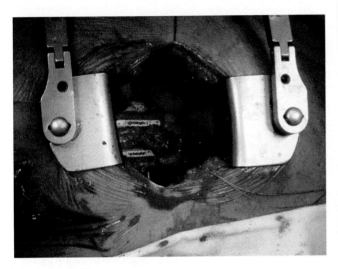

Fig. 32.3 Close-up of the LIMA-LAD anastomosis performed with the aid of the suction stabilizer device. Note the importance of placing the mini-thoracotomy incision directly over the area of the LAD where anastomosis will take place

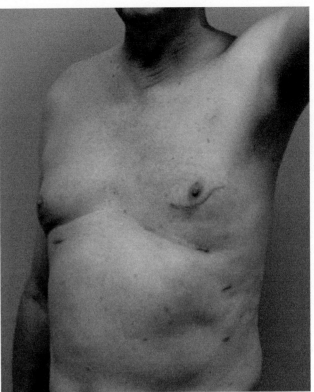

Fig. 32.4 Postoperative scars from multivessel robotically assisted MIDCAB. The patient in this image underwent LIMA-D1-LAD sequential grafting with robotic harvest of the LIMA. The physical proximity of the LAD and D1 allows for a relatively small anterior mini-thoracotomy

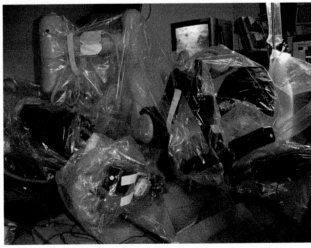

Fig. 32.5 The surgical robot is prepared and docked with a patient undergoing TECAB

that the patient does not tolerate positioning for an off-pump anastomosis, bypass may be initiated via peripheral cannulation.

Total Endoscopic Coronary Artery Bypass (TECAB)

Total endoscopic coronary artery bypass (TECAB) is performed similarly to robotic MIDCAB; however, the IMA to coronary artery anastomosis is performed in a totally endo-

scopic fashion with the aid of the robot (Fig. 32.5). Ports are placed in a similar location to that of robotic MIDCAB; however, after harvest of the IMA, tissue-stabilizing devices are placed via one to two additional ports. After satisfactory positioning of the stabilizer devices, the surgeon must decide whether to proceed on an arrested heart or beating heart. The decision to utilize CPB or arrest the heart must be made on a patient by patient basis with specific regard to surgeon experience, preference, and individual patient factors. Should the decision be made to proceed with the use of CPB, this is achieved peripherally with femoral arterial and venous cannulation, and if cardioplegic arrest is desired, it can be accomplished with a peripherally inserted endoaortic balloon or even a transthoracic aortic cross-clamp. After successful anastomosis, the heart is reperfused and cardiopulmonary bypass weaned. Importantly, in order to utilize the endoaortic balloon, a patient must have appropriately sized femoral vessels free of atherosclerosis and tortuosity such that they can accommodate the relatively large size of the balloon catheter.

There are several options for performing an IMA to coronary artery anastomosis in both MIDCAB and TECAB. Both techniques allow a skilled operator to perform a conventional suture anastomosis using polypropylene suture; however, this is a challenging procedure with a steep learning curve. Additional options for anastomosis include a sutureless anastomotic device that provides a rapid, automatic anastomosis using several interrupted micro-stell clips [17]. The use of automatic anastomotic devices or a traditional suture anastomosis requires considerable skill and specific expertise, and as a result only a small number of surgeons routinely choose to perform this technique. The relative difficulty of anastomosis is one reason for the lack of widespread popularity of TECAB.

Sequence and Timing of Hybrid Robotic Revascularization

In general, most surgeons who perform MIDCAB or TECAB do so with the intention of performing only a LIMA-LAD anastomosis. Therefore, the remainder of coronary lesions must be treated with PCI. The decision as to whether perform PCI prior to CABG, at the same time as CABG, or after CABG remains debated, with each approach carrying advantages and disadvantages.

In one-stage hybrid revascularization, PCI and CABG are performed in the same hybrid operating room in the same anesthesia setting. Typically, the LIMA-LAD anastomosis is performed first followed by PCI of the remaining lesions. When performed in this sequence, the LIMA-LAD bypass offers relative protection to the LAD territory during PCI and may allow for more complete revascularization via PCI [18]. Additionally, the patency of the LIMA-LAD anastomosis may be confirmed angiographically prior to leaving the operating room, and patients generally report a high level of satisfaction with a "one-stop" procedure [19]. Disadvantages of this technique include longer operative times, higher costs, higher risk of kidney injury, risk of stent thrombosis, and

higher bleeding risks [18]. The risk of bleeding is attributable to the use of dual antiplatelet agents (DAPT), while the risk of stent thrombosis is due to the proinflammatory and hypercoagulable state that occurs following surgery [20, 21].

The most commonly utilized sequence for a two-stage hybrid revascularization is CABG prior to PCI. When performed in this order, patients who can be fully heparinized for CABG are not on DAPT for prior stent placement and therefore have a lower risk of bleeding and have time to resolve the postsurgical inflammatory state [22] prior to PCI. Additionally, once PCI is performed, DAPT may be initiated and continued without interruption or increased risk of bleeding.

The performance of PCI prior to CABG is generally less preferable. It is often utilized for patients who present with an acute coronary syndrome with a non-LAD culprit. Advantages include prompt revascularization of culprit lesions and angiographic assessment of the LIMA; however, the disadvantages generally outweigh the advantages. These include a higher risk of bleeding as CABG is performed on DAPT and a higher risk of stent thrombosis given the proinflammatory and hypercoagulable state induced by surgery or protamine/platelet administration [22].

Patient Selection for MIDCAB/TECAB

There are few absolute contraindications to robotic MIDCAB or TECAB; however, in general sicker patients are best served by a traditional open revascularization procedure or PCI. Absolute contraindications to TECAB include cardiogenic shock, hemodynamic instability, inability to tolerate single lung ventilation, and ascending aortic aneurysm/concomitant cardiac pathology. Relative contraindications include significant intrathoracic space limitations secondary to chest wall deformities, intrathoracic adhesions, previous cardiac/thoracic surgery, intramyocardial coronary arteries, and peripheral arterial disease.

Outcomes

Evaluation of hybrid coronary revascularization (HCR) and minimally invasive CABG have been limited by the absence of a randomized, prospective, multicenter trial. Over the past two decades, the feasibility, safety, and efficacy of MIDCAB and TECAB have been evaluated largely through single-institution retrospective studies and meta-analyses. With respect to MIDCAB, from 1999 to 2009, 13 studies evaluated the safety and efficacy of hybrid coronary revascularization [19, 23–34]. Thirty-day mortality ranged from 0% to 1.4%, with most studies reporting a 0% 30-day mortality. Additionally, early outcomes were favorable with most studies reporting shorter intensive care stay, shorter duration of intubation, and shorter hospital stay. Recent studies have also confirmed these early results. Harskamp et al. compared both short- and midterm outcomes among patients undergoing hybrid coronary revascularization with patients undergoing traditional on-pump CABG. The incidence of a composite endpoint of death, MI, and stroke at 30 days was comparable between groups (3.3% vs 3.1%, $p = 0.85$); however, in-hospital morbidity (a combination of reoperation, renal failure, prolonged ventilation, and access-site infections) was markedly lower in the HCR group (8.5% vs 15.5%, $p = 0.005$) [13]. Additionally, the need for blood transfusion was significantly lower in the HCR group, a result that has been observed in several studies of HCR. These results have been further confirmed in a recent meta-analysis comparing HCR to conventional CABG. Among 6 observational studies including 1190 patients, 366 of whom underwent HCR, HCR was associated with lower in-hospital need for blood transfusions, shorter length of stay, and faster return to work [35]. Again, no significant difference was found in the composite endpoint of death, MI, stroke, or repeat revascularization during the index hospitalization. Midterm results of HCR were similarly encouraging, with 5-year survival >90% and similar angiographic patency to conventional CABG. Overall aesthetic outcomes are excellent, with patients pleased with the lack of sternotomy incision (Fig. 32.6).

Importantly, one limitation of these studies is the heterogeneity of technique in HCR. Although most contemporary groups utilized a robot to perform mammary artery harvest, several studies did not utilize robotics for any portion of the HCR procedure, thus limiting conclusions regarding the robotic contribution to these results. Additionally, although most groups performed only LIMA-LAD bypass, several groups did perform multiple vessel bypass with encouraging results. However, given the myriad technical challenges associated with this procedure, it is unlikely that the results may be broadly applicable within the cardiac surgical community.

Given the procedural novelty and relatively low utilization of TECAB, there is limited data regarding both short- and long-term outcomes. A meta-analysis by Seco and colleagues examined the outcomes of 14 studies evaluating TECAB [36]. A total of 880 beating heart TECABs (BHTECAB) and 360 arrested heart TECABs (AHTECAB) were examined, with 633 one-vessel operations and 357 two-vessel operations included. Within the BHTECAB and AHTECAB cohorts, the intraoperative conversion rate was 5.6% and 15.0%, all-cause mortality was 1.2% and 0.5%, stroke was 0.7% and 0.8%, myocardial infarction was 0.8% and 1.8%, and new-onset atrial fibrillation was 10.7% and 5.1%, respectively. Interpretation of this data is confounded by the significant learning curve and associated with TECAB. Recently Srivastava et al. published a report of 164 consecutive BHTECAB cases without a single intraoperative conversion and excellent postoperative outcomes, thus emphasizing the importance of procedural familiarity [37].

There is limited data regarding the angiographic patency of TECAB grafts in both the short and long term. Argenziano et al. performed a prospective multicenter trial of 98 patients undergoing AHTECAB. After exclusion of 13 patients intraop-

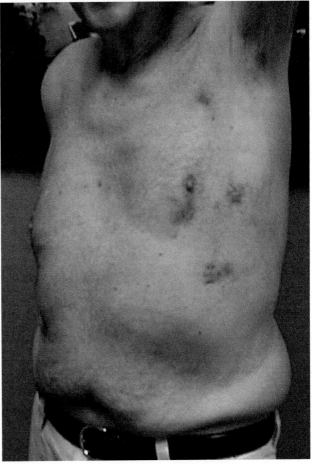

Fig. 32.7 Postoperative scars in a TECAB patient

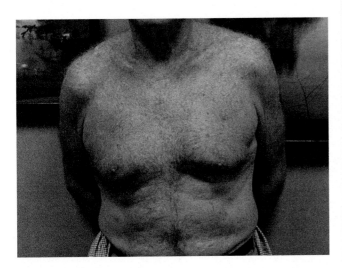

Fig. 32.6 Postoperative scar from robotically assisted MIDCAB (single-vessel LIMA-LAD). Note the small scar placed in the left inframammary fold

eratively, they demonstrated no mortality and a freedom from reintervention or angiographic failure at 3 months of 91% [38]. According to Secco et al., short-term patency of 659 grafts performed via BHTECAB was 98.3%, and 253 grafts performed via AHTECAB was 96.4% [36]. Long-term patency studies are limited by incomplete follow-up; however, Yang et al. compared 100 BHTECAB and 140 MINICAB patients and found a 3-year IMA patency rate of 97.1% in TECAB vs 96.4% in MINICAB patients [39]. These patency rates are comparable to those found in conventional CABG patients. The aesthetic outcomes from TECAB are impressive, as patients have only port-site incisions to heal (Fig. 32.7).

Conclusions

Despite the steep learning curve and myriad challenges associated with robotic CABG, it remains an excellent choice for patients with limited disease when performed at experienced centers. Given the advancements in minimally invasive technology, as well as patient preference for less invasive procedures, there is likely to be an increase in interest in robotic CABG. As this technique gains popularity, future studies are needed to better define both short-and long-term outcomes, as well as aid in patient selection. At present, the most promising application of this procedure is in hybrid coronary revascularization (HCR), which combines the long-term survival benefit of the LIMA-LAD bypass with the lesser invasiveness (and potentially better patency) of PCI for non-LAD lesions. We are currently enrolling patients in a prospective, randomized trial comparing HCR to multivessel PCI and expect that the results of this study will inform the choices of patients and physicians considering option for multivessel coronary revascularization.

References

1. Heron M. Deaths: leading causes for 2014. Natl Vital Stat Rep. 2016;65(5):1–96.
2. Organization WH. The top 10 causes of death. 2017 http://www.who.int/mediacentre/factsheets/fs310/en/. Accessed 14 Aug 2017.
3. Mueller RL, Rosengart TK, Isom OW. The history of surgery for ischemic heart disease. Ann Thorac Surg. 1997;63(3):869–78.
4. Tatoulis J, Buxton BF, Fuller JA. Patencies of 2127 arterial to coronary conduits over 15 years. Ann Thorac Surg. 2004;77(1):93–101.
5. Bonaros N, Schachner T, Wiedemann D, et al. Quality of life improvement after robotically assisted coronary artery bypass grafting. Cardiology. 2009;114(1):59–66.
6. Bonatti J, Ramahi J, Hasan F, et al. Long-term results after robotically assisted coronary bypass surgery. Ann Cardiothorac Surg. 2016;5(6):556–62.
7. Leyvi G, Forest SJ, Srinivas VS, et al. Robotic coronary artery bypass grafting decreases 30-day complication rate, length of stay, and acute care facility discharge rate compared with conventional surgery. Innovations. 2014;9(5):361–7. discussion 367
8. Oz MC, Argenziano M, Rose EA. What is 'minimally invasive' coronary bypass surgery? Experience with a variety of surgi-

cal revascularization procedures for single-vessel disease. Chest. 1997;112(5):1409–16.
9. Loulmet D, Carpentier A, d'Attellis N, et al. Endoscopic coronary artery bypass grafting with the aid of robotic assisted instruments. J Thorac Cardiovasc Surg. 1999;118(1):4–10.
10. Shennib H, Bastawisy A, McLoughlin J, Moll F. Robotic computer-assisted telemanipulation enhances coronary artery bypass. J Thorac Cardiovasc Surg. 1999;117(2):310–3.
11. Angelini GD, Wilde P, Salerno TA, Bosco G, Calafiore AM. Integrated left small thoracotomy and angioplasty for multivessel coronary artery revascularisation. Lancet. 1996;347(9003):757–8.
12. Halkos ME, Walker PF, Vassiliades TA, et al. Clinical and angiographic results after hybrid coronary revascularization. Ann Thorac Surg. 2014;97(2):484–90.
13. Harskamp RE, Vassiliades TA, Mehta RH, et al. Comparative effectiveness of hybrid coronary revascularization vs coronary artery bypass grafting. J Am Coll Surg. 2015;221(2):326–34. e321
14. Kofler M, Stastny L, Reinstadler SJ, et al. Robotic Versus Conventional Coronary Artery Bypass Grafting: Direct Comparison of Long-Term Clinical Outcome. Innovations. 2017;12:239–46.
15. Whellan DJ, McCarey MM, Taylor BS, et al. Trends in robotic-assisted coronary artery bypass grafts: a study of the Society of Thoracic Surgeons adult cardiac surgery database, 2006 to 2012. Ann Thorac Surg. 2016;102(1):140–6.
16. Langer NB, Argenziano M. Minimally invasive cardiovascular surgery: incisions and approaches. Methodist Debakey Cardiovasc J. 2016;12(1):4–9.
17. Canale LS, Mick S, Mihaljevic T, Nair R, Bonatti J. Robotically assisted totally endoscopic coronary artery bypass surgery. J Thorac Dis. 2013;5(Suppl 6):S641–9.
18. Ejiofor JI, Leacche M, Byrne JG. Robotic CABG and hybrid approaches: the current landscape. Prog Cardiovasc Dis. 2015;58(3):356–64.
19. Kon ZN, Brown EN, Tran R, et al. Simultaneous hybrid coronary revascularization reduces postoperative morbidity compared with results from conventional off-pump coronary artery bypass. J Thorac Cardiovasc Surg. 2008;135(2):367–75.
20. Bonatti J, Schachner T, Bonaros N, et al. Technical challenges in totally endoscopic robotic coronary artery bypass grafting. J Thorac Cardiovasc Surg. 2006;131(1):146–53.
21. Harskamp RE, Zheng Z, Alexander JH, et al. Status quo of hybrid coronary revascularization for multi-vessel coronary artery disease. Ann Thorac Surg. 2013;96(6):2268–77.
22. DeRose JJ. Current state of integrated "hybrid" coronary revascularization. Semin Thorac Cardiovasc Surg. 2009;21(3):229–36.
23. Cisowski M, Morawski W, Drzewiecki J, et al. Integrated minimally invasive direct coronary artery bypass grafting and angioplasty for coronary artery revascularization. Eur J Cardio-Thoracic Surg. 2002;22(2):261–5.
24. Davidavicius G, Van Praet F, Mansour S, et al. Hybrid revascularization strategy: a pilot study on the association of robotically enhanced minimally invasive direct coronary artery bypass surgery and fractional-flow-reserve-guided percutaneous coronary intervention. Circulation. 2005;112(9 Suppl):I317–22.
25. Gao C, Yang M, Wu Y, et al. Hybrid coronary revascularization by endoscopic robotic coronary artery bypass grafting on beating heart and stent placement. Ann Thorac Surg. 2009;87(3):737–41.
26. Gilard M, Bezon E, Cornily JC, et al. Same-day combined percutaneous coronary intervention and coronary artery surgery. Cardiology. 2007;108(4):363–7.
27. Katz MR, Van Praet F, de Canniere D, et al. Integrated coronary revascularization: percutaneous coronary intervention plus robotic totally endoscopic coronary artery bypass. Circulation. 2006;114(1 Suppl):I473–6.

28. Kiaii B, McClure RS, Stewart P, et al. Simultaneous integrated coronary artery revascularization with long-term angiographic follow-up. J Thorac Cardiovasc Surg. 2008;136(3):702–8.

29. Lloyd CT, Calafiore AM, Wilde P, et al. Integrated left anterior small thoracotomy and angioplasty for coronary artery revascularization. Ann Thorac Surg. 1999;68(3):908–11. discussion 911-902

30. Riess FC, Bader R, Kremer P, et al. Coronary hybrid revascularization from January 1997 to January 2001: a clinical follow-up. Ann Thorac Surg. 2002;73(6):1849–55.

31. Stahl KD, Boyd WD, Vassiliades TA, Karamanoukian HL. Hybrid robotic coronary artery surgery and angioplasty in multivessel coronary artery disease. Ann Thorac Surg. 2002;74(4):S1358–62.

32. Vassiliades TA Jr, Douglas JS, Morris DC, et al. Integrated coronary revascularization with drug-eluting stents: immediate and seven-month outcome. J Thorac Cardiovasc Surg. 2006;131(5):956–62.

33. Wittwer T, Cremer J, Boonstra P, et al. Myocardial "hybrid" revascularisation with minimally invasive direct coronary artery bypass grafting combined with coronary angioplasty: preliminary results of a multicentre study. Heart. 2000;83(1):58–63.

34. Zenati M, Cohen HA, Griffith BP. Alternative approach to multivessel coronary disease with integrated coronary revascularization. J Thorac Cardiovasc Surg. 1999;117(3):439–44. discussion 444-436

35. Harskamp RE, Brennan JM, Xian Y, et al. Practice patterns and clinical outcomes after hybrid coronary revascularization in the United States: an analysis from the society of thoracic surgeons adult cardiac database. Circulation. 2014;130(11):872–9.

36. Seco M, Edelman JJ, Yan TD, Wilson MK, Bannon PG, Vallely MP. Systematic review of robotic-assisted, totally endoscopic coronary artery bypass grafting. Annals of cardiothoracic surgery. 2013;2(4):408–18.

37. Srivastava S, Barrera R, Quismundo S. One hundred sixty-four consecutive beating heart totally endoscopic coronary artery bypass cases without intraoperative conversion. Ann Thorac Surg. 2012;94(5):1463–8.

38. Argenziano M, Katz M, Bonatti J, et al. Results of the prospective multicenter trial of robotically assisted totally endoscopic coronary artery bypass grafting. Ann Thorac Surg. 2006;81(5):1666–74. discussion 1674-1665

39. Yang M, Wu Y, Wang G, Xiao C, Zhang H, Gao C. Robotic Total arterial off-pump coronary artery bypass grafting: seven-year single-center experience and long-term follow-up of graft patency. Ann Thorac Surg. 2015;100(4):1367–73.

Robotic Pulmonary Lobectomy and Segmentectomy

Michael Zervos, Costas Bizekis, Benjamin Wei, and Robert Cerfolio

Introduction

Thoracic surgery has evolved since the initial published reports of pulmonary lobectomy by Drs. Norman Shenstone and Robert Janes from the Toronto General Hospital, in which they describe "a long incision... In the general direction of the ribs, passing just below the scapula," or via a thoracotomy [1]. Since then, surgeons have found ways to improve on minimally invasive options thereby optimizing postoperative morbidity, recovery time, and pain. Minimally invasive lobectomy has traditionally been performed using video-assisted thoracoscopic surgery (VATS) techniques. The first robotic lobectomies were reported in 2003 by Morgan et al. and Ashton et al. [2, 3] Since then, the use of robotic technology for lobectomy has become increasingly common. In 2015, over 6000 robotic lobectomies were performed in the United States, and over 8600 done worldwide.

Initial Evaluation

The evaluation of candidates for robotic lobectomy includes the standard preoperative studies for patients undergoing pulmonary resection. For patients with suspected or biopsy-proven lung cancer, whole-body PET-CT scan is currently the standard of care. Pulmonary function testing including measurement of diffusion capacity (DLCO) and spirometry is routine. Mediastinal staging can consist of either endobronchial ultrasound-guided fine-needle aspiration biopsy (EBUS-FNA) or mediastinoscopy, depending on expertise. Certain patients may warrant additional testing, including stress test, brain MRI if concern exists for metastatic disease, and/or dedicated computed tomography scan with intravenous contrast or MRI if concern exists for vascular or vertebral/nerve invasion, respectively.

Investigators have shown that thoracoscopic lobectomy is safe in patients with a predicted postoperative forced expiratory volume (FEV1) or DLCO <40% of predicted [4]. We consider robotic lobectomy feasible in these patients as well. At present, we view vascular invasion, locally invasive T4 lesions, Pancoast tumors, and massive tumor (>10 cm) as contraindications for a robotic approach to lobectomy. The need for reconstruction of the airway, chest wall invasion, the presence of induction chemotherapy and/or radiation, prior thoracic surgery, and hilar nodal disease are not contraindications for robotic-assisted lobectomy for experienced surgeons.

Contraindications

Robotic-assisted pulmonary lobectomy can be considered for any patient deemed fit to tolerate conventional lobectomy. The typical contraindications for lobectomy that apply to patients undergoing resection via thoracotomy would also apply to patients undergoing robotic lobectomy (e.g., prohibitive lung function or medical comorbidities, multi-station N2, gross N2 disease, or evidence of N3 disease). Team

M. Zervos (✉)
Division of Thoracic Surgery, New York University Medical Center, New York, NY, USA

Department of Cardiothoracic Surgery, New York University NYU Langone Medical Center, New York, NY, USA
e-mail: michael.zervos@nyumc.org

C. Bizekis
Division of Cardiothoracic Surgery, University of Alabama-Birmingham Medical Center, New York, NY, USA

B. Wei
Division of Thoracic Surgery, New York University Medical Center, New York, NY, USA

R. Cerfolio
Department of Cardiothoracic Surgery, New York University NYU Langone Medical Center, New York, NY, USA

training, familiarity with equipment, troubleshooting, and preparation are critical for the successful performance of robotic lobectomy. Similar to VATS lobectomy, robotic lobectomy is associated with decreased rates of blood loss, blood transfusion, air leak, chest tube duration, length of stay, and mortality compared to thoracotomy. Therefore, robotic lobectomy offers many of the same benefits in perioperative morbidity and mortality, as well as some additional advantages in terms of optics, dexterity, and surgeon ergonomics compared to VATS lobectomy.

Key Points on Anatomy

Excellent knowledge of pulmonary anatomy and specifically the relationship of the hilar structures are needed to perform any anatomic lung resection, whether via thoracotomy, VATS, or robotic techniques. The view of the pulmonary hilum is different depending on the angle of approach. Whereas during a thoracotomy the surgeon is viewing the hilum from either the anterior or posterior direction, typically in VATS and robotic lobectomy, the camera approaches the hilum from an inferior direction. Retraction of the lung can change the orientation of structures considerably. That said, the relationship between structures remains the same regardless of how structures are approached and/or retracted. Knowledge of what risk exists when performing particular steps and moves during an operation is critical to avoid injury. Avoiding misidentification of structures and attention to aberrant or variable anatomy is also of paramount importance during robotic lobectomy or segmentectomy, where an injury can force conversion to an open operation and negate the benefit of attempting minimally invasive surgery.

Conduct of Operation

Preparation

A well-trained team that communicates effectively is a priority for successful performance of robotic lobectomy. Criteria for a well-trained team include documented scores of 80% or higher on simulator exercises, certificate of robotic safety training and cockpit awareness, weekly access to the robot, familiarity with the robot and the instruments, and a mastery of the pulmonary artery from both an anterior and posterior approach.

Equipment

The da Vinci Surgical System is currently the only FDA-approved robotic system for lung surgery. The surgeon sits at a console some distance from the patient who is positioned on an operating table in close proximity to the robotic unit with its four robotic arms. The robotic arms incorporate remote center technology, in which a fixed point in space is defined, and about it, the surgical arms move so as to minimize stress on the thoracic wall during manipulations. The small proprietary EndoWrist instruments attached to the arms are capable of a wide range of high-precision movements. These are controlled by the surgeon's hand movements, via "master" instruments at the console. The "master" instruments sense the surgeon's hand movements and translate them electronically into scaled-down micro-movements to manipulate the small surgical instruments. Hand tremor is filtered out by a 6-Hz motion filter. The surgeon observes the operating field through console binoculars. The image comes from a maneuverable high-definition stereoscopic camera (endoscope) attached to one of the robot arms. The console also has foot pedals that allow the surgeon to engage and disengage different instrument arms, reposition the console "master" controls without the instruments themselves moving, and activate electric cautery. A second optional console allows tandem surgery and training. Da Vinci currently offers both the Xi and Si systems. The Xi system is the most recent edition of the robot and features an overhead boom that permits rotation of the instrument arms, allowing for greater flexibility. Compared to the Si, the Xi also has thinner instrument arms, longer instruments, lighter-weight camera with port hopping option, improved visualization, robotic stapling, integrated energy, near-infrared imaging, and stability of room setup. Currently, Xi is our preferred system for performing thoracic surgery.

Proper location of the robot should be established prior to the operation. If using a Xi system, the patient can remain with their head oriented toward the anesthesia station, and the robot can be driven in perpendicular to the patient's body as a side dock (Fig. 33.1). Currently Xi has completely negated the need for altering patient positioning which is a greatly advantageous to thoracic surgeons.

270° PATIENT ACCESS

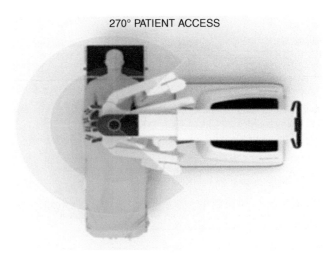

Fig. 33.1 Depiction of side-docking approach with Xi system

Patient Positioning/Port Placement

The patient is positioned in lateral decubitus with hips below the break of the operating table. Precise placement of the double-lumen endotracheal tube and the ability to tolerate single-lung ventilation should be established prior to draping the patient. Axillary rolls and arm boards are unnecessary (Fig. 33.2). The robotic ports are inserted in the 8th intercostal space for all lung resections unless size of patient dictates differently. Typical port placement is shown in Fig. 33.3 for a right robotic lung resection. The ports are placed as is shown in the diagram and are placed in the 8th interspace. All of the ports are 8 mm except for stapler port which is a 12 mm and the Airseal port which is a 5 mm or 12 mm port. The assistant port is triangulated behind the camera port and the most anterior robotic stapling port, usually over the 11th rib in the 10th interspace without disrupting the diaphragm. Dual stapler cannulation can be used for certain cases when both anterior and posterior stapling is required, i.e., right middle lobectomy and certain seg-

ments (Fig. 33.4). A zero-degree camera is used for most thoracic cases. A 30-degree up or down is helpful for certain cases, i.e., esophagectomy or lysis of adhesions. Insufflation with carbon dioxide is used to depress the diaphragm, decrease bleeding, and compress the lung, provide superior smoke evacuation and improved visualization. Our preference is to use the Airseal smoke evacuation-insufflation system (Conmed) as it is the most effective. When using this start at lower insufflation pressures of 5 mm Hg, and work your way up in order to avoid decreased venous return and hypotension.

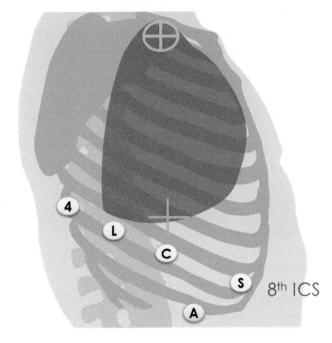

Fig. 33.3 Total port approach with four arm placements for right-sided pulmonary lobectomy with *da Vinci Xi:* camera (*C*), left arm (*L*), fourth arm(*4*) and access port (*A*), and (*S*) stapling port

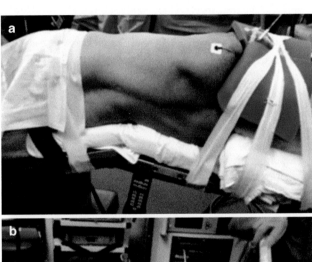

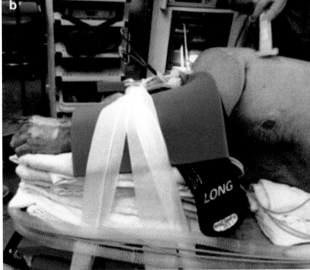

Fig. 33.2 A Posterior view of patient in lateral decubitus positioned with only foam and tape B Anterior view of patient in lateral decubitus positioned with only foam and tape

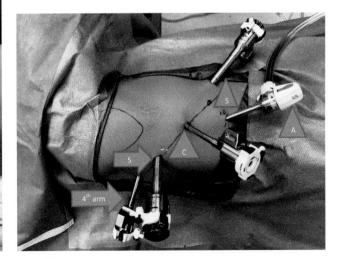

Fig. 33.4 Current port placement in 8th interspace with dual stapler cannulation, 4 arms, 5 mm air seal port. Camera (C), air seal 5 mm (A), 12 mm stapler(anterior), 12 mm stapler (posterior), fourth arm 8 mm

Mediastinal Lymph Node Dissection

After examining the pleura to confirm the absence of metastases, the next step when performing robotic lobectomy is removal of the mediastinal lymph nodes, for staging and also to help expose the structures of the hilum. Intrapulmonary lymph node dissection is clearly superior with robotic technology and facilitates anatomic sublobar lung resection.

- *Right side* – The inferior pulmonary ligament is divided. Lymph nodes at stations 9 and 8 are removed. The fourth robotic arm is used to retract the lower lobe medially and anteriorly in order to remove lymph nodes from subcarinal level 7. The fourth robotic arm is used to retract the upper lobe inferiorly during dissection of stations 2R and 4R, clearing the space between the SVC anteriorly, the esophagus posteriorly, and the azygos vein inferiorly. Avoiding dissection too far superiorly can prevent injury to the right recurrent laryngeal nerve that wraps around the subclavian artery.
- *Left side* – The inferior pulmonary ligament is divided to facilitate the removal of lymph node station 9. The nodes in station 8 are then removed. Station 7 is accessed in the space between the inferior pulmonary vein and lower lobe bronchus, lateral to the esophagus. The lower lobe is retracted medially/anteriorly with the fourth arm during this process. Absence of the lower lobe facilitates dissection of level 7 from the left. Finally, the fourth robotic arm is used to wrap around the left upper lobe and press it inferiorly to allow dissection of stations 5 and 6. Care should be taken while working in the aortopulmonary window to avoid injury to the left recurrent laryngeal nerve. Station 2 L cannot typically be accessed during left-sided mediastinal lymph node dissection due to the presence of the aortic arch, but the 4 L node is commonly removed.

Wedge Resection

Wedge resection of a nodule may be necessary to confirm the presence of cancer prior to proceeding with lobectomy. Because the current iteration of the robot does not offer tactile feedback, special techniques may be necessary to identify a nodule that is not obvious on visual inspection. An empty ring forceps may be used via the assistant port to palpate the nodule. Alternatively, preoperative marking of the nodule with a dye marker (methylene blue) or indocyanine green injected via navigational bronchoscopy can help facilitate localizing. Preoperative confirmation of a cancer diagnosis with tissue biopsy is helpful to avoid being unable to locate the nodule intraoperatively. In addition, near-infrared imaging of intravenously administered indocyanine green

can be used to detect lung nodules; this capability is integrated into the da Vinci Xi platform [5].

The Five Lobectomies [6]

A certain degree of adaptability is necessary for performance of robotic lobectomy. Structures may be isolated and divided in the order that the patient's individual anatomy permits. What follows is a description of an outline of the typical conduct of each lobectomy.

Right Upper Lobectomy

- Our preferred approach is what we consider to be "the posterior approach" through the fissure with division of the recurrent artery with anterior 30 ski tip robotic stapler followed by division of the right upper lobe bronchus with a 45 green stapler followed by removal of N1 nodes just anterior to the truncus. The truncus is divided next followed by division of the superior pulmonary vein. This approach avoids lung congestion and bleeding after vein has been divided. Fissures are completed and specimen removed with retrieval bag.

Alternatively a medial to lateral approach can be taken: retraction of the right upper lobe laterally and posteriorly with fourth robotic arm helps expose the hilum.

- The bifurcation between the right upper and middle lobar veins is developed by dissecting it off the underlying pulmonary artery.
- The 10R lymph node between the truncus branch and the superior pulmonary vein should be removed or swept up toward the lung, which exposes the truncus branch.
- The superior pulmonary vein is encircled with the vessel loop and then divided. The truncus branch is then divided.
- The right upper lobe is then reflected anteriorly to expose the bifurcation of the right main stem bronchus. There is usually a lymph node here that should be dissected out to expose the bifurcation. The right upper lobe bronchus is then encircled and divided. Care must be taken to apply only minimal retraction on the specimen in order to avoid tearing the remaining pulmonary artery branches.
- Finally the posterior segmental artery to the right upper lobe is exposed, the surrounding N1 nodes removed, and the artery encircled and divided.
- The upper lobe is reflected again posteriorly, and the anterior aspect of the pulmonary artery is inspected to make sure that there are no arterial branches remaining. If not, then the fissure between the upper and middle lobes, and the upper and lower lobes, is then divided. This is typically done from anterior to posterior but may be done in

the reverse direction if the space between the pulmonary artery and right middle lobe is already developed. During completion of the fissure, the right upper lobe should be lifted up to ensure that the specimen bronchus is included in the specimen.

Right Middle Lobectomy

- Retraction of the right middle lobe laterally and posteriorly with the accessory (4th) robotic arm helps expose the hilum.
- The bifurcation between the right upper and middle lobar veins is developed by dissecting it off the underlying pulmonary artery. The right middle lobe vein is encircled and divided.
- The fissure between the right middle and lower lobes, if not complete, is divided from anterior to posterior. Care should be taken to avoid transecting segmental arteries to the right lower lobe.
- The right middle lobe bronchus is then isolated. It will be running from left to right in the fissure. Level 11 lymph nodes are dissected from around it. It is encircled and divided, taking care to avoid injuring the right middle lobar artery that is located directly behind it.
- Dissection of the fissure should continue posteriorly until the branches to the superior segment are identified. Then the one or two right middle lobar segmental arteries are isolated and divided.
- Stapling of middle lobar structures may be facilitated by passing the stapler from posterior to anterior, to have a greater working distance.
- The fissure between right middle and upper lobes is then divided.
- Dual stapler cannulation facilitates middle lobectomy by optimizing angles from which structures are divided.

Right Lower Lobectomy

- The inferior pulmonary ligament should be divided to the level of the inferior pulmonary vein.
- The bifurcation of the right superior and inferior pulmonary veins should be dissected out. The location of the right middle lobar vein should be positively identified to avoid inadvertent transection.
- A subadventitial plane on the ongoing pulmonary artery should be established. If the major fissure is not complete, then it should be divided. The superior segmental artery and the right middle lobe arterial branches are identified. The superior segmental artery is isolated and divided. The common trunk to right lower lobe basilar segments may be taken as long as this does not compromise the middle lobar segmental artery/arteries; otherwise, dissection may

have to extend further distally to ensure safe division. Alternatively and preferably the pulmonary artery should be divided entirely to include basilar and superior segments. In the authors opinion, this is a safer approach.
- The inferior pulmonary vein is divided.
- The right lower lobe bronchus is isolated, taking care to visualize the right middle lobar bronchus crossing from left to right. The surrounding lymph nodes, as usual, are dissected and the bronchus divided. Ventilation of the lobe is generally unnecessary if proper stapler orientation is applied.

Left Upper Lobectomy

- Retraction of the left upper lobe laterally and posteriorly with fourth robotic arm helps expose the hilum.
- The presence of both superior and inferior pulmonary veins is confirmed, and the bifurcation dissected.
- The lung is then reflected anteriorly with fourth robotic arm, and interlobar dissection is started, going from posterior to anterior.
- If the fissure is not complete, then it will need to be divided. Reflecting the lung posteriorly again and establishing a subadventitial plane will be helpful. The branches to the lingula are encountered and divided in the fissure during this process. The posterior segmental artery is also isolated and divided. Division of the lingular artery or arteries can be done before or after division of the posterior segmental artery.
- The superior pulmonary vein is isolated then divided. Because the superior pulmonary vein can be fairly wide, it may require that the lingular and upper division branches be transected separately.
- Often the next structure that can be divided readily will be the left upper lobar bronchus, as opposed to the anterior and apical arterial branches to the left upper lobe. The upper lobe bronchus should be encircled and divided, often passing the stapler from the robotic arm anteriorly in order to avoid injuring the main pulmonary artery.
- Finally, the remaining arterial branches are encircled and divided.
- Alternatively the lingular and posterior branches are divided followed by division of the left upper bronchus then division of anterior apical trunk and leaving vein last. This prevents congestions and bleeding from the lung.

Left Lower Lobectomy

- The inferior pulmonary ligament should be divided to the level of the inferior pulmonary vein. The lower lobe is then reflected posteriorly by fourth robotic arm.

- The bifurcation of the left superior and inferior pulmonary veins should be dissected out.
- The lung is reflected anteriorly by fourth robotic arm. The superior segmental artery is identified. The posterior ascending arteries to the left upper lobe are frequently visible from this view also. The pulmonary artery to the lower lobe is divided with both basilar and superior segments. Similar to the right lower lobe, this is performed as we feel it to be a safer approach. The fissures should be completed.
- After division of the pulmonary artery, the lung is reflected again posteriorly. The inferior pulmonary vein is divided.
- The left lower lobe bronchus is isolated. The surrounding lymph nodes, as usual, are dissected and the bronchus divided.
- For left lower lobectomy, it may be simpler to wait until after resection is performed before targeting the subcarinal space for removal of level 7 lymph nodes.

Segmentectomies

Firefly or injection of indocyanine green can be used when performing any segmentectomy. It is helpful to establish perfused versus non-perfused lung during near-infrared imaging. This line is scored with bipolar to allow for more precise division of lung tissue.

Posterior Segmentectomy of Right Upper Lobe

- For a posterior segmentectomy of the right upper lobe and for a superior segment of the right lower lobe, the triangle between the bronchus intermedius and the right upper lobe bronchus is identified.
- The station 11 lymph node is removed, and the posterior segmental artery to the right upper lobe is identified. The fourth robotic arm is then used to retract the upper lobe inferiorly, while robotic arms are used to dissect out stations 2R and 4R, clearing the space between the superior vena cava anteriorly and the azygos vein.
- The 10R lymph node between the right main stem bronchus and the pulmonary artery is then removed.
- The appropriate interlobar lymph nodes are removed; especially the ones that are adjacent to the bronchus are to be removed. In patients with non-small cell lung cancer, these are sent for frozen section analysis, and if results are positive, a lobectomy is performed.
- If a posterior segmentectomy is performed, the posterior segmental artery is dissected free, taking care not to injure the posterior segmental vein of the right upper lobe that courses just under the artery in the posterior fissure.

- Once the artery is stapled or ligated, the posterior segmental vein is dissected free staying superior near the bronchus. It is encircled and then stapled or clipped.
- Now the bronchus can be dissected and the posterior segment and anterior-apical segments easily identified. The posterior bronchus is encircled and stapled, and it is then retracted cephalad by fourth robotic arm. This affords the pulmonary artery to the middle lobe and the lower lobe to be seen and preserved as the parenchyma is stapled to complete the segmentectomy.

Superior Segmentectomy

- If a superior segmentectomy on the right side is to be performed, the triangle between the bronchus intermedius and right upper lobe is identified. Bipolar dissection is carried down on the bronchus intermedius until the No. 11 lymph node is identified and removed.
- The superior segmental artery is seen medially under the No. 12 lymph node. The superior segmental artery is encircled and stapled after the posterior superior segmental bronchus is bluntly dissected.
- Before stapling the superior segmental bronchus, the lung should be retracted medially using fourth robotic arm, identifying the inferior pulmonary vein. The superior segmental branch of the inferior pulmonary vein is the most cephalad branch of the inferior pulmonary vein. It can be individually encircled and should be stapled or ligated first if it is seen. Alternatively it can be divided with the fissure.
- The stapler can then more easily pass around the superior segmental bronchus and be ligated now that the vein has been ligated.
- On the left side, the superior segmental bronchus is generally accessible after the superior segmental vein (or artery) is isolated and divided. The superior segmental artery can be approached via the fissure. The superior segmental vein is the cranial-most branch of the inferior pulmonary vein and is isolated while retracting the lung anteriorly.
- There is not infrequently a second superior segmental artery found in the left lower lobe.

Lingula-Sparing Upper Lobectomy

- A lingular artery-sparing trisegmentectomy (lingula-sparing upper lobectomy) is performed by removing the N2 lymph nodes and finding the pulmonary artery posteriorly, just cephalad to the inferior pulmonary vein after removal of the level 9, 8, and 7 lymph nodes.
- A complete fissure can be approached from the back by identifying the posterior segmental artery to the left upper lobe and dividing the artery and then working along the

pulmonary artery to identify the other branches and stapling the posterior fissure along the way.

- The lingular artery is identified and preserved, as is the lingular bronchus.
- The 11 L lymph node is removed and sent for frozen section analysis to ensure it is free of cancer.
- The lingular vein is identified and preserved, and the remaining pulmonary vein is then stapled. The left upper bronchus is now readily visible, and the lingular bronchus is easily identified and preserved.
- Once the anterior apical and posterior bronchi are all stapled concomitantly, the anterior apical pulmonary arterial trunk can be stapled typically before the airway. The operation is finished by stapling the pulmonary parenchyma from a posterior robotic approach.

Lingulectomy

- Lingulectomy can be performed with either a vein-first or artery-first technique.
- If performing a vein-first approach, the lung is retracted posteriorly, and the lingular vein is identified and divided. Then the lingular bronchus, which often is located fairly distally, is isolated and divided. Finally, the lingular arteries are then isolated and divided.
- The fissure may also be approached first during a lingulectomy. This provided the advantage of being able to assess the level 11 lymph node first, as if it is positive a lobectomy is a better oncologic operation if able to be

tolerated by the patient. If negative, then the vein-first approach can be taken. Alternatively, the lingular arteries can be accessed via the fissure and divided first. Then the bronchus is divided, and finally the vein.

Results

Robotic lobectomy can be performed with excellent perioperative and long-term outcomes. Our median length of stay following robotic lobectomy is 3 days [7]. We have demonstrated a 30-day mortality rate of 0.25%, 90-day mortality rate of 0.5%, and major morbidity rate of 9.6% in patients undergoing robotic lobectomy and segmentectomy [8]. Similar to VATS, robotic lobectomy is associated with decreased rates of blood loss, blood transfusion, air leak, chest tube duration, length of stay, and mortality compared to thoracotomy [9–11]. Conversion rates of <1% to thoracotomy may be achieved, although 3–5% is more typically reported [6]. Vascular injury is rare and, when it does occur, can occasionally be repaired without converting to a thoracotomy [12]. Lymph node upstaging rates and 5-year survival for robotic lobectomy are comparable to lobectomy via thoracotomy and possibly improved versus VATS [13, 14]. Table 33.1 shows results reported in series of robotic-assisted lobectomies.

Robotic segmentectomies have been considered a more demanding technical operation than robotic lobectomy. One investigator found longer operative times (219 min vs 175 min, $p < 0.01$) for robotic segmentectomy compared to robotic lobectomy. They found that patients undergoing

Table 33.1 Results reported in series of robotic-assisted lobectomies

	Year	n	Conversion rate	Morbidity	Perioperative mortality	Median LOS	Notes
Cerfolio et al. [11]	2016	520	12% (first 100 cases) → 3.3% (last 120 cases)	50% (first 100 cases) → 4.2% (last 120 cases)	0.19% (30-day), 0.57% (90-day)	3 days	
Yang et al. [15]	2016	172	9%	26%	0%	4 days	Equivalent OS and DFS at 5 years to VATS
Veronesi et al. [16]	2009	54	13%	20%	0%	4.5 days	
Gharagozloo et al. [17]	2009	100		21%	3%	4 days	
Echavarria et al. [18]	2016	208	9.6%	40.4%	1.44% (in hospital)	5 days	
Louie et al. [10] (STS database)	2016	1220	Not reported	No difference from VATS	0.3% (in hospital), 0.6% (30-day)	4 days	8.44% nodal upstaging
Toker et al. [19]	2016	102 (53% lobectomy)	4%	24%	2% (60-day)	5 days (mean)	104 min mean operative time
Adams et al. [20]	2014	116	3.3%	No difference from VATS	0% (30-day)	4.7 days (mean)	
Melfi et al. [21]	2014	229	10.5% (first 69 cases), 5.6% (next 160 cases)	22% and 15%	1.4% and 0%	4.4 days and 3.8 days (mean)	

LOS length of stay, *QOL* quality of life, *OS* overall survival, *DFS* disease-free survival

robotic segmentectomies were more likely to have an effusion or empyema, and pneumothorax after chest tube removal, than patients undergoing robotic lobectomy. We have demonstrated that robotic segmentectomy can be performed with excellent technical and perioperative results (100 patients, 88 minutes median operative time, 7% conversion rate, 10% major postoperative complication rate, 0% 30-day and 90-day mortality rate) [22]. Two other series of 21 and 17 patients also support the safety and feasibility of robotic segmentectomy; both authors commented on the subjective advantages of lymphadenectomy using robotic techniques [23, 24]. The oncologic sequelae of and indications for performing segmentectomy as opposed to lobectomy remain active areas of study for both VATS and robotic techniques.

One disadvantage of robotic lung resection compared to VATS lung resection is cost. On average, a robotic lobectomy can cost an additional $3000–5000 per case due to the use of disposable instruments and the additional sunk cost of the robot itself and the maintenance plans required for employing the robot [15, 25]. Even with this additional cost, however, each robotic lobectomy yields an estimated median profit margin of around $3500 per patient [26].

Conclusion

Robotic lobectomy and segmentectomy have been demonstrated to be safe operations that can be done expeditiously and with low conversion rates. Perioperative morbidity and mortality are similar to VATS lobectomy/segmentectomy and improved compared to lung resection via thoracotomy. Long-term oncologic outcomes for robotic lobectomy mirror those demonstrated following VATS and open lobectomy. Improved optics, increased dexterity of the instruments, and better ergonomics can yield subjective advantages to the surgeon. With proper training and experience, robotic lobectomy can become part of the fundamental armamentarium of the modern thoracic surgeon.

References

1. Shenstone NS, Janes RM. Experiences in pulmonary lobectomy. Can Med Assoc J. 1932;27:138–45.
2. Morgan JA, Ginsburg ME, Sonett JR, et al. Advanced thoracoscopic procedures are facilitated by computer-aided robotic technology. Eur J Cardiothorac Surg. 2003;23:883–7.
3. Ashton RC, Connery CP, Swistel DG, DeRose JJ. Robot-assisted lobectomy. J Thorac Cardiovasc Surg. 2003;126:292–3.
4. Burt BM, Kosinski AS, Shrager JB, et al. Thoracoscopic lobectomy is associated with acceptable morbidity and mortality in patients with predicted postoperative forced expiratory volume in 1 second or diffusing capacity for carbon monoxide less than 40% of normal. J Thorac Cardiovasc Surg. 2014;148:19–28.
5. Okusanya OT, Holt D, Heitjian D, et al. Intraoperative near-infrared imaging can identify pulmonary nodules. Ann Thorac Surg. 2014;98:1223–30.
6. Cerfolio RJ, Cichos KH, Wei B, Minnich DJ. Robotic lobectomy can be taught while maintaining quality patient outcomes. J Thorac Cardiovasc Surg. 2016;152:991–7.
7. Cerfolio RJ, Bryant AS, Skylizard L, Minnich DJ. Initial consecutive experience of completely portal robotic pulmonary resection with 4 arms. J Thorac Cardiovasc Surg. 2011;142:740–6.
8. Adams RD, Bolton WD, Stephenson JE, et al. Initial multicenter community robotic lobectomy experience: comparisons to a national database. Ann Thorac Surg. 2014;97:1893–8.
9. Kent M, Want T, Whyte R, et al. Open, video-assisted thoracic surgery, and robotic lobectomy: review of a national database. Ann Thorac Surg. 2014;97:236–42.
10. Louie BE, Wilson JL, Kim S, et al. Comparison of video-assisted thoracoscopic surgery and robotic approaches for clinical stage I and stage II non-small cell lung cancer using the Society of Thoracic Surgeons database. Ann Thorac Surg. 2016;102:917–24.
11. Cerfolio RJ, Bess KM, Wei B, Minnich DJ. Incidence, results, and our current intraoperative technique to control major vascular injuries during minimally invasive robotic thoracic surgery. Ann Thorac Surg. 2016;102:394–9.
12. Toosi K, Velez-Cubian FO, Glover J, et al. Upstaging and survival after robotic-assisted thoracoscopic lobectomy for non-small cell lung cancer. Surgery. 2016;160(5):1211–8.
13. Park BJ, Melfi F, Mussi A, et al. Robotic lobectomy for non-small cell lung cancer (NSCLC): long-term oncologic results. J Thorac Cardiovasc Surg. 2012;143:383–9.
14. Cerfolio RJ, Watson C, Minnich DJ, et al. One hundred planned robotic segmentectomies: early results, technical details, and preferred port placement. Ann Thorac Surg. 2016;101:1089–96.
15. Yang H, Woo KM, Sima CS, et al. Long-term survival based on the surgical approach to lobectomy for clinical stage I nonsmall cell lung cancer. Ann Thorac Surg. 2016 (in press).
16. Veronesis G, Galetta D, Maisonneuve P, et al. Four-arm robotic lobectomy for the treatment of early-stage lung cancer. J Thorac Cardiovasc Surg. 2010;140:19–25.
17. Gharagozloo F, Margolis M, Tempesta B, et al. Robot-assisted lobectomy for early-stage lung cancer: report of 100 consecutive cases. Ann Thorac Surg. 2009;88:380–4.
18. Echavarria MF, Cheng AM, Velez-Cubian FO, et al. Comparison of pulmonary function tests and perioperative outcomes after robotic-assisted pulmonary lobectomy vs segmentectomy. Am J Surg. 2016 (in press);212:1175.
19. Toker A, Ozyurtkan MO, Kaba E, et al. Robotic anatomic lung resections: the initial experience and description of learning in 102 cases. Surg Endosc. 2016;30:676–83.
20. Adams RD, Bolton WD, Stephenson JE, et al. Initial multicenter community robotic lobectomy experience: comparisons to a national database. Ann Thorac Surg. 2014;97:1893–900.
21. Melfi FM, Fanucchi O, Davini F, et al. Robotic lobectomy for lung cancer: evolution in technique and technology. Eur J Cardiothorac Surg. 2014;46:626–31.
22. Pardolesi A, Park B, Petrella F, et al. Robotic anatomic segmentectomy of the lung: technical aspects and initial results. Ann Thorac Surg. 2012;94:929–34.
23. Toker A, Ayalp K, Uyumaz E, et al. Robotic lung segmentectomy for malignant and benign lesions. J Thorac Dis. 2014;6:937–42.
24. Deen SA, Wilson JL, WIshire CL, et al. Defining the cost of care for lobectomy and segmentectomy: a comparison of open, video-assisted thoracoscopic, and robotic approaches. Ann Thorac Surg. 2014;9:1000–7.
25. Swanson SJ, Miller DL, McKenna RJ, et al. Comparing robot-assisted thoracic surgical lobectomy with conventional video-assisted thoracic surgical lobectomy and wedge resection: results from a multihospital database. J Thorac Cardiovasc Surg. 2014;147:929–37.
26. Nasir BS, Bryant AS, Minnich DJ, et al. Performing robotic lobectomy and segmentectomy: cost, profitability, and outcomes. Ann Thorac Surg. 2014;98:203–8.

Robotic Esophagectomy

34

Roman V. Petrov, Charles T. Bakhos, and Abbas E. Abbas

Anatomy

The esophagus is a tubular structure that connects the pharynx to the stomach. On its way it traverses three body areas and cavities – the neck, the chest, and the abdomen. It has a multi-layered architecture, consisting of the mucosa with squamous epithelium, the submucosa (a strong layer of connective tissue and vasculature), and the muscularis propria, consisting of internal circular, and outer longitudinal layers. The esophagus has no serosal lining, except in the very distal intraabdominal portion, proximal to the gastroesophageal junction (GEJ) and is otherwise surrounded by an adventitia and mediastinal fat.

History

Esophagectomy is most commonly performed for malignancy and, occasionally, for end-stage benign diseases. The first successful esophagectomy for cancer was performed by Dr. Franz Torek in 1913 in New York. The author removed the thoracic esophagus, closed the distal end, and connected a cervical esophagostomy to a gastrostomy with an extracorporeal rubber tube. The patient, a 67-year-old female, survived for more than 11 years on a pureed diet [1]. Since then, more sophisticated approaches have been introduced with immediate reconstruction of alimentary tract continuity.

Definition and Classification

Esophagectomy is a complex surgical procedure, involving the removal of part of the esophagus and replacing it with a suitable conduit, most commonly, a gastric tube.

Esophagectomy can be classified by several parameters, such as:

- Surgical approach to the esophagus for resection (i.e., transthoracic vs. transhiatal)
- Location of the anastomosis (neck, chest, abdomen)
- Type of the conduit – the stomach (whole or tubularized), colon, small bowel, or skin tubes
- Route of the conduit placement (native – posterior mediastinal bed, left or right chest, substernal or subcutaneous)
- Timing of the reconstruction (immediate vs. delayed)

Classic Esophagectomy Procedures

Several classical esophagectomy procedures have been described. We will discuss the history of esophageal resection, with immediate or delayed reconstruction using a tubularized gastric conduit. We will also review the current state of robotic-assisted esophagectomy.

Transhiatal Esophagectomy (THE)

Transhiatal esophagectomy performed via laparotomy and a left cervical incision were reported as early as 1933 by Dr. Turner, who used an ante-thoracic skin tube to connect the esophageal stump and stomach in a second-stage procedure [2]. This approach was popularized by Dr. Orringer in 1978 in his initial report on 26 patients [3]. Until the development of minimally invasive port-based techniques, this procedure was regarded as "minimally invasive," due to decreased pulmonary morbidity by avoiding thoracotomy. It was, however, challenged by a decrease in the lymph node (LN) yield, as well as increased risk of airway and cardiac injury from the blunt dissection, neck morbidity (specifically recurrent laryngeal nerve (RLN) paralysis), and higher incidence of anastomotic leaks. On the other hand, it was praised for the ease of management of leaks by simply opening of the wound and external drainage [4, 5].

R. V. Petrov · C. T. Bakhos · A. E. Abbas (✉)
Thoracic Medicine and Surgery, Temple University Hospital, Philadelphia, PA, USA
e-mail: abbas.abbas@tuhs.temple.edu

Ivor Lewis Esophagectomy (ILE)

This procedure combines a laparotomy for the preparation of the gastric conduit, followed by right thoracotomy for esophageal resection and esophagogastrostomy, first described by Dr. Ivor Lewis in 1946 [6]. Its benefits include visual-guided dissection with a higher lymph node yield, lower incidence of anastomotic leaks due to shorter conduit, and avoidance of the neck morbidity. However, traditionally, intrathoracic leaks are harder to manage, and there is increased pulmonary morbidity. Proponents of this approach argue that although the proximal margin is shorter, it is usually sufficient, especially for GEJ adenocarcinomas. Another disadvantage is the full commitment to resection with division of the stomach prior to chest exploration, where surgeon can stumble upon unresectable malignancy, despite a thorough preoperative workup. Incomplete resection or esophageal bypass might be performed as a bailout plan in these circumstances [5, 7].

McKeown Esophagectomy (MKE)

Described by K. C. McKeown [8], this approach combines right thoracotomy, laparotomy, and a left cervicotomy. This allows visual control of intrathoracic dissection, minimizes sequelae of intrathoracic leaks, and allows better proximal margin, especially for more proximal squamous cell cancers. It also allows a three-field lymphadenectomy, with a potential for a higher LN yield [7, 8]. However, it combines the morbidity of both the transthoracic and cervical approaches [9, 10].

Left Thoracoabdominal Esophagectomy (TAE) (Sweet Esophagectomy)

Described by Richard Sweet in 1947 [11], this procedure is infrequently performed nowadays. It is performed via a left thoracoabdominal incision in the 9th interspace across the costal margin toward the umbilicus and usually requires division of the diaphragm. Due to limitation of the exposure by the aortic arch in the left chest, resection is limited to the middle and lower esophagus, potentially compromising proximal oncologic margin [12].

Left Thoracoabdominal Esophagectomy with Neck Anastomosis (Hugo Matthews Esophagectomy)

This modification combines a left cervicotomy for the proximal margin and left thoracoabdominal approach for visual control and mediastinal dissection. It combines the benefits and complications of both procedures. It was introduced into clinical practice by H.R. Matthews in 1976 and was reported

in 1987 [13]. It has declined in clinical applications since the development of minimally invasive techniques.

Minimally Invasive and Robotic Approaches

Since the introduction of minimally invasive techniques towards the end of the last century, it was natural to expect expansion of these approaches in an attempt to decrease the morbidity and mortality of this complex procedure [9, 14, 15]. A multitude of the approaches have been described with different combinations of laparoscopy, thoracoscopy and open approaches (hybrid techniques), or purely minimally invasive techniques to replicate the classical procedures [9, 16–18]. The robotic technology further advanced the field of minimally invasive surgery by offering superior dexterity and visualization, tremor filtration, improved ergonomics, and additional technologies with potential impact on outcomes, such as the near-infra red autoflourescence [18–23]. This, in turn, produced yet another multitude of different combinations of robotics, traditional thoracoscopy, and laparoscopy and sometimes opens approaches, sometimes complicating analysis of outcomes, and meaningful comparison.

Anesthesia Consideration

Esophagectomy is a major procedure and is performed under general anesthesia with endotracheal intubation. Single lung ventilation is necessary for the thoracic portion and usually is achieved with double-lumen endotracheal tube [16, 19].

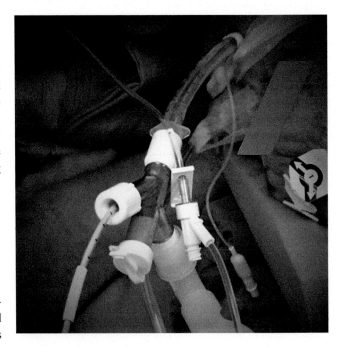

Fig. 34.1 Lung isolation with single-lumen endotracheal tube with bronchial blocker

In order to maximize working space and exposure positive pressure by capnothorax is usually employed in port-based techniques. Maintaining the intrathoracic pressure at 8–10 mmHg displaces the mediastinum and diaphragm, maximizing the working space without negative hemodynamic effects. That also facilitates lung atelectasis, and our group prefers to use single-lumen tube with bronchial blocker in that setting (Fig. 34.1).

Preoperative Evaluation

Before undergoing an esophagectomy for cancer, patients require an extensive workup that is beyond the scope of this chapter. However, before committing to resection, an intraoperative endoscopy should be performed for clear anatomic definition of the tumor extent with potential implication on the surgical approach, location of the anastomosis, and choice of the conduit. For example, a high proximal tumor extension might require a neck anastomosis even for surgeons who prefer a transthoracic (TTE) approach. Extension of the tumor onto the cardia and further onto the lesser curvature might render the stomach unusable and require the use of alternative conduit [16, 24]. Bronchoscopy is also performed on the table to clear tracheobronchial secretions and confirm absence of airway invasion by the esophageal tumor.

Surgical Technique

Robotic McKeown Esophagectomy

Thoracic Part of the Procedure: Right Robotic-Assisted Thoracoscopic Surgery (RATS)

The patient is positioned in the left lateral decubitus position with slight flexion and 45° anterior tilting in a "semi-prone" position. A total of four 8 mm ports are placed (Fig. 34.2).

The first is the "assistant port" placed at the seventh intercostal space (ICS), just anterior to the anterior axillary line. Capnothorax to a pressure of 8–10 mmHg is created. A 5 mm thoracoscope is placed and utilized for visual control of the placement of the remaining three ports. The camera port is placed at the sixth ICS, midaxillary line to be at the midpoint of the thoracic esophagus, about 2 inches below the azygos vein arch. Following this, another port is placed in the third ICS, midaxillary line for the right arm, and the final port is placed in the 9th ICS at the posterior axillary line for the left arm. Port placement can be verified with injection needle for fine-tuning of the precise location. To avoid robotic arm collision, the port should be spaced at least 10 cm for the Si platform and 8 cm for the Xi.

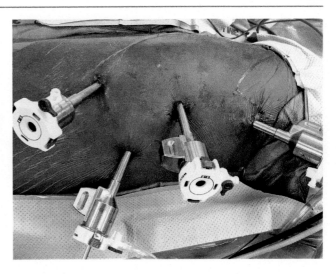

Fig. 34.2 Thoracic port placement for the robotic McKeown esophagectomy

For the dissection in the thoracic cavity, Vessel Sealer is placed in the right arm, while the left arm will use a bipolar fenestrated or Cadiere forceps. Bedside assistant will utilize initial assistant port to apply suction and in passing sutures, drains and controlling staplers if necessary.

Steps of the Thoracic Part of the Procedure

The lung is retracted anteriorly, and the inferior pulmonary ligament is divided. The mediastinal pleura is divided longitudinally anterior and posterior to the esophagus up to the level of the azygos vein arch. At this point, the esophagus is encircled with Penrose drain, which facilitates the retraction. The vein is then dissected free and usually left intact unless the tumor is large (Fig. 34.3). Above the azygos vein, parietal pleura is kept intact to remain as a "tent," covering the eventual conduit. This may help to "wall off" any cervical anastomotic leak from the chest. Both vagus nerves are divided bilaterally below the recurrent laryngeal nerve takeoff. The esophagus with all the lymph nodes and fatty tissue in between the azygous vein, aorta, and pericardium is then dissected circumferentially. The Vessel Sealer is especially useful in controlling bleeding from the aorto-esophageal blood vessels. All lymph nodes in subcarinal, periesophageal, and inferior pulmonary ligament stations are dissected with the esophagus. Superior and inferior paratracheal lymph nodes are dissected and removed separately. After completing esophageal dissection, Penrose drains are used to encircle the esophagus at both the thoracic inlet and the diaphragm (Fig. 34.4) and are tucked under the tissue to help in identifying the esophagus in the neck and in the hiatus. A flexible 24 French drain is placed next along the posterior esophageal gutter. The instruments are then removed, the robot is undocked, and the incisions are closed. The bronchial blocker is removed as the remainder of the procedure does not require lung isolation.

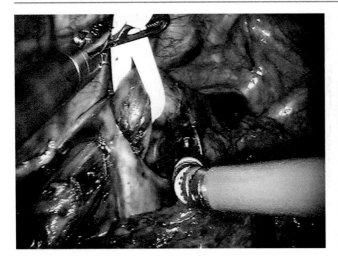

Fig. 34.3 The esophagus is encircled with the Penrose drain to aid with the retraction and exposure

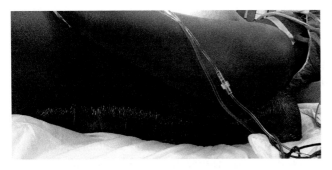

Fig. 34.4 Positioning of the patient for the abdominal and cervical part of the procedure

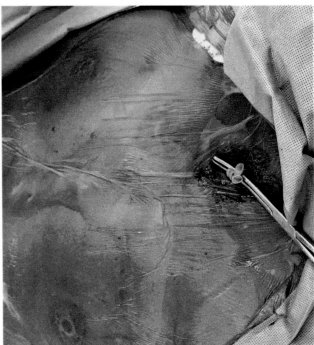

Fig. 34.5 Identification and delivery of the upper Penrose drain into the cervicotomy wound

Left Cervicotomy

The patient is repositioned into the supine position and a long soft medium size gel roll is placed under the left flank and left shoulder (Fig. 34.4). This facilitates both the placement of the most lateral port in the abdomen and the cervical esophageal exposure. The head is turned to the right, and the skin is prepped from the abdomen to the neck in one field.

Cervicotomy is performed simultaneously with abdominal part through a 4 centimeter incision along the inferior anterior border of the left sternomastoid muscle. Carotid sheath and internal jugular vein are dissected laterally, and the prevertebral plain is developed. The Penrose drain around the esophagus from thoracic dissection is identified and delivered into the wound (Fig. 34.5). This facilitates the circumferential dissection of the cervical esophagus keeping the left recurrent laryngeal nerves away from the harm ways.

Abdominal Part of the Procedure: Robotic-Assisted Laparoscopic Surgery (RALS)

Pneumoperitoneum is created either with a Veress needle through the umbilicus or after the placement of the optical 5 mm trocar. Next, a 12 mm port is placed in the linea alba just below the umbilicus and used for visual control via a regular laparoscope for correct placement of the robotic ports. The left-hand port is placed at the right midclavicular line, a hand width below the costal margin, few centimeters above the umbilicus. The camera port is positioned at the left paramedian line, an inch above the level of the umbilicus and below the lowest point of the greater curve of the stomach. Two remaining ports are placed on the same level – an inch above umbilicus. Right-hand port is located in the left midclavicular line and hand width below the costal margin. Retraction port is placed maximally laterally in the flank, few centimeters below costal margin. For liver retraction we use a flexible retractor through a 5 mm port in the right flank which is secured in place with table mount (Fig. 34.6). Before robot docking, the patient is transitioned into steep reverse Trendelenburg position to use gravity in retraction of the omentum and the loops of bowel and facilitate the exposure.

During the dissection, the right flank arm is used mainly for retraction utilizing a non-traumatic double fenestrated or tip-up fenestrated grasper. The right-hand port is used for majority of the dissection and will mainly use the Vessel Sealer, which, with some practice, can be also used as a needle driver and suture cutter. During pyloromyotomy, this arm is switched for the bipolar Maryland forceps for fine dissection of the layers of the gastric wall. The left arm will mainly use the Fenestrated Bipolar or Cadiere Forceps to assist in dissection and retraction.

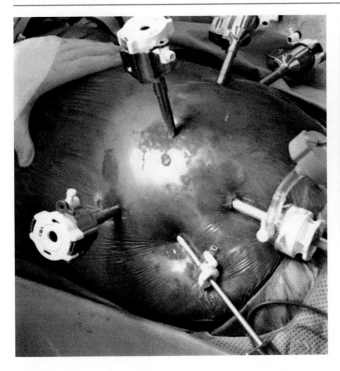

Fig. 34.6 Placement of the abdominal robotic ports, the assistant port, and the liver retractor

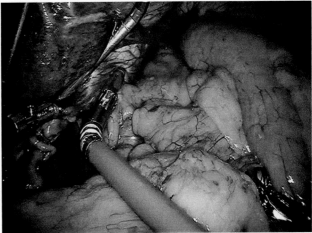

Fig. 34.7 Dissection of the gastrohepatic ligament on exposure of the hiatus

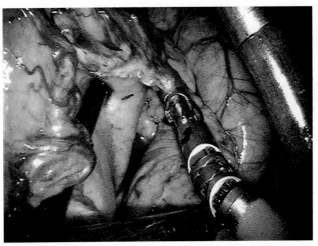

Fig. 34.8 Mobilization of the greater curvature of the stomach with division of the short gastric vessels

Steps of the Abdominal Part of the Procedure

Gastric dissection and conduit preparation begun by dividing the gastrohepatic ligament and dissection of the diaphragmatic hiatus (Fig. 34.7). At this stage to avoid entrance to the chest with loss intraperitoneal pressure and complicated exposure, the phrenoesophageal ligament was left intact until the end of the gastric mobilization. The gastrocolic ligament is then opened at the level of the mid-body, dividing the short gastric vessels toward the fundus for complete mobilization (Fig. 34.8). An omental flap, based on the shot gastric vessels, can be harvested at this stage for the later use in anastomotic coverage. After clearly identifying the location of the gastroepiploic pedicle, the greater omentum is divided, while keeping the pedicle intact, in a caudal direction toward the pylorus to the takeoff of the gastroepiploic artery from the gastroduodenal artery (Fig. 34.9). Extreme diligence is required during this stage, especially in obese individuals with excessive omental fat deposits, as injury to the vascular pedicle will render the stomach unusable as the conduit.

The attachments of the hepatic flexure are divided to allow exposure of the duodenum. Gentle "kocherization" is completed next by dividing lateral retroperitoneal attachments of the duodenum. The goal is to achieve tension-free transposition of the pylorus to the level of the hiatus. This promotes a tension-free conduit placement. The pylorus is identified and can be dealt with according to the surgeon's preference. We perform classical pyloromyotomy that is facilitated by a magnification and depth perception of the robotic platform. Stitch is applied to the pyloric muscle, and with the use of bipolar Maryland grasper, pyloric fibers are divided to the submucosal plane, which is developed without mucosotomy (Fig. 34.10).

The stomach is then retracted superiorly to expose retrogastric adhesions which are divided until the left gastric pedicle is identified. A complete nodal dissection is accomplished by mobilizing the lymphatic nodal tissue along the celiac artery toward the specimen. The left gastric artery is then divided with the linear stapler at its takeoff from the celiac artery (Fig. 34.11).

At this point, division of the phrenoesophageal ligament allows delivery of the Penrose drain into the abdomen, traction on which facilitated complete circumferential dissection of the gastroesophageal junction (Fig. 34.12). Attention at this point is turned to the formation of the gastric conduit. Nasogastric tube is pulled until into the thoracic esophagus. The stomach

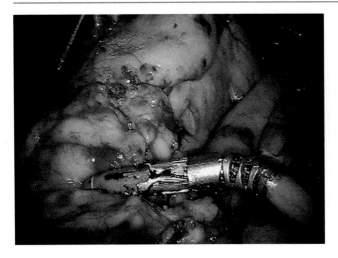

Fig. 34.9 Division of the gastrocolic ligament caudally for complete mobilization of the greater curvature up to the takeoff of the gastroepiploic artery

is divided with a linear stapler, starting at the incisura and running along the greater curvature to the fundus to form a narrow, 5 cm gastric tube (Fig. 34.13). Attention is paid to avoid the common mistake of stapling too close to the esophagogastric junction (EGJ) as this might compromise lateral margin at the GEJ and might also have negative impact on the final conduit length. Perfect aligning of the tissue is required at this stage by stretching the stomach with all robotic arms to avoid spiraling of the staple line and folding of the posterior wall. After completing the conduit, its proximal end is secured to the distal end of the specimen with a silk stitch.

Under vigilant visual control from the surgeon on the console to assure appropriate conduit placement without axial torsion, the assistant delivers the esophagogastric specimen along with the attached conduit into the cervicotomy wound by constant gentle traction (Fig. 34.14). After surgeon is satisfied with conduit placement, diaphragmatic hiatus is closed

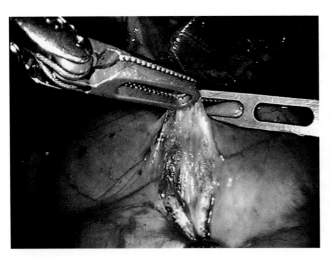

Fig. 34.10 Robotic pyloromyotomy

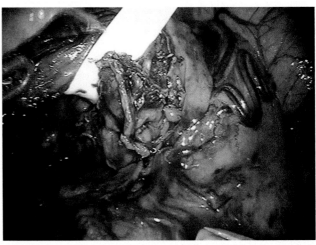

Fig. 34.12 Circumferential esophageal dissection after delivery of lower thoracic Penrose drain into the abdomen

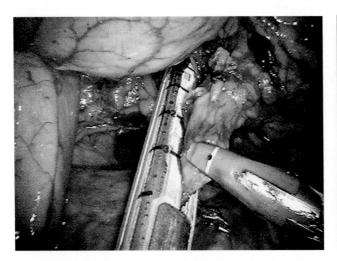

Fig. 34.11 Division of the left gastric pedicle

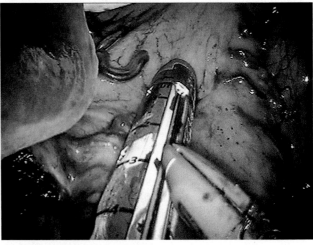

Fig. 34.13 Formation of the narrow gastric tube

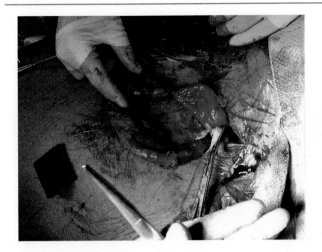

Fig. 34.14 Delivery of the specimen and the conduit into the cervicotomy wound

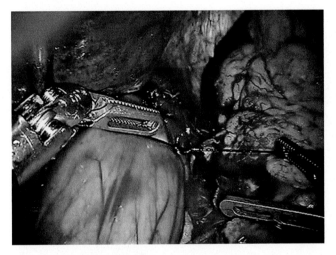

Fig. 34.15 Closure of the hiatus around the conduit

Fig. 34.16 Extraction of the specimen and proximal division of the esophagus

around the conduit to avoid visceral herniation (Fig. 34.15). The robot is then undocked, and the surgeon returns to the operating table to complete the procedure.

The cervical anastomosis is completed according to surgeon's preference. We prefer linear completely stapled side-to-side technique, which is illustrated in the following images (Figs. 34.16, 34.17, and 34.18).

A laparoscopic feeding jejunostomy with 14 Fr jejunostomy tube with the balloon is performed using a percutaneous Seldinger technique after undocking the robot (Figs. 34.19 and 34.20).

Robotic Ivor Lewis Esophagectomy

The initial steps, including anesthesia, intubation, endoscopy, and positioning for abdominal part of the procedure are identical to previously described steps.

Abdominal Part of the Procedure: Robotic-Assisted Laparoscopic Surgery (RALS)

The robotic gastric dissection and preparation of the gastric conduit is also identical to that described above. The exception is that since the conduit remains in the abdomen, it is not possible to close the hiatus, and thus it has to be accomplished later on from the chest. At the conclusion of the abdominal part, jejunostomy is placed if indicated.

Thoracic Part of the Procedure: Right Robotic-Assisted Thoracic Surgery (RATS)

After completion of the abdominal dissection, the patient is transitioned into left lateral decubitus position for thoracic part. However, due to higher complexity of the thoracic part,

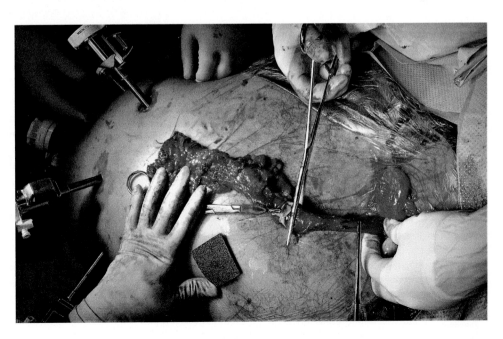

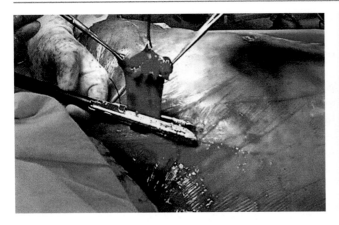

Fig. 34.17 Advancement of the NGT after creation of the linear anastomosis

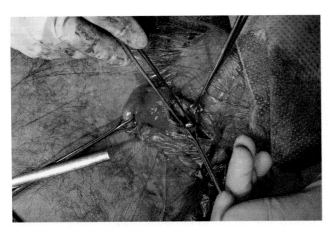

Fig. 34.18 Closure of the enterotomy with creation of the triangular anastomosis and resection of the excessive gastric conduit

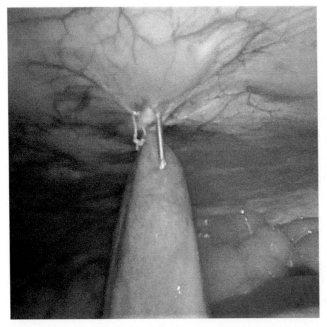

Fig. 34.19 Jejunostomy. Placement of access needle

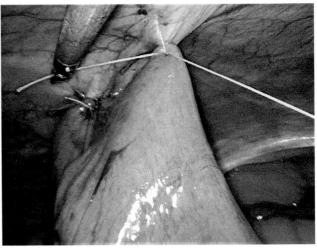

Fig. 34.20 Final view of the feeding jejunostomy with antitorsion stitch

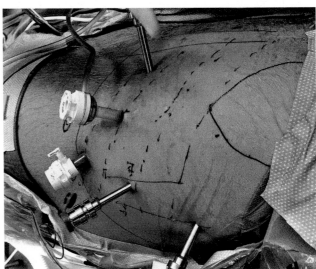

Fig. 34.21 Placement of the robotic ports for the thoracic part of Ivor Lewis esophagectomy

because of creation of the anastomosis, as opposed to the simple dissection, the location and number of ports differs from McKeown modification (Fig. 34.21). If robotic stapler is available, a 12 mm robotic stapling port is placed in the 8th ICS anterior axillary line. Two other robotic 8 mm ports are then placed also in the 8th ICS at the posterior axillary line and lateral to the paraspinal muscles. A third robotic 8 mm port is placed in the fifth ICS midaxillary line for retraction. If the plan is for robotic linear stapled anastomosis, we only place an 8 mm assistant port at the 9th ICS at the midclavicular line. However, if bedside stapling is planned, a 15 mm port is placed in the anterior axillary line through the diaphragm attachments below the costal margin.

The superior robotic arm is used mainly for retraction, utilizing an atraumatic double fenestrated or tip-up fenestrated forceps. The right hand will use mainly the bipolar Vessel Sealer, alternating with the robotic stapler. The left arm will mainly use the bipolar fenestrated or Cadiere forceps to assist in dissection, exposure, and hemostasis.

Steps of the Thoracic Procedure

The lung is retracted anteriorly and the inferior pulmonary ligament is divided. The mediastinal pleura is opened longitudinally both anterior and posterior to the esophagus up to the level of the azygos vein arch. The vein is then circumferentially dissected free and divided with the robotic or handheld linear vascular stapler. The thoracic esophagus is then mobilized circumferentially with all the surrounding lymphatics and fatty tissue in between the azygos vein, aorta, and pericardium including a complete mediastinal nodal dissection. The vagus nerve is divided bilaterally below the recurrent laryngeal nerve takeoff.

After completing the circumferential dissection of the esophagus, the specimen and attached to it conduit are delivered into the chest, until the caudal end of conduit staple line is visible above the diaphragm (Fig. 34.22). Attention is paid to maintain proper orientation of the conduit to avoid axial torsion during the conduit delivery. The NGT is pulled back to 20 cm, and the esophagus is divided with a linear stapler just above the azygos vein arch (Fig. 34.23). The specimen is placed anteriorly to the lung until completion of the anastomosis.

There are different techniques for the formation of the anastomosis. We prefer a robotic side-to-side linear stapler technique. The conduit is placed in the native esophageal bed and medial to the esophageal stump. The conduit is secured to the medial aspect of the esophagus with two 2-0 silk sutures. The stapled end of the esophagus is opened at the medial end of the staple line. Likewise, a gastrotomy is created in the lateral aspect of the conduit. A 45 mm robotic linear stapler is advanced into the lumen of the esophageal stump and gastric conduit and fired, creating the anastomosis (Fig. 34.24). Under direct vision the NGT is advanced into the caudal portion of the conduit. The enterotomy of the esophagogastrostomy is approximated with 2-0 silk stitches and then reinforced by firing another linear stapler (Fig. 34.25).

Another technique of the esophagogastrostomy is utilizing a circular stapler for the creation of the end-to-side anastomosis. The entire esophageal staple line is resected using the Vessel Sealer. The assistant port is removed and enlarged to accommodate EEA anvil which is then passed inside the esophageal lumen. A purse-string running suture is applied

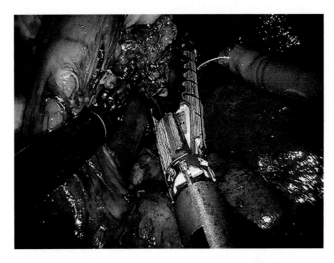

Fig. 34.23 Proximal division of the esophagus with the linear stapler

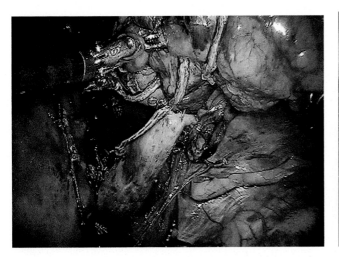

Fig. 34.22 Delivery of the specimen and attached to it conduit into the chest

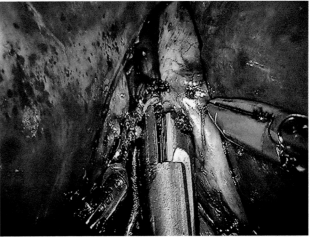

Fig. 34.24 Placement of the linear stapler for the esophagogastric anastomosis

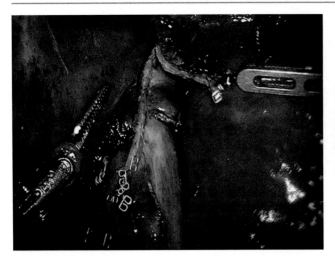

Fig. 34.25 Closure of the esophagogastrostomy with linear stapler

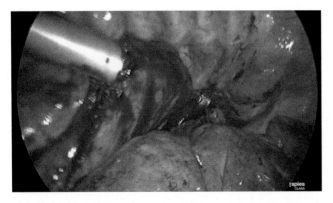

Fig. 34.26 Technique of esophagogastrostomy with circular EEA stapler

around it with 3-0 Prolene. A gastrotomy is made at the tip of the conduit, and the EEA stapler is advanced into the lumen. The spike is pushed through the conduit wall, opposite to the staple line, engaged to the anvil, tightened, and then fired, creating a circular anastomosis (Fig. 34.26). The tip of the conduit, containing the opening, is then transected with a linear stapler, providing closure. Specimen is retrieved in the plastic bag.

Alternatively, OrVil can be used for the placement of the EEA anvil. It represents an anvil, attached to the long plastic tube, which can be advanced transorally. Whereas it facilitated the placement by avoiding the need of the purse-string stitch, it comes in smaller sizes (not large than 25 mm) that potentially can contribute to stricture formation and in author's experience can fail to deploy appropriately for firing.

The diaphragmatic hiatus is closed with interrupted silk stitches around the conduit which is sutured to the right crus with 2-0 silk.

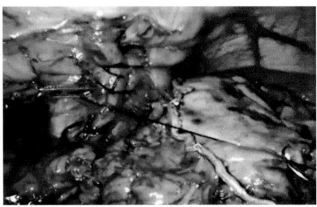

Fig. 34.27 Closure of the hiatus with nonabsorbable sutures

Finally, a flexible 24 French flexible drain is placed along the posterior esophageal gutter. The robotic instruments are then removed, the robot is undocked, and the incisions are closed.

Extra-anatomic Substernal Reconstruction

Immediate reconstruction after esophagectomy almost always positions conduit in the native, posterior mediastinal bed. In cases of delayed reconstruction, when native bed is scarred and obliterated, palliative resection and esophageal bypass alternative routes might be employed. Among those, substernal route is most commonly utilized.

Patient is placed in supine position with the neck hyperextended and the head turned to the right. If jejunostomy was previously established, left flank ports need to be placed superior and medial to jejunostomy loop.

Abdominal Part of the Procedure

Initial port placement and conduit dissection is similar to previously described. Hiatus is dissected, and the esophagus is mobilized maximally high into posterior mediastinum if it hasn't been done before. The esophagus is divided with linear stapler as high as in the mediastinum as possible. Hiatus then is completely closed in the interrupted fashion with nonabsorbable stitches (Fig. 34.27).

Sternal part of the diaphragm is dissected off of the posterior table of the sternum for approximately 5 cm. With blunt and sharp dissection with both working arms, pericardium and mediastinal tissue is mobilized off of the sternum, creating retrosternal tunnel.

Left Cervicotomy

Neck dissection is started simultaneously and performed as previously described. In delayed reconstruction cases, esophagostomy is dissected from the skin, and esophagus is

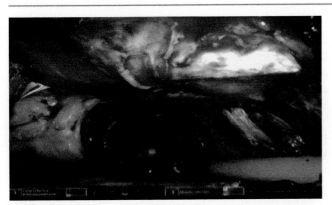

Fig. 34.28 Connection of the cervical and substernal dissection planes with surgeon digit identified in the tunnel

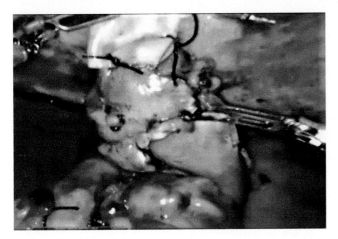

Fig. 34.29 Conduit is secured to the Penrose drain and is delivered to the neck

mobilized for the sufficient distance for the anastomosis. Resection of the left sternoclavicular junction is performed next to prevent conduit compression and obstruction. Digital dissection is carried caudally, over the aortic arch to meet the dissection plane from the abdomen (Fig. 34.28).

Delivery of the Conduit and Anastomosis

Umbilical tape is advanced from the cervicotomy wound into the abdomen through the tunnel and secured to the specimen, which is removed. At this point (Fig. 34.29), cervical anastomosis is performed in one of the previously described fashions.

Postoperative Management

Patients typically remain in the hospital until their thoracic and nasogastric drains are removed. This is usually achieved by postoperative days 4–5. They are discharged on enteral

nutrition via the jejunal tube. A water-soluble esophagram is performed as an outpatient procedure on postoperative days 10–14. When an esophageal leak is ruled out, the patient's diet is advanced to oral fluids and later soft food. The diet is progressively advanced until full calorie intake is met via oral route. At this point, enteral nutrition is ceased, and if the patient maintains weight and oral intake, the jejunostomy tube is removed several weeks later. Postoperatively patients require rigorous support and are advised of lifestyle and diet modification with small frequent meals, avoiding eating before bedtime, sleeping with the head of bed elevated, and remaining on proton pump inhibitors (PPI) twice a day for life [25, 26].

Early Postoperative Complications

Cardiac Arrhythmias

Cardiac arrhythmias, especially atrial fibrillation, are common after thoracic surgical interventions. Development of the arrhythmia has been associated with anastomotic leaks. Rate and rhythm control is usually achieved with beta blockers and calcium channel blockers and amiodarone. Anticoagulation can be started when it is safe from surgical standpoint [27–29].

Anastomotic Leaks

Anastomotic leak is defined as disruption of the integrity of the anastomosis, resulting in transposition of luminal content outside of the confines of the esophagus. Anastomotic leaks can be classified as grade 1/subclinical (radiological, biochemical), not requiring change in management; grade II/clinical minor, requiring conservative management without anastomotic intervention; grade III/clinical major, requiring reintervention; and grade IV/conduit necrosis, requiring surgical diversion [30].

Anastomotic leaks usually present after the fifth postoperative day and could be as late as 3–4 weeks postoperatively. Once identified, endoscopy is performed to evaluate the extent of the dehiscence and rule out gastric tip necrosis. The leak is treated according to the extent of the anastomotic dehiscence. In cases of disruption of less than 50% of the circumference, conservative management with simple drainage or exclusion with covered stent is utilized [31, 32]. In cases of cervical anastomosis, the incision is opened to allow drainage of infection. Serial esophageal dilation to prevent structuring and distal obstruction seems to facilitate healing as well [4, 30]. Cases with complete disruption of the anastomosis are treated as gastric tip necrosis [30, 33, 34]. Application of new endoscopic suturing overstitch device has been reported for the closure of fistulas, however, was less successful for management of anastomotic leaks [35].

Gastric Tip (Conduit) Necrosis

This is a rare but potentially lethal complication related to ischemia of the gastric conduit. This usually requires take-down of the anastomosis with resection of the ischemic por-tion and diversion of the esophagus with a cervical esophagostomy [30]. The remaining healthy portion of the stomach is repositioned into the abdomen, and the hiatus is closed. Delayed reconstruction with either preserved rem-nant of gastric conduit or alternative conduit can be per-formed. It is recommended to perform gastrostomy to the tip of the conduit with bolus feeds postoperatively to avoid gas-tric conduit contraction. It is necessary to identify these cases early to avoid the onset of sepsis [16, 19, 33, 34]. Firefly technology helps in assessment of the conduit perfusion and has a potential of decreasing incidence of the anastomotic leaks [20, 21].

Airway Injury

It is a devastating complication, regardless of the approach. Intraoperative occurrence usually immediately detected. Presentation in early postoperative period is believed due to thermal injury to the posterior membra-nous portions of the airway during mediastinal dissec-tion. Once identified, it requires swift and radical intervention as delay leads to the development of the con-duit airway fistula and results in severe lung soilage, sep-sis, and unsalvageable situation. Repair requires thoracotomy with muscle flap buttressing of the airway and usually a takedown of the conduit with diversion esophagectomy and delayed reconstruction via extra-anatomic routes [36–38]. Attempts of palliating with stents usually only delay the inevitable [39].

Chylothorax

Prevention is the best management of thoracic duct injury. Preoperative administration of either heavy cream or vegeta-ble oil has been shown to improve identification of the duct and decreased incidence of injury [40]. Some authors advo-cate routine thoracic duct ligation to prevent this occurrence [41]. Although low-volume chylothorax, presumably due to small side branch injury, can be successfully treated with conservative measures such as fasting, octreotide, and TPN, most will require definitive intervention. Delayed repair may predispose to malnutrition, immunodeficiency, and dehydra-

tion. Ligation of the thoracic duct can be performed surgi-cally via right chest approach. Administration of cream or olive via jejunostomy tube helps in identifying the source of chyle leak [42]. Alternatively, cisterna chyli embolization can be attempted, but this requires robust IR support and has various degree of success [43].

Vocal Cord Paralysis

Although this complication is secondary to retraction and is usually self-limited, it may impact on the patient's abil-ity to clear pulmonary secretions and predispose patient to aspirations. Thorough speech pathologist evaluation is required postoperatively. If patient is aspirating, oral intake can be safely postponed with enteral nutrition until patient can undergo medialization or thyroplasty [5, 44, 45].

Conduit Obstruction

Early conduit obstruction is due to technical errors during conduit positioning and creation of the anastomosis. Axial torsion or kinking of the conduit can occur. As such, the best management is prevention of this occurrence with meticu-lous attention to details during this part of the procedure. If identified early, especially intraoperatively, the best course of action is takedown and redo of the anastomosis. Many surgeons believe that conduit obstruction and subsequent leak can be due to pylorospasm as a consequence of denerva-tion and routinely perform either full pyloroplasty or medical pyloromyotomy. Others avoid pyloric draining procedures in consideration of later complications such as dumping and bile reflux [32, 46, 47].

Late Complications

Anastomotic Stricture

Typically, patients present with late-onset dysphagia up to a year postoperatively. It is more common in patients who experienced anastomotic leak postoperatively. Usually, this can be managed endoscopically by serial endoscopic dilations. Repeat and maintenance procedures might be required. Refractory strictures may be ameliorated with temporary self-expanding covered stents, placed for 4–6 weeks. In severe cases, endoscopic incision or surgi-cal structureless can be considered [48, 49]. Endoscopic injection of the steroids has been shown to decrease rate of restricturing and number of the repeat interventions [50, 51].

Hiatal Hernia (Paraconduit Hernia)

This occurrence seems to be unique after minimally invasive esophagectomies believed to be related to inadequate hiatal closure and diminished adhesions formation postoperatively. These hernias do not have a sack, and significant portions of small and large bowel can translocate into the chest, compromising respiratory mechanics and increasing the risk of strangulation. Surgical repair may be approached by means of a thoracotomy on the side of the herniation or laparotomy. Minimally invasive approaches have been reported successful as well [52–54].

Delayed Conduit Emptying

This can lead to stasis in the conduit, chronic aspiration, and malnutrition. Thorough investigation is required to determine the cause of the problem. If pyloric drainage procedure has not been performed, pyloric obstruction can be the cause. Initially, endoluminal interventions (balloon dilation, botulinum toxin injection) can be trialed. Definitive drainage can be achieved with surgical pyloroplasty. Promising results have been reported with gastric peroral endoscopic myotomy (GPOEM) procedure [55].

Conduit Redundancy

This is a consequence of a long-standing vagotomized conduit in the negative pressure environment of the chest, leading to conduit elongation and dilation with tortuosity and kinking. Patients present with dysphagia, chronic aspiration, and malnutrition, usually many years after the procedure. Distal obstruction from pylorospasm might play a role and needs to be addressed. Reoperation might be the only option in severe cases. Careful dissection with preservation of vascular pedicle of the conduit is necessary. After complete intrathoracic conduit mobilization, abdominal part commences with careful dissection of the hiatus. Subsequently, conduit is straightened by pulling down to eliminate redundancy. The hiatus is closed and pexy of the conduit to the hiatus is performed. Re-resection of the conduit with anastomosis at proximal end is rarely required. Retubularization of dilated conduit along previous stapling line might be performed [53, 56].

Tracheoesophageal Fistula (TEF)

This is a serious complication, and when it occurs, careful evaluation for malignancy recurrence is required. Endoscopic palliation with covered stents or endoscopic fistula closure is possible. In severe cases conduit takedown and extra-anatomic reconstruction might be undertaken [35–37, 57].

Reflux and Barrett's Esophagus

After esophagectomy with gastric conduit reconstruction, patient requires regular surveillance endoscopy to monitor for recurrence and development of Barrett's esophagus due to acid reflux. Lifelong diet and lifestyle modification and chronic maximal dose PPI use are required. If patient develops Barrett's esophagus, aggressive endoscopic treatment is required to prevent progression to metachronous malignancy [58, 59]. In cases of uncontrolled debilitating reflux, conversion to Roux-en-Y or colon interposition has been described [60]. The use of pyloric drainage procedure was associated with increased prevalence of reflux esophagitis [46, 47].

Recurrent or Metachronous Malignancy

Esophageal cancer usually recurs systemically with distant metastasis. However, even local recurrence carries poor prognosis. Recurrent malignancy usually develops within the first 3 years and occurs from regrowth of tumor deposits in the surrounding tissues and lymph nodes. It is rarely salvageable; however, long-term survival has been reported in select group of patients [61, 62]. Usually, palliative interventions for lumen restoration and enteral access are undertaken with savage chemoradiation.

Metachronous malignancy usually develops many years later and, due to mucosal origin, sometimes might be re-resected. In cases of previously low anastomosis with enough length of esophageal stump, repeat resection and potential diversion or even extra-anatomic reconstruction may be feasible. For early-stage malignancies, endoscopic resection can be undertaken [63].

Outcomes of Robotic Esophagectomy

Published Robotic Esophagectomy Series (Table 34.1)

The application of laparoscopic and thoracoscopic techniques in esophageal cancer surgery has been well established [16]. The robotic technology with its included digital processing offers additional advantages, particularly depth perception due to tridimensional view, wristed motion, magnification, Firefly, and surgeons' total control of all arms including camera and the stapler. The first robotic thoracoscopic mobilization of the esophagus was reported by Bodner and coauthors in 2004 in four patients along with the other procedures [64].

In 2007 Kernstine et al. reported one of the early series of totally robotic McKeown esophagectomy. Of 14 patients, 8 had completely robotic procedures. Total average operating

Table 34.1 Outcomes of published robotic esophagectomy series

Author and year	Number of patients	Surgical approach	Procedure type	LOS	OR time total/consol	LN yield	Morbidity	Mortality (30 days/90 days)	Leak rate/conduit necrosis
Kernstine, 2007	14	RT, RL – (8)	MKE	8–72	11.1 (9.5–13.2)/5.0 (4.2–5.9), hrs	18 (10–32)	93% (minor), 29% (major)	0/7.1%	14.3%/–
Sarkaria, 2013	21	RT, RL	ILE – 17, MKE – 4	10 (7–70)	556 (395–807)	20 (10–49)	24%	/4.9%	14%/0
Abbas, 2013	33	RT, RL	MKE	7 (4–31)	310 (270–340)	16 (7–44)	39	3/3	6%/
Dylewski, 2013	20	RT, RL	–	9	303	–	–	/10%	15%/
Carrera, 2015	32	RT, RL	MKE – 11, ILE – 21	12	Console time 218 (190–285)	16	28.1	3.1%/	21.875% /3.125%
Cerfolio, 2015	85	RT (85), CL (79), RL (5), OL (1), (conversion)	ILE	8	361 (283–489)	22	36.4%	3.5/10.6	4.3%/2.3
Hodari, 2015	54	RT, CL	ILE	12.9 (7–37)	362 (260–516)	16 (3–35)	–	0/1.8%	5.5% + 1.8% (staple line)
Park, 2016	114	RT, CL/OL	MKE	16	419.6 ± 7.9 (consol time 206.6 ± 5.2)	49 ± 1.9	–	3.5%/2.5%	14.9%
Chiu, 2017	20	RT, OL (2), CL (18). Exteriorized conduit	MKE	13 ± 6	499 ± 70	18 ± 13	–	–	15%/
Okusanya, 2017	25	RT, RL. Conversion (CT 3, OL 1)	ILE	8 (6–20)	661 (503–902)	26 (11–78)	–	4%	0/0
Amaral, 2017	237	RT, RL/CL	ILE	9	–	–	–	–	15% (4% clinical)
Luketich, 2012	1011	CT, CL,	MKE 481, ILE 530	8 IQR (6-14)		21	–	1.7% total, 2.5% MKE, 0.9% ILE /2.8% total,3.95% MKE, 1.7% ILE	

NB. Last study is presented for comparison as the largest minimally invasive esophagectomy series

MKE McKeown esophagectomy, *ILE* Ivor Lewis esophagectomy, *RT* Robotic thoracoscopy, *RL* Robotic laparoscopy, *CT* conventional thoracoscopy, *CL* conventional laparoscopy, *OT* open thoracotomy, *OL* open laparotomy

room time was 11.1 h with console time of 5.0 h. Major complications occurred in four (29%) of the patients – thoracic duct leak (one), severe pneumonia (one), anastomotic leak (two), and bilateral vocal cord paresis (one). There was one intraoperative right main stem bronchus injury. One patient died on POD 72 [65].

In another series by Sarkaria and colleagues, 16 (76%) out of 21 patients had received induction therapy. An R0 resection rate was achieved in 17 (81%) patients, and the median operative time was 556 min (range, 395–807 min), which decreased to 414 min (range, 405–543 min) for the last 5 cases in the series. The median number of lymph nodes resected was 20 (range, 10–49). Five patients (24%) had major complications. One (5%) died of complications on postoperative day 70, and three (14%) had clinically significant anastomotic leaks (grade II or greater). Three patients (14%) in this early experience developed airway fistulas [36].

Cerfolio and coauthors reported on his series of 92 patients, undergoing robotic Ivor Lewis Esophagectomy. Seven initial patients were excluded due to open abdominal part of the procedure. Of 85 patients with robotic thoracic part, laparoscopy was used in 79 (92.9%), robotic approach in 5 (5.9%), and conversion to laparotomy was required in 1 (1.2%) patient due to stapling failure. Total procedure time (skin to skin) was 360 min with average blood loss on 35 ml and no intraoperative transfusions. Median lymph node yield was 22 and R0 resection was achieved in 99% (84/85). Median hospital stay was 8 days (5–46 days). Morbidity occurred in 31 (36.4%) patients. Four patients had anastomotic leak and two had conduit necrosis requiring surgical intervention. Leaks occurred on average on POD 8 [4–15]. Thirty day in-hospital mortality was 3 (3.5%), and 90 days mortality was 9 (10.6%) [19].

Carrera and coauthors report on their experience of robotic esophagectomy. Of 51 cases of minimally invasive esophagectomy, 32 patients underwent robotic esophagectomy. There was 11 MKE and 21 ILE. Tumors located below 30 cm from incisors were treated with TTE and above that with MKE. Twenty-nine patients received induction therapy. The thoracic part was performed in the prone position, and hand-sewn anastomosis was performed. Average console time was 218 min (190–285). Blood loss was 170 min. One (3%) patient died from cardiac causes. Major complications (Dindo-Clavien grade II and up) occurred in nine (28%) patients. Mean LOS was 12 [8–50] days. All patients had R0 resection, and median LN yield was 16 [2–23]. In 21 patients with ILE, 4 (19%) patients developed grade I leak, all treated with covered stent placement. One (5%) patient developed grade IV leak, failing stenting and requiring surgical diversion. There were four (19%) cases of chylothorax, two of which required surgical reintervention. In the 11 patients of MKE group, 2 (18%) patients developed grade II leak, treated conservatively, and 1 (9%) grade IV leak, requiring diversion [66].

Hodari et al. reported on their experience with hybrid ILE in 54 patients. Authors performed laparoscopic abdominal part of the procedure with robotic thoracic part. Authors estimated that with the need of robot docking and undocking, robotic abdominal part will extend the total timing of the procedure for up to an hour. Forty-six (85%) had adenocarcinoma and 3 (6%) had squamous cell carcinoma histology. Thirty-eight (70%) patients underwent induction therapy. Authors utilized Firefly technology for real-time perfusion assessment of the conduit. Of the total 3 (20%) leaks, all happened in first 15 patients, prior to the use of perfusion assessment. One leak was traumatic due to reintubation and perforation by nasogastric tube, requiring surgical closure with muscle flap. One more leak from conduit staple line was due to technical error of stapling the NGT, requiring hand-sewn closure. Mean ICU stay was 4.6 days and hospital stay of 12.9 days. All patients had R0 resection. Average LN yield was 16.2 (range 3–35) [21].

Park with coauthors summarized his experience in robotic-assisted thoracoscopic esophagectomy (RATE) vs standard thoracoscopic esophagectomy. Authors utilized robotic thoracoscopic mobilization with lymphadenectomy and laparoscopic (84 (73.7%) or open (30 (26.3%) abdominal part in McKeown esophagectomy. In the group of 114 patients, 110 patients had squamous cell carcinoma. Fifteen (13%) received induction therapy. All but one patient underwent RATE. Five patients had salvage esophagectomy. Total operation time was 419.6 ± 7.9 min with robot console time of 206.6 ± 5.2 min. Pulmonary complications developed in 11 patients (9.6%). Seven patients (6%) needed reintubation or prolonged ventilator therapy in the ICU. RLN palsy was observed in 30 patients (26.3%): unilateral in 27 patients (23.7%) and bilateral in 3 patients (2.6%). Anastomotic leak developed in 17 patients (14.9%), and most of these were treated by drainage only. Reoperation was required in five patients (4.4%). Ninety-day mortality was 2.6% due to pneumonia [18].

In 2017 Park et al. in a follow-up analysis reported on the oncologic feasibility of his technique. Three years overall survival for the group was 85% and recurrence-free survival 79.4%. Subgroup analysis demonstrated 3-year OS was 94.4% in patients with stage I disease, 86.2% in patients with stage II disease, 77.8% in patients with stage IIIA disease, and 37.5% in patients with stage IIIB/C disease. The 3-year RFS was 96.2% in patients with stage I disease, 80.1% in patients with stage II disease, and 79.5% in patients with stage IIIA disease. Tumor recurrence within 2 years after operation developed in more than 80% of patients with stage IIIB/C disease. Authors believe these excellent outcomes related to high rate of R0 resection (97.4%) and high lymph nodes yield [49, 67].

Reporting on the Moffitt Cancer Center experience, Amaral and coauthors analyzed results of the 237 patients, undergoing robotic-assisted esophagectomy [68]. Fifteen percent of the patients developed anastomotic leak; however, only 4% required an intervention.

Senior author of this chapter has published his experience of 33 robotic esophagectomies in 2013 [24]. All patients underwent robotic-assisted MKE. Postoperative complications developed in 39% of patients, with anastomotic leaks and chylothorax in 6% each. Mortality occurred in one (3%) patient on POD 12 due to mesenteric ischemia. Since that time the group experience has expanded, and presently an analysis of outcomes is underway.

Currently there is a monocenter randomized controlled trial underway, comparing result of robotic assisted vs open esophagectomy [69]. Publication of the results is anxiously awaited.

In summary, robotic surgery appears to offer advantages in surgical management of patient with esophageal cancer and benign conditions, requiring esophagectomy. Thorough staging workup is still obviously required. Meticulous surgical technique, diligent postoperative care, and timely intervention for management of complications are required for the best outcomes. In the foreseeable future, with rising adoption and increased affordability of the robotic technology, we fully expect near universal adoption of the robotics in the area of esophagectomy.

References

1. Torek F. The first successful case of resection of the thoracic portion of the esophagus for carcinoma. Surg Gynecol Obst. 1913;16:614.
2. Turner G. Excision of thoracic oesophagus for carcinoma with construction of extra-thoracic gullet. Lancet. 1933;2:1315.
3. Orringer MB, Sloan H. Esophagectomy without thoracotomy. J Thorac Cardiovasc Surg. 1978;76(5):643–54.

4. Orringer MB, Lemmer JH. Early dilation in the treatment of esophageal disruption. Ann Thorac Surg. 1986;42(5):536–9.

5. Colvin H, Dunning J, Khan OA. Transthoracic versus transhiatal esophagectomy for distal esophageal cancer: which is superior? Interact Cardiovasc Thorac Surg. 2011;12(2):265–9.

6. Lewis I. The surgical treatment of carcinoma of the oesophagus; with special reference to a new operation for growths of the middle third. Br J Surg. 1946;34:18–31.

7. D'Amico TA. Mckeown esophagogastrectomy. J Thorac Dis. 2014;6(Suppl 3):S322–4.

8. McKeown KC. Trends in oesophageal resection for carcinoma with special reference to total oesophagectomy. Ann R Coll Surg Engl. 1972;51(4):213–39.

9. Bakhos CT, Fabian T, Oyasiji TO, Gautam S, Gangadharan SP, Kent MS, et al. Impact of the surgical technique on pulmonary morbidity after esophagectomy. Ann Thorac Surg. 2012;93(1):221–6; discussion 226–7

10. Raymond DP, Seder CW, Wright CD, Magee MJ, Kosinski AS, Cassivi SD, et al. Predictors of major morbidity or mortality after resection for esophageal cancer: a Society of Thoracic Surgeons general thoracic surgery database risk adjustment model. Ann Thorac Surg. 2016;102(1):207–14.

11. Sweet RH. Carcinoma of the esophagus and the cardiac end of the stomach immediate and late results of treatment by resection and primary esophagogastric anastomosis. J Am Med Assoc. 1947;135(8):485–90.

12. Zhang H, Wang J, Wang W, Zhou L, Chen J, Yang B, et al. A meta-analysis of esophagectomy: the comparative study of Ivor-Lewis operation and Sweet operation. Zhonghua Wei Chang Wai Ke Za Zhi. 2014;17(9):892–7.

13. Matthews HR, Steel A. Left-sided subtotal oesophagectomy for carcinoma. Br J Surg. 1987;74(12):1115–7.

14. Palazzo F, Rosato EL, Chaudhary A, Evans NR 3rd, Sendecki JA, Keith S, et al. Minimally invasive esophagectomy provides significant survival advantage compared with open or hybrid esophagectomy for patients with cancers of the esophagus and gastroesophageal junction. J Am Coll Surg. 2015;220(4):672–9.

15. Zhou C, Zhang L, Wang H, Ma X, Shi B, Chen W, et al. Superiority of minimally invasive oesophagectomy in reducing in-hospital mortality of patients with resectable oesophageal cancer: a meta-analysis. PLoS One. 2015;10(7):e0132889.

16. Luketich JD, Pennathur A, Awais O, Levy RM, Keeley S, Shende M, et al. Outcomes after minimally invasive esophagectomy: review of over 1000 patients. Ann Surg. 2012;256(1):95–103.

17. Ben-David K, Kim T, Caban AM, Rossidis G, Rodriguez SS, Hochwald SN. Pre-therapy laparoscopic feeding jejunostomy is safe and effective in patients undergoing minimally invasive esophagectomy for cancer. J Gastrointest Surg. 2013;17(8):1352–8.

18. Park S, Hwang Y, Lee HJ, Park IK, Kim YT, Kang CH. Comparison of robot-assisted esophagectomy and thoracoscopic esophagectomy in esophageal squamous cell carcinoma. J Thorac Dis. 2016;8(10):2853–61.

19. Cerfolio RJ, Wei B, Hawn MT, Minnich DJ. Robotic esophagectomy for cancer: early results and lessons learned. Semin Thorac Cardiovasc Surg. 2016;28(1):160–9.

20. Yukaya T, Saeki H, Kasagi Y, Nakashima Y, Ando K, Imamura Y, et al. Indocyanine green fluorescence angiography for quantitative evaluation of gastric tube perfusion in patients undergoing esophagectomy. J Am Coll Surg. 2015;221(2):e37–42.

21. Hodari A, Park KU, Lace B, Tsiouris A, Hammoud Z. Robot-assisted minimally invasive Ivor Lewis esophagectomy with real-time perfusion assessment. Ann Thorac Surg. 2015;100(3):947–52.

22. Weksler B, Sharma P, Moudgill N, Chojnacki KA, Rosato EL. Robot-assisted minimally invasive esophagectomy is equivalent to thoracoscopic minimally invasive esophagectomy. Dis Esophagus. 2012;25(5):403–9.

23. Salami A, Abbas AE, Petrov R, Jhala N, Bakhos CT. Comparative analysis of clinical, treatment, and survival characteristics of basaloid and squamous cell carcinoma of the esophagus. J Am Coll Surg. 2018;226(6):1086–92.

24. Abbas AE, Dylewski MR. Robotic assisted minimally invasive esophagectomy. In: Kim KC, editor. Robotics in general surgery. New York: Springer; 2014. https://doi.org/10.1007/978-1-4614-8739-5_4.

25. Fujita T, Iida Y, Tanaka C, Nakamura K, Yamanaka K, Ueno J, et al. Development and evaluation of an "interdisciplinary postoperative support program" in outpatient clinics after thoracic esophagectomy. Int J Surg. 2017;43:58–66.

26. Schmidt HM, Gisbertz SS, Moons J, Rouvelas I, Kauppi J, Brown A, et al. Defining benchmarks for transthoracic esophagectomy: a multicenter analysis of Total minimally invasive esophagectomy in low risk patients. Ann Surg. 2017;266(5):814–21.

27. Riber LP, Larsen TB, Christensen TD. Postoperative atrial fibrillation prophylaxis after lung surgery: systematic review and meta-analysis. Ann Thorac Surg. 2014;98(6):1989–97.

28. Berry MF, D'Amico TA, Onaitis MW. Use of amiodarone after major lung resection. Ann Thorac Surg. 2014;98(4):1199–206.

29. Zhao BC, Huang TY, Deng QW, Liu WF, Liu J, Deng WT, et al. Prophylaxis against atrial fibrillation after general thoracic surgery: trial sequential analysis and network meta-analysis. Chest. 2017;151(1):149–59.

30. Lerut T, Coosemans W, Decker G, De Leyn P, Nafteux P, van Raemdonck D. Anastomotic complications after esophagectomy. Dig Surg. 2002;19(2):92–8.

31. van den Berg MW, Kerbert AC, van Soest EJ, Schwartz MP, Bakker CM, Gilissen LP, et al. Safety and efficacy of a fully covered large-diameter self-expanding metal stent for the treatment of upper gastrointestinal perforations, anastomotic leaks, and fistula. Dis Esophagus. 2016;29(6):572–9.

32. Sutcliffe RP, Forshaw MJ, Tandon R, Rohatgi A, Strauss DC, Botha AJ, et al. Anastomotic strictures and delayed gastric emptying after esophagectomy: incidence, risk factors and management. Dis Esophagus. 2008;21(8):712–7.

33. Dickinson KJ, Blackmon SH. Management of conduit necrosis following esophagectomy. Thorac Surg Clin. 2015;25(4):461–70.

34. Schaheen L, Blackmon SH, Nason KS. Optimal approach to the management of intrathoracic esophageal leak following esophagectomy: a systematic review. Am J Surg. 2014;208(4):536–43.

35. Sharaiha RZ, Kumta NA, DeFilippis EM, Dimaio CJ, Gonzalez S, Gonda T, et al. A large multicenter experience with endoscopic suturing for management of gastrointestinal defects and stent anchorage in 122 patients: a retrospective review. J Clin Gastroenterol. 2016;50(5):388–92.

36. Sarkaria IS, Rizk NP, Finley DJ, Bains MS, Adusumilli PS, Huang J, et al. Combined thoracoscopic and laparoscopic robotic-assisted minimally invasive esophagectomy using a four-arm platform: experience, technique and cautions during early procedure development. Eur J Cardiothorac Surg. 2013;43(5):e107–15.

37. Morita M, Saeki H, Okamoto T, Oki E, Yoshida S, Maehara Y. Tracheobronchial fistula during the perioperative period of esophagectomy for esophageal cancer. World J Surg. 2015;39(5):1119–26.

38. Arnold PG, Pairolero PC. Intrathoracic muscle flaps. An account of their use in the management of 100 consecutive patients. Ann Surg. 1990;211(6):656–60; discussion 660–2

39. Koshenkov VP, Yakoub D, Livingstone AS, Franceschi D. Tracheobronchial injury in the setting of an esophagectomy for cancer: postoperative discovery a bad omen. J Surg Oncol. 2014;109(8):804–7.

40. Shen Y, Feng M, Khan MA, Wang H, Tan L, Wang Q. A simple method minimizes chylothorax after minimally invasive esophagectomy. J Am Coll Surg. 2014;218(1):108–12.

41. Crucitti P, Mangiameli G, Petitti T, Condoluci A, Rocco R, Gallo IF, et al. Does prophylactic ligation of the thoracic duct reduce chylothorax rates in patients undergoing oesophagectomy? A systematic review and meta-analysis. Eur J Cardiothorac Surg. 2016;50(6):1019–24.

42. Pillay TG, Singh B. A review of traumatic chylothorax. Injury. 2016;47(3):545–50.

43. Cope C, Salem R, Kaiser LR. Management of chylothorax by percutaneous catheterization and embolization of the thoracic duct: prospective trial. J Vasc Interv Radiol. 1999;10(9):1248–54.

44. Sato Y, Kosugi S, Aizawa N, Ishikawa T, Kano Y, Ichikawa H, et al. Risk factors and clinical outcomes of recurrent laryngeal nerve paralysis after Esophagectomy for thoracic esophageal carcinoma. World J Surg. 2016;40(1):129–36.

45. Wright CD, Zeitels SM. Recurrent laryngeal nerve injuries after esophagectomy. Thorac Surg Clin. 2006;16(1):23–33. v

46. Antonoff MB, Puri V, Meyers BF, Baumgartner K, Bell JM, Broderick S, et al. Comparison of pyloric intervention strategies at the time of esophagectomy: is more better? Ann Thorac Surg. 2014;97(6):1950–7; discussion 1657–8

47. Arya S, Markar SR, Karthikesalingam A, Hanna GB. The impact of pyloric drainage on clinical outcome following esophagectomy: a systematic review. Dis Esophagus. 2015;28(4):326–35.

48. Manfredi MA. Endoscopic management of anastomotic esophageal strictures secondary to esophageal atresia. Gastrointest Endosc Clin N Am. 2016;26(1):201–19.

49. Kinoshita Y, Udagawa H, Tsutsumi K, Ueno M, Mine S, Ehara K. Surgical repair of refractory strictures of esophagogastric anastomoses caused by leakage following esophagectomy. Dis Esophagus. 2009;22(5):427–33.

50. Williams VA, Watson TJ, Zhovtis S, Gellersen O, Raymond D, Jones C, et al. Endoscopic and symptomatic assessment of anastomotic strictures following esophagectomy and cervical esophagogastrostomy. Surg Endosc. 2008;22(6):1470–6.

51. Kochhar R, Makharia GK. Usefulness of intralesional triamcinolone in treatment of benign esophageal strictures. Gastrointest Endosc. 2002;56(6):829–34.

52. Vallbohmer D, Holscher AH, Herbold T, Gutschow C, Schroder W. Diaphragmatic hernia after conventional or laparoscopic-assisted transthoracic esophagectomy. Ann Thorac Surg. 2007;84(6):1847–52.

53. Kent MS, Luketich JD, Tsai W, Churilla P, Federle M, Landreneau R, et al. Revisional surgery after esophagectomy: an analysis of 43 patients. Ann Thorac Surg. 2008;86(3):975–83; discussion 967–74

54. Sutherland J, Banerji N, Morphew J, Johnson E, Dunn D. Postoperative incidence of incarcerated hiatal hernia and its prevention after robotic transhiatal esophagectomy. Surg Endosc. 2011;25(5):1526–30.

55. Malik Z, Kataria R, Modayil R, Ehrlich AC, Schey R, Parkman HP, et al. Gastric per oral endoscopic myotomy (G-POEM) for the treatment of refractory gastroparesis: early experience. Dig Dis Sci (2018). https://doi.org/10.1007/s10620-018-4976-9.

56. Rove JY, Krupnick AS, Baciewicz FA, Meyers BF. Gastric conduit revision postesophagectomy: management for a rare complication. J Thorac Cardiovasc Surg. 2017;154(4):1450–8.

57. Lee P, Kupeli E, Mehta AC. Airway stents. Clin Chest Med. 2010;31(1):141–50. Table of Contents

58. Dunn LJ, Shenfine J, Griffin SM. Columnar metaplasia in the esophageal remnant after esophagectomy: a systematic review. Dis Esophagus. 2015;28(1):32–41.

59. El-Serag HB, Naik AD, Duan Z, Shakhatreh M, Helm A, Pathak A, et al. Surveillance endoscopy is associated with improved outcomes of oesophageal adenocarcinoma detected in patients with Barrett's oesophagus. Gut. 2016;65(8):1252–60.

60. Gasparri MG, Tisol WB, Haasler GB. Roux-en-Y diversion for debilitating reflux after esophagectomy. Am Surg. 2005;71(8):687–9.

61. Schieman C, Wigle DA, Deschamps C, Nichols FC 3rd, Cassivi SD, Shen KR, et al. Salvage resections for recurrent or persistent cancer of the proximal esophagus after chemoradiotherapy. Ann Thorac Surg. 2013;95(2):459–63.

62. Schipper PH, Cassivi SD, Deschamps C, Rice DC, Nichols FC 3rd, Allen MS, et al. Locally recurrent esophageal carcinoma: when is re-resection indicated? Ann Thorac Surg. 2005;80(3):1001–5; discussion 1005–6

63. Knabe M, May A, Ell C. Endoscopic resection for patients with mucosal adenocarcinoma of the esophagus. Minerva Gastroenterol Dietol. 2016;62(4):281–95.

64. Bodner J, Wykypiel H, Wetscher G, Schmid T. First experiences with the da Vinci operating robot in thoracic surgery. Eur J Cardiothorac Surg. 2004;25(5):844–51.

65. Kernstine KH, DeArmond DT, Shamoun DM, Campos JH. The first series of completely robotic esophagectomies with three-field lymphadenectomy: initial experience. Surg Endosc. 2007;21(12):2285–92.

66. Trugeda Carrera MS, Fernandez-Diaz MJ, Rodriguez-Sanjuan JC, Manuel-Palazuelos JC, de Diego Garcia EM, Gomez-Fleitas M. Initial results of robotic esophagectomy for esophageal cancer. Cir Esp. 2015;93(6):396–402.

67. Park SY, Kim DJ, Do YW, Suh J, Lee S. The oncologic outcome of esophageal squamous cell carcinoma patients after robot-assisted thoracoscopic esophagectomy with total mediastinal lymphadenectomy. Ann Thorac Surg. 2017;103(4):1151–7.

68. Amaral M, Pimiento J, Fontaine JP. Robotic esophagectomy: the Moffitt Cancer Center experience. Ann Cardiothorac Surg. 2017;6(2):186–9.

69. van der Sluis PC, Ruurda JP, van der Horst S, Verhage RJ, Besselink MG, Prins MJ, et al. Robot-assisted minimally invasive thoraco-laparoscopic esophagectomy versus open transthoracic esophagectomy for resectable esophageal cancer, a randomized controlled trial (ROBOT trial). Trials. 2012;13:230. https://doi.org/10.1186/1745-6215-13-230.

Part VI

Plastic Surgery

Robotic Telemicrosurgery

35

Juan José Hidalgo Diaz, Nicola Santelmo, Fred Xavier,
and Philippe Liverneaux

Introduction

Microsurgery was developed in the 1960s from experimental work in animals. The first vascular microsurgical anastomosis was performed in a rat in 1960 [1] and the first ear replantation in a rabbit in 1966 [2]. Very quickly, applications were described in humans, and the first replantation of the thumb was published in 1965 [3]. Numerous applications have subsequently been described in human clinical practice, including vascular microsurgery and peripheral nerve microsurgery. As regards vascular microsurgery, technical advances have made it possible to successively perform replantations, free flaps, pedicled flaps, and more recently, perforator flaps [4]. Regarding microsurgery of the peripheral nerves, technical advances have made it possible to successively perform nerve sutures and nerve grafts, brachial plexus reconstructions, nerve transfers, and recently terminolateral nerve sutures [5].

Since the 1960s, microsurgery has undergone considerable development in its surgical indications, but no major technical advances have been observed, either visually or instrumentally. Although the operating microscopes are now digital, their magnification has not changed. These are always exoscopes that cannot penetrate inside the body. The instruments are now made of titanium, but their handling has not changed. They are always bulky instruments that cannot penetrate inside the body. A technological leap is observed in all industrial fields every 50 years. It is a safe bet that robotics will be the technological leap of microsurgery for two main reasons: optical and instrumental. Robotics allows the use of endoscopes that can penetrate inside the body through minimally invasive routes. Robotics allows the use of miniaturized instruments to subtract the physiological tremor and reduce the movements by the microsurgeon.

Robot-assisted microsurgery or telemicrosurgery offers two major advantages over conventional microsurgery: the minimally invasive surgical approaches and the use of more ergonomic hand gestures by reducing the movements.

Literature Review

Robot-assisted microsurgery is of interest in the two major applications of microsurgery: vascular microsurgery [6] and peripheral nerve microsurgery [7]. Although many prototypes have been recently designed, the da Vinci® robot is currently the only one used in clinical practice [8]. Microsurgery-specific instruments have been developed, such as the Black Diamond® clamps and the Pott® scissors, as well as microsurgical imaging devices such as a micro-Doppler for detecting inframillimetric vessels [9]. Using these instruments and devices requires a learning curve [10]. The learning of robot-assisted microsurgery follows rules identical to those of conventional microsurgery and specific rules [11], validated by precise evaluation methods [12, 13].

Regarding vascular microsurgery, many experimental techniques have been described. The feasibility of microsurgical vascular anastomoses has been demonstrated in the artery of the rat tail [14], the forearm arteries of the human anatomical subject [15]. Pedicled flaps have been described by hand [16, 17]. Live pig feet replantation has been successfully performed [18]. The main clinical applications of robot-assisted vascular microsurgery are free flaps [19] for breast reconstruction [20], rectus abdominis [21–23], and latissimus dorsi [24–27]. Some have performed venous

J. J. Hidalgo Diaz · P. Liverneaux (✉)
Department of Hand Surgery, SOS Main, CCOM, University Hospital of Strasbourg, FMTS, University of Strasbourg, Illkirch, France
e-mail: Philippe.liverneaux@chru-strasbourg.fr

N. Santelmo
Department of Thoracic Surgery,
University Hospital of Strasbourg, FMTS, Strasbourg, France

F. Xavier
Orthopedic Surgery, Biomedical Engineering,
Cincinnati, OH, USA

Spine Surgery, Dalhousie University, Halifax, NS, Canada

© Springer Nature Switzerland AG 2019
S. Tsuda, O. Y. Kudsi (eds.), *Robotic-Assisted Minimally Invasive Surgery*, https://doi.org/10.1007/978-3-319-96866-7_35

grafts to reconstruct the ulnar artery as part of a hypothenar hammer syndrome [28].

Concerning nerve microsurgery of peripheral nerves, many experimental techniques have been described. The feasibility of microsurgical nerve anastomoses has been demonstrated in the rat sciatic nerve [7] and numerous nerve transfers in brachial plexus palsies such as intercostal nerve [29], phrenic nerve [30], the contralateral transfer of the C7 root of the brachial plexus by two approaches [31] and a minimally invasive technique [32], the description of new approaches for the lower brachial plexus [33], the axillary nerve, and the nerve of the long head triceps [34] in the human anatomical subject.

The main clinical applications of robot-assisted peripheral nerve microsurgery are direct brachial plexus repairs by root [35] and indirect nerve transfusions of the long triceps nerve on the axillary nerve [36, 37] and of a motor fascicle of the ulnar nerve on the motor branch of the musculocutaneous nerve [38]. Some neurolyses have been proposed, such as the lateral femoral cutaneous nerve in the course of a meralgia paresthetica [39] or the median nerve in the carpal tunnel [40], as well as resection of nerve tumors [41, 42].

Preoperative Planning

The robot-assisted microsurgery described herein by way of example relates to the peripheral nerves. The aim of this procedure is to recover the most important function in the event of complete paralysis of the brachial plexus: active flexion of the elbow. This is the robot-assisted transfer of intercostal nerves to the motor branch of the musculocutaneous nerve for the biceps muscle by intrathoracic minimally invasive approaches. The conventional technique for harvesting intercostal nerves requires a very extensive incision of dozens of centimeters [43]. The advantage of robot-assisted microsurgical techniques is to use only four incisions of 1 cm each for the placement of the tubes and the exit of the intercostal nerves from the thorax.

There is no specific planning for robotics in this indication. A trained thoracic surgeon must do the trocar placement. A history of major thoracic trauma that could have caused intercostal nerve damage on the side to be operated is a relative contraindication.

Setup

The procedure is performed in two stages: the first in lateral decubitus to harvest the intercostal nerves and the second in supine position to carry out the nerve transfer.

At the first stage, the patient is placed in lateral decubitus, on the opposite side to the surgical site. General anesthesia is performed with contralateral unipulmonary ventilation by selective intubation using a Carlens probe to clear the intrathoracic workspace. The incisions for the tubes are drawn against the eighth intercostal space so that all the instruments and endoscope can converge on the third and fourth intercostal spaces (Fig. 35.1). The endoscopic camera trocar is installed first. A da Vinci SI® (Intuitive Surgical™, Sunnyvale, CA, USA) robot is placed at the patient's head, and its arms are deployed in such a way that the amplitude of movement of the instruments and of the endoscopic camera allow access to the full length of the intercostal nerves to be taken, that is, to say from the mammary artery, in the front, to the pleural dome, in the rear (Fig. 35.2). An insufflation of approximately 12 mmHg is done on the endoscopic camera trocar to enlarge the workspace and reduce the parietal bleeding. During the nerve harvesting phase, a bipolar Maryland® forceps and a pair of curved scissors are used.

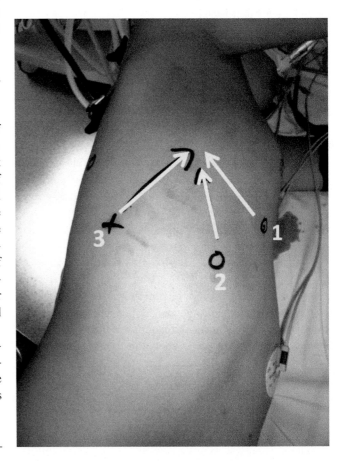

Fig. 35.1 Preparation of surgical approaches. The patient is placed in the left lateral decubitus. Three incisions of 1 cm each are drawn along the eighth intercostal space in front of the axillary line (1), opposite the axillary line (2), and behind the axillary line (3). Incisions 1 and 3 are designed to accommodate the instrumental tubes and incision 2 the camera trocar of the da Vinci® robot. The tubes must allow the instruments and the camera to stay in the workspace, along the third and fourth intercostal spaces

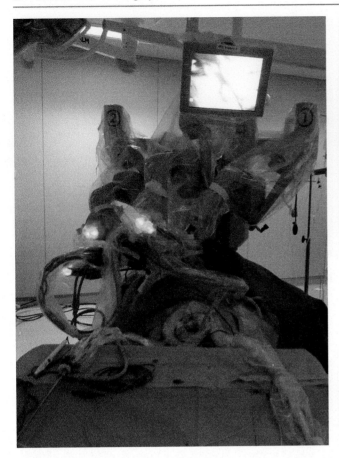

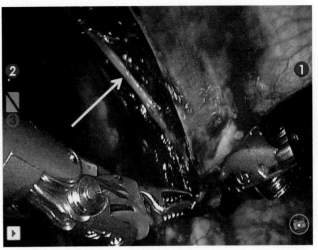

Fig. 35.3 Intrathoracic view. Beginning of dissection of the nerve of the fourth intercostal space (arrow). The instruments cut the parietal pleura along the fourth intercostal space to reveal the nerve

Fig. 35.2 Installation of the da Vinci® robot. The patient is placed in the left lateral decubitus. The da Vinci® robot is placed at the patient's head

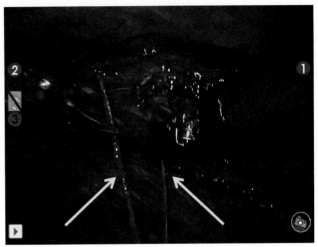

Fig. 35.4 Intrathoracic view. End of the dissection of the nerves of the third and fourth intercostal spaces (arrows). The nerves have been severed at their anterior extremity and remain. The instruments look for the point of entry of the trocar intended to remove the intercostal nerves from their posterior extremities

In the second stage, the patient is placed in supine position and the upper limb to operate rests on a surgical arm table. The incision is drawn on the medial side of the arm to give access to the motor branch of the musculocutaneous nerve for the biceps muscle. The da Vinci® robot is placed at the side edge of the patient's arm, and the arms of the robot are deployed so that the instruments work on the medial edge of the patient's arm. During the microsurgical suture phase of the intercostal nerves with the motor branch of the musculocutaneous nerve, two Black Diamond® clamps and a pair of Pott® scissors are used.

Procedure

In the first stage, the dissection begins with the most cranial intercostal nerve, in order to prevent the bleeding of the caudal nerve from flowing over the most cranial nerve and interfere with its dissection. In the present case, the dissection of the intercostal nerve of the fourth space will begin before that of the third space. The parietal pleura is then carefully

opened at the lower edge of the rib to identify the nerve to be harvested without any damage (Fig. 35.3). As soon as the nerve is located, the parietal pleura is incised all along the nerve path, from the mammary artery to the pleural dome. The nerve is then freed from all its attachments along its length, and its sensory branches are severed. When the intercostal nerves and third and fourth spaces are completely released, the anterior extremities of the two nerves are cut near their anterior end (Fig. 35.4). A trocar is inserted between the two nerves at their posterior ends in the axilla to recover their anterior ends and to make them leave the thorax with the aid of an atraumatic forceps. The two intercostal

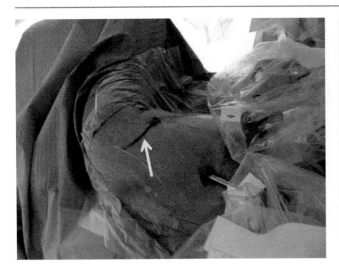

Fig. 35.5 Extrathoracic view. The nerves of the third and fourth intercostal spaces have been removed from the thorax by their anterior extremity (arrows)

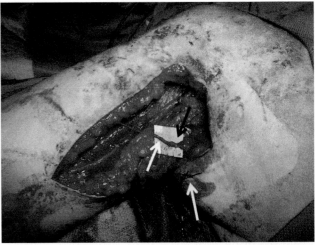

Fig. 35.6 Axillary view. The incision out of the thorax nerves of the third and fourth intercostal spaces was closed (yellow arrow). Result of the robot-assisted microsurgical suture of the two intercostal nerves (black arrow) with the motor branch of the biceps nerve (white arrow)

nerves are then exposed on the skin, wrapped in a moist compress, all applied hermetically by an adhesive dressing to avoid damage during the patient's position change (Fig. 35.5). A thoracic drain is placed before modifying the lateral decubitus to supine position.

In the second stage, after change of position, dissection begins with the musculocutaneous nerve whose motor branch for the biceps muscle is individualized as near as possible and then cut into the axilla to obtain a maximum length. A subcutaneous tunnel is made using a long clamp to connect the incision from the thorax of the intercostal nerves to the incision of the arm to the axilla. The nerve ends on the one hand of the motor branch of the musculocutaneous nerve for the biceps muscle and on the other hand of the two intercostal nerves which are confronted and then sutured using the robot da Vinci SI® with 2 points of nylon 10/0 (Fig. 35.6). Biological glue is applied all around the suture area. The incisions are closed in a cutaneous plane without drainage.

Postoperative Care

The operated upper limb is immobilized in a vest elbow to the body to avoid stressing the nerve suture and failure. The thoracic drain is removed on the second day, and the patient can return home on the third day. The patient is seen again in the third week to remove the elbow to the body, the dressing, and the sutures. The rehabilitation of maintenance of joint mobility is undertaken for 6 weeks, and the patient is reviewed at the sixth month postoperative, to watch for the first signs of nerve recovery. The active flexion of the elbow is generally obtained at the end of the first year (Figs. 35.7 and 35.8).

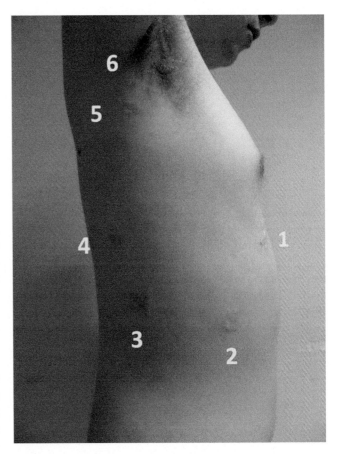

Fig. 35.7 Result after 1 year. The scars are hardly visible. The scars 1-2-3 correspond to the instrumental and optical trocars, the scar 4 corresponds to the exit point of the thoracic drain, the scar 5 corresponds to the point of exit of the nerves of the third and fourth intercostal spaces, and the scar 6 corresponds to the axillary part of the scar of nerve anastomosis between the two intercostal nerves and the motor branch of the biceps nerve

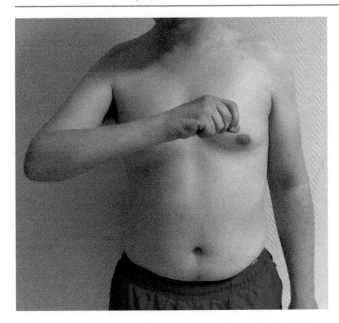

Fig. 35.8 Result after 1 year. The flexion of the elbow is recovered

Conclusion

The advantage of robotics in microsurgery is the increase in ergonomics for the surgeon and the reduction of scars for the patient.

The disadvantage of robotics in microsurgery is the absence of a dedicated device on the market and the abandonment of the motion reduction in the most recent versions of the da Vinci® robot's instrumentation.

Conflicts of Interest Philippe Liverneaux has conflicts of interest with Newclip Technics, Argomedical, Biomodex, Zimmer Biomet

None of the other authors have conflicts of interest

References

1. Jacobson JH, Suarez EL. Microsurgery in anastomosis of small vessels. Surg Forum. 1960;11:243–5.
2. Buncke HJ, Schulz WP. Total ear reimplantation in the rabbit utilizing microminiature vascular anastomosis. Br J Plast Surg. 1966;19:15–22.
3. Komatsu S, Tamai S. Successful replantation of a completely cut-off thumb. Plast Reconstr Surg. 1968;42:374–7.
4. Koshima I, Soeda S. Inferior epigastric skin flaps without rectus abdominis muscle. Br J Plast Surg. 1989;42:645–8.
5. Viterbo F, Trindade JC, Hoshino K, Mazzoni NA. End-to-side neurorrhaphy with removal of the epineurial sheath: an experimental study in rats. Plast Reconstr Surg. 1994;94:1038–47.
6. Saleh DB, Syed M, Kulendren D, Ramakrishnan V, Liverneaux PA. Plastic and reconstructive robotic microsurgery – a review of current practices. Ann Chir Plast Esthet. 2015;60:305–12.
7. Nectoux E, Taleb C, Liverneaux P. Nerve repair in telemicrosurgery: an experimental study. J Reconstr Microsurg. 2009;25:261–5.
8. Mattos LS, Caldwell DG, Peretti G, Mora F, Guastini L, Cingolani R. Microsurgery robots: addressing the needs of high-precision surgical interventions. Swiss Med Wkly. 2016;26:1–14.
9. Brahmbhatt JV, Gudeloglu A, Liverneaux P, Parekattil SJ. Robotic microsurgery optimization. Arch Plast Surg. 2014;41:225–30.
10. Ramdhian RM, Bednar M, Mantovani GR, Facca SA, Liverneaux PA. Microsurgery and telemicrosurgery training: a comparative study. J Reconstr Microsurg. 2011;279:537–42.
11. Liverneaux PA, Hendriks S, Selber JC, Parekattil SJ. Robotically assisted microsurgery: development of basic skills course. Arch Plast Surg. 2013;40:320–6.
12. Alrasheed T, Liu J, Hanasono MM, Butler CE, Selber JC. Robotic microsurgery: validating an assessment tool and plotting the learning curve. Plast Reconstruct Surg. 2014;134:794–803.
13. Alrasheed T, Selber JC. Robotic microsurgical training and evaluation. Semin Plast Surg. 2014;28:5–10.
14. Taleb C, Nectoux E, Liverneaux PA. Telemicrosurgery: a feasibility study in a rat model. Chir Main. 2008;27(2–3):104–8.
15. Robert E, Facca S, Atik T, Bodin F, Bruant-Rodier C, Liverneaux P. Vascular microanastomosis through an endoscopic approach: feasibility study on two cadaver forearms. Chir Main. 2013;323:136–40.
16. Huart A, Facca S, Lebailly F, Garcia JC, Liverneaux PA. Are pedicled flaps feasible in robotic surgery? Report of an anatomical study of the kite flap in conventional surgery versus robotic surgery. Surg Innov. 2012;191:89–92.
17. Maire N, Naito K, Lequint T, Facca S, Berner S, Liverneaux P. Robot-assisted free toe pulp transfer: feasibility study. J Reconstr Microsurg. 2012;287:481–4.
18. Taleb C, Nectoux E, Liverneaux P. Limb replantation with two robots: a feasibility study in a pig model. Microsurgery. 2009;293:232–5.
19. Selber JC, Pederson JC. Muscle flaps. In: Liverneaux PA, Berner SH, Bednar MS, et al., editors. Telemicrosurgery: robot assisted microsurgery. Paris: Springer; 2013. p. 145–57.
20. Van der Hulst R. Microvascular anastomosis: is there a role for robotic surgery? J Plast Reconstr Aesthet Surg. 2007;60:101–2.
21. Pedersen J, Song DH, Selber JC. Robotic, intraperitoneal harvest of the rectus abdominis muscle. Plast Reconstr Surg. 2014;134:1057–63.
22. Ibrahim AE, Sarhane KA, Pederson JC, Selber JC. Robotic harvest of the rectus abdominis muscle: principles and clinical applications. Semin Plast Surg. 2014;28:26–31.
23. Patel NV, Pedersen JC. Robotic harvest of the rectus abdominis muscle: a preclinical investigation and case report. J Reconstr Microsurg. 2012;28:477–80.
24. Ichihara S, Bodin F, Pedersen JC, Porto de Melo P, Garcia JC Jr, Facca S, Liverneaux PA. Robotically assisted harvest of the latissimus dorsi muscle: a cadaver feasibility study and clinical test case. Hand Surg Rehabil. 2016;352:81–4.
25. Selber JC, Baumann DP, Holsinger CF. Robotic harvest of the latissimus dorsi muscle: laboratory and clinical experience. J Reconstr Microsurg. 2012;28:457–64.
26. Selber JC, Baumann DP, Holsinger FC. Robotic latissimus dorsi muscle harvest: a case series. Plast Reconstr Surg. 2012;129:1305–12.
27. Clemens MW, Kronowitz S, Selber JC. Robotic-assisted latissimus dorsi harvest in delayed-immediate breast reconstruction. Semin Plast Surg. 2014;28:20–5.
28. Facca S, Liverneaux P. Robotic assisted microsurgery in hypothenar hammer syndrome: a case report. Comput Aided Surg. 2010;15(4–6):110–4.
29. Miyamoto H, Serradori T, Mikami Y, Selber J, Santelmo N, Facca S, Liverneaux P. Robotic intercostal nerve harvest: a feasibility study in a pig model. J Neurosurg. 2016;1241:264–8.

30. Porto De Melo P, Miyamoto H, Serradori T, Ruggiero Mantovani G, Selber J, Facca S, Xu WD, Santelmo N, Liverneaux P. Robotic phrenic nerve harvest: a feasibility study in a pig model. Chir Main. 2014;335:356–60.

31. Jiang S, Ichihara S, Prunières G, Peterson B, Facca S, Xu WD, Liverneaux P. Robot-assisted C7 nerve root transfer from the contralateral healthy side: a preliminary cadaver study. Hand Surg Rehabil. 2016;352:95–9.

32. Bijon C, Chih-Sheng L, Chevallier D, Tran N, Xavier F, Liverneaux P. Endoscopic robot-assisted C7 nerve root retrophalangeal transfer from the contralateral healthy side: a cadaver feasibility study. Ann Chir Plast Esthet. 2018;63(1):86–90. https://doi.org/10.1016/j.anplas.2017.05.004. Epub 2017 Jun 16. PubMed. PMID: 28624267.

33. Tetik C, Uzun M. Novel axillary approach for brachial plexus in robotic surgery: a cadaveric experiment. Minim Invasive Surg. 2014;2014:927456.

34. Porto De Melo PM, Garcia JC, Montero EF, Atik T, Robert EG, Facca S, Liverneaux PA. Feasibility of an endoscopic approach to the axillary nerve and the nerve to the long head of the triceps brachii with the help of the da Vinci robot. Chir Main. 2013;324:206–9.

35. Garcia JC Jr, Lebailly F, Mantovani G, Mendonca LA, Garcia J, Liverneaux P. Telerobotic manipulation of the brachial plexus. J Reconstr Microsurg. 2012;287:491–4.

36. Miyamoto H, Leechavengvongs S, Atik T, Facca S, Liverneaux P. Nerve transfer to the deltoid muscle using the nerve to the long head of the triceps with the da Vinci robot: six cases. J Reconstr Microsurg. 2014;306:375–80.

37. Facca S, Hendriks S, Mantovani G, Selber JC, Liverneaux P. Robot-assisted surgery of the shoulder girdle and brachial plexus. Semin Plast Surg. 2014;281:39–44.

38. Naito K, Facca S, Lequint T, Liverneaux PA. The oberlin procedure for restoration of elbow flexion with the Da Vinci robot: four cases. Plast Reconstr Surg. 2012;1293:707–11.

39. Bruyere A, Hidalgo Diaz JJ, Vernet P, Salazar Botero S, Facca S, Liverneaux PA. Technical feasibility of robot-assisted minimally-invasive neurolysis of the lateral cutaneous nerve of thigh: about a case. Ann Chir Plast Esthet. 2016;616:872–6.

40. Guldmann R, Pourtales MC, Liverneaux P. Is it possible to use robots for carpal tunnel release? J Orthop Sci. 2010;153:430–3.

41. Tigan L, Miyamoto H, Hendriks S, Facca S, Liverneaux P. Interest of Telemicrosurgery in peripheral nerve tumors: about a series of seven cases. Chir Main. 2014;331:13–6.

42. Lequint T, Naito K, Chaigne D, Facca S, Liverneaux P. Mini-invasive robot-assisted surgery of the brachial plexus: a case of Intraneural Perineurioma. J Reconstr Microsurg. 2012;287:473–576.

43. Fleury M, Lepage D, Pluvy I, Pauchot J. Nerve transfer between the intercostal nerves and the motor component of the musculocutaneous nerve. Anatomical study of feasibility. Ann Chir Plast Esthet. 2017;62(3):255–60. https://doi.org/10.1016/j.anplas.2016.11.004. Epub 2016 Dec 29.

Richard C. Baynosa

Introduction

Robotic surgery has gained wide popularity over the last decade because of the improved visualization and access to smaller and tighter body areas with more maneuverable and precise instrumentation than that available via endoscopic and laparoscopic methods. For multiple surgical subspecialties including general surgery, surgical oncology, bariatric surgery, urology, colorectal, gynecology, thoracic surgery and otolaryngology, robotic techniques are becoming more widespread and quickly becoming the standard for many different procedures.

The specialty of plastic surgery involves the rearrangement and transfer of tissues to repair and reconstruct defects resulting from trauma, congenital anomalies, or tumor extirpation for cancer. Because many of these defects are external and associated with open wounds or large open surgical incisions, the field of plastic surgery has necessarily relied on open approaches to achieve its goals. Minimally invasive techniques have been limited to approaches such as minimizing incision length, masking the location of the incisions, percutaneous injections of fat and/or filler to fill volume deficits, and the occasional use of the endoscope.

Reconstructive surgeons are continually presented with new and varying complex defects that continue to change with advancements in surgical treatments. With the advent and popularity of robotic surgery, new challenges have been presented to the plastic surgeon to provide reconstructive options while minimizing the morbidity of additional incisions and donor sites. This chapter presents the rationale and technique for incorporating the robotically harvested rectus abdominis muscle flap for reconstruction of a variety of defects after robotic pelvic surgery.

R. C. Baynosa
Division of Plastic Surgery, Plastic Surgery Residency Program, UNLV School of Medicine, Las Vegas, NV, USA
e-mail: Richard.baynosa@unlv.edu

Rationale

The rectus abdominis flap has long been a workhorse for reconstructive surgery in the pelvis [1–14]. The rectus flap can be harvested as a muscle only flap or including an overlying skin paddle such as in the vertical rectus abdominis musculocutaneous (VRAM) flap. The rectus flap is a robust flap with a consistent and long axial pedicle that allows for the flap to be transferred down as a pedicled flap to almost any region in the pelvis [15–20]. The primary disadvantage of the rectus flap has been the requirement for an oftentimes long open incision with sacrifice of the anterior rectus fascia, which is a primary strength layer of the abdominal wall.

It is well established that repair of perineal wounds and fistulas from the colon/rectum to the vagina, urethra, or bladder in the previously irradiated pelvis benefits from well-vascularized coverage to promote tissue healing [21–27]. In particular, irradiated defects after abdominoperineal resection (APR) have been shown to have better outcomes when vascularized tissue is used to reinforce the perineal incision and obliterate the rectal dead space [28–30]. The literature demonstrates consistent lower rates of major complications including major wound dehiscence, pelvic abscess, and fistula formation when immediate reconstruction of the pelvic defects was reinforced with well-vascularized muscle flaps [31, 32]. Additionally, while the gracilis muscle flap from the thigh has been used as an alternative reconstructive option in the deep pelvis and perineum, the rectus muscle flap has been shown to be clearly superior to the gracilis flap likely secondary to its greater mass and bulk as well as a much more robust and less tenuous blood supply [33].

The theoretical advantages of an intraperitoneal harvest of the rectus muscle compared to the standard open approach are numerous. The most obvious benefit is the lack of the long incision that is routinely needed to harvest the muscle. While this is not an issue with open pelvic surgery, when these procedures are performed minimally invasively using the surgical robot, then the open incision adds unnecessary increased morbidity and negates many of the benefits of the

© Springer Nature Switzerland AG 2019
S. Tsuda, O. Y. Kudsi (eds.), *Robotic-Assisted Minimally Invasive Surgery*, https://doi.org/10.1007/978-3-319-96866-7_36

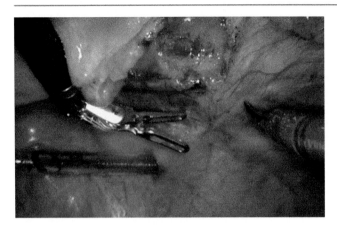

Fig. 36.1 Intraperitoneal view of the deep inferior epigastric vascular pedicle. The left side of the vessel has the peritoneum dissected free, but the continuation to the right (superiorly) is still readily seen through the intact peritoneum and posterior rectus fascia

robotic surgery. In addition to eliminating the morbidity of a long access incision for harvest, the intraperitoneal approach leaves the anterior rectus sheath, which serves as a significant layer for abdominal wall strength, preserved and intact. Last but not least, the intraperitoneal approach provides superior visualization of the rectus muscle along its entire course through the thin posterior rectus sheath. This is in stark contrast to the poor visualization through the thick anterior rectus sheath. Most importantly, the intraabdominal approach allows excellent visualization of the deep inferior epigastric vascular pedicle through the transparent peritoneum prior to the dissection and harvest of the muscle flap (Fig. 36.1).

Robotic Rectus Flap Technique

The benefits of robotic surgery beyond minimal access incisions are numerous and include superhuman precision with tremor elimination and motion scaling; clear, magnified, and high-resolution 3D stereoscopic views; enhanced exposure with the use of multiple robotic arms for precise traction; and the ability for wristed movements and retroflexing of the camera and instruments that is not possible with laparoscopy. The continued advancement in robotic surgery by numerous specialties has necessitated innovative approaches by plastic surgeons to solve these new reconstructive challenges.

The robotically harvested rectus muscle flap was first described and published in 2010 [34]. Subsequent publications have demonstrated the safety and feasibility of this technique for numerous different applications [35–37]. In our practice, the use of the robotic rectus flap arose with the introduction and incorporation of the robotic abdominoperineal resection (APR) as the standard approach to low-lying rectal and anal cancers where the anal sphincter could not be

preserved. By incorporating robotic techniques for the muscle flap harvest, we have significantly minimized the morbidity associated with the open approaches of the typical reconstructive options including the vertical rectus abdominis musculocutaneous (VRAM) flap and the gracilis flap. There has been less pain from the flap harvest, and this has eliminated the potential for donor site infection because the harvest is completed entirely through an intraperitoneal approach.

As with the integration of any novel technique, the mainstay to achieving good outcomes is dependent on the development of good inclusion and exclusion criteria for patient selection. Patients that are suitable for a robotic APR are often good candidates for a robotic rectus flap, but it should be noted that in the early portion of the learning curve, operative times can be significantly longer and patients should have minimal comorbidities that would preclude them from undergoing a prolonged anesthetic. Although long-term data and outcomes still need to be analyzed, in theory the decreased pain, narcotic use, hospital stay, and overall decreased morbidity should justify the initially longer operative time. Additionally as the surgeon's experience in the robotic harvest increases, the average operative time for a robotic rectus harvest will be typically less than 1 h [36].

Exclusion criteria for this procedure include a significant soft tissue defect requiring reconstruction with a large skin paddle. These patients would be more appropriately treated with a VRAM flap and/or gracilis musculocutaneous flap. Resurfacing of posterior vaginal defects, however, should not be considered a contraindication to robotic rectus harvest. In fact, we feel that the peritoneum and posterior rectus fascia provide an ideal tissue substitute for resurfacing the mucosa of the vagina. The literature has shown that these tissues readily mucosalize and provide a good reconstructive option in this area [38]. We will also exclude obese patients with excessive BMI and large intraabdominal fat components as we have seen an increased rate of postoperative bulge in these patients when the rectus flap is harvested and the posterior rectus fascia is weakened and/or incorporated into the reconstruction. We recommend repair of the posterior rectus fascia after harvest and now routinely incorporate biologic mesh to repair the defect and provide additional soft tissue support in an underlay fashion. The use of mesh and preservation of the anterior rectus fascia helps to minimize the development of an abdominal bulge in these patients postoperatively.

Technique

Robotic harvest of the rectus muscle can be readily accomplished with three 8 mm robotic ports, although a 12 mm camera port was required in our early experience. When working in conjunction with the colorectal surgeon for post-APR perineal reconstruction, insufflation will have already been achieved. When planning the rectus flap harvest for free tissue transfer, however, standard Veress needle technique should be used to obtain insufflation. After achieving appropriate insufflation, the ports are then placed in the hemiabdomen contralateral from the rectus muscle to be harvested and as far lateral as possible to allow for dissection of the muscle off of the posterior rectus fascia at the midline. When this flap is performed for post-APR reconstruction, the muscle will typically be the right-sided rectus muscle to allow maturing of the end colostomy in the standard left lower quadrant position through the left rectus muscle.

Accurate port placement is critical to obtaining the exposure necessary to harvest the flap as well as having the freedom of movement of the robotic arms to harvest the entire length of the rectus muscle. The central camera port should be placed approximately 2–3 cm or two finger breadths posterior the anterior axillary line at the midpoint between the costal margin superiorly and the anterior superior iliac spine (ASIS) inferiorly. The two robotic working ports are then placed 2 cm inferior to the costal margin and 2 cm superior to the ASIS, respectively (Fig. 36.2). When the rectus flap is done in conjunction with the colorectal surgeon for robotic APR, proper preoperative planning and communication will allow one of the ports to be incorporated as one of the colorectal surgeon's working ports to minimize the number of necessary port sites and incisions. Additionally, the use of the AirSeal insufflation system (CONMED, Utica, NY) will assist in maintaining the appropriate amount of intraperitoneal insufflation, particularly after removal of the specimen and creation of the perineal defect. After placement of the ports, the surgical table is oriented with the right (harvest side) up and slight Trendelenburg. After proper positioning to allow the abdominal contents to fall away from the operative site, the robot is docked in the standard fashion.

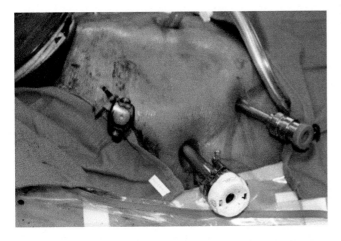

Fig. 36.2 Standard port placement at the contralateral hemiabdomen in an early case with 12 mm camera port on the DaVinci Si robot. Newer applications allow three 8 mm ports throughout

After all ports are docked, a 30° camera is then placed to allow improved visualization of the posterior abdominal wall. Harvest of the flap is performed with Hot Shears/monopolar curved scissors (Intuitive Surgical) in the dominant working arm and a Cadiere or ProGrasp Forceps (Intuitive Surgical) in the nondominant arm. Attention is first turned to the right lower quadrant to identify and preserve the deep inferior epigastric pedicle. The pedicle is readily visualized through the overlying peritoneum, which is sharply divided, and dissection is performed from the lateral rectus muscle to several centimeters laterally to allow ease of transposition of the muscle flap. Although usually not necessary, the pedicle vessels may be dissected to their origin at the external iliac vessels if there is any tension, kinking, or twisting of the pedicle.

After the pedicle has been identified, dissection of the posterior rectus sheath is performed. At the level of the inferior epigastric pedicle, the peritoneum is sharply incised transversely across the entirety of the posterior surface of the rectus muscle from lateral to the medial edge of the muscle. This allows not only transposition of the rectus muscle flap to be reflected down into the pelvis but also identifies the medial and lateral borders of the rectus muscle for subsequent dissection. The dissection begins medially by making a vertical incision just lateral to the medial border of the rectus muscle and continuing this cranially. This is typically the most difficult part of the dissection as the camera and instruments are positioned directly up almost at the midline and the working area is fairly tight. The incision is then continued superiorly to the costal margin. It is helpful to have the robotic tech or assistant palpate and identify the costal margin externally as this level is often difficult to identify from the intraperitoneal surface. Dissecting the muscle to this level will allow the flap to easily reach down to the perineum.

Attention is then turned to the lateral border of the muscle. The dissection again begins at the caudal portion of the rectus muscle at the level of the transverse incision in the peritoneum. The vertical incision is made at least 1 cm medial to the lateral border of the rectus muscle. This ensures that the insertion of the transversalis and oblique muscles to the lateral portion of the rectus sheath is not disrupted. The dissection is then carried superiorly in the same fashion as the medial dissection. Care is taken to identify and cauterize the neurovascular pedicles entering laterally into the rectus muscle from the intercostal system. The dissection is continued to the same level as the medial dissection superiorly (Fig. 36.3).

At the level of the costal margin, the medial and lateral dissection points are joined by dividing the peritoneum, posterior rectus fascia, and rectus muscle transversely with electrocautery (Fig. 36.4). Care is taken to ensure hemostasis of the muscle and to identify and control the superior epigastric vessels. The rectus muscle is now dissected from distal to proximal. Extreme care is taken to identify all large perforators to

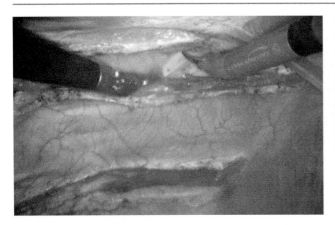

Fig. 36.3 Intraperitoneal view of medial and lateral borders (superior and inferior aspects of the figure, respectively) of the rectus muscle dissected

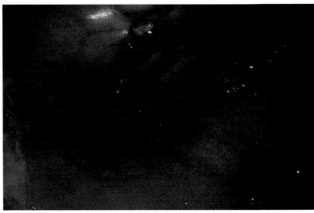

Fig. 36.5 Intraperitoneal view of the rectus muscle transposed through the rectal vault

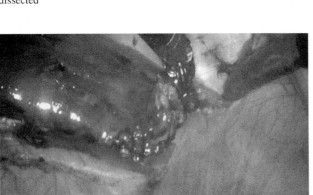

Fig. 36.4 Intraperitoneal view of the superior rectus muscle (distal flap) being divided with electrocautery

minimize the risk of avulsion and bleeding. Most perforators can be controlled by electrocautery, but large perforators should be identified and controlled with medium Weck Hem-o-lok clips (Intuitive Surgical) and divided. Caution must also be employed when dissecting the rectus muscle from the anterior rectus sheath at the level of the tendinous inscriptions so as not to damage either the muscle or the inscriptions. Poor dissection of the inscriptions will lead to large defects in the anterior rectus sheath and further weaken the remaining strength layer of the abdominal wall and increase the risk of bulge and/or hernia. The dissection of the rectus muscle off of the anterior rectus sheath continues until the level of the entrance of the deep inferior epigastric pedicle. The rectus muscle insertion to the pubis is left intact so as to not allow excessive tension on the vascular pedicle.

This technique of muscle harvest necessarily leaves a strip of posterior rectus fascia and peritoneum attached to the posterior surface of the rectus muscle. This strip of fascia allows the rectus muscle to be secured to the proper position needed. Directly securing the muscle with sutures leads to tearing of the muscle and inadequate positioning of the flap. Additionally,

the peritonealized posterior rectus fascia is the ideal tissue to use in resurfacing posterior vaginal wall defects. The peritoneum on the posterior rectus fascia quickly mucosalizes and also brings well-vascularized tissue to areas that are questionable. When the rectus muscle and posterior rectus sheath are harvested, it is recommended to reinforce the posterior abdominal wall with a biologic mesh to minimize the development of hernia or bulge. We recommend synthetic mesh due to the potential for contamination in APR or fistula surgery.

After complete harvest of the flap and reconstruction of the posterior abdominal wall donor site, the robot is undocked and placed back into the standard pelvic position for re-docking and securing the muscle between the areas of fistula repair. Alternatively in post-APR reconstruction, the inset is done from the open pelvis, and the muscle can be brought down through the rectal vault to the perineum manually (Fig. 36.5). This can be done under laparoscopic visualization to ensure that there is no twisting or kinking of the pedicle. The flap may be secured just under the skin or to the posterior vaginal wall if needed for reconstruction after tumor extirpation. A drain is left adjacent to the flap and exited through the buttock in these cases. In situations where the rectus muscle flap is buttressing the fistula repair, a drain can be placed and exited through the robotic port.

Postoperatively, the patients are restricted from sitting directly on the perineal incision for 4 weeks in the cases of post-APR reconstruction. They are allowed to lie down, stand, walk, or sit on a circular donut cushion to prevent pressure on the perineum and the distal end of the flap. When the flap is inset deeper in the pelvis, no pressure restriction is necessary.

Discussion

The robotic rectus muscle flap is a novel technique that allows a minimally invasive approach to harvest a workhorse vascularized tissue flap from an intraperitoneal approach.

This technique, like many techniques in plastic surgery, was borne out of necessity as robotic techniques became more prevalent in colorectal surgery, gynecology, and urology. With advanced minimally invasive techniques for deep pelvic surgery minimizing morbidity and the documented benefit of vascularized tissue transfer to fill dead space and improve healing in radiation-damaged tissue, the morbidity of open reconstructive approaches to these cases becomes increasingly harder to justify.

As with the adoption of any new procedure, there is a learning curve when incorporating the robotic rectus flap harvest into one's surgical repertoire. The learning curve is steep, however, and with experience the flap harvest itself can be readily performed in less than an hour. Additionally, recent literature has supported the safety and feasibility of this technique for a wide range of applications [35–37].

Complications of robotic rectus muscle harvest include the possibility of bleeding, hernia, and/or bulge in the donor site. Early reports in the literature suggested that maintaining the anterior rectus sheath intact was protective of true hernia, but our experience has demonstrated that significant bulge does occur in certain instances. We have noted increased risk of bulge in patients with higher BMI and/or large intraabdominal fat component as the pressure from the intraabdominal contents produces significant tension on the single anterior rectus sheath. It is therefore recommended to reinforce and/or repair the posterior rectus sheath with biologic mesh.

Conclusion

With the advent of continually advancing minimally invasive robotic techniques for abdominopelvic surgery, the need and importance of developing and adopting robotic methods of pelvic reconstruction are becoming paramount. We have presented our institution's preferred technique for use of the robotically harvested rectus abdominis muscle flap as a workhorse for minimally invasive pelvic reconstruction. Incorporation of both tumor extirpation and/or fistula repair combined with reconstructive surgery using minimally invasive techniques employing the surgical robot provides patients with the potential for improved outcomes with minimal morbidity in complex pelvic surgery.

References

1. Mathes SJ, Bostwick J 3rd. A rectus abdominis myocutaneous flap to reconstruct abdominal wall defects. Br J Plast Surg. 1977;30(4):282–3.
2. Parkash S, Bhandari M. Rectus abdominis myocutaneous island flap for bridging defect after cystectomy for bladder exstrophy. Urology. 1982;20(5):536–7.
3. Hartrampf CR, Scheflan M, Black PW. Breast reconstruction with a transverse abdominal island flap. Plast Reconstr Surg. 1982;69(2):216–25.
4. Giampapa V, Keller A, Shaw WW, Colen SR. Pelvic floor reconstruction using the rectus abdominis flap. Ann Plast Surg. 1984;13(1):56–9.
5. Bunkis J, Walton RL, Mathes SJ. The rectus abdominis free flap for lower extremity reconstruction. Ann Plast Surg. 1983;11(5):373–80.
6. Shukla HS, Hughes LE. The rectus abdominis flap for perineal wounds. Ann R Coll Surg Engl. 1984;66(5):337–9.
7. Logan SE, Mathes SJ. The use of a rectus abdominis myocutaneous flap to reconstruct a groin defect. Br J Plast Surg. 1984;37(3):351–3.
8. Sbitany U, Wray RC Jr. Use of the rectus abdominis muscle flap to reconstruct an elbow defect. Plast Reconstr Surg. 1986;77(6):988–9.
9. Robertson CN, Riefkohl R, Webster GD. Use of the rectus abdominis muscle flap in urological reconstructive procedures. J Urol. 1986;135(5):963–5.
10. Ford TD. Rectus abdominis myocutaneous flap used to close a median sternotomy chest defect. A case report. S Afr Med J. 1985;68(2):115–6.
11. Tobin GR, Day TG. Vaginal and pelvic reconstruction with distally based rectus abdominis myocutaneous flaps. Plast Reconstr Surg. 1988;81(1):62–73.
12. McCraw J, Kemp G, Given F, Horton CE. Correction of high pelvic defects with the inferiorly based rectus abdominis myocutaneous flap. Clin Plast Surg. 1988;15(3):449–54.
13. Horton CE, Sadove RC, Jordan GH, Sagher U. Use of the rectus abdominis muscle and fascia flap in reconstruction of epispadias/exstrophy. Clin Plast Surg. 1988;15(3):393–7.
14. Young WA, Wright JK. Scrotal reconstruction with a rectus abdominis muscle flap. Br J Plast Surg. 1988;41(2):190–3.
15. Bunkis J, Fudem GM. Rectus abdominis flap closure of ischiosacral pressure sore. Ann Plast Surg. 1989;23(5):447–9.
16. Kroll SS, Pollock R, Jessup JM, Ota D. Transpelvic rectus abdominis flap reconstruction of defects following abdominal-perineal resection. Am Surg. 1989;55(10):632–7.
17. Shepherd JH, Van Dam PA, Jobling TW, Breach N. The use of rectus abdominis myocutaneous flaps following excision of vulvar cancer. Br J Obstet Gynaecol. 1990;97(11):1020–5.
18. Tobin GR, Pursell SH, Day TG Jr. Refinements in vaginal reconstruction using rectus abdominis flaps. Clin Plast Surg. 1990;17(4):705–12.
19. Skene AI, Gault DT, Woodhouse CR, Breach NM, Thomas JM. Perineal, vulvar and vaginoperineal reconstruction using the rectus abdominis myocutaneous flap. Br J Surg. 1990;77(6):635–7.
20. Kluger Y, Townsend RN, Paul DB, Diamond DL. Rectus muscle flap for the reconstruction of disrupted pelvic floor. J Am Coll Surg. 1994;179(3):344–6.
21. Young MR, Small JO, Leonard AG, McKelvey ST. Rectus abdominis muscle flap for persistent perineal sinus. Br J Surg. 1988;75(12):1228.
22. McDonald MW, Elliott LF 2nd, Sullivan JW, Ortenberg J. Repair of vesicocutaneous fistula by rectus abdominis myocutaneous flap. Br J Urol. 1991;67(4):445.
23. Brough WA, Schofield PF. The value of the rectus abdominis myocutaneous flap in the treatment of complex perineal fistula. Dis Colon Rectum. 1991;34(2):148–50.
24. Cox MR, Parks TG, Hanna WA, Leonard AG. Closure of persistent post-proctectomy perineal sinus using a rectus muscle flap. Aust N Z J Surg. 1991;61(1):67–71.
25. Salup RR, Julian TB, Liang MD, Narayanan K, Finegold R. Closure of large postradiation vesicovaginal fistula with rectus abdominis myofascial flap. Urology. 1994;179(3):344–6.
26. Krasniak CL. Retroperitoneal transfer of a transverse rectus abdominis musculocutaneous flap for closure of a sacral radiation ulcer. Ann Plast Surg. 1995;34(3):332–4.

27. Viennas LK, Alonso AM, Salama V. Repair of radiation-induced vesicovaginal fistula with a rectus abdominis myocutaneous flap. Plast Reconstr Surg. 1996;97(2):455–9.

28. Erdmann MW, Waterhouse N. The transpelvic rectus abdominis flap: its use in the reconstruction of extensive perineal defects. Ann R Coll Surg Engl. 1995;77(3):229–32.

29. Loessin SJ, Meland NB, Devine RM, Wolff BG, Nelson H, Zincke H. Management of sacral and perineal defects following abdomino-perineal resection and radiation with transpelvic muscle flaps. Dis Colon Rectum. 1995;38(9):940–5.

30. De Haas WF, Miller MJ, Temple WJ, Kroll SS, Schusterman MA, Reece GP, Skibber JM. Perineal wound closure with the rectus abdominis musculocutaneous flap after tumor ablation. Ann Surg Oncol. 1995;2(5):400–6.

31. Butler CE, Gundeslioglu AO, Rodriguez-Bigas MA. Outcomes of immediate vertical rectus abdominis myocutaneous flap reconstruction for irradiated abdominoperineal resection defects. J Am Coll Surg. 2008;206(4):694–703.

32. Chessin DB, Hartley J, Cohen AM, Mazumdar M, Cordeiro P, Disa J, Mehrara B, Minsky BD, Paty P, Weiser M, Wong WE, Guillem JG. Rectus flap reconstruction decreases perineal wound complications after pelvic chemoradiation and surgery: a cohort study. Ann Surg Oncol. 2005;12(2):104–10.

33. Nelson RA, Butler CE. Surgical outcomes of VRAM versus thigh flaps for immediate reconstruction of pelvic and perineal cancer resection defects. Plast Reconstr Surg. 2009;123(1):175–83.

34. Patel NV, Pedersen JC. Robotic harvest of the rectus abdominis muscle: a preclinical investigation and case report. J Reconstr Microsurg. 2012;28(7):477–80.

35. Ibrahim AE, Sarhane KA, Pedersen JC, Selber JC. Robotic harvest of the rectus abdominis muscle: principles and clinical applications. Semin Plast Surg. 2014;28(1):26–31.

36. Pedersen JC, Song DH, Selber JC. Robotic, intraperitoneal harvest of the rectus abdominis muscle. Plast Reconstr Surg. 2014;134(5):1057–63.

37. Singh P, Teng E, Cannon LM, Bello BL, Song DH, Umanskiy K. Dynamic article: tandem robotic technique of extralevator abdominoperineal excision and rectus abdominis muscle harvest for immediate closure of the pelvic floor defect. Dis Colon Rectum. 2015;58(9):885–91.

38. Wu LC, Song DH. The rectus abdominis musculoperitoneal flap for the immediate reconstruction of partial vaginal defects. Plast Reconstr Surg. 2005;115(2):559–62.

Robotic Thyroidectomy

Mark S. Sneider and Peter S. Dahlberg

Introduction

Robotic thyroidectomy is a novel approach that avoids an anterior neck incision. Since the introduction of robotic surgery, several authors have described various techniques for remote-access robotic thyroidectomy. The initial description and most widely known technique was described by Chung and colleagues in Korea, which involves a gasless, single-incision, transaxillary approach [1]. Since then, several other techniques have been described, including transaxillary gas insufflation techniques, bilateral axillo-breast approach (BABA), and the retroauricular approach (RA).

The standard technique for open thyroidectomy was described between 1873 and 1893 by Billroth and Kocher [2], which is essentially unchanged to this day. The advent of endoscopic surgery made it feasible to perform thyroid surgery through a smaller neck incision. In 1996, Gagner was the first to describe endoscopic techniques for parathyroid surgery [3], and a year later, Hüscher first implemented them for thyroidectomy [4]. Over time, a diversity of other endoscopic techniques have been described, and they can be divided into cervical or extracervical (remote access) approaches [5].

The endoscopic approach has resulted in improved cosmetic outcomes; however, the limited working space in the neck makes the procedure more challenging. The adoption of the daVinci surgical system has further revolutionized the surgical treatment of thyroid disease. It provides many advantages over both traditional open and endoscopic thyroidectomy, including improved access and visualization, decreased tremor, superior range of motion, and improved ergonomics [6]. However, it also introduces a new set of potential complications, not typically associated with thyroid surgery, related to a new approach to the surrounding anatomy, such as stretch injury to the brachial plexus, esophageal perforation, and injury to the carotid artery and/or internal jugular vein. Furthermore, at this point, the use of the daVinci surgical system for thyroidectomy is not FDA approved and remains off-label [7]. It is critical to stress that with these additional set of risks and those associated with the learning curve, performing robotic thyroidectomy requires a thoughtful approach for its adoption. Several authors have recommended a framework for its safe implementation, with the following suggested elements: being a skilled surgeon with expertise in the standard approach to thyroidectomy, adequate education and training of the surgeon and staff, data collection, appropriate patient selection, and undergoing preceptored cases [8].

Literature Review

Overall there are a limited amount of published randomized controlled trials with regard to robotic thyroidectomy. However, there are detailed descriptions in the literature regarding the different robotic approaches to thyroidectomy as well as several meta-analysis that compare robotic thyroidectomy vs non-robotic approaches.

In 2013 Jackson and colleagues reported on the safety of robotic thyroidectomy, reporting that patients who underwent robotic surgery had greater cosmetic satisfaction. Robotic operative times were longer as compared to conventional open techniques but shorter than endoscopic approaches. Furthermore, all procedures had similar risks and rates of complications. The authors concluded that robotic thyroidectomy is as safe, feasible, and efficacious as conventional cervical and endoscopic thyroidectomy, with superior patient cosmetic satisfaction [6].

Sun published a meta-analysis comprised of 11 studies with 726 patients undergoing robotic transaxillary or bilateral axillo-breast approach thyroidectomy and 1205 undergoing open thyroidectomy. Again these authors found that operative times were longer for the robotic approach, while there

M. S. Sneider (✉) · P. S. Dahlberg
Department of Surgery, Allina Health, United Hospital, St. Paul, MN, USA
e-mail: mark.sneider@allina.com

© Springer Nature Switzerland AG 2019
S. Tsuda, O. Y. Kudsi (eds.), *Robotic-Assisted Minimally Invasive Surgery*, https://doi.org/10.1007/978-3-319-96866-7_37

was no significant difference in the length of hospital stay. Similarly, no differences were noted in hematoma, seroma, recurrent laryngeal nerve injury, hypocalcemia, or chyle leak rates. Overall the robotic groups reported improved cosmetic outcomes. The authors concluded that robotic and open approaches to thyroidectomy had similar complication rates; although, robotic approaches introduced the risk of new complications and require longer operative times, they were associated with better cosmetic outcomes [7].

Another systematic review publication by Lang et al. compared surgical and oncologic outcomes between robotic and non-robotic endoscopic thyroidectomy. These authors concluded that the robotic approach was associated with fewer recurrent laryngeal nerve injury rates, shorter length of hospital stay, and retrieval of a greater number of central neck lymph nodes during the procedure [9]. With similar findings, Kandil and colleagues report that robotic thyroid surgery is safe and feasible and provides similar perioperative complications and oncologic outcomes when compared to both conventional cervical and endoscopic approaches but is associated with longer operative times [10].

Pan and colleagues recently published a systematic review and meta-analysis that analyzed robotic versus conventional open thyroidectomy for thyroid cancer. They found that the robotic approach was associated with similar rates of several specific complications as well as equivalent surgical completeness including postoperative radioactive iodine (RAI) ablation rate, number of RAI ablation sessions, mean total RAI dose, and post-ablation stimulated thyroglobulin levels. They concede that robotic thyroidectomy for differentiated thyroid cancer is as safe as the conventional open approach [11].

To date there are four described robotic thyroidectomy approaches. They include the single-incision, gasless transaxillary approach, the bilateral axillo-breast (BABA) approach, the retroauricular approach, and the gas insufflation, transaxillary approach.

The single-incision, gasless transaxillary approach was the first described technique [1] and has been the most widely published. The patient is placed in a supine position on a small shoulder roll with the neck slightly extended. The arm on the operative side is raised naturally as to avoid brachial plexus injury. A 6-cm-long incision is made along the border of the pectoralis major muscle in the axilla; a flap is created along the subplatysmal plane until the bifurcation of the sternocleidomastoid (SCM) muscle is reached. The space between the sternal and clavicular heads of the SCM is opened superiorly, and the strap muscles are elevated from the thyroid gland. In order to maintain exposure, a spatula-shaped external retractor is placed under the strap muscles. The camera and robotic instruments are all inserted as spread out as possible through the single incision. Typically a four-instrument procedure is done, using the camera, ProGrasp,

Maryland dissector, and ultrasonic curved shears. The thyroid is removed maintaining the same principles as in the conventional open approach. The described limitations of this technique are the loss to tactile feedback, significant difficulty in performing a total thyroidectomy through a unilateral approach and costs [12].

The bilateral axillo-breast approach (BABA) was also first described in Korea by Lee and colleagues [13]. In 2004 they described this technique for endoscopic surgery, which soon after was combined with the daVinci system. This technique has the distinct advantage over a transaxillary approach of having the ability to perform a total thyroidectomy. Several publications have demonstrated the safety and efficacy of this approach; furthermore, Lee and colleagues have described 968 cases of total thyroidectomy with this approach for thyroid cancer, with adequate surgical completeness and low complication rates and recurrence [13–15]. The procedure involves four stages: creation of a working space, robot docking, console time, and closure. Incisions are made bilaterally at the areola skin line and at the axillary folds bilaterally. Working space flap is created and robotic trocars are inserted. The flap covers an area from the thyroid cartilage superiorly to 2 cm below the clavicles. The working space is maintained by low-pressure CO_2 gas insufflation. Instruments used include the robotic camera, ultrasonic shears, ProGrasp, and Maryland dissector. The midline strap muscles are identified and opened, the thyroid isthmus is divided, and total thyroidectomy is able to be done following the standard surgical principles.

A third described technique is the retroauricular approach. Terris et al. identified some of the limitations with single-incision, transaxillary thyroidectomy, so they developed and reported the feasibility and safety of the robotic facelift thyroidectomy [16, 17]. Kandil and colleagues have also described their results with this approach, concluding that thyroid lobectomy and parathyroidectomy can be safe and feasible [18]. In addition, Byeon et al. have described performing a robotic total thyroidectomy with a modified radical neck dissection via a unilateral retroauricular approach [19]. The procedure begins with an incision behind the ear, followed by elevation of the subplatysmal flap. A self-retaining retractor is placed, and robotic-assisted neck dissection is carried out, followed by ipsilateral thyroidectomy, central neck dissection, and finally contralateral thyroidectomy. A 30° robotic camera is used, along with a grasper and ultrasonic shears.

Lastly, there is a modified robotic unilateral axillo-breast approach using gas insufflation. This is the technique that is mainly performed by the authors. It involves placing trocars in the areola skin line and along the axillary folds at the edge of the pectorals major muscle. A subcutaneous pocket is created up to the heads of the SCM muscle, and the 2 heads are divided. The strap muscles are then retracted medially, and the thyroid gland is exposed. The working space is maintained with low-flow gas insufflation, and thyroid lobectomy is performed.

Preoperative Preparation

Robotic thyroidectomy has traditionally been utilized as a surgical tool to treat unilateral benign or indeterminate disease. Ideal patients have benign or indeterminate nodules that are less than 5 cm in size without signs of extensive thyroiditis. As guidelines for the treatment of well-differentiated thyroid cancers have evolved, the procedure has become an option for patients with malignant disease as well [20]. This would include tumors <4 cm in size without gross extra thyroidal extension or clinically apparent nodal disease. For low-risk papillary and follicular lesions <1 cm in size in the absence of prior neck radiation, or a familial cancer syndrome, lobectomy alone should be adequate treatment. For 1–4 cm tumors, lobectomy may be an option provided the treating team is not planning on postoperative use of radioiodine. In our series, only three patients had malignant disease, all diagnosed after lobectomy and isthmusectomy. Two patients had a contralateral robotic completion thyroidectomy with central node dissection, whereas one chose to have traditional open procedure.

Early in our series, we did not offer robotic thyroid procedures to patients with a BMI > 30. However, as we gained experience, we found that the operation is often easier to perform in larger BMI patients. Concomitant neck disease, previous ipsilateral clavicular fracture, upper outer quadrant breast surgery or radiation, and axillary hidradenitis are relative contraindications to the robotic procedure. Severe COPD is uncommon in this patient population, but CO_2 retention from gas insufflation would likely be problematic.

Preoperative imaging and evaluation are identical to other patient populations with thyroid disease. We use office ultrasound to characterize nodules and to identify the location and characteristics of parathyroid glands. Laboratory testing too is used to check for hyperthyroidism, hypothyroidism, or hypercalcemia. FNA and molecular testing are used when indicated [20]. Physical examination focuses on the neck, but also examines the axilla, and the breast. Placement of incisions is discussed with the patient. Preoperative vocal cord examination is used when indicated by an abnormal character of the voice. Informed consent is obtained at the time of the office visit and affirmed prior to the procedure. Complications specific to the robotic procedure include possible numbness of the anterior upper chest skin and injury to the subclavian vessels or even the brachial plexus due to a postoperative hematoma [8]. A plan for management of the contralateral thyroid lobe in the event of malignancy is also outlined during the preoperative consultation.

Setup

There are a few anesthetic concerns that are specific to the robotic thyroid operation. Access to the airway may be limited during the procedure depending on the room configuration and the robotic platform in use. The bedside surgeon may also encroach upon the anesthetist's space, and a preoperative discussion about ET tube and monitoring line access is necessary. Recurrent nerve monitoring is routinely performed and requires accurate placement and testing of the NIM tube. Hyperventilation may be necessary due to CO_2 retention during longer procedures using insufflation gas. If available preoperative injection of indocyanine green may be useful to identify normal parathyroid glands and to assess their vascular status after thyroid removal [21].

Patient positioning has evolved as we gained experience and altered the technique used during the robotic operation. Initially our patients were placed in a supine position with the neck extended and rotated away from the side of the lesion, and the arm was retracted above the operating table as described by Chung. However, injury to the brachial plexus has been described due to the arm positioning, and by using the complete trocar approach that will be described, it is not necessary to suspend the arm. It can be extended from the table at 90° in a neutral position. This avoids any risk of brachial plexus injuries. Lines, tubing, and cords follow the extended arm to the anesthesia working space and are accessible as necessary. A slight roll under the shoulder helps to open the working space that is obtained by hyperextension alone. The surgical field is prepped from the mandible to the costal margin. The initial dissection begins with one surgeon on each side of the arm board.

Early in our experience, we used a Chung's retractor with a sizable 7 cm axillary incision to create a tunnel into the space between the insertions of the sternal and clavicular heads of the sternocleidomastoid muscle. Although somewhat hidden from site in the axilla, the incision was larger than that necessary for a traditional thyroid operation, and postoperative pain was considerable. As others have also described, our procedure has evolved to a totally endoscopic, gas-assisted, and robotic operation.

Operative Dissection

The first key step in the operation is selection of sites for the trocars (Fig. 37.1). Breast and axillary skin fold creases are marked in the preoperative suite, and a convenient fold about midway between the nipple and the axillary fold is chosen for the camera port. If using laparoscopic trocars for the camera, either balloon ports or screw ports work well to prevent gas escape. The size of the incision matches the impression of the empty trocar on the skin. Before inserting the port, dissection is carried down to the pectoralis muscle, and the fat plane anterior to the muscle is bluntly developed with an instrument or the operating fingertip. At this point a dissecting balloon or more blunt finger dissection can be used to develop the space anterior to the muscle toward the sternal notch, superiorly toward the clavicle and inferiorly toward the nipple or other robotic operating port site chosen for the procedure. It is helpful to mark the tunneling space to be created on the skin. An 8 mm robotic port is inserted into the dissected space near the acromion. A second 8 mm robotic port is placed at the lateral nipple/areolar complex or on the upper mid part of the breast. Placing these ports before inserting the 12 mm port is helpful in guiding them to the most useful positions. Gas is connected at 10–15 mm Hg and at low flow, and then a laparoscope is inserted to finish creating the working space with a long hand-actuated cautery extension. Conversely, the robot can be docked at this point, and the procedure is initiated robotically.

Care must be taken as the clavicle is approached. It is quite possible to confuse the subclavius muscle for one of the heads of the SCM and dive too deeply and into trouble. It is safest to dissect to the sternal notch, then work back along the clavicle and identify the tendinous insertion of the sternal head of the SCM. Most, but not all patients will have a small gap between heads of the SCM, and this is the point through which the thyroid should be approached (Fig. 37.2a). In other patients there is simply a thinning in the number of fibers, and the space can be easily created by gently separating the fibers. Sensory branches of the ansa cervicalis and of the intercostal nerves are often identified and can usually be spared. This decreases the chance of postoperative sensory dysesthesias and numbness. The most critical structure to identify is the internal jugular vein, which should be lateral to the direction of approach to the thyroid (Fig. 37.2b). Close by and more posterior to the vein will be the carotid artery and the vagus nerve. The omohyoid muscle may be divided to facilitate exposure of the upper pole vessels at this point, which is also the time to transition to robotic dissection. At

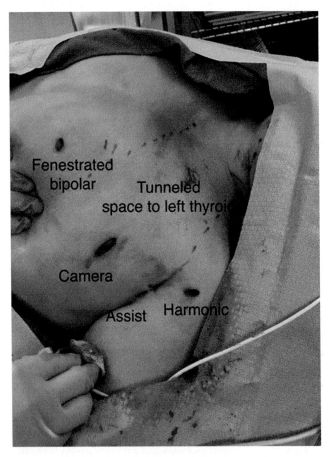

Fig. 37.1 View of trocar and instrument placement

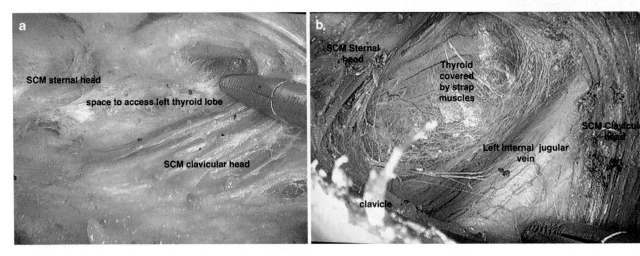

Fig. 37.2 (**a**, **b**) View of landmarks through the subcutaneous tunnel

this point the middle thyroid vein may be visible as will be the strap muscles covering the thyroid gland.

After docking the robot, a fenestrated bipolar instrument is placed through the left arm port and a harmonic scalpel through the right arm port. Robotic vessel sealers have more dexterity, but their bulk makes the operation more difficult to perform. A 5 mm assist port is placed after docking and inserting instruments in an accessible location for the bedside surgeon, usually slightly below and toward the back from the camera port. A "cigar" rolled sponge is placed to facilitate any urgent control of bleeding that may be necessary.

Dissection of the thyroid usually begins at the upper pole vessels beneath the strap muscles (Fig. 37.3a). The superior pole artery can be found by following the jugular vein in a cephalad direction. The vessels are divided and secured using the harmonic instrument (Fig. 37.3b). We have found that the robotic vessel sealer is too bulky to easily use for the dissection and sealing of vessels that is necessary. Next, we search for the upper parathyroid and the recurrent nerve. The trachea and the cricopharyngeus muscle can usually be identified. A very small incision with an 11 blade is made to introduce the nerve stimulator (Fig. 37.3c). A bloodless field greatly facilitates identification of the nerve in the tracheoesophageal groove. Once the nerve has been identified, the lower pole vessels can be safely divided, and the lower parathyroid is identified. Finally the division of the isthmus and of Berry's ligament begins from the upper pole of the gland, and the thyroid is removed through the 12 port in a laparoscopic bag. No drain is left, and the port site incisions are closed in one or two layers.

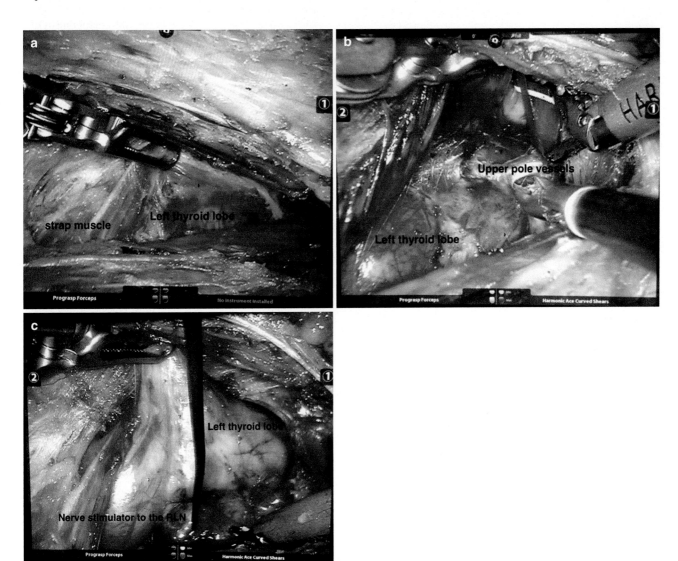

Fig. 37.3 (a–c) View of thyroid and surrounding structures anatomy; use of laryngeal nerve monitoring

Outcomes

To date we have completed 64 modified robotic unilateral axillo-breast approach thyroid lobectomies using gas insufflation. We have had no conversions to open, and complication rates are similar to what is reported in the literature for conventional thyroidectomy. We have had two transient laryngeal nerve palsies and one postop hematoma that did not require operative intervention. Patients have minimal to no complaints of chest wall numbness and dysesthesias in long-term follow-up.

In summary, there are several approaches to robotic thyroidectomy. As described, many studies have demonstrated its efficacy. Adhering to sound surgical principles is essential to ensure a successful outcome for these procedures.

References

1. Kang SW, Jeong JJ, Yun JS, et al. Robot-assisted endoscopic surgery for thyroid cancer: experience with first 100 patients. Surg Endosc. 2009;23:2399–406.
2. Ellis H. Thyroid and parathyroid. The Cambridge illustrated history of surgery. Cambridge, MA: Cambridge University Press; 2009. p. 195–209.
3. Gagner M. Endoscopic subtotal parathyroidectomy in patients with primary hyperparathyroidism. Br J Surg. 1996;83:875.
4. Hüscher CS, Chiodini S, Napolitano C, et al. Endoscopic right thyroid lobectomy. Surg Endosc. 1997;11:877.
5. Lee J, Chung WY. Robotic thyroidectomy and neck dissection. Past, present and future. Cancer J. 2013;19:151–61.
6. Jackson NR, Yao L, Tufano R, et al. Safety of robotic thyroidectomy approaches: meta-analysis and systematic review. Head Neck. 2014;36:137–43.
7. Sun GH, Peress L, Pynnonen MA. Systematic review and meta-analysis of robotic vs conventional thyroidectomy approaches for thyroid disease. Otolarygol Head Neck Surg. 2014;150(4):520–32.
8. Perrier ND, Randolph GW, Inabnet WB. Robotic thyroidectomy: a framework for new technology assessment and safe implementation. Thyroid. 2010;20:1327–32.
9. Lang BH, Wong C, Tsang J, et al. A systematic review and meta-analysis comparing outcomes between robotic-assisted thyroidectomy and non-robotic endoscopic thyroidectomy. JSR. 2014;191:389–98.
10. Kandil E, Hammad A, Walvekar R, et al. Robotic thyroidectomy versus nonrobotic approaches: a meta-analysis examining surgical outcomes. Surg Innov. 2016;23(3):317–25.
11. Pan J, Zhou H, Ding H. Robotic thyroidectomy versus conventional open thyroidectomy for thyroid cancer: a systematic review and meta-analysis. Surg Endosc. 2017;31:3985–4001.
12. Lee J, Chung W. Current status of robotic thyroidectomy and neck dissection using a gasless transaxillary approach. Curr Opin Oncol. 2012;24:7–15.
13. Lee KE, Kim E, Koo DH. Robotic thyroidectomy by bilateral axillo-breast approach: review of 1026 cases and surgical completeness. Surg Endosc. 2013;27:2955–62.
14. Lee KE, Koo DH, Im HJ, et al. Surgical completeness of bilateral axillo-breast approach robotic thyroidectomy: comparison with conventional open thyroidectomy after propensity score matching. Surgery. 2011;150(6):1266–74.
15. Lee KE, Koo DH, Kim SJ, et al. Outcomes of 109 patients with papillary thyroid carcinoma who underwent robotic total thyroidectomy with central node dissection via the bilateral axillo-breast approach. Surgery. 2010;148(6):1207–13.
16. Terris DJ, Singer MC, Seybt MW. Robotic facelift thyroidectomy: II. Clinical feasibility and safety. Laryngoscope. 2011;121:1636–41.
17. Terris DJ, Singer MC, Seybt MW. Robotic fecelift thyroidectomy: patient selection and technical considerations. Surg Laparosc Endosc Percutan Tech. 2011;21:237–42.
18. Alshehri M, Mohamed HE, Moulthrop T, et al. Robotic thyroidectomy and parathyroidectomy: an initial experience with the retroauricular approach. Head Neck. 2017;39(8):1568–72.
19. Byeon HK, Holsinger C, Tufano R, et al. Robotic total thyroidectomy with modified radical neck dissection via unilateral retroauricular approach. Ann Surg Oncol. 2014;21:3872–5.
20. Haugen BR, Alexander EK, Bible KC, et al. 2015 American Thyroid Association management guidelines for adult patients with thyroid nodules in differentiated thyroid cancer. Thyroid. 2016;26:1–133.
21. Lavazza M, Liu X, Wu C, et al. Indocyanine green-enhanced fluorescence for assessing parathyroid perfusion during thyroidectomy. Gland Surg. 2016;5(5):512–21.

Part VIII

Future of Robotic Surgery

Upcoming Robotic Systems

38

Daniel M. Herron and Matthew Dong

Introduction

Ever since there was work to do, humans have been endeavoring to use machines to augment and improve our ability to do that work. Surgery, with its need for precise and often repetitive movements, seems particularly well-suited for robotic augmentation or automation. Due to the complex nature of the field, however, robotics has only relatively recently made any inroads, and still in limited settings.

Current-generation robots confer several theoretical advantages compared to traditional open surgical or laparoscopic techniques covered in greater detail elsewhere in this book, including enhanced visualization, improved surgeon ergonomics, increased degrees of freedom with wristed instruments, and the capability to operate remotely. Still, penetrance into surgery has been limited mostly to certain fields – in particular, urology, gynecology, and pelvic colorectal surgery – and has been very modest in other surgical subspecialties. There are several drawbacks to currently available robotic platforms that may account for some of this slow adoption, including increased setup time, significant capital investments, and the requirement to utilize at a high rate to make up for operational costs, bulky equipment, the lack of haptic feedback, and concerns about trainee education.

Since coming to market in the late 1990s and early 2000s, Intuitive Surgical, Inc. (Sunnyvale, CA, USA) has been the dominant force in the field of surgical robotics, and it has seen rapid growth in market penetration in recent years. In the United States, most patents last 20 years from their earliest effective filing date, and many patents associated with Intuitive's technology are expiring or will be expiring in the coming years. As such, many competitors are expected to attempt to take advantage of the rapidly expanding, multi-billion-dollar market of surgical robotics. With any luck, this will result in increased innovation, reduced costs, and ultimately improved patient outcomes.

There are several forthcoming robot systems and modifications of existing systems that seek to extend upon some of the advantages and ameliorate the disadvantages of robotic surgery. The industry is primed for increased competition, which will ideally result in rapid innovation and ultimately improved patient outcomes in the coming years.

Enhancements to Current Systems

Da Vinci: Single Port

The da Vinci Xi Surgical System (Intuitive Surgical, Inc. Sunnyvale, CA, USA) is the most recent iteration of what is the industry standard robotic surgical platform. Prior to the release of the Xi, Intuitive demonstrated a prototype da Vinci SP (single port), with a deployable 3D camera, and three instruments with wristed motion. Intuitive has continued to develop this platform and is currently in the testing stages.

The currently available generation of the da Vinci single-site platform, compatible with the da Vinci Si, does not feature wristed motion, thus limiting triangulation and retraction. The instruments and camera cross within the port to allow for some degree of triangulation and to minimize interference between the working arms.

As compared to conventional single-incision solutions, robotic platforms eliminate some of the issues with instruments that collide or require the surgeon to manipulate instruments on the opposite side from their hands.

D. M. Herron · M. Dong (✉)
Department of Surgery, The Mount Sinai Hospital,
New York, NY, USA
e-mail: matthew.dong@mountsinai.org

© Springer Nature Switzerland AG 2019
S. Tsuda, O. Y. Kudsi (eds.), *Robotic-Assisted Minimally Invasive Surgery*, https://doi.org/10.1007/978-3-319-96866-7_38

Haptic Feedback

Intuitive is also developing a mechanism for haptic feedback, utilizing sensors already built in to the hardware of the Xi system, which could be deployed via a software-only update. While directly addressing one of the major drawbacks of robotic platforms in general, the utility of such an update would be greatly dependent upon the quality of its implementation. An ideal haptic feedback system would allow the surgeon to detect arm collisions and problem shoot them with minimal bedside assistance, reduce off screen visceral injuries, and improve feel while performing fine motor tasks such as suturing or manipulating fragile structures.

New Systems

TransEnterix

At the time of the writing of this chapter, Senhance Surgical Robotic System (Fig. 38.1), developed by TransEnterix (Morrisville, NC, USA), is approved by the FDA for colorectal and gynecologic surgery and has been submitted for approval for gallbladder and inguinal hernia surgery. To date, the company has sold a total of three systems, one in the United States [7]. Its key differentiating features include an open console system, utilizing polarized glasses for its three-dimensional display, eye tracking to move the camera, robotic instruments housed in independent arms, and haptic force feedback through controllers that are designed similarly to conventional laparoscopic instrument handles. Most

of the instruments do not have increased degrees of freedom, but a wristed needle driver is available. The company claims cost containment is a priority of this system, but quantitative assessments are not available.

AVRA Medical

AVRA Medical Robotics (Orlando, FL, USA), in partnership with the University of Central Florida, is developing a robotic platform with small, light, modular arms that can be attached to the patient bed, bedside cart, or a rail system mounted to the operating room itself. The company hopes to offer increased flexibility, reduced bulk, and reduced cost. The company is developing integrated image guidance combined with machine learning in hopes of creating an autonomous or semiautonomous robotic instrument that could be used in the office as well as the operating room [2]. Their marketing materials generally target the aesthetic surgery market. AVRA's current models and concepts bear more resemblance to robotic manufacturing than robotic surgical instruments, and some utilize instruments from Intuitive's da Vinci robot. Additionally, they hope to integrate their system with operating room lights, patient tables, surgical instruments, and a training platform.

Titan Medical

The SPORT Surgical System (Titan Medical, Inc., Toronto, ON, Canada), being developed by a publically traded Canadian firm, is a single-port surgical robot, with a deployable 3D

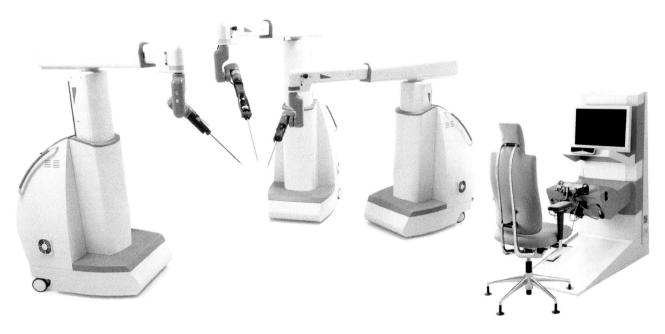

Fig. 38.1 Senhance surgical robotic system. (Courtesy of TransEnterix, Inc.)

camera and two replaceable wristed motion instruments. Currently in the prototype phase, the robot is mounted in a single stalk on a mobile tower with a boom. The instruments are controlled from a remote, open configuration workstation [6].

Auris Health

Auris Health (San Carlos, CA, USA), based in Silicon Valley, has recently gained FDA approval for its Monarch Platform (formerly ARES – Auris Robotic Endoscopy System) for use as a bronchoscopy diagnostic and therapeutic platform [1]. It is controlled with a remote design similar to a video gaming console. Although the company has yet to provide many public details, they possess several patents pertaining to endoluminal surgery, and its founder is a veteran of Intuitive Surgical, Mako Surgical, and Hansen Medical. The company's recent purchase of Hansen Medical, which produces robotic catheter-based tools for treating cardiac arrhythmias, suggests an expansion of its market, but it has made no public statements about future plans in that area.

Medrobotics

The Flex Robotic System, developed by Medrobotics (Raynham, MA, USA), is a robotic platform mounted on a flexible endoscope with two articulating 3 mm instruments, such as retractors, scissors, monopolar cautery, or a needle driver [4]. The endoscope has a telescopic inner core stabilizer to maintain the spatial orientation of the proximal scope. It is designed for transoral surgery, particularly oropharyngeal, hypopharyngeal, and laryngeal surgery. The company also produces a colorectal apparatus called the Flex Colorectal Drive, similarly designed for natural orifice surgery in the anus, rectum, and colon. Control of the instruments is via a hand piece directly connected to the instrument at the patient's bedside.

Mazor Robotics

Medtronic (Parsippany, NJ, USA) has been making substantial financial investments in Mazor Robotics (Caesarea, Israel), to distribute its surgical robotic guidance system, the Mazor X and its image-based guidance system, Renaissance. Mazor Robotics has a background in image-based, preplanned robotic guidance for spine and brain surgery. To date, Medtronic has invested $72 million in three separate disbursements in exchange for 10.6% of fully diluted shares of Mazor and distribution rights for Mazor's existing Mazor X Surgical Assurance Platform. As of Q1 2018, the company claimed 33,000 procedures performed with Mazor systems but would not add additional details [5].

Verb Surgical

Ethicon (subsidiary of Johnson and Johnson, New Brunswick, NJ, USA) is invested in a joint venture with Verily Life Sciences (a part of Alphabet, Inc., Mountain View, CA, USA the parent company of Google) called Verb Surgical, which is in the development stages of a surgical robot, or what it terms digital surgery. The company's goal is to democratize surgery, with its stated pillars of robotics, visualization, advanced instrumentation, data analytics, and connectivity, increasing access to technology and information, improving outcomes and reducing cost [8]. Given Alphabet's background in data analytics and machine learning and Ethicon's background in medical device manufacturing, this is an intriguing partnership, but specific details have not been made public at the time of this chapter's writing. The company's goal is to bring a product to market in 2020 [3].

Several truly autonomous robotic surgical devices and implantable remote-controlled instruments currently in various stages of research and development are beyond the scope of this chapter but are described elsewhere in this textbook.

Minimally invasive surgery, and surgical robotics in particular, has always been a rapidly developing field, but the expiration of many of the initial patents for surgical robot technologies and subsequent entrance of several new players to the field is likely to result in accelerated growth in the number of options, ideally leading to improved choice, reduced cost, and ultimately improved patient outcomes.

References

1. Auris Health. Auris health. Retrieved May 15, 2018, from Auris health unveils the FDA-cleared monarch platform, ushering in a new era of medical intervention. 2018, March 23. https://www.aurishealth.com/about/press/monarch-bronchoscopy-auris-health-fda-clearance.
2. AVRA Medical Robotics, Inc. AVRA Medical Robotics. 2018. Retrieved 15 May 2018, from Our Technology: https://www.avra-medicalrobotics.com/our-technology/.
3. Farr C. CNBC. 2018, March 15. Retrieved 15 May 2018, from Why Google co-founder Sergey Brin was using a robot to put sutures in synthetic tissue: https://www.cnbc.com/2018/03/15/alphabet-verily-joint-venture-verb-health-tech.html.
4. Medrobotics. Medrobotics. 2018. Retrieved 15 May 2018, from Flex® robotic system: expanding the reach of surgery®: https://medrobotics.com/gateway/flex-robotic-system/?c=US.
5. Motley Fool Staff. The Motley Fool, LLC. 2018, May 15. Retrieved 15 May 2018, from Mazor Robotics (MZOR) Q1 2018 Earnings Conference Call Transcript: https://www.fool.com/earnings/call-transcripts/2018/05/15/mazor-robotics-mzor-q1-2018-earnings-conference-ca.aspx.
6. Titan Medical, Inc. Titan Medical. 2018. Retrieved 15 May 2018, from Technology: https://titanmedicalinc.com/technology/.
7. TransEnterix, Inc. TransEnterix, Inc. Reports operating and financial results for the first quarter 2018. 2018, May 8. Retrieved May 15, 2018, from TransEnterix.com: http://ir.transenterix.com/news-releases/news-release-details/transenterix-inc-reports-operating-and-financial-results-first.
8. Verb Surgical Inc. Our story. 2017. Retrieved 10 16, 2017, from Verb Surgical: http://www.verbsurgical.com/about/.

Robert B. Lim and Dmitry Oleynikov

Abbreviations

CMAS   Canadian Centre for Minimal Access Surgery
CSH   Combat support hospital
DARPA   Defense Advanced Research Programs Agency
FST   Forward surgical team
NASA   National Aeronautics and Space Administration
TATRC   Telemedicine and Advanced Technology Research Center
HIFU   High-intensity focused ultrasound

Introduction

Like the rest of the world, military surgeons are using robots to assist with laparoscopic surgery in their hospitals. Currently 13 military treatment facilities in the US Department of Defense use robot assistance for their elective and sometimes acute cases. Most cases are done by general surgeons with urologists following as a close second. There is a lot of research and work being done using military funding to explore two more specific areas where robotic usage is integral: on the battlefield and in the area of noninvasive surgery.

On the battlefield, there are several advantages that could be gained by the use of robots. It may allow for fewer humans to be positioned in the far forward more austere and dangerous settings thereby assuming less risk to human life. With robots, teleconsultation and telesurgery capability would be increased allowing not only cognitive assistance to a remote surgeon but also physical assistance. In the past few years, a

R. B. Lim (✉)
Uniformed Services University of the Health Sciences, Bethesda, MD, USA

Department of Surgery, Tripler Army Medical Center, Honolulu, HI, USA

D. Oleynikov
University of Nebraska Medical Center, Omaha, NE, USA
e-mail: doleynik@unmc.edu

concept to deploy 5–8-person highly mobile surgical teams has gained popularity. The thought is that such teams will be even more mobile than the traditional 20-person forward surgical teams (FST). However the effectiveness of these smaller teams is in question as their capability is not equivalent to even a ¼ or ½ FST due to personnel and equipment limitations. In fact, the died of wounds rate from combat is believed to have increased during the conflict in the Middle East, and these smaller teams may be one reason why.

Biomodulation is the concept of manipulating tissue at the cellular level, and its accuracy requires the use of robotics. With the use of robots, the application of light, sound, or other energy sources could be used to stop bleeding, diagnose diseases, and even treat cancerous cells without needing to make an incision. The use of robots allows accuracy and faster real-time calculations so that individual cells can be treated while avoiding damage to normal cells and without the use of surgery.

The military's Defense Advanced Research Projects Agency (DARPA) funds many projects in both the military and civilian sector. As such, many advances made in the civilian sector are funded by the Department of Defense in hopes of having future use in the military. The purpose of this chapter will be to describe the current state of robotics both in the military and those robotic research activities funded by the military with a focus on the battlefield and in the area of cellular biomodulation.

Literature Review

Battlefield Medicine

To understand the use of robots on the battlefield, one has to understand the levels of care concept that the military employs. In contrast to the civilian trauma center designations, I–III, where a level I trauma center offers the highest level of care and capability, the military increases care capability as the number of the level increases [1]. Level I in the military is considered the basics of battlefield care or essen-

© Springer Nature Switzerland AG 2019
S. Tsuda, O. Y. Kudsi (eds.), *Robotic-Assisted Minimally Invasive Surgery*, https://doi.org/10.1007/978-3-319-96866-7_39

tially what a fellow soldier or field medic/corpsman would do to an injured soldier or service member. Similar to an emergency medical technician in the civilian world, their job is to stop bleeding, establish an airway, and assist with breathing. Their second function would be to rapidly triage the casualties. To do so, they would have to identify the persons who would most likely benefit from faster evacuation to the next level of care. More specifically, they would have to identify those patients whose bleeding would need urgent surgical control and give them priority in evacuation.

At the military level II, an FST or medical company would be present to assist with medical care, including resuscitation or damage control surgery. This level would be close to the actual combat and typically within 60 min of travel time. The FST is a 20-person team capable of performing about 30 operations before resupply is needed. A team would be at level II to provide life-saving damage control surgery only. Evacuation at this level is also paramount, so that stabilized patients would be quickly evacuated to level III.

At level III, there is a combat support hospital (CSH), which would have a full complement of surgical and medical staff along with radiologic support like computed tomography, laboratory assets, and intensive care unit capabilities. The CSH is still within the confines of the battlefield but further away from the actual fighting. More definitive care could be done at the CSH, but the seriously injured would still need evacuation to a higher level (level IV) for continued critical care. Level IV care is outside of the combat zone.

The current robotic research has been designed to augment the battlefield at levels I and II. At this time, all of the published research is mostly theoretical or on animal models only. The Coremicro® Robotic System described by Wong et al. uses ultrasound to detect internal injuries and infrared imaging to detect internal bleeding [2]. The placement of the robot requires human assistance, but with it, the provider could identify internal injuries like a pneumothorax, an injured liver, or a damaged spleen using robot-controlled ultrasound and an actively bleeding vessel using infrared light. This system would help the medic triage the patients more accurately. Infrared imaging has been studied in the civilian setting and described to have great potential in evaluating bleeding for cerebral perfusion and ischemia from coronary lesions [3, 4]; and attempts have been made to use it in the civilian trauma setting to evaluate tissue perfusion [5]. At this time, though, infrared imaging for trauma has been successful in a swine model, but this robot has not been tested under battlefield or in austere conditions [2]. Therapeutic options using robots will be discussed later.

For level II, robot prototypes have been designed to perform telesurgery. Rentschler et al.'s work involves minirobots deployed inside the abdominal cavity. There are two basic robot types: fixed-based and mobile. A small 12–15 mm × 50–75 mm robot that expands to 15 mm × 60 mm during retraction with its own laparoscope is inserted into the abdominal wall through a laparoscopic port. This puts the camera inside the abdomen, and the camera can be controlled to rotate around to provide visualization for surgery. The mobile model involves placing a 110 mm × 20 mm camera into the abdominal cavity to provide telementoring [6]. In this model, the camera can move freely around the abdominal cavity to provide visualization. In an environment 20 m underwater, astronauts did simulated surgical tasks in a study sponsored by the National Aeronautics and Space Administration (NASA), the Telemedicine and Advanced Technology Research Center (TATRC), the University of Nebraska, and the Canadian Center for Minimal Access Surgery (CMAS) using in vivo robots. On a simulation platform, astronauts were able to perform some basic surgical tasks [6]. In humans, a similar concept has been used for an elective cholecystectomy, using telesurgery over the Internet [7, 8].

Reichenbach et al. have expanded on the wireless concept and developed a model whereby a robot is placed using a platform similar to a single-incision laparoscopic port. The robot, as well as the surgical arms, has several degrees of motion similar to the flexible-tip laparoscopes of the robotic arms of the da Vinci model (Fig. 39.1). Once the port is placed locally, the scope and the arms can be operated from anywhere in the world using a wireless connection [9] (Fig. 39.2).

Lum et al.'s HAPs/MRT (high-altitude platforms/mobile robotic telesurgery) robot was deployed to Simi Valley, CA, to simulate hot and dusty conditions. Using wireless remote control only, similar to an unmanned armed vehicle, two surgeons were able to perform surgical tasks from 100 m away [10].

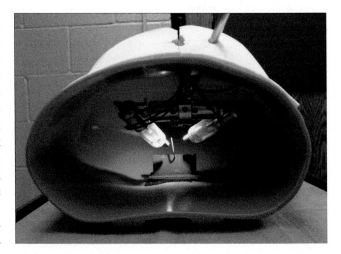

Fig. 39.1 Robot platform is inserted into the abdomen in this model. When expanded, it will have two working arms and a camera, each with its own range of motion

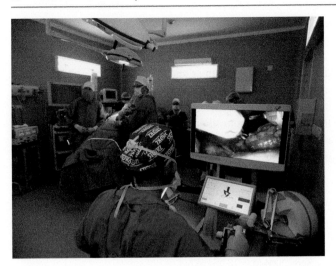

Fig. 39.2 Here the surgeon (author) sits at a console, while the bedside surgeon inserts the robot platform. The console surgeon can then conduct the operation. This could be done with the console surgeon at a remote location and via wireless connectivity

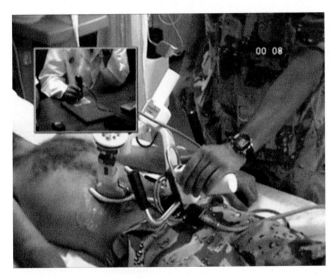

Fig. 39.3 In this image, the bedside provider is in Afghanistan applying the ultrasound probe, while the radiologist manipulates the probe and interprets the scan from Spain

In addition to telesurgical skills, other specialties have been added to provide consultation to the providers at level II to aid in patient care. The Spanish Army utilizes a 24-h per day consultation service for its forward deployed teams. Teleradiology consultation has been described, and using a robotic platform, a radiologist in Spain was able to control the ultrasound probe in Afghanistan to help perform echocardiograms and abdominal ultrasound exams on patients [11] (Fig. 39.3).

Since level II is close to the actual combat fighting and the personnel have to be highly mobile and able to function in austere settings, adding a robotic surgeon with telementoring and telesurgical skills would increase the capability of the

surgical team without deploying more personnel to a high-risk environment. This model would be a force multiplier in that two surgeons could be used to perform this type of surgery: one locally and one via telesurgery. This has a second-order effect in that it may reduce the frequency at which an actual surgeon deploys, thereby reducing the chance for his or her non-trauma surgical skills to degrade.

Biomodulation

As stated earlier, biomodulation is the manipulation of tissue at the cellular level. The concept has been around for almost two decades. This type of manipulation can be done to individual cells down to the level of 3–8 microns. As such, collateral injury to normal cells can be avoided while simultaneously destroying diseased or cancerous cells. Again this is an area that military funding has supported. The area of treated cells is so small, and because calculations for energy delivery have to be done in real time, this type of treatment requires robots for precision and tireless repetition of the tedious and delicate task.

The initial transdermal work focused on the control of bleeding. High-intensity focused ultrasound (HIFU) uses heat to induce coagulation necrosis at vessel injury sites to control bleeding [12]. The focusing of this heat enabled minimal destruction to surrounding tissue (including the vessel itself) to prevent thrombosis and pseudoaneurysm formation. HIFU has been used in a number of clinical settings to control bleeding and treat tumors using direct application of a device on the lesion [13]. In the trauma setting, it has been studied for hemostasis and pneumostasis for lung injuries but only in animal models [14].

The HIFU concept has since been applied to a transdermal approach as well but testing so far has been limited to the animal model. With a transdermal approach, the unit would not only determine if vessel bleeding was present as previously discussed, it would also calculate the depth of the injury to concentrate the HIFU therapy there in order to halt bleeding without damage to surrounding organs [15]. The role of robotics in this circumstance is in the automatic calculation of this equation and adjustments in real time. Additionally, the HIFU probe could be manipulated from remote areas to assist with the hemorrhage control. For the medic on the battlefield then, internal bleeding could be determined and treated with remote assistance. This would allow the field medic the ability to triage his or her patients faster, treat internal injuries, and focus his attention on other patients when multiple patients are injured.

In regards to biomodulation of cancers, most of the work has been done in urologic malignancies, and it involves direct robotic placement of interstitial brachytherapy. Using image guidance via ultrasound or magnetic resonance imaging, there are several robot platforms that assist with the application of brachytherapy to the prostate and lung [13]. While robots have demonstrated varying degrees of automation and autonomy, the most advanced ones can be given a task and then adjust independently during therapy to compensate for patient movement. The advantages of the robot platform include better accuracy of seed placement, decreased surgical trauma, and decreased radiation exposure to the clinical staff [13]. Clinical studies are lacking on long-term efficacy, and these robots are not yet commercially available.

Federally funded research has also focused on the manipulation of diseased or cancerous cells at the cellular level transdermally or without having direct contact with the tumor. In order to identify these cells and treat each individually, the clinician would have to be accurate down to the microscopic level. This, of course, is not possible with the human hand alone. Robot platforms are being developed to do just this. The work of Yuan et al. in the identification of cancerous brain cells has been able to use plasmonic gold nanostars to label and identify diseased cells with accuracy to 80 nanomicrons in mice [16]. The scientists at the University of Washington, using the Raven II surgical robot, have been able to adopt a similar concept of labeling tumor cells and ablating them using the robotic accuracy in a simulated environment [17]. While these concepts are still in their infancy phase, the development of this technology effectively means that the cancerous cells could be removed without needing an incision or, in the case of brain tumors, a craniotomy.

Future

At this point we can only guess what the future of robotics on the battlefield and in the area of noninvasive biomodulation will be; but with the research and advances described, there is no harm in dreaming about what these entities can do. Robotics has already been described with helping amputees regain full function of extremities using a robotic nerve interface that allows the patient to control his or her prosthesis more naturally [18]. For brain injuries, robotics has been used to assist with the cognitive recovery of patients. The US Army will soon be deploying robotic legs for its infantry. The legs will allow soldiers to run a mile in 4–5 min. It will also allow the wearer to carry more weight, and consequently, a medic could lift a much heavier person to take them out of harm's way [19]. All of these concepts have been funded by DARPA.

Now imagine identifying every cancer cell in the body and treating them directly without performing surgery and without risk to the healthy, normal cells. Imagine a medic under fire controlling cavitary bleeding from a traumatic injury in the chest, the skull, or the abdomen without needing to use a knife to enter the body. Imagine deploying one surgeon to the forward edge of the battlefield but having the physical capability of two. Imagine also that that surgeon on the battlefield has an entire staff of surgical specialists, from all over the world, able to provide consultation in real time and to first-assist in the surgical procedure. While many of these concepts seem like science fiction, the surgical world may be a lot closer to achieving them with the advancements of robotic surgery and medicine.

References

1. Beekley AC, Watts DM. Combat trauma experience with the United States Army 102nd Forward Surgical Team in Afghanistan. Am J Surg. 2004 May;187(5):652–4.
2. Wong KH, Lob SC, Lin CF, Lasser B, Mun SK. Imaging components for a robotic casualty evaluation system. Conf Proc IEEE Eng Med Biol Soc. 2009;2009:467–70.
3. Xu L, Tao X, Liu W, Li Y, Ma J, Lu T, et al. Portable near-infrared rapid detection of intracranial hemorrhage in Chinese population. J Clin Neurosci. 2017;40:136–46.
4. Matsumura M, Mintz GS, Kang SJ, Sum ST, Madden SP, Burke AP, et al. Intravascular ultrasound and near-infrared spectroscopic features of coronary lesions with intraplaque haemorrhage. Eur Heart J Cardiovasc Imaging. 2017 Nov;18(11):1222–8.
5. Ward KR, Ivatury RR, Barbee RW, Terner J, Pittman R, Filho IP, et al. Near infrared spectroscopy for evaluation of the trauma patient: a technology review. Resuscitation. 2006 Jan;68(1):27–44.
6. Rentschler ME, Platt SR, Berg K, Dumpert J, Oleynikov D, Farritor SM. Miniature in vivo robots for remote and harsh environments. IEEE Trans Inf Technol Biomed. 2008 Jan;12(1):66–75.
7. Anvari M, McKinley C, Stein H. Establishment of the world's first telerobotic remote surgical service: for provision of advanced laparoscopic surgery in a rural community. Ann Surg. 2005 Mar;241(3):460–4.
8. Marescaux J, Leroy J, Rubino F, Smith M, Vix M, Simone M, et al. Transcontinental robot-assisted remote telesurgery: feasibility and potential applications. Ann Surg. 2002 Apr;235(4):487–92.
9. Reichenbach M, Frederick T, Cubrich L, Bircher W, Bills N, Morien M, et al. Telesurgery With Miniature Robots to Leverage Surgical Expertise in Distributed Expeditionary Environments. Mil Med. 2017 Mar;182(S1):316–21.
10. Lum MJ, Rosen J, King H, Friedman DC, Donlin G, Sankaranarayanan G, et al. Telesurgery via Unmanned Aerial Vehicle (UAV) with a field deployable surgical robot. Stud Health Technol Inform. 2007;125:313–5.
11. Lim RB, Hernandez-Abadia A, Trigueros Martin JL, Del Real Colomo A. Effectiveness of Telemedicine in a Forward Combat Environment (poster presentation).
12. Zderic V, Keshavarzi A, Noble ML, Paun M, Sharar SR, Crum LA, et al. Hemorrhage control in arteries using high-intensity focused ultrasound: a survival study. Ultrasonics. 2006 Jan;44(1):46–53.
13. Podder TK, Beaulieu L, Caldwell B, Cormack RA, Crass JB, Dicker AP, et al. AAPM and GEC-ESTRO guidelines for image-guided robotic brachytherapy: report of Task Group 192. Med Phys. 2014 Oct;41(10):101501.
14. Vaezy S, Zderic V, Karmy-Jones R, Jurkovich GJ, Cornejo C, Martin RW. Hemostasis and sealing of air leaks in the lung using high-intensity focused ultrasound. J Trauma. 2007 Jun;62(6):1390–5.
15. Sekins KM, Barnes SR, Fan L, Hopple JD, Hsu SJ, Kook J, et al. Deep Bleeder Acoustic Coagulation (DBAC)-part II: in vivo test-

ing of a research prototype system. J Ther Ultrasound. 2015;3:17. https://doi.org/10.1186/s40349-015-0038-3. eCollection 2015

16. Yuan H, Wilson CM, Xia J, Doyle SL, Li S, Fales AM, et al. Plasmonics-enhanced and optically modulated delivery of gold nanostars into brain tumor. Nanoscale. 2014 Apr 21;6(8):4078–82.

17. Hu D, Gong Y, Hannaford B, Seibel EJ. Semi-autonomous Simulated Brain Tumor Ablation with RavenII Surgical Robot using Behavior Tree. IEEE Int Conf Robot Autom. 2015 May;2015:3868–75.

18. Miranda RA, Casebeer WD, Hein AM, Judy JW, Krotkov EP, Laabs TL, et al. DARPA-funded efforts in the development of novel brain-computer interface technologies. J Neurosci Methods. 2015 Apr 15;244:52–67.

19. DARPA. http://www.darpa.mil/our-research. Available at: http://www.darpa.mil/our-research. Accessed 23 April 2017.

Future Robotic Systems: Microrobotics and Autonomous Robots

40

Erica Dolph, Crystal Krause, and Dmitry Oleynikov

Introduction

Current methods for robotic minimally invasive surgery (MIS) offer many advantages over their traditional laparoscopic counterparts; however, these advantages come with many trade-offs [1]. With the collective push toward single-incision or incisionless surgery comes the need for increasingly dexterous and untethered robots. Current surgical robots have limited degrees of freedom (DOF) and external power supplies, making them difficult to maneuver in hard-to-reach body cavities and bulky in the operating room [2]. Due to these limitations, minimally invasive surgeries entail more complex motions to compensate for the reduced mobility of the robot, leading to greater surgeon fatigue [3]. This necessitates either the creation of robots capable of autonomously completing surgical tasks or the creation of robots with increased DOF. Additionally, it is important to both miniaturize the surgical robots and also make the robots affordable for a wider range of hospital settings [4, 5]. Research groups have been working toward robots for MIS that are smaller and more dexterous and require less manipulation of the body to help combat these shortfalls. These robots will lead to safer and less costly procedures for patients resulting in less rehabilitation time, surgical complications, and surgeon fatigue [6, 7]. Current trends toward smaller, more mobile, autonomous robots could have applications in a variety of procedures, including endoscopy, biopsy, incisionless surgery, and autonomous MIS. This would allow for surgery to not only be more efficient in the operating room but could also extend surgery to more rural areas and even for use in disaster scenarios through remote telestration [6, 8]. This chapter will discuss prominent innovations in the field of MIS robotics within the last 5 years. Each of the robots presented in this chapter represents a novel approach to alleviating some of the current shortcomings in robotic MIS.

Colonoscopy Robot

Colonoscopies are imperative in the diagnosis of many conditions affecting the colon. The current method of colonoscopy using a flexible scope can be painful for the patient due to the deformation of the colon wall and other complications that may occur as a result of the procedure. Dehghani et al. have developed a robot with a less invasive approach to alleviate these negative side effects [9]. Their colonoscopy robot (Fig. 40.1) uses a pneumatic driving system to gently traverse the colon. The robot consists of four separate parts: the robotic tip, latex tubing, a tethered camera, and anal fixture. It achieves movement through a pneumatic circuit that inflates the latex tubing, moving the robotic tip further into the colon. Currently, the tubing is manually inflated as the robot moves; however, in the future, the hope would be to automate the inflation of the tubing to produce a semiautonomous robot. As the robot traverses the colon, the spiraled camera tether is slowly released from the camera tip and remains stationary inside the colon. This resolves the friction that occurs when dragging a mobile cable through the colon.

In testing, the robot was able to traverse a simulated colon with 90° turns in ten out of fourteen trials. One of the trials failed due to balloon rupture, and the other failures were due to malfunctions in the tip of the robot. In an ex vivo experiment using pig colons with acute angles, the robot was able to successfully move through the colon ten out of eleven times, with the failed trial due to an anomaly in the pig's colon that would not be found in a human. The robot held an average speed of 28 mm/s, making it much faster than the traditional scope. Tests were also performed to ensure the

E. Dolph · C. Krause
Department of Surgery, Center for Advanced Surgical Technology, University of Nebraska Medical Center, Omaha, NE, USA

D. Oleynikov (✉)
Department of Surgery, Center for Advanced Surgical Technology, University of Nebraska Medical Center, Omaha, NE, USA

Department of Surgery, University of Nebraska Medical Center, Omaha, NE, USA
e-mail: doleynik@unmc.edu

© Springer Nature Switzerland AG 2019
S. Tsuda, O. Y. Kudsi (eds.), *Robotic-Assisted Minimally Invasive Surgery*, https://doi.org/10.1007/978-3-319-96866-7_40

a

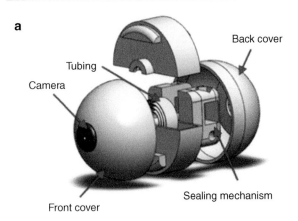

b

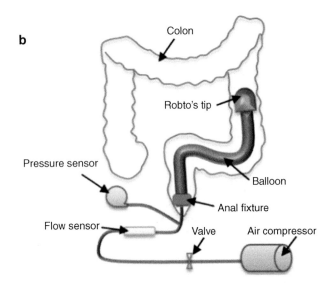

Fig. 40.1 (**a**) The robotic tip of the colonoscopy robot contains a camera, sealing mechanism, and coiled tubing which is released from the tip as the robot traverses the colon. (**b**) The robotic tip progresses through the colon as the latex balloon is inflated by the air compressor. The anal fixture holds the tubing in place, and the sensors allow for dynamic force and pressure control. (Unpublished figure provided by Dr. Hossein Dehghani)

pressure and temperature did not exceed safe values. In these tests, the pressure remained well below typically accepted values, meaning the colonoscopy robot could greatly decrease the pain and deformation that occurs in a typical colonoscopy. The temperature of the tip of the robot was 43 degrees during the tests, which was one degree above the temperature they considered to be safe. In future, the temperature of the tip of the robot would need to be dynamically controlled. Additionally in a stress test of the balloon, where they forced rupture of the balloon, substantial injuries were sustained to the pig colon. To ensure safety for the patient in case of an anomaly causing the balloon to break, they are considering using a noncompressible fluid as a safer alternative. Ultimately, even though improvements are needed for this robot, it does offer a safer, skill-independent, less invasive alternative to the traditional colonoscopy. The robot

exerted less force than a traditional scope and was able to greatly decrease the time necessary to move through the colon, showing great promise toward improving colonoscopy procedures [9].

UNL Single-Incision Robots

Our robotics team at UNL has also been working toward developing robots for use in single-incision surgeries. These robots are made with the intent to be completely enclosed within the abdomen during surgery, allowing for improved surgeon dexterity and resulting in fewer incisions and less pain for the patient [5, 10, 11]. Each robot employs a similar design, including a robot base attached to two dexterous arms with varying DOF, allowing for manipulation, cautery, and grasping within the body cavity. Each is operated using a master-slave configuration. These robots each represent a fundamental step toward improving laparoscopic single-incision surgery and making it a feasible alternative to traditional, multi-port procedures.

In 2012, we presented a robot with two six-DOF arms, which allow for an almost infinite array of motions to improve dexterity from within the body [10]. This robot was actuated using cordless, permanent magnet, direct-current motors and was tested in five single-incision pig colectomies. At least one robot malfunction occurred each surgery; however, even with these technical errors, the robot was still able to perform the key sections of a colectomy the majority of the time. In 2013, we developed a new model of the robot with two four-DOF arms that could be inserted through a single 30 mm incision (Fig. 40.2) [11]. This robot was tested on a porcine model and to our knowledge was the first robot to successfully perform an entire in vivo robotic single-incision colectomy.

Two recent designs under development implement the Geomagic Touch system to incorporate haptic feedback [5]. Additionally, these robots have been developed using a custom software platform allowing for rapid development and incorporation of future robots. The software is built on a . NET Framework and offers core robot services via a "plug-in" type of infrastructure. This allows for reusability and versatility of the software, supporting a broad range of future robots. One robot design in development has four DOF per arm and is equipped with a two-DOF elbow joint with a small port for a laparoscopic camera, a wrist joint, and an elbow joint, giving it a sufficient workspace for MIS. Because of the two independent shoulder joints, the arms can fold inward to allow for insertion through a small hole in the abdomen. This robot was subjected to testing in both in vivo and ex vivo experiments to ensure feasibility. Through these tests, revisions were made to ensure the robot could securely enter into a pressurized body cavity, and the robot's speed, dexterity, grasping force, and end-effector reliability were also evaluated. It had some

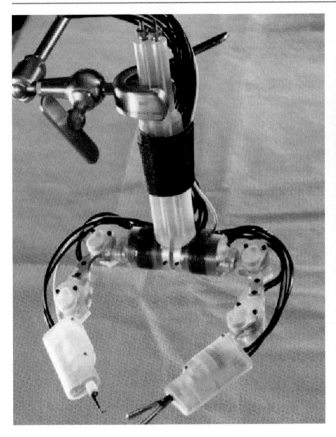

Fig. 40.2 The UNL robot developed in 2013 has two six-DOF arms that allow for maneuverability inside the body cavity. It was developed for use in single-incision colectomies and designed to be completely enclosed in the abdomen and teleoperated by an external console. This robot was the first of its kind to perform a single-incision in vivo porcine colectomy. (Figure originally published in [11], © 2018 IEEE. Reprinted, with permission, from Wortman et al. [11])

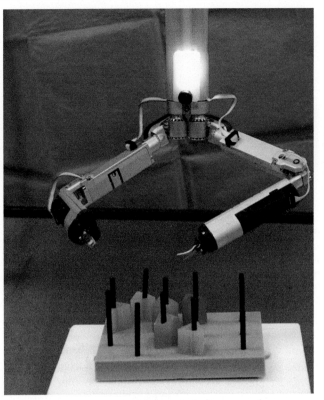

Fig. 40.3 The most recent iteration of the UNL robot is small enough to enter the body cavity through a singular port but maintains dexterity through its two-armed, five-DOF design. The figure depicts the robot performing a peg transfer task while being teleoperated. (Unpublished figure provided by Lou Cubrich)

shortcomings in target velocities around the edges of the workspace and the monopolar cautery shielding and grounding but proved successful in the other areas.

Another robot was also created to improve upon the previous model (Fig. 40.3). This robot has a five-DOF design with a structure very similar to the previous robot but including a three-DOF shoulder joint. This extra degree of freedom nearly doubled the robot's available workspace. Each joint contained within the robot is actuated by its own motor control module but shares one bus for power and data, simplifying the cable system. Additionally, this robot implements a custom camera system to allow for further miniaturization of the shoulder joint, enabling entry through a smaller port. There has been limited testing of this module, but it shows great promise of increased agility for use in single-incision surgery. These robots could allow a surgeon to operate with more mobility while greatly decreasing the number of patient incisions required. With additional revisions and testing, these robots could make single-incision surgery an easier, safer, more feasible alternative to current laparoscopic methods [5].

HeartLander

MIS is most prominent in gastrointestinal procedures, but MIS robots are also being developed in alternate fields. Petronik et al. have been developing a robot for use in minimally invasive heart surgery, the HeartLander (Fig. 40.4) [13]. The original robot had a miniaturized design and was made to be inserted into a small incision below the sternum. The robot implemented a tandem-body structure to achieve an inchworm-like motion actuated by a suction mechanism to allow for movement on a beating heart [13]. Due to the surface properties of the heart and because it is in constant motion, the suction mechanism employed by the HeartLander robot would have to exert a significant amount of suction force on the tissue at the heart surface in order to maintain contact, which could lead to complications, including tissue deformation.

The group has since been working on ways to improve the attachment of the robot onto the heart. In 2012, they investigated using gecko-inspired bio-fibers to improve the hold on the epicardial tissue [12]. The group used mushroom-tipped microstructures composed of a two-part polyurethane elastomer to mimic the feet of a gecko inside of the

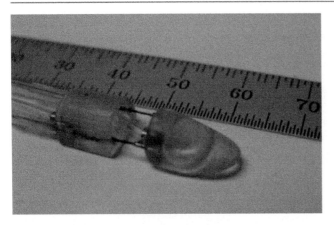

Fig. 40.4 The dual-chamber body of the HeartLander robot allows for it to move along the heart via an inchworm-like motion actuated through a suction mechanism. The small design allows for insertion via a small incision below the sternum and applications in minimally invasive heart surgery. (Courtesy of Cameron Riviere, from Tortora et al. [12])

suction chamber. Through the ex vivo testing, the force on the tissue was determined to be significantly better with the fibers, giving a 57.3% improvement in the attachment to the tissue sample. The addition of these fibers shows promise for the robot to safely travel on the heart without risk of deforming the tissue, but further testing is needed to investigate the necessary acclimation period of the fibers on the heart. This advancement could have diverse applications for low-risk adhesion and movement of surgical robotics made for various different regions of the body [12].

Four-DOF Origami Grasper

A major issue regarding surgical microrobotics is the trade-off that occurs between miniaturization and force exertion. The team of Salerno et al. has developed a robotic tip for use on larger robotic arm to enhance dexterity without having to considerably compromise on either term [14]. Their inspiration comes from paper origami and the idea of three-dimensional objects having the ability to fold down into two dimensions. Their robotic tip uses this idea to implement foldable triangular laser-cut carbon fiber to allow for rotational and translational movement. The robot consists of a three-DOF folding parallel module, passive twisting modules, and a compliant one-DOF gripper. The parallel module houses shape memory alloy (SMA) helical spring linear actuators which allow for foldability and motion. The design supports miniaturization while still allowing the grippers to exert large forces up to 2000 times its own weight because of its origami-like features. In external testing, the robot was able to exert a force of around 5 N and achieve over 6 mm of translational movement and a sufficient amount of tilting movement. This equips the robot with enough movement

and force for use in clinical applications. Though this design is still in the early stages of development, it offers a unique approach to combining actuation and miniaturization. The foldable structure is a novel advancement toward allowing for extensive gripping and actuating capabilities in microrobots [14].

Active Locomotion Intestinal Capsule Endoscope (ALICE)

Capsule endoscopy has become an emerging trend among MIS because of the increased visibility and control it allows a physician. Numerous research teams have developed capsule endoscopes with the ability to view and biopsy tubular organs, but many don't provide a mechanism for active locomotion and instead rely on the passive movement through the body. Le et al. have developed an active locomotion intestinal capsule endoscope (ALICE) that is able to be swallowed and can be actively guided by an operator to different areas in the digestive tract [15]. The group then adapted this capsule to have the ability to biopsy a lesion area inside the body [16]. The active locomotion allows the biopsy instrument to take precise biopsies in both tubular and non-tubular organs throughout the digestive system. Movement is achieved via a permanent magnet embedded in the robot, and it is steered using electromagnetic actuation, allowing the robot a full five DOF. A notable problem associated with this smooth type of capsule design is the decreased mobility in a collapsed colon, which could be accommodated for in the future with an expanding device [17]. The biopsy tool employed by the robot is controlled by a micro-reed switch, which is triggered by a higher-intensity electromagnetic field. It contains a sharp razor and torsional spring to obtain a biopsy of around 5 mm^3. When tested in simulation, the robot was able to navigate to a target lesion accurately, and the micro-reed switch was able to be activated. In ex vivo testing using a fresh pig intestine, 12 trials were ran, and the robot was able to obtain a biopsy 100% of the time, with an average biopsy volume of 4.5 mm^3. In future, the applications of this capsule could be further expanded to be utilized for tattooing inside of the body and position recognition for use in MIS [16].

Motor-Based Capsule

Gao et al. also created a capsule endoscope that uses active locomotion to traverse the digestive track [17]. This capsule is 13 by 28 mm, with two expanding leg-based devices to promote movement in a collapsed intestine. Previous groups have created similarly structured robots with expanding legs, but these earlier designs did not incorporate a sealing mechanism around the expanders to prevent the robot from taking up fluid or tissue from the body. Gao's design uses two O-rings to seal the inner chamber of the robot. These O-rings, though they cause a small amount of torque loss for the robot, improve the overall safety and functionality of the robot. A sealed expanding chamber is used to facilitate movement of the robot through promoting an inchworm-like pattern of motion. This movement is powered by a wireless power transmission consisting of a one-dimensional transmission coil and three-dimensional receiving coil. The power supply did cause some stalling in ex vivo testing, but this issue was overcome by a recording-restoring gait which allowed the robot to continue without resetting each time there was a lull in the supply. Additionally, they performed waterproof and acid-proof testing, which verified the sealing ability of the O-rings. Ex vivo tests were also performed in a collapsed porcine intestine, and the robot was able to successfully traverse it. This robot shows promise toward the reduction of pain and discomfort in endoscopy and has the potential to allow the physician to have more control over the endoscope. Future work would include incorporating other functional modules into the capsule such as a drug chamber, grasper, and a biopsy device to make a more robust capsule endoscope [17].

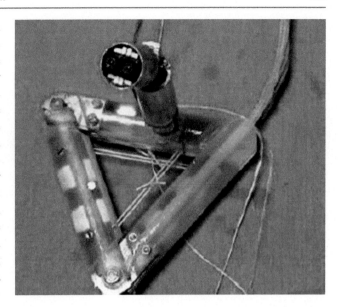

Fig. 40.5 The modular magnetic robot has a detachable triangular base for esophageal insertion and magnetic anchoring inside the body. It can house up to three two-DOF mini-surgical tools, such as the camera shown in the figure. (Courtesy of Dr. Tognarelli, from Tognarelli et al. [18])

Modular Magnetically Anchored Robot

Tognarelli et al. are developing a robot that takes an entirely different approach to NOTES. Their robot implements a magnetically anchored triangular frame built to house mini surgical robots (Fig. 40.5) [18]. This frame design was created specifically to maximize the magnetic anchoring potential in patients with larger abdominal walls while still maintaining a safe level of force on the skin. This robot can support a weight of 500 g when assuming an abdominal thickness of around 25 mm. The frame consists of three SMA-actuated docking stations, each capable of housing an individual surgical tool. The frame was built in a manner that allows for insertion and extraction in a linear fashion, thus allowing for entry through the esophagus. Each of the surgical tools is also small enough in size for esophageal insertion. These tools implement a modular design with interchangeable end-effectors equipped with two DOF. Currently, the camera module is the most developed, and a full set of surgical tools is under development. The prototype robot uses an external power supply but in future work would implement a wireless design for additional mobility. This robot has been tested in an in vivo porcine model. For the insertion of the robot, an 18 mm port was needed, and the insertion took around 4–5 min. The robot was able to be successfully deployed, maneuvered through the gastric wall to the abdominal wall, and anchored. The camera module was inserted through a separate trocar opening and was able to be anchored to the frame in order to test the motion of the camera and external handle. This study concluded that the magnetically anchored frame proved to be a feasible option for NOTES surgery in the future. Their ability to apply a magnetic anchoring system to cases of thick abdominal walls without damaging the tissue is an integral step toward making magnetic anchoring robots a reality in gastrointestinal MIS [18].

Stiffness Controllable Flexible and Learnable Manipulator for Surgical Operations (STIFF-FLOP)

The Stiffness Controllable Flexible and Learnable Manipulator for Surgical Operations (STIFF-FLOP) robot design (Fig. 40.6) is inspired by the fluid but strong motion of an octopus arm [20]. This robot is built to eliminate the divide between force and dexterity and marry the two together, creating a robot capable of being used as both a retractor and a grasper in MIS. The robot is cylindrical, consisting of three fluid-actuated inner chambers housed in a larger elastomeric cylinder, complete with braiding to prevent outward expansion and promote elongation. In the central portion of the robot, there is a stiffening channel filled with granular material to be used in a granular jamming mechanism, allowing the robot to stiffen upon command.

In testing, the robot was able to bend to an angle of 120 degrees, elongate by 86.3%, and apply a force of 46.1 N,

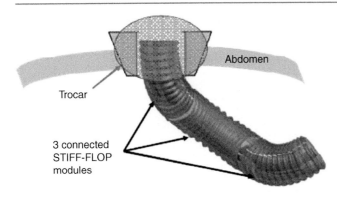

Fig. 40.6 The modular STIFF-FLOP robot can be inserted through a trocar port and used for MIS in hard-to-reach body cavities. The cylindrical chamber provides the ability for fluid motion, while a jamming mechanism allows the robot to stiffen when activated, allowing for both grasping and retracting applications. (Courtesy of Matteo Cianchetti, from Cianchetti et al. [19])

which were all deemed acceptable for surgical tasks. The robot was able to significantly stiffen when the jamming mechanism was actuated, but it is not yet capable of complete shape-locking [19, 21]. Upon testing, there were some issues with the expansion of the inner tubes, but in a subsequent prototype, these issues were subdued by adding a braided structure to the inner channels, preventing them from excessive outward expansion [20]. With improvements in the jamming mechanism, this robot could allow for improved agility in surgery with enough strength to still perform surgical tasks. This could greatly increase the mobility for the surgeon and allow for surgery in hard-to-reach body cavities. Additionally, in follow-up studies led by outside groups, this robot has been used to automate reaching and targeting behaviors, further showing its utility toward improving robotic MIS [22, 23].

Autonomous Suturing

One of the most tedious and redundant tasks involved in MIS is suturing. This process is both fatiguing and time-consuming for the surgeon. For this reason, a major focus of surgical robotics research is the development of automation for the process of surgical knot tying and tissue piercing. Mayer et al. has been working to automate the process of MIS suturing using numerous techniques [24]. In 2008, they investigated using the Endoscopic Partial Autonomous Robot (EndoPAR) and recurrent neural networks to achieve an autonomous knot-tying action. The EndoPAR is an experimental robot that uses four ceiling-mounted arms to operate in a semiautonomous fashion. This learning approach produced knot tying at four times the demonstration speed. In 2012, they investigated using skill transfer with a scaffolded framework on surgical arms originally deployed by the da

Vinci system [25]. This learning approach allowed the robot the ability to tie a knot in a new environment, which is incredibly useful for the dynamic environment present in the operating room [24, 25].

In 2010, the authors evaluated using a laser pointer to guide a robot to automatically pierce the tissue in preparation for suturing [26]. They used six-DOF arms that were previously employed by the da Vinci System, one of which was equipped with a laser pointer to allow the surgeon to select where to guide the robot to pierce the tissue. They used position-based alignment to guide the needle to the laser pointer and then switched to image-based alignment to zero in on the exact location. The needle could then execute a bite of the tissue and follow-through in a circular motion. In testing, the position-based alignment was able to guide the needle within 10 mm of the laser pointer, and after the image-based alignment, the error was only around 1 mm. They performed the piercing action on both a piece of phantom tissue and ex vivo tissue. The phantom tissue trials were successful, but the robot was not able to successfully pierce the ex vivo tissue because it was too soft and the laser point was diffused. However, this study presented a novel method to use a laser guidance system to direct tissue piercing, and in the future, lasers could be employed as part of a larger automated suturing system. Though the execution still has flaws, these studies show significant advancement toward automating the suturing process and diminishing surgeon fatigue in MIS [26].

Interchangeable Surgical Instrument System

In the operating room, it can expend valuable time to continually remove the instruments for cleaning and exchanging outside of the body cavity. A group of researchers at Berkeley, led by McKinley, has developed a fleet of end-effector tools, with the potential to be automated for tool change within the body [27]. The end-effectors created were built to be used with the da Vinci Research Kit in an automated tumor resection simulation. They designed a specific instrument tip mount that attaches onto surgical retractors, allowing the tool tips to be easily mounted and dismounted from the instrument. Once the feasibility of this mounting system is assessed, the future goal is to implement an interchangeable tool-tip attachment to allow for autonomous tool change during surgeries. The authors have developed a novel tool-changing adapter (TCA) that can be mounted to a needle driver to assist in the removal and attachment of different tool tips. Using this method, the TCA could carry a new tool tip to the receiving arm and then attach it to the end of the arm, all while inside the body cavity. In testing, the team evaluated the feasibility of the mounts during an autonomous tumor resection. The robot was able to carry out an autonomous tumor resection with the novel tool tips, only requiring human interaction to switch out the tool tips. In the future, the switching of the end-effectors would be implemented as an autonomous feature allowing for the ease of use and time-savings during the operation [27].

Conclusion

Each of the robots presented in this chapter takes a unique approach to improving various aspects of MIS. With the future of surgical robots leaning toward the creation of untethered, dexterous, autonomous microrobots, these advancements are crucial moving forward. In the future, robots could be capable of carrying out complex surgeries with limited human intervention, performing single-cell surgery, and working in swarms to address problems from within the body [4]. The applications of microrobots will continue to grow as researchers create robots capable of more advanced procedures and interventions. This will allow for great improvements in the quality of care for patients and extend the reach of advanced medicine to more people [6].

References

1. Huda MN, Yu H, Cang S. Robots for minimally invasive diagnosis and intervention. Robot Comput Integr Manuf. 2016;41:127–44.
2. Moustris G, Hiridis S, Deliparaschos K, Konstantinidis K. Evolution of autonomous and semi-autonomous robotic surgical systems: a review of the literature. Int J Med Robot Comput Assisted Surg. 2011;7(4):375–92.
3. Keshavarz Panahi A, Cho S. Prediction of muscle fatigue during minimally invasive surgery using recurrence quantification analysis. Minim Invasive Surg. 2016;2016:1–8.
4. Vikram Singh A, Sitti M. Targeted drug delivery and imaging using mobile milli/microrobots: a promising future towards theranostic pharmaceutical design. Curr Pharm Des. 2016;22(11):1418–28.
5. Cubrich LP. Design of a flexible control platform and miniature in vivo robots for laparo-endoscopic single-site surgeries. Lincoln: University of Nebraska; 2016.
6. Costarides V, Zygomalas A, Giokas K, Koutsouris D. Robotics in surgical techniques robotics in surgical techniques: present and future trends. In: Design, development, and integration of reliable electronic healthcare platforms. Hershey: IGI Global; 2016. p. 86.
7. Díaz CE, Fernández R, Armada M, García F. A research review on clinical needs, technical requirements, and normativity in the design of surgical robots. Int J Med Robot Comput Assisted Surg 2017;13(4):1–10.
8. Zygomalas A, Kehagias I, Giokas K, Koutsouris D. Miniature surgical robots in the era of NOTES and LESS: dream or reality? Surg Innov. 2015;22(1):97–107.
9. Dehghani H, Welch CR, Pourghodrat A, Nelson CA, Oleynikov D, Dasgupta P, et al. Design and preliminary evaluation of a self-steering, pneumatically driven colonoscopy robot. J Med Eng Technol. 2017;41(3):223–36.
10. Wortman TD, Meyer A, Dolghi O, Lehman AC, McCormick RL, Farritor SM, et al. Miniature surgical robot for laparoendoscopic single-incision colectomy. Surg Endosc. 2012;26(3):727–31.
11. Wortman TD, Mondry JM, Farritor SM, Oleynikov D. Single-site colectomy with miniature in vivo robotic platform. IEEE Trans Biomed Eng. 2013;60(4):926–9.
12. Tortora G, Glass P, Wood N, Aksak B, Menciassi A, Sitti M, Riviere C. Investigation of bioinspired gecko fibers to improve adhesion of HeartLander surgical robot. Conf Proc IEEE Eng Med Biol Soc (EMBC). 2012;2012:908–11.
13. Patronika NA, Rivierea CN, El Qarrab S, Zenatia MA. The HeartLander: a novel epicardial crawling robot for myocardial injections. Int Congr Ser Elsevier. 2005;1281:735–9.
14. Salerno M, Zhang K, Menciassi A, Dai JS. A novel 4-DOF origami grasper with an SMA-actuation system for minimally invasive surgery. IEEE Trans Robot. 2016;32(3):484–98.
15. Lee C, Choi H, Go G, Jeong S, Ko SY, Park J, et al. Active locomotive intestinal capsule endoscope (ALICE) system: a prospective feasibility study. IEEE/ASME Trans Mechatron. 2015;20(5):2067–74.
16. Le VH, Jin Z, Leon-Rodriguez H, Lee C, Choi H, Go G, et al. Electromagnetic field intensity triggered micro-biopsy device for active locomotive capsule endoscope. Mechatronics. 2016;36:112–8.
17. Gao J, Yan G, Wang Z, He S, Xu F, Jiang P, et al. Design and testing of a motor-based capsule robot powered by wireless power transmission. IEEE/ASME Trans Mechatron. 2016;21(2):683–93.
18. Tognarelli S, Salerno M, Tortora G, Quaglia C, Dario P, Schurr MO, et al. A miniaturized robotic platform for natural orifice transluminal endoscopic surgery: in vivo validation. Surg Endosc. 2015;29(12):3477–84.
19. Cianchetti M, Ranzani T, Gerboni G, De Falco I, Laschi C, Menciassi A. STIFF-FLOP surgical manipulator: mechanical design and experimental characterization of the single module. IEEE/RSJ international conference on intelligent robots and systems (IROS); 2013.
20. Fras J, Czarnowski J, Macia M, Główka J, Cianchetti M, Menciassi A. New STIFF-FLOP module construction idea for improved actuation and sensing. IEEE international conference on robotics and automation (ICRA); 2015.
21. Cianchetti M, Ranzani T, Gerboni G, Nanayakkara T, Althoefer K, Dasgupta P, et al. Soft robotics technologies to address shortcomings in today's minimally invasive surgery: the STIFF-FLOP approach. Soft Robot. 2014;1(2):122–31.
22. Bruno D, Calinon S, Caldwell DG. Learning autonomous behaviours for the body of a flexible surgical robot. Auton Robot. 2017;41(2):333–47.
23. Calinon S, Bruno D, Malekzadeh MS, Nanayakkara T, Caldwell DG. Human–robot skills transfer interfaces for a flexible surgical robot. Comput Methods Prog Biomed. 2014;116(2):81–96.
24. Mayer H, Gomez F, Wierstra D, Nagy I, Knoll A, Schmidhuber J. A system for robotic heart surgery that learns to tie knots using recurrent neural networks. Adv Rob. 2008;22(13–14):1521–37.
25. Knoll A, Mayer H, Staub C, Bauernschmitt R. Selective automation and skill transfer in medical robotics: a demonstration on surgical knot-tying. Int J Med Robot Comput Assist Surg. 2012;8(4):384–97.
26. Staub C, Osa T, Knoll A, Bauernschmitt R. Automation of tissue piercing using circular needles and vision guidance for computer aided laparoscopic surgery. IEEE international conference on robotics and automation (ICRA); 2010.
27. McKinley S, Garg A, Sen S, Gealy DV, McKinley JP, Jen Y, Guo M, Boyd D, Goldberg K. An interchangeable surgical instrument system with application to supervised automation of multilateral tumor resection. IEEE international conference on automation science and engineering (CASE); 2016.

Index

Printed by Printforce, the Netherlands